Chapter	Chapter Title	Video Contributor	Video Title
2	Diagnostic Arthroscopy and Loose Body Removal	Larry Field, MD	Diagnostic Elbow Arthroscopy and Loose Body Removal
3	Lateral Epicondylitis: Debridement, Repair, Evaluation of Associated Pathology	Champ L. Baker, Jr., MD and Champ L. Baker III, MD	Lateral Epicondlyitis
4	PLICA Synovialis of the Elbow	Bernard F. Morrey, MD	Elbow PLICA Arthroscopic Debridement
10	Arthroscopic Radial Head Excision	Graham J. W. King, MD, MSc, FRCSC	Arthroscopic Radial Head Resection for Post-Traumatic Arthritis
11	Arthroscopic Synovectomy for Inflammatory Arthritis	Graham J. W. King, MD, MSc, FRCSC	Arthroscopic Synovectomy for Inflammatory Arthritis
12	Arthroscopic Management of Postero-Lateral Instability	Buddy Savoie, MD	Posterolateral Reconstruction
19	Wrist Arthroscopy: Setup, Anatomy and Portals	Larry Field, MD	Diagnostic Wrist Arthroscopy: Anatomy and Portals
21	Triangular Fibrocartilage Complex Injuries	Thomas Trumble, MD	Radial TFCC Repair with Anchor
		Thomas Trumble, MD	Arthroscopic Ulnar TFCC Repair
22	Triangular Fibrocartilage Debridement and Arthroscopically Assisted Ulnar Shortening	Daniel J. Nagle, MD	Arthroscopically Assisted Ulnar Shortening Set Up
		Daniel J. Nagle, MD	TFCC Debridement and Arthroscopically Assisted Ulnar Shortening
25	Midcarpal Instability	David J. Slutsky, MD	Midcarpal Instability
28	Carpal, Metacarpal, and Phalangeal Fractures	Sidney M. Jacoby, MD	Arthroscopic Probing of Stable "Die Punch" Fracture
		Sidney M. Jacoby, MD	Probing Intra-articular Fracture of a Metacarpal Head
32	Arthroscopy of the Metacarpophalangeal and Proximal Interphalangeal Joints for Degenerative Joint Disease	Alejandro Badia, MD	Arthroscopic Debridement/ Shrinkage for Chronic Ulnar Collateral Thumb MCP Tear

AANA Advanced Arthroscopy

The Elbow and Wrist

Series Editor

Richard K. N. Ryu, MD
President (2009-2010)
Arthroscopy Association of North America
Private Practice
Santa Barbara, California

Other Volumes in the AANA Advanced Arthroscopy Series

The Foot and Ankle

The Hip

The Knee

The Shoulder

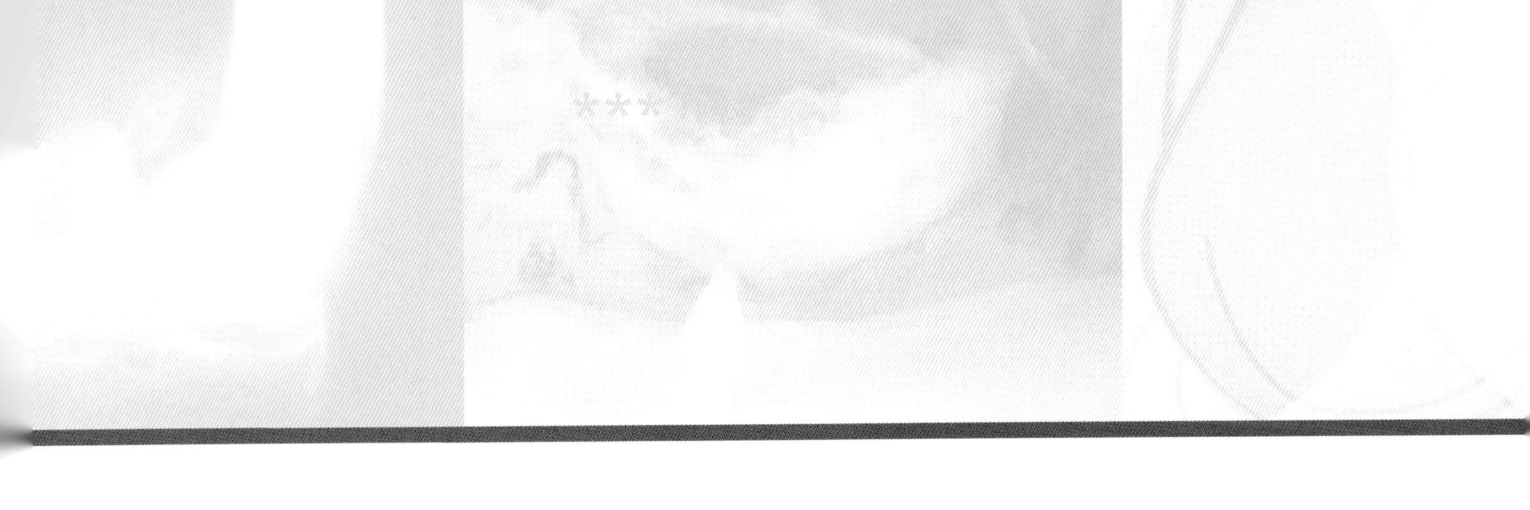

AANA Advanced Arthroscopy

The Elbow and Wrist

Felix H. Savoie III, MD
Lee Schlesinger Professor of Clinical Orthopaedic Surgery
Tulane University
New Orleans, Louisiana

Larry D. Field, MD
Director, Upper Extremity Service
Mississippi Sports Medicine and Orthopaedic Center
Clinical Instructor
University of Mississippi School of Medicine
Jackson, Mississippi

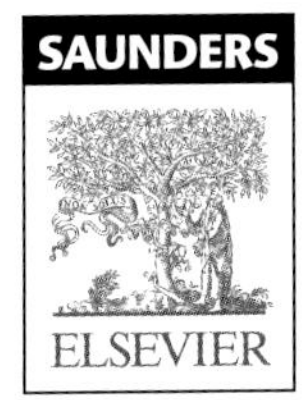

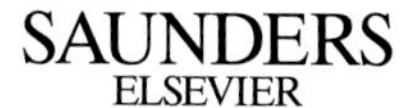

1600 John F. Kennedy Blvd.
Ste 1800
Philadelphia, PA 19103-2899

AANA Advanced Arthroscopy: The Elbow and Wrist

ISBN: 978-1-4377-0705-2

Notice

Knowledge and best practice in this field are constantly changing. As new research and experience broaden our knowledge, changes in practice, treatment and drug therapy may become necessary or appropriate. Readers are advised to check the most current information provided (i) on procedures featured or (ii) by the manufacturer of each product to be administered to verify the recommended dose or formula, the method and duration of administration, and contraindications. It is the responsibility of the practitioner, relying on their own experience and knowledge of the patient, to make diagnoses, to determine dosages and the best treatment for each individual patient, and to take all appropriate safety precautions. To the fullest extent of the law, neither the Publisher nor the Authors assumes any liability for any injury and/or damage to persons or property arising out of or related to any use of the material contained in this book.

The Publisher

Library of Congress Cataloging-in-Publication Data
AANA advanced arthroscopy. The wrist and elbow / [edited by] Larry D. Field, Felix H. Savoie III.
-- 1st ed.
p. ; cm.
Includes bibliographical references.
ISBN 978-1-4377-0705-2
1. Wrist--Endoscopic surgery. 2. Elbow--Endoscopic surgery. I. Savoie, Felix H. III. II. Field, Larry D. III. Arthroscopy Association of North America. IV. Title: Advanced arthroscopy. V. Title: Wrist and elbow.
[DNLM: 1. Wrist Joint--surgery. 2. Arthroscopy--methods. 3. Elbow Joint--surgery. WE 830 A112 2010] RD559.A255 2010
617.5'740597--dc22 2010011089

Publishing Director: Kim Murphy
Developmental Editor: Ann Ruzycka Anderson
Publishing Services Manager: Frank Polizzano
Senior Project Manager: Peter Faber
Design Direction: Ellen Zanolle

Printed in China

Last digit is the print number: 9 8 7 6 5 4 3 2 1

DEDICATION

To my wonderful wife, Amy, and our great family,

Chris, Michelle, Rob, Skyler, John, and Taylor.

Thanks for your patience, support and understanding,

which allowed me to do this project.

Buddy Savoie, MD

To my wife, Cindy, and our three children, Eric, Evelyn and Adam.

Your love and support make everything possible.

Larry D. Field, MD

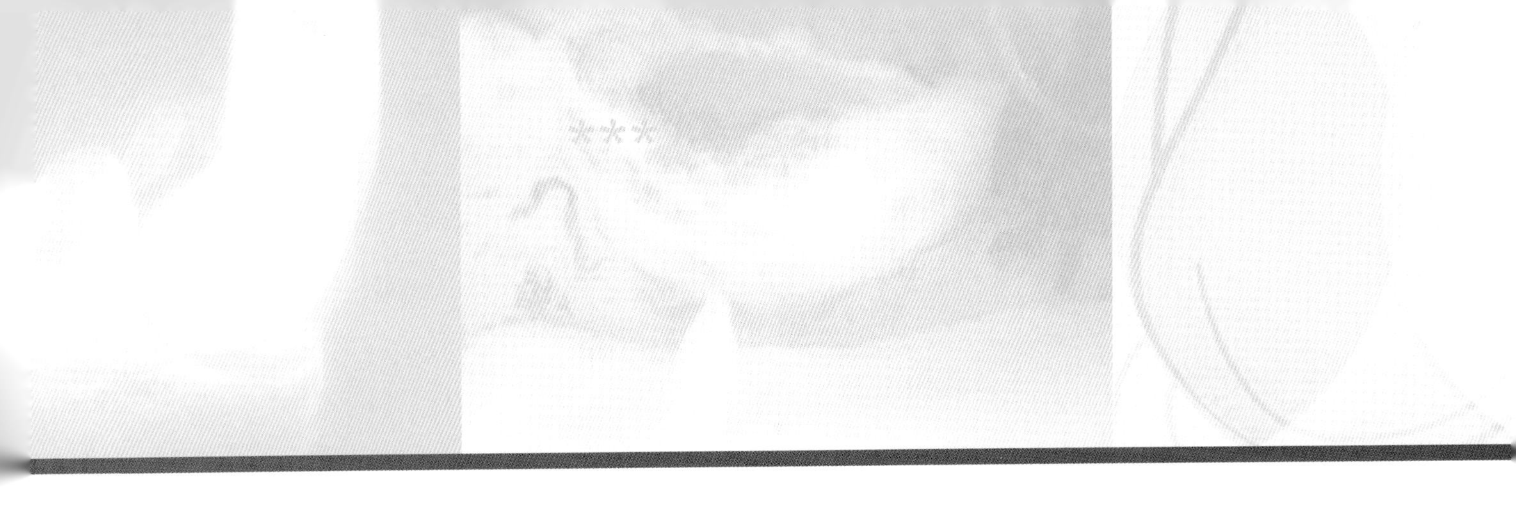

Contributors

Julie E. Adams, MD, MS
Assistant Professor of Orthopaedic Surgery, University of Minnesota Medical School, Minneapolis, Minnesota
The Stiff Elbow: Degenerative Joint Disease; Trapezial Metacarpal Arthritis

Christopher S. Ahmad, MD
Associate Professor of Clinical Orthopaedic Surgery, Columbia University College of Physicians and Surgeons; Associate Attending Orthopaedic Surgeon, New York–Presbyterian/Columbia University Medical Center, New York, New York
Osteochondritis Dissecans of the Elbow

Justin Alexander
Modbury Public Hospital, Adelaide, Australia
Wrist Arthroscopy: The Future

David W. Altchek, MD
Professor of Orthopaedic Surgery, Weill Cornell Medical College; Co-Chief, Sports Medicine and Shoulder Service, Hospital for Special Surgery, New York, New York
Arthroscopy in the Throwing Athlete

Kane Anderson, MD, MS
Durango Orthopedic Associates, Durango, Colorado
Injuries to the Triangular Fibrocartilage Complex

Alejandro Badia, MD
Hand and Upper Extremity Surgeon, Badia Hand to Shoulder Center, Doral; Chief of Hand Surgery, Baptist Hospital, Miami, Florida
Degenerative Disease of the Metacarpophalangeal and Proximal Interphalangeal Joints

Gregory I. Bain, PhD, MB BS
Associate Professor, Department of Orthopaedic Surgery, University of Adelaide School of Medicine; Senior Visiting Orthopaedic Surgeon, Royal Adelaide Hospital, Adelaide, South Australia; Senior Visiting Orthopaedic Surgeon, Modbury Hospital, Modbury, South Australia, Australia
Endoscopic Distal Biceps Repair; New Techniques in Elbow Arthroscopy; Wrist Arthroscopy: The Future

Champ L. Baker, Jr., MD
Clinical Assistant Professor, Department of Orthopaedics, Medical College of Georgia, Augusta; Staff Physician, The Hughston Clinic, Columbus, Georgia
Lateral Epicondylitis: Débridement, Repair, and Associated Pathology

Champ L. Baker III, MD
Staff Physician, The Hughston Clinic, Columbus, Georgia
Lateral Epicondylitis: Débridement, Repair, and Associated Pathology

Eric J. Balaguer, MD
Chief of Hand Surgery, Plancher Orthopaedics & Sports Medicine, New York, New York
Wrist Arthritis: Arthroscopic Synovectomy, Abrasion Chondroplasty, and Radial Styloidectomy of the Wrist

Matthew J. Boardman, DO
Fellow, Hand and Upper Extremity Surgery, University of Pittsburgh Medical Center, Pittsburgh, Pennsylvania
Arthroscopic Proximal Row Carpectomy

James C. Y. Chow, MD
Clinical Assistant Professor, Southern Illinois University School of Medicine, Springfield; Founder, Orthopaedic Research Foundation of Southern Illinois, Mt. Vernon, Illinois
Endoscopic Carpal Tunnel Release: Chow Technique

James Campbell Chow, MD
Orthopaedic Surgeon, Arizona Center for Bone and Joint Disorders; Orthopaedic Surgeon, St. Luke's Medical Center, Phoenix, Arizona
Endoscopic Carpal Tunnel Release: Chow Technique

Mark S. Cohen, MD
Professor and Director, Orthopaedic Education; Director, Hand and Elbow Section, Department of Orthopaedic Surgery, Rush University Medical Center, Chicago, Illinois
The Stiff Elbow: Arthrofibrosis

Randall W. Culp, MD
Professor, Orthopaedic, Hand, and Microsurgery, Jefferson Medical College of Thomas Jefferson University; Partner, Philadelphia Hand Center, King of Prussia, Pennsylvania
Carpal, Metacarpal, and Phalangeal Fractures; Arthroscopic Proximal Row Carpectomy

Phani K. Dantuluri, MD
Assistant Clinical Professor, Department of Orthopaedic Surgery, Jefferson Medical College of Thomas Jefferson University; Attending Orthopaedic Surgeon, Philadelphia Hand Center, Philadelphia, Pennsylvania
Carpal, Metacarpal, and Phalangeal Fractures

D. Nicole Deal, MD
Assistant Professor, Department of Orthopaedic Surgery, University of Virginia School of Medicine, Charlottesville, Virginia
Complications of Wrist Arthroscopy

Robert Dews, MD
Orthopaedic Surgeon, Jackson, Mississippi
Diagnostic Wrist Arthroscopy

Christopher C. Dodson, MD
Assistant Professor of Orthopaedic Surgery, Jefferson Medical College of Thomas Jefferson University; Attending Orthopaedic Surgeon, Sports Medicine Service, Rothman Institute, Philadelphia, Pennsylvania
Arthroscopy in the Throwing Athlete

Raymond R. Drabicki, MD
Fellow, Mississippi Sports Medicine and Orthopaedic Center, Jackson, Mississippi
Diagnostic Elbow Arthroscopy and Loose Body Removal

Scott Edwards, MD
Associate Professor, Georgetown University School of Medicine; Chief, Division of Hand and Elbow Surgery, Georgetown University Hospital, Washington, DC
Arthroscopic Excision of Dorsal Ganglions

Neal S. ElAttrache, MD
Clinical Instructor, Department of Orthopaedic Surgery, University of Southern California Keck School of Medicine; Director, Sports Medicine Fellowship, Kerlan-Jobe Orthopaedic Clinic, Los Angeles, California
Osteochondritis Dissecans of the Elbow

Larry D. Field, MD
Director, Upper Extremity Service, Mississippi Sports Medicine and Orthopaedic Center, Clinical Instructor, University of Mississippi School of Medicine, Jackson, Mississippi
Diagnostic Elbow Arthroscopy and Loose Body Removal; Arthroscopic and Open Radial Ulnohumeral Ligament Reconstruction for Posterolateral Rotatory Instability of the Elbow; Arthroscopic Triceps Repair; Arthroscopic Treatment of Elbow Fractures; Complications of Elbow Arthroscopy; Wrist Arthroscopy: Setup, Anatomy, and Portals; Diagnostic Wrist Arthroscopy

William B. Geissler, MD
Professor and Chief, Sports Medicine and Shoulder Programs, Department of Orthopaedic Surgery, University of Mississippi Medical Center, Jackson, Mississippi
Displaced Intra-articular Distal Radius Fractures; Acute Scaphoid Fractures in Nonunions

Guillem Gonzalez-Lomas, MD
Sports Fellow, Kerlan-Jobe Orthopaedic Clinic, Los Angeles, California
Osteochondritis Dissecans of the Elbow

Jeffrey A. Greenberg, MD, MS
Clinical Assistant Professor, Department of Orthopaedic Surgery, Indiana University School of Medicine; Partner and Fellowship Director, Indiana Hand to Shoulder Center, Indianapolis, Indiana
Volar Carpal Ganglion Cysts

Daniel J. Gurley, MD
Orthopaedic Surgeon, Kansas City, Missouri
Arthroscopic and Open Radial Ulnohumeral Ligament Reconstruction for Posterolateral Rotatory Instability of the Elbow

Sidney M. Jacoby, MD
Assistant Professor of Orthopaedic Surgery, Jefferson Medical College of Thomas Jefferson University, Philadelphia; Attending Physician, Philadelphia Hand Center, King of Prussia, Pennsylvania
Carpal, Metacarpal, and Phalangeal Fractures

Luke Johnson
Modbury Public Hospital, Adelaide, Australia
Endoscopic Distal Biceps Repair

Graham J. W. King, MD, MSc, FRCSE
Professor, Department of Surgery, University of Western Ontario Faculty of Medicine; Chief of Orthopaedics, St. Joseph's Health Centre, London, Ontario, Canada
Arthroscopic Radial Head Resection; Arthroscopic Synovectomy for Inflammatory Arthritis

Mark Morishige, MD
Orthopaedic Surgeon, Wichita, Kansas
Wrist Arthroscopy: Setup, Anatomy, and Portals

Bernard F. Morrey, MD
Professor, Department of Orthopaedics, Mayo Clinic, Rochester, Minnesota
Plica Synovialis of the Elbow

Michael J. Moskal, MD
Orthopaedic Surgeon, Sellersburg, Indiana
Lunotriquetral Tears

Daniel J. Nagle, MD, FACS
Professor of Clinical Orthopedics, Northwestern Feinberg School of Medicine; Attending Physician, Northwestern Memorial Hospital, Chicago, Illinois
Triangular Fibrocartilage Débridement and Arthroscopically Assisted Ulnar Shortening

Michael O'Brien, MD
Assistant Professor of Clinical Orthopaedics, Division of Sports Medicine, Tulane University School of Medicine, New Orleans, Louisiana
Arthroscopic Triceps Repair

Shawn W. O'Driscoll, PhD, MD
Professor of Orthopedics, Mayo Clinic, Rochester, Minnesota
Osteocapsular Arthroplasty of the Elbow

Darrell J. Ogilvie-Harris, MB ChB, BSc (Hons), FRCS
Associate Professor, Department of Surgery, University of Toronto Faculty of Medicine; Consultant Surgeon in Orthopaedics, University Health Network, Toronto, Ontario, Canada
Arthroscopic Resection of the Olecranon Bursa

A. Lee Osterman, MD
Professor of Orthopaedics and Hand Surgery, Jefferson Medical College of Thomas Jefferson University, Philadelphia; President, Philadelphia Hand Center, King of Prussia, Pennsylvania
Arthroscopic Excision of Dorsal Ganglions; Carpal, Metacarpal, and Phalangeal Fractures

Wayne S. O. Palmer, MB BS, KM (Ortho)
Lecturer, University of the West Indies at Mona; Consultant, Orthopaedic Surgeon, University Hospital of the West Indies, Kingston, Jamaica, West Indies
Arthroscopic Resection of the Olecranon Bursa

Athanasios A. Papachristos, MD
Fellow, Orthopaedic Research Foundation of Southern Illinois, Mt. Vernon, Illinois
Endoscopic Carpal Tunnel Release: Chow Technique

Robert L. Parisien, BA
Medical Student, Tufts University School of Medicine, Boston, Massachusetts
Arthroscopy in the Throwing Athlete

John P. Peden, MD
Clinical Assistant Professor, Florida State University College of Medicine—Fort Pierce Regional Campus, Fort Pierce; Vero Orthopaedics and Neurology, Vero Beach, Florida
Arthroscopic Treatment of Elbow Fractures

Kevin D. Plancher, MD
Associate Clinical Professor, Department of Orthopaedics, Albert Einstein College of Medicine of Yeshiva University, Bronx; Fellowship Director, Plancher Orthopaedics & Sports Medicine, New York, New York; Chairman, Orthopaedic Foundation for Active Lifestyles, Cos Cob, Connecticut
Wrist Arthritis: Arthroscopic Synovectomy, Abrasion Chondroplasty, and Radial Styloidectomy of the Wrist

Gary G. Poehling, MD
Professor of Orthopaedics, Wake Forest University School of Medicine; Orthopaedic Surgeon, North Carolina Baptist Hospital, Winston Salem; Orthopaedic Surgeon, Stokes Reynolds Memorial Hospital, Danbury, North Carolina
Complications of Wrist Arthroscopy

Felix H. Savoie III, MD
Lee Schlesinger Professor of Clinical Orthopaedic Surgery, Tulane University, New Orleans, Louisiana
Diagnostic Elbow Arthroscopy and Loose Body Removal; Arthroscopic and Open Radial Ulnohumeral Ligament Reconstruction for Posterolateral Rotatory Instability of the Elbow; Arthroscopic and Open Radial Ulnohumeral Ligament Reconstruction for Posterolateral Rotatory Instability of the Elbow; Arthroscopic Triceps Repair; Arthroscopic Treatment of Elbow Fractures; Complications of Elbow Arthroscopy; Wrist Arthroscopy: Setup, Anatomy, and Portals

Kush Shrestha
Modbury Public Hospital, Adelaide, Australia
Wrist Arthroscopy: The Future

David J. Slutsky, MD, FRCS(C)
Assistant Professor of Orthopedics, David Geffen School of Medicine at UCLA; Chief of Reconstructive Hand Surgery, Harbor-UCLA Medical Center, Los Angeles; Orthopedic Surgeon, Hand and Wrist Center, Torrance, California
Midcarpal Instability

Scott P. Steinmann, MD
Professor of Orthopedic Surgery, Mayo Clinic College of Medicine, Rochester, Minnesota
Plica Synovialis of the Elbow; The Stiff Elbow: Degenerative Joint Disease; Trapezial Metacarpal Arthritis

William B. Stetson, MD
Associate Clinical Professor of Orthopaedic Surgery, University of Southern California Keck School of Medicine, Los Angeles; Stetson Powell Orthopaedics and Sports Medicine, Burbank, California
Elbow Arthroscopy: Positioning, Setup, Anatomy, and Portals

Richard J. Thomas, MD
Attending Physician, Medical Center of Central Georgia and Macon Northside Hospital, Macon, Georgia
Complications of Elbow Arthroscopy

Thomas Trumble, MD
Professor, Department of Orthopaedics and Sports Medicine, University of Washington School of Medicine; Chief, University of Washington Hand Surgery Institute, Seattle, Washington
Injuries to the Triangular Fibrocartilage Complex

Tony Wanich, MD
Assistant Professor of Orthopaedic Surgery, Albert Einstein College of Medicine of Yeshiva University; Orthopaedic Surgeon, Montefiore Medical Center, Bronx, New York
Osteochondritis Dissecans of the Elbow

Adam C. Watts, BSc, MB BS
Hand and Upper Limb Fellow, Wrightington Hospital, Lancashire, United Kingdom
Endoscopic Distal Biceps Repair; New Techniques in Elbow Arthroscopy; Wrist Arthroscopy: The Future

Darryl K. Young, MD, FRCSC
Orthopaedic Surgeon, Queensway Carleton Hospital, Ottawa, Ontario, Canada
Arthroscopic Radial Head Resection; Arthroscopic Synovectomy for Inflammatory Arthritis

Preface

The Arthroscopy Association of North America (AANA) is a robust and growing organization whose mission, simply stated, is to provide leadership and expertise in arthroscopic and minimally invasive surgery worldwide.

Towards that end, this five-volume series represents the very best that AANA has to offer the clinician in need of a timely, authoritative, and comprehensive arthroscopic textbook. These textbooks covering the shoulder, elbow and wrist, hip, knee, and foot and ankle were conceived and rapidly consummated over a 15-month timeline. The need for an up-to-date and cogent text as well as a step-by-step video supplement was the driving force behind the rapid developmental chronology. The topics and surgical techniques represent the cutting edge in arthroscopic philosophy and technique, and the individual chapters follow a reliable and helpful format in which the pathoanatomy is detailed and the key elements of the physical examination are emphasized in conjunction with preferred diagnostic imaging. Indications and contraindications are followed by a thorough discussion of the treatment algorithm, both nonoperative and surgical, with an emphasis on arthroscopic techniques. Additionally, a Pearls and Pitfalls section provides for a distilled summary of the most important features in each chapter. A brief annotated bibliography is provided in addition to a comprehensive reference list so that those who want to study the most compelling literature can do so with ease. The supporting DVD meticulously demonstrates the surgical techniques, and will undoubtedly serve as a critical resource in preparing for any arthroscopic intervention.

I am most grateful for the outstanding effort provided by the volume editors: Rick Angelo and Jim Esch (shoulder), Buddy Savoie and Larry Field (elbow and wrist), Thomas Byrd and Carlos Guanche (hip), Rob Hunter and Nick Sgaglione (knee), and Ned Amendola and Jim Stone (foot and ankle). Their collective intellect, skill, and dedicaton to AANA made this series possible. Furthermore, I sincerely thank all the chapter contributors whose expertise and wisdom can be found in every page. Elsevier, and in particular Kim Murphy, Ann Ruzycka Anderson, and Kitty Lasinski, was a delight to work with, and deserves our gratitude for a job well done. I would be remiss if I did not acknowledge that the proceeds of this five-volume series will go directly to the AANA Education Foundation, from which ambitious and state-of-the-art arthroscopic educational initiatives will be funded.

Richard K.N. Ryu, MD
Series Editor

Contents

PART

I

The Elbow

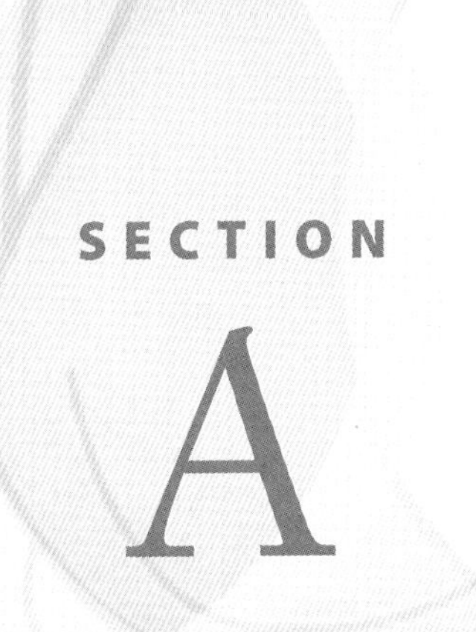

SECTION A

Basics

CHAPTER

1

Elbow Arthroscopy: Positioning, Setup, Anatomy, and Portals

William B. Stetson

Elbow arthroscopy is a technically demanding procedure, and extensive hands-on training and supervised experience are needed to acquire proficiency. When performed with appropriate judgment and technique, elbow arthroscopy is an excellent tool for the correction of many lesions of the elbow joint with minimal risk.[1] However, it poses greater technical challenges and neurologic risks than knee or shoulder arthroscopy. Arthroscopy of the elbow joint is perhaps the most hazardous in terms of its potential for causing injury to nearby nerves and vessels because of the complex relationship of these structures to the joint (Fig. 1-1).[2] Because of the surrounding neurovascular structures, familiarity with the normal elbow anatomy and portals can decrease the risk of damage to important structures.[3] Elbow arthroscopy provides an opportunity for diagnostic and therapeutic intervention with little morbidity.

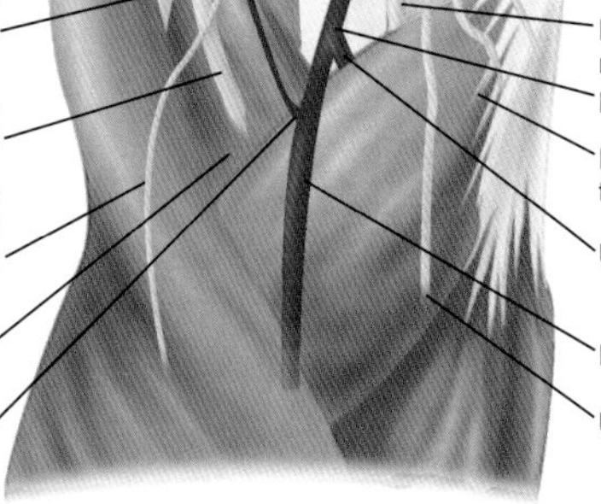

FIGURE 1-1 The antecubital fossa with important neurovascular structures

Burman[4] first described elbow arthroscopy in 1931, but he stated that the elbow is "... unsuitable for examination since the joint is so narrow for the relatively large needle." In 1932, he revised his opinion based on the arthroscopic examination of 10 cadaveric elbows.[5] After Burman's studies were published, a small number of reports appeared in the German and Japanese literature, but it was not until the middle to late 1980s that reports began to appear in the American literature.[6,7]

In 1985, Andrews and Carson[7] described the patient-supine technique and the use of various portals for elbow arthroscopy. In 1989, Poehling and colleagues[8] described the patient-prone position for elbow arthroscopy. Since then, the techniques and indications for elbow arthroscopy have expanded, and there have been many more reports describing variations in operative technique.

This chapter provides an overview of the positioning, setup, anatomy, and portals used for elbow arthroscopy.

ANATOMY

A clear understanding of the anatomy of the elbow is important before proceeding with arthroscopy. Important bony anatomic landmarks that should be palpated include the lateral and medial epicondyles, olecranon process, and radial head (Fig. 1-2). On the lateral side, the lateral epicondyle, olecranon process, and radial head form a triangle. Located in the center of this triangle is a soft spot called the *anconeus triangle*. It often is used to inflate the joint with fluid before introducing instruments or cannulas, and it can be the landmark for a direct lateral portal (Fig. 1-3). Posteriorly, important structures include the triceps muscle, tendon, and tip of the olecranon.

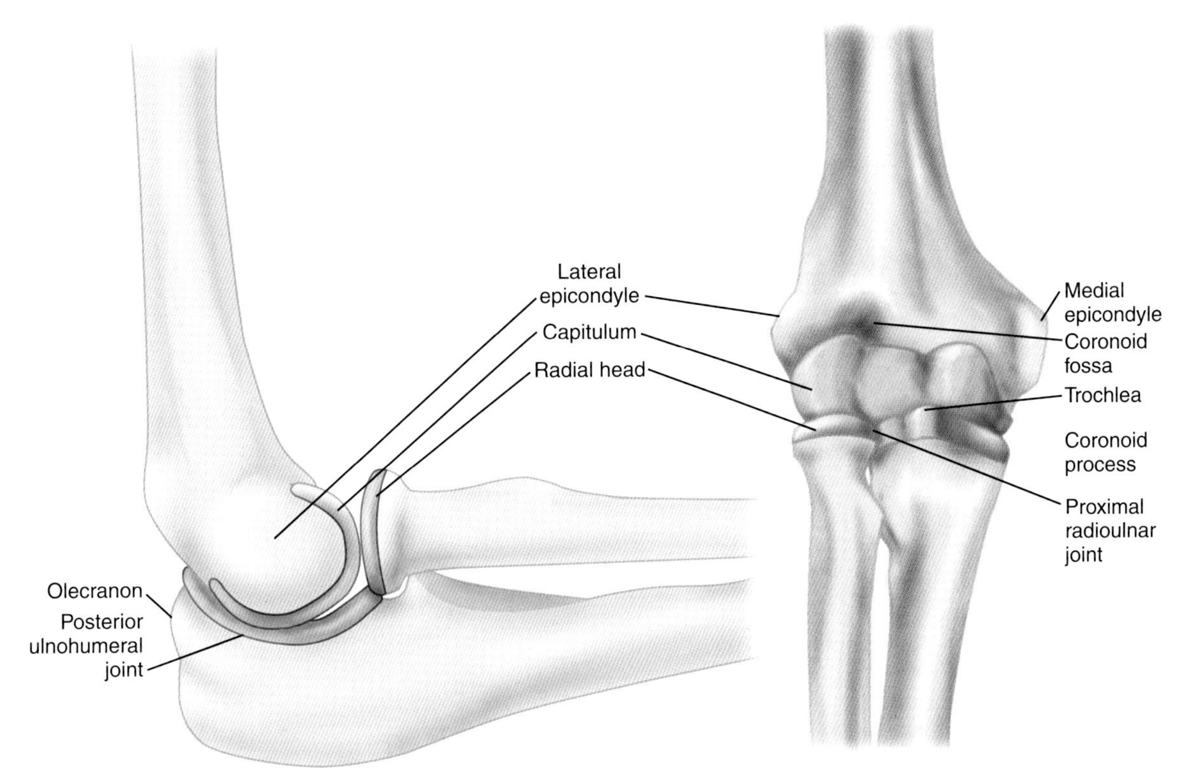

FIGURE 1-2 Bony landmarks of the elbow joint.

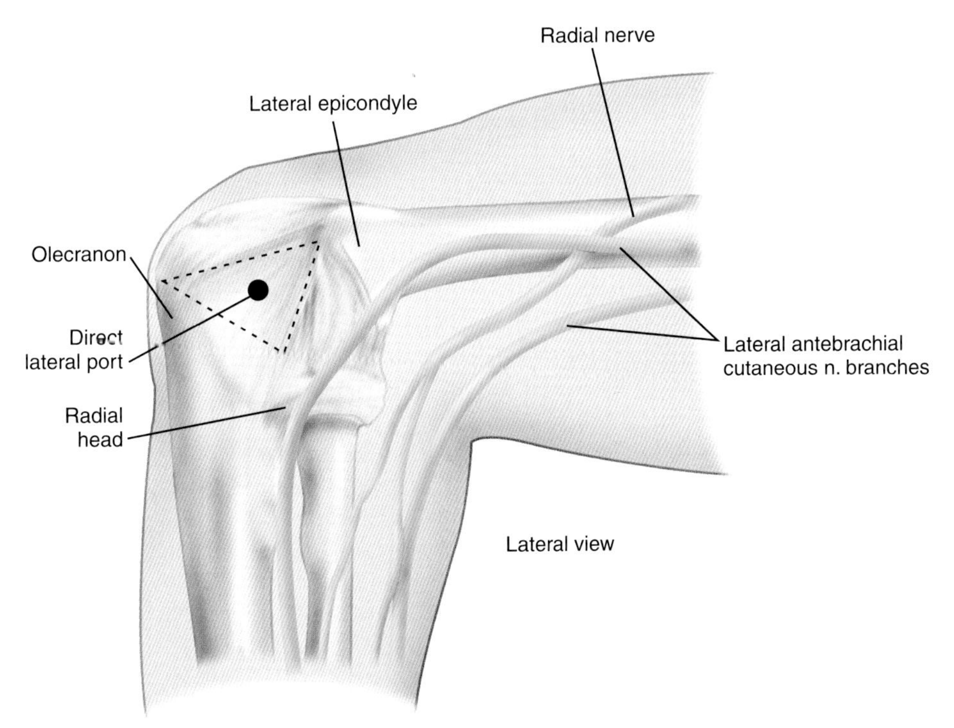

FIGURE 1-3 Lateral view in the prone position

Anteriorly, the antecubital fossa is formed by three muscular borders: laterally by the mobile wad of three—the brachioradialis, the extensor carpi radialis brevis, and the extensor carpi radialis longus muscles; medially by the pronator teres muscle; and superiorly by the biceps muscle. The anconeus muscle, which is located on the posterolateral aspect of the joint, originates on the lateral epicondyle and posterior elbow capsule and inserts on the proximal ulna.

Sensory nerves around the elbow include the medial brachial cutaneous, the medial antebrachial cutaneous, the lateral antebrachial cutaneous, and the posterior antebrachial cutaneous nerves.[9] The medial brachial cutaneous nerve penetrates the deep fascia midway down the arm on the medial side, and it supplies skin sensation to the posteromedial aspect of the arm to the level of the olecranon. The medial antebrachial cutaneous nerve supplies sensation to the medial side of the elbow and forearm. The lateral antebrachial cutaneous nerve is a branch of the musculocutaneous nerve, which exits between the biceps and brachialis muscles laterally to supply sensation to the elbow and lateral aspect of the forearm. The posterior antebrachial cutaneous nerve branches from the radial nerve and courses down the lateral aspect of the arm to supply sensation to the posterolateral elbow and posterior forearm.[6]

The main neurovascular structures about the elbow are the median nerve, radial nerve, ulnar nerve, and brachial artery.[9] The radial nerve spirals around the posterior humeral shaft, penetrates the lateral intermuscular septum, and descends anteriorly to the lateral epicondyle between the brachioradialis and brachialis muscles. The radial nerve then branches to form the superficial radial nerve, which supplies sensation to the dorsoradial wrist and posterior surface of the radial three and one-half digits, and the posterior interosseous nerve, which provides motor branches to the wrists, thumb, and finger extensors. The ulnar nerve penetrates the medial intermuscular septum in the distal one third of the arm, courses posteriorly to the median epicondyle, and then descends distally between the flexor carpi ulnaris and flexor digitorum superficialis muscles. The brachial artery courses just medial to the biceps tendon in the antecubital fossa and then descends to the level of the radial head, where it bifurcates into the radial and ulnar arteries (see Fig. 1-1).[6]

PATIENT EVALUATION

History

A comprehensive history should be taken, including the occupation of the patient, whether he or she is right or left handed, and the duration of symptoms. It is also important to determine the details of whether their symptoms started with a single traumatic event or resulted from repetitive activities. The physician should inquire about the presence and character of the pain, swelling, and locking and catching episodes, which can indicate intra-articular loose bodies. The location of the pain is important, because medial pain is most often medial epicondylitis but can also be caused by a medial epicondyle avulsion fracture, a medial collateral ligament sprain, ulnar neuritis, or ulnar nerve subluxation. Symptoms in the lateral region of the elbow may be indicative of radiocapitellar chondromalacia, osteochondral loose bodies, radial head fracture, osteochondritis dissecans (OCD) lesions, and most commonly lateral epicondylitis.

The differential diagnosis for symptoms of the anterior elbow includes distal biceps tendon rupture, which can be partial or complete; anterior capsular strain; and brachioradialis muscle strain.[10] Symptoms in the posterior compartment can reflect valgus extension overload syndrome, posterior impingement, osteochondral loose bodies, triceps tendonitis, triceps tendon avulsion, or olecranon bursitis.[11] Deep, aching pain in the posterior region of the elbow may indicate an olecranon stress fracture.[12]

A careful neurovascular history is also important as ulnar nerve paresthesias can be the result of cubital tunnel syndrome, a subluxing ulnar nerve, or a traction injury from valgus instability.[6]

Throwing athletes are a unique patient population, and it is important to gather information about prior injury and any changes in the throwing mechanism or rehabilitation regimen.[10] A patient whose symptoms are related to throwing and are located medially may have an injury to the medial collateral ligament. Throwing athletes who report lost velocity and control or an inability "to let the ball go" may have pain posterior on forced extension, which may signify posterior olecranon impingement caused by a medial collateral ligament injury. The typical patient is a baseball pitcher in his mid-20s who has posterior elbow pain during the acceleration and follow-through phases of pitching and complains of the inability to fully extend the elbow.[6] Young throwing athletes (<18 years) with OCD lesions often report progressive lateral elbow pain during late acceleration and follow-through phases, with loss of extension and episodes of locking.[11]

Physical Examination

A careful physical examination of all three compartments of the elbow is critical to determine the correct diagnosis. Each compartment should be examined individually to fully evaluate the elbow. The physical examination starts with careful inspection of the skin and soft tissues to make sure there are no scars, swelling, ecchymosis, soft tissue masses, or bony abnormalities. The alignment of the elbow should be inspected, noticing any significant varus or valgus deformities. Range of motion of the elbow in flexion, extension, supination, and pronation should be observed and compared with the contralateral side. Those with posteromedial impingement or valgus extension overload may reveal a flexion contracture and pain over the posteromedial olecranon tip.[6]

Pain along the medial aspect in response to palpation at the medial epicondyle usually indicates medial epicondylitis with provocative testing, with the elbow extended and resisted wrist flexion reproducing the pain. In adolescents, pain medially can suggest a medial epicondyle avulsion fracture. It is important to differentiate medial epicondylitis from an injury to the ulnar or medial collateral ligament. Pain just distal to the medial epicondyle along the medial collateral ligament usually indicates an injury to the ligament. Palpation of the proximal flexor-pronator mass can indicate tendinopathy. The ulnar nerve should be palpated, and Tinel's sign demonstrates ulnar neuropathy. The elbow is also flexed and extended as the nerve is palpated to determine whether the nerve subluxates.

The examiner should test for valgus instability with the elbow flexed to 30 degrees to relax the anterior capsule and free the olecranon from its bony articulation in the olecranon fossa. A valgus stress is then applied with the elbow in full supination. Discomfort along the medial aspect of the elbow can indicate ulnar collateral ligament injury. Valgus laxity, however, is often difficult to discern, particularly if there is tearing of the undersurface of the ulnar collateral ligament.[13] Comparison with the contralateral elbow can help differentiate physiologic laxity from pathologic instability.[14]

The triceps muscle insertion and the posterolateral and posteromedial joint areas are palpated to assess for tenderness, bone spurs, and posterior impingement lesions. The so-called clunk test is performed to demonstrate posterior olecranon impingement.[15] The upper arm is grasped and stabilized as the elbow is brought into full extension. Reproduction of pain at the posteromedial aspect of the joint suggests compression of the olecranon into the fossa and indicates valgus extension overload.

The lateral epicondyle and extensor origin are palpated to assess for lateral epicondylitis. The radiocapitellar joint is palpated while the forearm is pronated and supinated to elicit crepitus or catching, which can be caused by chondromalacial lesions or impingement from a lateral synovial fringe.[16] The soft spot is also inspected to determine whether there is synovitis or an effusion in the elbow joint.[6]

Stability can be assessed with O'Driscoll's posterolateral rotatory instability test.[17] The test is best done under general anesthesia because of the patient's apprehension while awake, which may give a false-negative result. However, it can be done with the patient awake with the extremity over the patient's head and the shoulder in full external rotation. During the test, a valgus, supination, and axial compression load is applied to the elbow, which is flexed approximately 20 to 30 degrees. With the elbow in extension, subluxation or dislocation of the radius and of the proximal ulna creates a posterior prominence and sulcus sign. When the elbow is flexed, radiohumeral and ulnohumeral joints are visibly or palpably reduced.[6] Details of this technique can be found in Chapter 11.

A careful neurovascular examination should be done on every patient, paying close attention to the ulnar nerve medially to differentiate cubital tunnel syndrome from concomitant medial epicondylitis or a medial collateral ligament injury.

Diagnostic Imaging

Routine diagnostic radiographs include an anteroposterior view with the elbow in full extension and a lateral view with the joint in 90 degrees of flexion. An axial view can be obtained to outline the olecranon and its medial and lateral articulations. This is the best view for identifying and assessing a posteromedial osteophyte. When there is a history of trauma, an oblique view should be done, and careful attention should be paid to the radial head and the coronoid process for subtle fracture lines. Radiographs should be reviewed for more obvious anterior or posterior elbow dislocations, along with more subtle degenerative changes, osteophytes, and loose bodies. However, plain radiographs are not always able to demonstrate all loose bodies.[18]

A gravity stress test radiograph can be used to detect valgus laxity of the elbow.[19] The patient is placed in a supine position, and the shoulder is abducted and brought to maximum external rotation so that the elbow is parallel to the floor. If there is an injury to the ligament or bony attachment, increased joint space can be seen on radiographs.[6]

Magnetic resonance imaging (MRI) and computed tomography (CT) arthrography (CTA) have are accurate in diagnosing a complete tear of the ulnar collateral ligament.[13] However, in early studies, CTA was more sensitive in detecting a partial undersurface tear of the ulnar collateral ligament.[20] This was described as a *T-sign lesion* by Timmerman and Andrews, who said that it represents "...dye leaking around the detachment of the deep portion of the ulnar collateral ligament from its bony insertion, but remaining within the intact superficial layer, ulnar collateral ligament, and capsule."[13]

MRI is useful for evaluating osteochondral lesions in the radiocapitellar joint[21,22] and for demonstrating early vascular changes that are not yet apparent on plain radiographs, and it can be used to assess the extent of the lesion and displacement of fragments.[6] MRI is also helpful for evaluating the soft tissue structures of the elbow, including the tendinous insertions of the flexor and extensor musculature to help in diagnosing medial and lateral epicondylitis, the triceps insertion and associated musculature to evaluate for triceps tendonitis, and the medial and lateral collateral ligaments for possible tears. However, MRI may not demonstrate subtle undersurface tears of the ulnar collateral ligament. Magnetic resonance arthrography with saline contrast or gadolinium can increase the sensitivity for detecting undersurface tears of the ulnar collateral ligament and has become the test of choice to detect these tears.[13]

TREATMENT

Indications and Contraindications

In 1992, O'Driscoll and Morrey described the early indication for elbow arthroscopy, which was pain or symptoms that were substantial enough to interfere with work, daily activities, sports, or sleep and that did not resolve after conservative treatment.[23] In this early study, they analyzed the results of 71 elbow arthroscopies as the indications for such a procedure were evolving. Not surprising, the best early results were seen for arthroscopic removal of loose bodies, assessment of undiagnosed snapping, idiopathic flexion contractures, local débridement of damaged articular surfaces, and synovectomy. They found that the patients least likely to benefit were the ones in whom there was a disparity between objective and subjective findings.[23]

Since then, the indications for elbow arthroscopy have evolved. In 1994, Poehling further refined the indications, which included its use for the diagnosis of intra-articular lesions of the elbow, the removal of loose and foreign bodies, irrigation of the joint, débridement of an infected joint, excision of osteophytes, synovectomy, capsular release, excision of the radial head, and treatment of acute fractures of the elbow.[1]

Several investigators have since reported the usefulness of elbow arthroscopy for the removal of loose bodies,[6,7,18,23-25] and this continues to be the primary indication for elbow arthroscopy. Several pathologic processes may initiate the formation of a loose body, including trauma and synovial chondromatosis. Regardless of the cause, the patients usually present with swelling, locking, pain, and loss of motion, all of which can be improved with the removal of loose bodies. These loose bodies can be found in the anterior and posterior compartments and in the posterior medial gutter, and removing them can be a technically demanding procedure. Further details and helpful hints can be found in Chapter 2.

Elbow arthroscopy can be an effective tool if the diagnosis of an infection is made or suspected. It is a less invasive way to enter into the joint with minimal trauma to confirm the diagnosis of an infection, irrigate the joint, débride infected tissue, and assess the condition of the underlying bone, cartilage, and synovial tissue.[1]

The presence of osteophytes, or osseous spurs, is another condition that lends itself to arthroscopic management and removal.[23-26] A true lateral radiograph of the elbow is useful for the identification of osteophytes that may limit full extension of the elbow with impingement of the posterior olecranon spur in the olecranon fossa.[1,23] An axial view may also show a posteromedial osteophyte,[6] which can be easily removed arthroscopically.

The term *valgus extension overload* was coined[27] to describe the findings that can be identified in baseball pitchers and other overhead athletes. The tremendous repetitive valgus forces generated during the acceleration and follow-through phases of pitching, as the elbow goes into extension, can result in osteochondral changes in the olecranon and distal humerus. A significant osteophyte forms on the posteromedial aspect of the olecranon fossa with continued pitching or overhead activities, creating an area of chondromalacia.[6] The use of elbow arthroscopy in the throwing athlete, including evaluation of the medial collateral ligament, is addressed in Chapter 12. The inability to reliably visualize the anterior bundle of the medial collateral ligament with the arthroscope limits the value of the arthroscope when assessing medial collateral ligament injuries.[28,29] The management of posterolateral instability is discussed in Chapter 11.

Chronic synovitis caused by inflammatory arthritis that does not respond to nonoperative management and when there is minimal joint destruction can be an indication for elbow arthroscopy. Synovectomy can provide considerable relief of pain.[23,30,31] Diagnostic elbow arthroscopy can also be used for synovial biopsy to establish the diagnosis of rheumatoid arthritis or other inflammatory arthritides or a monoarticular or polyarticular arthritis of unknown origin.[23] The elbow joint is affected in approximately 20% to 50% of patients with rheumatoid arthritis, and 50% of these patients develop pain and associated loss of motion.[23,32] Lee and Morrey achieved a 93% rate of good or excellent results in a short-term follow-up assessment of 14 arthroscopic synovectomies in 11 patients. However, only 57% of their patients maintained good or excellent results at an average of 42 months after surgery.[31] When performing elbow arthroscopy and synovectomy for rheumatoid arthritis and other inflammatory arthritides, it is important to set realistic expectations for the patient because the symptoms can recur.

OCD of the capitellum is characterized by pain, swelling, and limitation of motion, and it usually occurs during adolescence or young adulthood in a throwing athlete or gymnast.[33] The underlying cause of this lesion is most likely repetitive microtrauma to a vulnerable epiphysis with a precarious blood supply.[33] The lesion may progress to joint incongruity, loose body formation, and a locked elbow with chronic pain, all of which are indications for elbow arthroscopy when conservative measures fail. The procedure involves the arthroscopic removal of osteophytes, excision of loose or detached cartilage, and curettement and drilling of the base of the lesion.[34]

Panner's disease is an osteochondrosis of the entire capitellum in children and adolescents, and it may represent an early stage of OCD.[6] Reconstitution of the capitellum usually occurs with rest and without late sequelae or limitations.[33] More information about OCD can be found in Chapter 7.

The indications for arthroscopic débridement of the elbow for degenerative osteoarthritis are similar to those described for loose body removal, valgus extension overload, and OCD. Pain associated with swelling and mechanical symptoms of catching and locking respond well to arthroscopic débridement.[24-26] Removal of loose bodies and osteophytes from the olecranon, olecranon fossa, and coronoid process can reduce pain, increase range of motion, and eliminate mechanical-like symptoms.[24-26] Elbow arthroscopy has limited value in primary degenerative arthrosis when there are no significant osteophytes, loose bodies, or mechanical-like symptoms. The arthritic elbow is addressed in Chapter 9.

Arthrofibrosis of the elbow treated arthroscopically can be a technically demanding procedure with an increased risk of complications because of the limited ability to distend the arthrofibrotic capsule and the proximity of many neurovascular structures.[1,6,24] Loss of elbow joint motion can be a result of bone or soft tissue problems caused by trauma and degenerative or inflammatory arthritides. Patients can have a loss of flexion or extension, or both. It is important to attempt to determine the cause of the contracture because this can influence treatment.[6] If a nonoperative treatment of nonsteroidal anti-inflammatory drugs (NSAIDs), stretching exercises, splinting, and other modalities fail, arthroscopic release and thorough joint débridement may be indicated in properly selected patients.[24,35,36] The details of this technically demanding procedure can be found in Chapter 8.

The indications for elbow arthroscopy have been extended to include the treatment of lateral epicondylitis. When conservative measures fail, arthroscopic release offers several potential advantages over open techniques.[6] It preserves the common extensor origin by addressing the lesion directly,[37] and it allows for intra-articular examination for possible chondral lesions, loose bodies, and other disorders, such as an inflamed lateral synovial fringe. It also permits a shorter postoperative rehabilitation period and an earlier return to work or sports.[6] The details of the technique of the treatment of arthroscopic lateral epicondyle release can be found in Chapter 3.

Radial head excision can be performed arthroscopically for post-traumatic arthritis of the radiocapitellar joint caused by a radial head fracture.[1,6,24,38] Advantages of arthroscopic treatment include more complete visualization of the articular surface of the elbow and associated chondral lesions or ligamentous disruptions.[6] In addition to the entire radial head, as much as 2 or 3 mm of the radial neck can be removed. To maintain stability at the proximal radioulnar joint, the annular ligament must be left intact.[1] More information about this technique can be found in Chapter 10.

The arthroscopic management of selected fractures around the elbow with percutaneous pins and screws is evolving and includes the treatment of radial head fractures, capitellum fractures, and coronoid fractures. The arthroscopic-assisted treatment of coronoid fractures has shown promise in a small study group of 7 patients.[39] More information about the arthroscopic treatment of fractures of the elbow can be found in Chapter 15. New frontiers of elbow arthroscopy include the treatment of olecranon bursitis (Chapter 5), endoscopic repair of a torn distal biceps tendon (Chapter 13), arthroscopic triceps repair (Chapter 14), and arthroscopic ulnar nerve release (Chapter 16).

The primary contraindication to elbow arthroscopy is any significant distortion of normal bony or soft tissue anatomy that precludes safe entry of the arthroscope into the joint.[23,9] For example, a previous ulnar nerve transposition that was submuscular or subcutaneous would interfere with safe proximal, anteromedial portal placement and is a relative contraindication for safe introduction of the arthroscope through the medial side of the elbow.[6,40] In these cases, identification of the ulnar nerve is necessary before establishing a medial portal.[40]

Another relative contraindication is a severely ankylosed joint that may distort normal anatomy and place important neurovascular structures at risk. This may not allow for adequate joint distention and may not allow proper displacement of neurovascular structures away from portal sites and within the joint from instrumentation.[6] Localized infection in the area of portal placement is also a contraindication to elbow arthroscopy.

Conservative Management

Appropriate conservative measures should always be tried before making the decision to proceed with elbow arthroscopy. However, the diagnosis often is not clear until the time of diagnostic arthroscopy, because loose bodies, articular cartilage damage, or other pathology cannot always be detected by physical examination, radiographs, or MRI.

Elbow Arthroscopy

When conservative measures have failed, elbow arthroscopy is a useful tool in the treatment of simple and complex disorders of the elbow. However, it does not replace a careful history, physical examination, diagnostic testing, or an adequate course of nonoperative treatment. When the decision is made to proceed with elbow arthroscopy, it is important to discuss with the patient the risks and benefits of the procedure, including the remote risk of blood vessel and nerve damage, and what realistic results can be expected after the surgery. Documentation of this discussion in the medical record and proper informed consent are essential before proceeding with this or any other surgical procedure.

Anesthesia

Most surgeons prefer to use general endotracheal anesthesia for patients undergoing elbow arthroscopy because it provides total muscle relaxation and is more comfortable for the patient.[6,40] The use of regional anesthesia is advocated by some, including the use of an axillary nerve block or an interscalene nerve block. These blocks can be administered safely and successfully by a trained anesthesiologist, but there is still inherent risk in these blocks not seen with general anesthesia.

There is apprehension among some surgeons about using local and intravenous blocks because the patient's postoperative neurologic status cannot be assessed and may be compromised by an extended axillary or interscalene nerve block.[6] If there is a neurologic deficit found after the procedure, it may be difficult to determine how it occurred, and there may be finger pointing between the anesthesiologist and the surgeon.

Local anesthetics for postoperative pain control are not commonly used because of the difficulty in assessing the patient's postoperative neurologic status. However, there is no hard and fast rule against the use of local anesthetics for postoperative pain control, and it should be left to the discretion of the operating surgeon.

Positioning

Traditionally, elbow arthroscopy was performed with the patient resting supine on the operating table,[7] until use of the prone position was introduced in 1989 by Poehling.[8] The prone position improves the mobility of the arthroscope within the joint, facilitates manipulation of the joint, provides for a more complete intra-articular inspection (especially in the posterior aspect of the joint), and eliminates the need for an overhead suspension device to support the elbow. The main disadvantage to this position is a more difficult access to the patient's airway.[1]

After an appropriate level of anesthesia (i.e., general endotracheal or axillary block) has been achieved, the patient is placed prone, with large chest rolls under the torso. The chest rolls must bee large enough to raise the patient's torso up from the operating table. If these rolls are not large enough, it makes it difficult to position the arm and elbow to access the proximal anteromedial portal. An arm board is placed on the operative side of the table and parallel to it. To increase the mobility of the upper extremity intraoperatively, a sandbag, block, or firm bump of towels is placed under the shoulder to further elevate the arm away from the table. The forearm is then allowed to hang in a dependent position over the arm board at 90 degrees (Fig. 1-4). A sterile tourniquet may be placed around the proximal aspect of the arm to help to control bleeding during the procedure, but it is not always necessary to inflate when using a mechanical irrigation system.[1] After the extremity is prepared and draped, a large sterile bump is placed under the arm proximal to the elbow to keep the shoulder abducted to 90 degrees and to keep the elbow at approximately 90 degrees of flexion (Fig. 1-5).

Some surgeons prefer the lateral decubitus position because they feel it provides improved stability of the extremity, is more

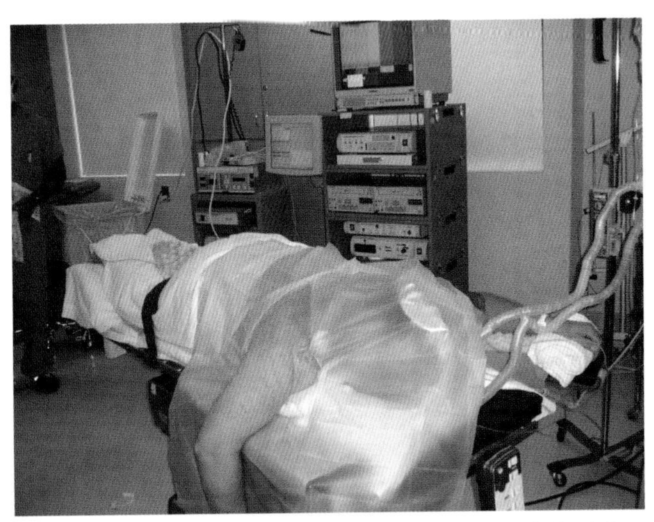

FIGURE 1-4 The patient is placed in the prone position with the right elbow resting over an arm board, which is parallel to the operating room table. A nonsterile U-drape is placed proximally. A sterile bump is placed under the arm for support after the extremity is prepared.

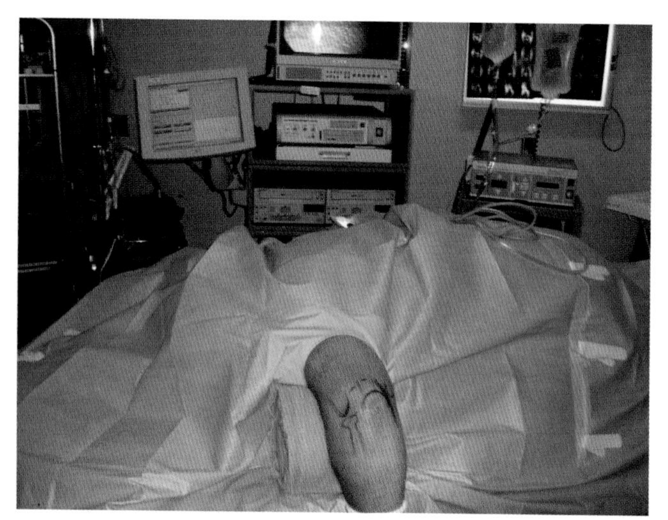

FIGURE 1-5 A left elbow is shown in the prone position. Anesthesia is left of the head of the patient, and all equipment is on the opposite side of the table. Notice the sterile bump under the arm that helps to stabilize the elbow during the procedure. It rests on the arm board, which has been placed parallel to the table.

convenient for the anesthesiologist, and allows posterior elbow joint access without compromising airway access.[23,40] O'Driscoll and Morrey prefer the lateral decubitus position because it has the advantages of the prone positioning without compromising the anesthesiologist's access to the airway.[23] The patient is placed in the lateral decubitus position with the involved extremity facing upward. The arm is then supported on a well-padded bolster, with the forearm hanging free and the elbow flexed to 90 degrees. In this position, the elbow is supported in front of the surgeon, who then has access to the various portal sites.

Whether using the prone or lateral decubitus position, the forearm is prepared from the proximal arm to the tip of the fingers, and the extremity is wrapped with an elastic bandage from the fingers to just below the elbow to minimize fluid extravasation into the forearm.[40]

Operating Room Setup

When using the prone position, anesthesia is positioned at the head of the table, the surgeon stands directly lateral to the flexed elbow, and the assistant stands toward the head of the patient. The ancillary scrub personnel stand toward the foot of the patient or behind the surgeon and the assistant. One Mayo stand is placed behind the surgeon, and the other Mayo stand is on the opposite side of the table. All tubing and electrical cords run from this Mayo stand to the video monitor, recorder, light source, camera, fluid bags, and mechanical irrigation system, which are placed on the opposite side of the patient (see Fig. 1-5).

Instrumentation

A standard 4.0-mm, 30-degree arthroscope enables excellent visualization of the elbow joint. A smaller, 2.7-mm arthroscope usually is unnecessary but can be useful for viewing small spaces, such as the lateral compartment from the direct lateral portal and for arthroscopy in adolescent patients.[6,40] The use of cannulas allows the surgeon to switch viewing and working portals without repeated joint capsule injuries. This also minimizes the risk of injury to neurovascular structures and decreases the chance of fluid extravasation into the soft tissues, swelling, and possible compartment syndrome.[6] A metal cannula typically is used for the arthroscope, and the working portal is usually a disposable plastic cannula with a diaphragm that allows instruments to be introduced without loss of joint distention.

Side-vented inflow cannulas should be avoided in elbow arthroscopy because the distance between the skin ad the joint capsule is often very slight. With side-vented cannulas, the cannula can be intra-articular while the side vents remain extra-articular, resulting in fluid extravasation into the surrounding soft tissues. Inflow cannulas should be devoid of side vents, with fluid flow occurring directly at the end of the cannula.[41]

All trocars should be conical and blunt tipped to decrease the possibility of neurovascular and articular cartilage injury. A variety of handheld instruments, such as probes, grasping forceps, and punches, and motorized instruments, such as synovial resectors and burrs, are used during elbow arthroscopy.[6,40]

If a mechanical pump is used, an inflow pressure of 35 mm Hg is usually used to maintain joint distention.[6] Some surgeons prefer the use of gravity inflow and think it gives adequate joint distention without the risk of fluid extravasation. If a tourniquet is used, it can be set at 250 mm Hg and inflated if needed.

General Surgical Technique

Elbow arthroscopy has a significant potential for complications, particularly neurovascular injury.[6] The key to avoiding complications is to have a clear understanding of the relationship of the neurovascular structures to the soft tissue and bony anatomy. With the patient positioned in the lateral decubitus or prone position, it is important to identify and mark landmarks. They include the tip of the olecranon, the medial and lateral epicondyles, the radial head, the soft spot of the elbow, the medial intermuscular septum, and the ulnar nerve (Fig. 1-6). Some sur-

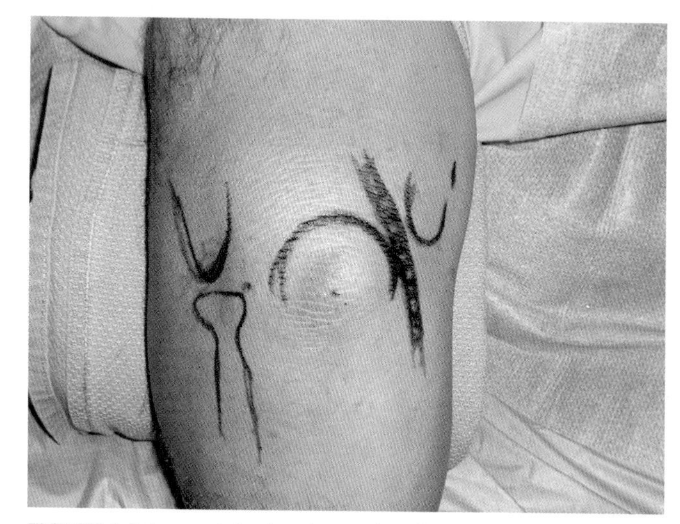

FIGURE 1-6 Anatomic landmarks are identified on the left elbow in the prone position, including the medial epicondyle *(right)*, the lateral epicondyle *(left)*, the radial head, the olecranon, and the ulnar nerve *(dark blue line on right)*. The intermuscular septum is identified on the medial aspect of the elbow, just anterior to the medial epicondyle.

geons recommend distending the joint with 20 to 40 mL of fluid through the lateral soft spot before establishing the initial portal.[42] Cadaveric studies have demonstrated that joint insufflation significantly increases the distance between the joint surfaces and neurovascular structures, helping to protect them from injury during joint entry.[43]

In a different cadaveric study looking at the role of joint insufflation before portal placement, Miller and coworkers.[44] demonstrated that there was a small distance (as narrow as 6 mm) between the joint capsule and neurovascular structures and that joint insufflation did not increase the capsule-to-nerve distance. My colleagues and I have found joint insufflation unnecessary before making the proximal anteromedial portal, the first portal that we typically establish. If the surgeon pays close attention to anatomic landmarks, the elbow joint can be safely entered into without having to inflate the joint with fluid.

When creating portals, the surgeon should avoid penetrating the subcutaneous tissue, thereby helping to prevent injury to the superficial cutaneous nerves. A hemostat or mosquito clamp should be used to spread tissues down to the capsule.[6] When the arthroscope is introduced, the elbow should be flexed to 90 degrees to relax and protect the anterior neurovascular structures,[43] and only blunt trocars should be used.

Whether the anteromedial or anterolateral portal should be created first has been an issue of some debate. Many surgeons create a lateral portal initially and then establish a medial portal with a spinal needle by direct visualization from within the joint. Alternatively, an inside-out technique may be employed in which a switching stick is used to establish the medial portal from inside the joint.[45] Other surgeons, using the same techniques, establish the medial portal first, and cadaveric studies have found that it is safer to establish the proximal anteromedial portal first than the lateral portal.[46]

Other surgeons and I think the proximal anteromedial portal should be created first, because it is the safest approach as long as the surgeon has identified and outlined the important soft tissue and bony landmarks, including the intermuscular septum.[6,40,45,46] There is less fluid extravasation when starting medially, because a superomedial portal traverses predominately tendinous tissue and a tough portion of the forearm flexor muscles.[9,38] The thicker tissues minimize fluid extravasation more effectively than the softer, thinner radial capsule.[9,38] Most elbow disorders are located in the lateral compartment, which is best visualized from the proximal anteromedial portal.[6]

Portal Placement

Anterior Compartment. The proximal anteromedial portal is established first, and it was first described by Poehling.[8] It is located approximately 2 cm proximal to the medial epicondyle and just anterior to the intermuscular septum (Fig. 1-7). Before establishing this portal, the location and the stability of the ulnar nerve should be assessed. The prevalence rate of ulnar nerve subluxation anterior to the cubital tunnel is approximately 17%. Blunt dissection is carried out until the anterior aspect of the humerus is palpated while staying anterior to the intermuscular septum. The arthroscopic sheath is then inserted anterior to the intermuscular septum while maintaining contact with the anterior aspect of the humerus and directing the trocar toward the radial head. Use of the anterior surface of the humerus as a constant guide helps to prevent injury to the median nerve and the brachial artery, which are anterior to the capsule. The ulnar nerve is located approximately 3 to 4 mm from this portal and posterior to the intermuscular septum (Fig. 1-8). Palpating the septum and making sure that the portal is established anterior to the

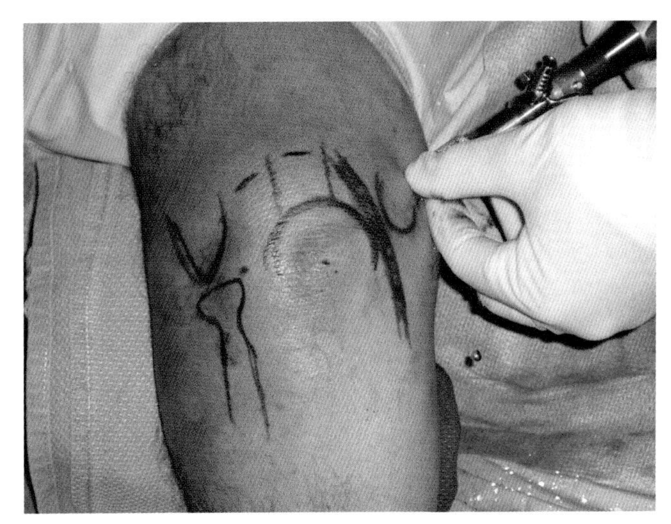

FIGURE 1-7 The proximal anteromedial portal is the first to be established. It is located just anterior to the intermuscular septum and 2 cm proximal to the medial epicondyle.

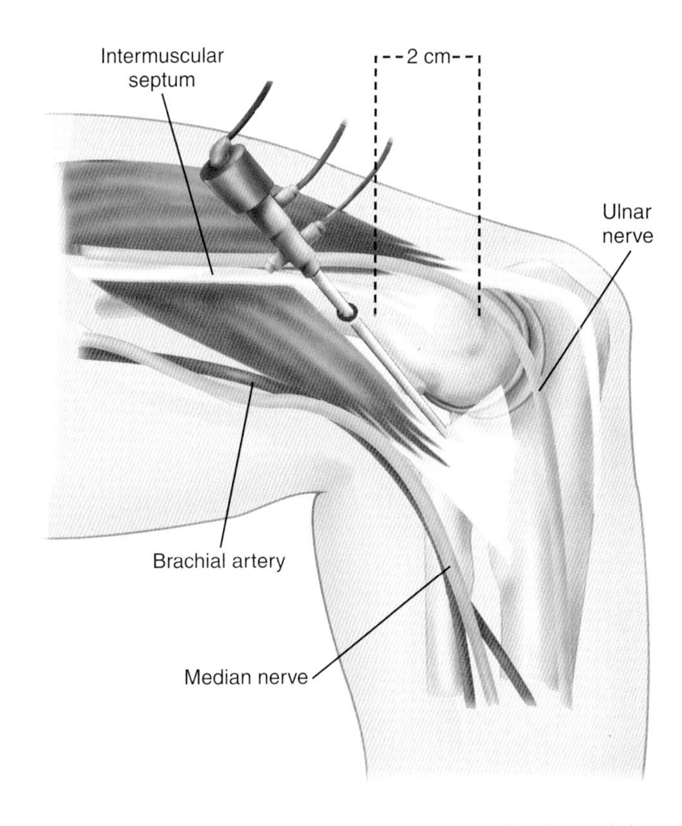

FIGURE 1-8 The arthroscope is inserted 2 cm proximal to the medial epicondyle and just anterior to the intermuscular septum on the medial aspect of the arm. In the prone position, the brachial artery and median nerve fall away from the joint capsule, allowing safe portal placement.

septum minimizes the risk of injury to the nerve while providing excellent visualization. This portal provides excellent visualization of the anterior compartment of the elbow, particularly the radiocapitellar joint, the humeroulnar joints, the coronoid fossa, and superior joint capsule.[1,6]

Careful attention should be paid to the medial aspect of the elbow, and the ulnar nerve should be carefully examined to make sure the ulnar nerve does not subluxate. If there is any question, the ulnar nerve should be dissected out and identified, and the trocar should then be placed carefully around it. Another option is for two lateral portals to be used, or a trans-fossa portal with a 70-degree scope to view into the anterior compartment can be used.

The anteromedial portal as described by Lynch and associates[47] is located 2 cm distal and 2 cm anterior to the medial epicondyle, and it is at or near the distal extent of the elbow capsule. Because of the location of this portal, the cannula can enter the joint only by being advanced straight laterally, toward the median nerve.[46] Because of this, the proximal anteromedial portal is recommended; it is safer because the more proximal position allows the arthroscope to be directed distally, resulting in the arthroscope being almost parallel to the median nerve in the anteroposterior plane.[6,46]

The anterolateral portal was originally described by Carson and Andrews as being located 3 cm distal and 2 cm anterior to the lateral epicondyle.[7] However, this portal location places the radial nerve at significant risk for iatrogenic injury.[47] Lindenfeld demonstrated the radial nerve could be as close as 3 mm to this portal.[46] To decrease risk of injury to the radial nerve, several investigators have stressed the importance of avoiding the distal placement of this portal in favor of a more proximal placement of the anterolateral portal.[2,42] Field and colleaues[42] compared three lateral portals: a proximal anterolateral portal (located 2 cm proximal and 1 cm anterior to the lateral epicondyle), a distal anterolateral portal (as described by Carson and Andrews), and a middle anterolateral portal (located 1 cm directly anterior to the lateral epicondyle). The investigators found that the proximal anterolateral portal was the safest and that the radiohumeral joint visualization was most complete and technically easiest using this most proximal portal.

After creating the proximal anteromedial portal and using it as viewing portal, we think creating this proximal anterolateral portal is done best using an outside-in technique and localizing the position with a spinal needle. This portal is created 2 cm proximal and 1 cm anterior to the lateral epicondyle, as described by Field and coworkers.[42] The exact entry depends on the pathology to be addressed. From the proximal anteromedial portal, the lateral capsule is visualized, and palpation of the skin helps to localize the exact location of the spinal needle to aid in portal placement (Fig. 1-9). It is important to direct the cannula toward the humerus while penetrating the capsule so that the portal placement is not too far anterior and medial.[3] From the proximal anteromedial portal, the radiocapitellar joint is easily visualized (Fig. 1-10). The trochlea and the coronoid process can be seen from the proximal anteromedial portal (Fig. 1-11).

The proximal anterolateral portal is often a working portal and is ideal for arthroscopic lateral epicondyle release and for

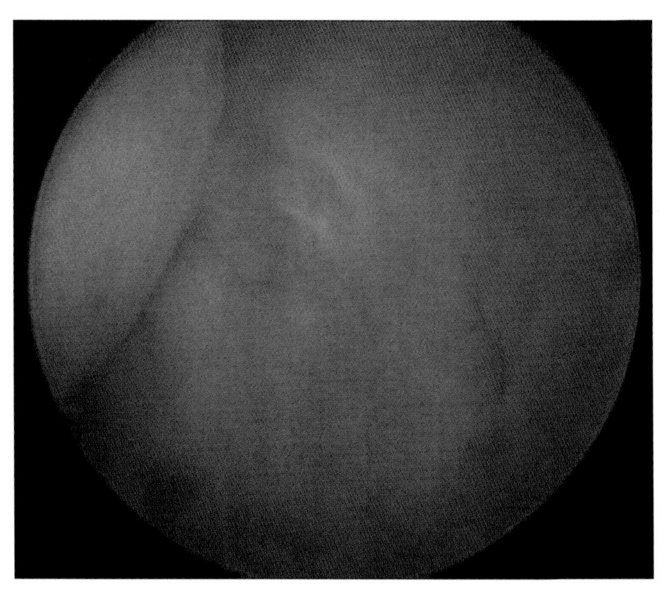

FIGURE 1-9 The lateral capsule is seen from the proximal anteromedial portal. A spinal needle is introduced in this location for the proximal anterolateral portal.

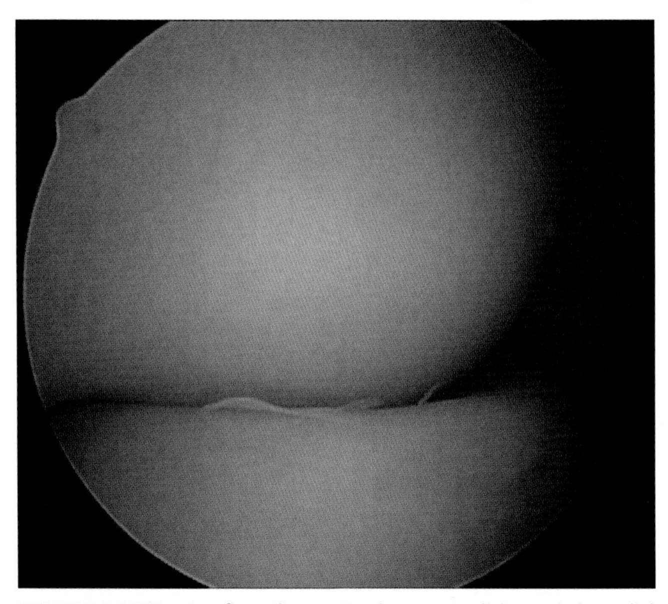

FIGURE 1-10 Viewing from the proximal anteromedial portal, the radial head and the capitellum are easily visualized.

débridement of the radiocapitellar joint. Viewing from this portal permits visualization of the anterior compartment (Fig. 1-12) and is particularly good for evaluating medial structures, such as the trochlea, coronoid tip, and the medial capsule (Fig. 1-13).

Posterior Compartment. The straight posterior portal is located 3 cm proximal to the tip of the olecranon and can be used as a viewing portal or as a working portal. When it is the first portal created, a cannula with a blunt trocar is inserted. The cannula pierces the triceps muscle just above the musculotendinous junction and is bluntly maneuvered in a circular motion, manipulating the soft tissues from the olecranon fossa for better visualization. When used as a working portal, it is helpful for removal of

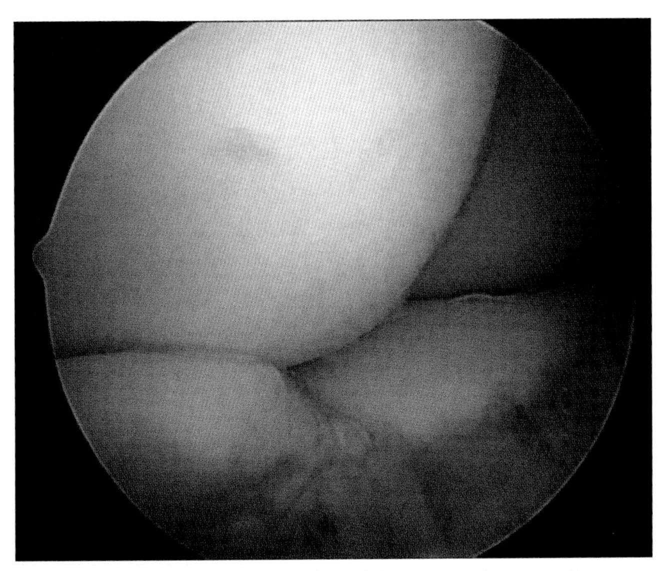

FIGURE 1-11 The trochlea *(top left)* and the coronoid process *(lower left)* can be seen from the proximal anteromedial portal.

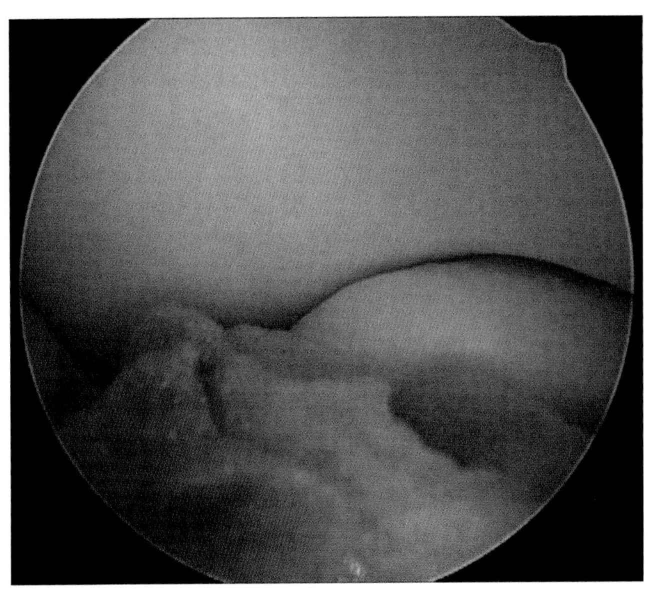

FIGURE 1-13 Viewing from the proximal anterolateral portal, the trochlea and the coronoid process can be seen.

impinging olecranon osteophytes and loose bodies from the posterior elbow joint.[45] It is also needed for a complete synovectomy of the elbow.[6] The straight posterior portal passes within 25 mm of the ulnar nerve and within 23 mm of the posterior antebrachial cutaneous nerve.[9]

The posterolateral portal is located 2 to 3 cm proximal to the tip of olecranon at the lateral border of the triceps tendon. This is created while visualizing from the straight posterior portal and using a spinal needle directed toward the olecranon fossa (Fig. 1-14). Initial visualization is often difficult due to scar, fat pad hypertrophy, and synovitis. A trocar is then directed toward the olecranon fossa, passing through the triceps muscle to reach the capsule. A shaver is introduced to improve visualization of the posterior compartment. This portal permits visualization of the olecranon tip, olecranon fossa, and the posterior trochlea, and it can be used as a working portal to remove osteophytes and loose bodies from the posterior compartment (Fig. 1-15). However, the posterior capitellum is not seen well from this portal.[6] The medial and posterior antebrachial cutaneous nerves are the two neurovascular structures at most risk; they are an average of 25 mm from this portal.[47] The ulnar nerve is approximately 25 mm from this portal, but as long as the cannula is kept lateral to the posterior midline, the nerve is not at risk for injury.[9]

The posterolateral anatomy of the elbow allows for portal placement anywhere from the proximal posterolateral portal to

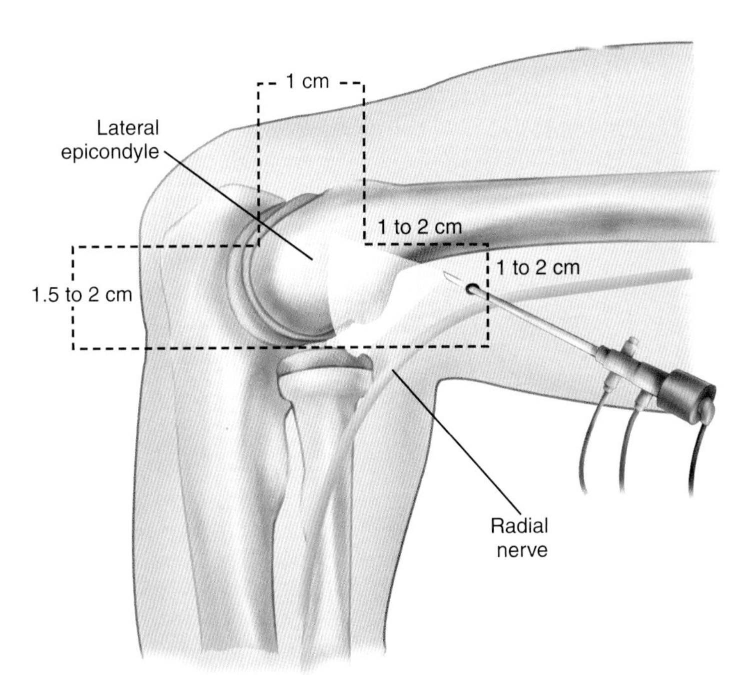

FIGURE 1-12 The proximal anterolateral portal is created 1 to 2 cm proximal to the lateral epicondyle and 1 to 2 cm anterior to the lateral epicondyle. Placing the arthroscope in the proximal anterolateral portal allows visualization of the anterior compartment looking medially.

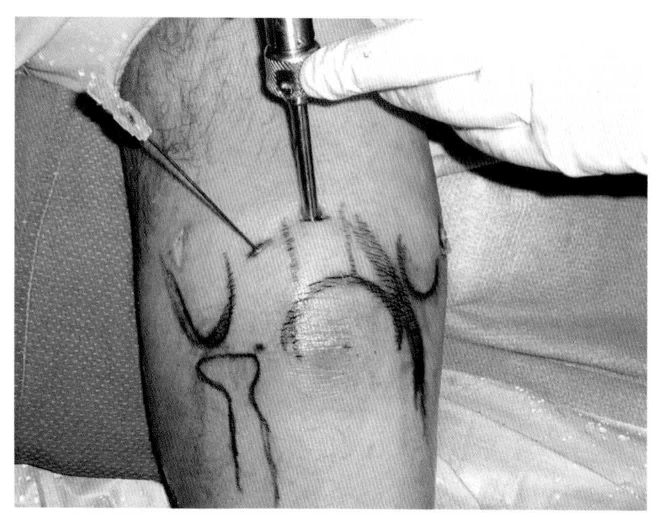

FIGURE 1-14 The arthroscope is introduced into the posterior compartment using a straight posterior portal at 3 cm proximal from the tip of the olecranon. A spinal needle is introduced lateral to the triceps tendon toward the olecranon fossa for the posterolateral portal.

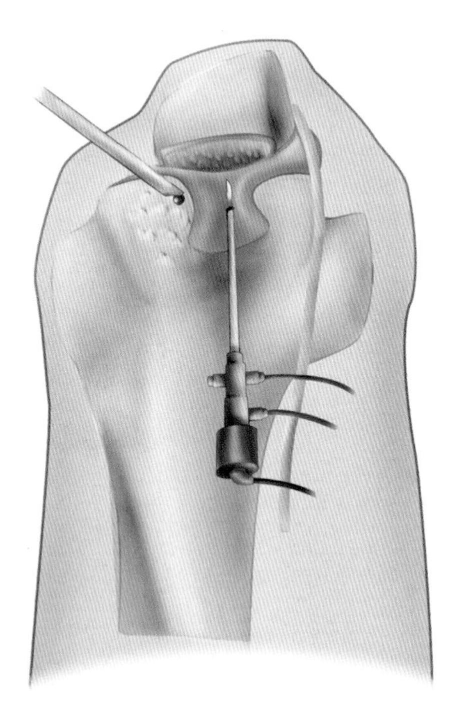

FIGURE 1-15 The posterior lateral portal is used as a working portal to remove osteophytes and loose bodies from the posterior compartment.

the lateral soft spot. Altering the portal position along the line between the posterolateral portal and lateral soft spot changes the orientation of the portal relative to the joint.[40] These portals are particularly useful for gaining access to the posterolateral recess.

The direct lateral portal is located at the soft spot, which is the triangle formed by the radial head, lateral epicondyle, and olecranon. It is developed under direct visualization using a spinal needle. It is useful as a viewing portal for working in the posterior compartment and viewing the radiocapitellar joint and as a working portal for radial head resection.[24] This is the only portal that provides easy access to the posterior capitellum and radioulnar joint, and it can be useful for lesions of the radiocapitellar joint.[6]

DIAGNOSTIC ARTHROSCOPY

Diagnostic arthroscopy is useful when the clinical diagnosis is unclear and other studies have failed to lead to a diagnosis. Unexpected synovitis, osteoarthritis, loose bodies, and chondral defects may be discovered. It can also be used for the management of arthrofibrosis, osteoarthritis, removal of olecranon spurs, OCD, fractures, and lateral epicondylitis. Diagnostic arthroscopy and the details of specific arthroscopic elbow procedures are discussed in the following chapters.

COMPLICATIONS

Complications due to elbow arthroscopy can be minimized if the surgeon has a sound knowledge of the anatomy of the elbow and uses proper equipment and meticulous operative technique.[1] One of the most common complications is neurologic injury,[1,47,48] including transient nerve palsies involving the radial nerve, posterior interosseous nerve, and ulnar nerve. Injury can be caused by direct laceration of a nerve by a knife penetrating deeply beneath the skin or from the cannula trocar.[10] Compression from a cannula, from fluid extravasation, or from the use of local anesthetics has caused neurologic injuries[23] but was usually transient. Transection of the posterior interosseous nerve, median nerve, ulnar nerve, and radial nerve has been reported. In a 1986 review of 569 elbow arthroscopic procedures performed by members of the Arthroscopy Association of North America (AANA), only one neurovascular complication, a radial nerve injury, was reported.[49] In a 2001 report of 473 elbow arthroscopies performed by experienced arthroscopists, four types of minor complications, including infection, nerve injury, prolonged drainage, and contracture, were identified in 50 cases. The most common complication was persistent portal drainage,[48] especially from the lateral portal. There is little subcutaneous tissue separating the skin from the capsule. Portal drainage can be reduced by using a side box stay suture, which closes the portal securely and minimizes drainage.

Many of the complications associated with elbow arthroscopy are the result of inexperience, poor technique, and lack of knowledge regarding elbow anatomy. The surgeon who wishes to perform elbow arthroscopy safely and effectively must adhere to strict surgical technique and portal placement to avoid preventable complications.[10]

PEARLS & PITFALLS

PEARLS

- A thorough physical and neurovascular examination is essential before performing elbow arthroscopy. Pay attention to the medial aspect of the elbow, and carefully examine the ulnar nerve to ensure it does not subluxate. If there is any question about its position, the ulnar nerve should be dissected out and identified, and a trocar should be placed carefully around it.

- Identify and mark landmarks of the elbow joint. This includes the tip of the olecranon, the medial and lateral epicondyle, the radial head, the soft spot of the elbow, the medial intermuscular septum, and the ulnar nerve.
- Know and review the superficial anatomy of the elbow before beginning elbow arthroscopy. The bony landmarks provide the key to avoiding damage to important neurovascular structures.
- The prone or the lateral decubitus position is the preferred patient positioning for elbow arthroscopy. Both positions allow easy access to the anterior and posterior compartments.
- The proximal anteromedial portal is established first and is located approximately 2 cm proximal to the medial epicondyle and just anterior to the intermuscular septum. Palpate the intermuscular septum, because this is the guide to safe portal placement. The arthroscopic sheath is then inserted anterior to the intermuscular septum while maintaining contact with the anterior aspect of the humerus and directing the trocar toward the radial head.
- The proximal anterolateral portal, which is located 2 cm proximal and 1 cm anterior to the lateral epicondyle, is safest and provides excellent visualization of the radiohumeral joint.
- Initial visualization of the posterior compartment can be difficult because of synovitis, scar tissue, and fat pad hypertrophy. Patiently triangulate with the arthroscope and shaver within the olecranon fossa to débride tissues to gain adequate visualization. The tip of the olecranon is one of the first landmarks to be identified.
- Alternatively, two lateral portals may be used, or a trans-fossa portal can be used with a 70-degree arthroscope to view into the anterior compartment.

PITFALLS

- Failure to identify the important bony and neurovascular landmarks can lead to iatrogenic nerve or blood vessel injury. The most important landmark is the medial intermuscular septum because it protects the ulnar nerve, and by staying anterior to it, the nerve is safe.
- If the trocar is placed posterior to the intermuscular septum, injury to the ulnar nerve can occur.
- A subluxating ulnar nerve or a previous ulnar nerve transposition places the ulnar nerve at risk with proximal anteromedial portal placement.
- Without having a thorough understanding of the anatomy of the elbow, improper portal placement can cause significant harm to neurovascular structures.
- The anterolateral portal, which is located 3 cm distal and 2 cm anterior to the lateral epicondyle, places the radial nerve at significant risk, and it should be avoided.
- Blindly débriding in the posterior compartment and straying outside of the olecranon fossa can cause severe iatrogenic nerve injury.
- The supine position should be avoided because it makes it difficult to access the posterior compartment.

CONCLUSIONS

Arthroscopic surgery of the elbow is a technically demanding procedure. Attention to detail, including careful portal placement, is necessary to avoid iatrogenic injury to neurovascular structures around the elbow joint. In every clinical case, the bony anatomy should be drawn on the patient's elbow, and an 18-gauge spinal needle should be used to confirm the correct portal location before introducing larger arthroscopic instruments.[10]

With innovations in techniques and technology, it is possible to treat a variety of lesions of the elbow. As with any operative procedure, careful preoperative planning, including a detailed history, physical examination, and proper imaging studies, must be combined with sound clinical judgment to ensure a successful procedure.

REFERENCES

1. Poehling GG, Ekman EF. Arthroscopy of the Elbow. *J Bone Joint Surg Am.* 1994;76A:1265-1271.
2. Strothers D, Day B, Regan WR. Arthroscopy of the elbow: anatomy, portal sites, and description of the proximal lateral portal. *Arthroscopy.* 1995;11:449-457.
3. Moskal MJ. Advanced arthroscopic management of common elbow disorders. Presented at the Arthroscopy Association of North America 24th Annual Meeting, May 2005; Vancouver, Canada.
4. Burman MS. Arthroscopy or the direct visualization of the joints: an experimental cadaveric study. *J Bone Joint Surg.* 1931;13:669-695.
5. Burman MS. Arthroscopy of the elbow joint. A cadaver study. *J Bone Joint Surg.* 1932;14:349-350.
6. Baker CL, Grant LJ. Arthroscopy of the elbow. *Am J Sports Med.* 1999; 27:251-264.
7. Andrews JR, Carson WG. Arthroscopy of the elbow. *Arthroscopy.* 1985; 1:97-107.
8. Poehling GG, Whipple TL, Sisco L, Goldman B. Elbow arthroscopy: a new technique. *Arthroscopy.* 1989;5:220-224.
9. Baker CL, Brooks AA. Arthroscopy of the elbow. *Clin Sports Med.* 1996; 15:261-281.
10. Dodson CC, Nho SJ, Williams RJ, Altchek DW. Elbow arthroscopy. *J Am Acad Orthop Surg.* 2008;16:574-585.
11. Yadao MA, Field LD, Savoie FH III. Osteochondritis dissecans of the elbow. *Instr Course Lect.* 2004;53:599-606.
12. Cain EL, Dugas JR, Wolf RS, Andrews JR. Elbow injuries in throwing athletes: a current concepts review. *Am J Sports Med.* 2003;31:621-635.
13. Timmerman LA, Schwartz ML, Andrews JR. Preoperative evaluation of the ulnar ligament by magnetic resonance imaging and computed tomography arthrography. Evaluation in 25 baseball players with surgical confirmation. *Am J Sports Med.* 1994;22:26-32.
14. Jobe FW. *Operative Techniques in Upper Extremity Sports Injuries.* St. Louis, MO: Mosby–Year Book; 1996.
15. Baker CL. The Elbow. In: Whipple TL, ed. *Arthroscopic Surgery: The Shoulder and Elbow.* Philadelphia, PA: JB Lippincott; 1993:239-300.
16. Clarke RP. Symptomatic, lateral synovial fringe (plica) of the elbow joint. *Arthroscopy.* 1988;4:112-116.
17. O'Driscoll SW, Bell DF, Morrey BF. Posterolateral rotatory instability of the elbow. *J Bone Joint Surg Am.* 1991;73A:440-446.
18. Oglivie-Harris DJ, Schemitsch E. Arthroscopy of the elbow for removal of loose bodies. *Arthroscopy.* 1993;9:5-8.
19. Bennett JB, Hulles HS. Ligamentous and articular cartilage injuries in the athlete. In: Money BF, ed. *The Elbow and its Disorders.* Philadelphia, PA: WB Saunders; 1985:502-522.
20. Timmerman LA, Andrews JR. Undersurface tear of the ulnar collateral ligament in baseball players. A newly recognized lesion. *Am J Sports Med.* 1964;22:33-36.
21. Jaraw PM, Hessen U, Hirsch G. Osteochondral lesion in the radiocapitellar joint in the skeletally immature: radiographic MRI and arthroscopic findings in 13 conservative cases. *J Pediatr Orthop.* 1997;17: 311-314.
22. Takahara M, Shundo M, Kondo M, et al. Early Detection of Osteochondritis dissecans of the capitellum in young baseball players: report of three cases. *J Bone Joint Surg Am.* 1998;80A:892-897.
23. O'Driscoll SW, Morrey BF. Arthroscopy of the elbow. Diagnostic and therapeutic benefits and hazards. *J Bone Joint Surg Am.* 1992;74A:84-94.
24. Savoie FH, Nunley PD, Field LD. Arthroscopic management of the arthritic elbow: indications, technique and results. *J Shoulder Elbow Surg.* 1999;8:214-219.
25. Thal R. Osteoarthritis. In: Savoie FH, Field LD, eds. *Elbow Arthroscopy.* New York, NY: Churchill Livingstone; 1996.
26. Steinmann SP, King GJ, Savoie FH. Arthroscopic treatment of the arthritic elbow. *J Bone Joint Surg Am.* 2005;87A:2114-2121.

27. Wilson FD, Andrews JR, Blackburn TA, et al. Valgus extension overload in the pitching elbow. *Am J Sports Med.* 1983;11:83-88.
28. Field LD, Callaway GH, O'Brien SJ, et al. Arthroscopic assessment of the medial collateral ligament complex of the elbow. *Am J Sports Med* 1995;.23:396-400.
29. Field LD, Altchek DW. Evaluation of the arthroscopic valgus instability test of the elbow. *Am J Sports Med.* 1996;24:177-181.
30. Angelo RL. Advances in elbow arthroscopy. *Orthopedics.* 1993;16: 1037-1046.
31. Lee BPH, Morrey BF. Arthroscopic synovectomy of the elbow for rheumatoid arthritis: a prospective study. *J Bone Joint Surg Br.* 1997;79B: 770-772.
32. Nestor BJ. Surgical treatment of the rheumatoid elbow: an overview. *Rheum Dis Clin J North Am.* 1998;24:83-99.
33. Schenck RC Jr, Goodnight JM. Osteochondritis dissecans. *J Bone Joint Surg Am.* 1996;78:439-456.
34. Ruch DS, Poehling GG. Arthroscopic treatment of Panner's disease. *Clin Sports Med.* 1991;10:629-636.
35. Timmerman LA, Andrews JR. Arthroscopic treatment of posttraumatic elbow pain and stiffness. *Am J Sports Med.* 1994;22:230-235.
36. Phillips BB, Strasburger S. Arthroscopic treatment of arthrofibrosis of the elbow joint. *Arthroscopy.* 1998;14:38-44.
37. Baker CL, Cummings PD. Arthroscopic management of miscellaneous elbow disorders. *Oper Tech Sports Med.* 1998;6:121-129.
38. McLaughlin RE, Savoie FH, Field LF, Ramsey JR. Arthroscopic treatment of the arthritic elbow due to primary radiocapitellar arthritis. *Arthroscopy.* 2006;22:63-69.
39. Adams JE, Merten SM, Steinmann SP. Arthroscopic assisted treatment of coracoid fractures. *Arthroscopy.* 2007;23:1060-1065.
40. Abboud JA, Ricchette ET, Tjoumakaris F, Ramsey ML. Elbow arthroscopy: basic set-up and portal placement. *J Am Acad Orthop Surg.* 2006; 14:312-318.
41. Ramsey ML, Naranja RJ. Diagnostic arthroscopy of the elbow. In: Baker CL Jr, Plancher DL, eds. *Operative Treatment of Elbow Injuries.* New York, NY: Springer-Verlag; 2002:162-169.
42. Field LD, Altchek DW, Warren RF, et al. Arthroscopy anatomy of the lateral elbow: a comparison of 3 portals. *Arthroscopy.* 1994;10:602-607.
43. Adolfsson L. Arthroscopy of the elbow joint: a cadaveric study of portal placement. *J Shoulder Elbow Surg.* 1994;3:53-61.
44. Miller CD, Jobe CM, Wright MH. Neuroanatomy in elbow arthroscopy. *J Shoulder Elbow Surg.* 1995;4:168-174.
45. Andrews JR, St Pierre RK, Carson WG. Arthroscopy of the elbow. *Clin Sports Med.* 1986;5:653-662.
46. Lindenfeld TN. Medial approach in elbow arthroscopy. *Am J Sports Med.* 1990;18:413-417.
47. Lynch GJ, Meyers JF, Whipple TL, Caspari RB. Neurovascular anatomy and elbow arthroscopy: inherent risks. *Arthroscopy.* 1986;2:190-197.
48. Kelly EW, Morrey BF, O'Driscoll SW. Complications of elbow arthroscopy. *J Bone Joint Surg Am.* 2001;83:25-34.
49. Small NC. Complications in arthroscopy: the knee and other joints. *Arthroscopy.* 1986;2:253-258.

CHAPTER

2

Diagnostic Elbow Arthroscopy and Loose Body Removal

Raymond R. Drabicki • Larry D. Field • Felix H. Savoie III

Advances in elbow arthroscopy have enabled surgeons to treat a broad spectrum of disorders that were once thought to be unsafe using arthroscopic techniques.[1] Although technically demanding, advances in surgical technique and arthroscopic equipment and an improved understanding of neurovascular and joint anatomy have made this procedure safer and more effective than its initial applications.

The indications for elbow arthroscopy continue to evolve. In previous years, elbow arthroscopy was mainly used for removal of loose bodies,[2-8] synovectomy,[9,10] lysis of adhesions,[11,12] excision of osteophytes,[13,14] débridement of osteochondritis dissecans lesions,[6,15-17] radial head resection,[18] plica excision,[19,20] instability,[21] septic arthritis,[22] and diagnostic arthroscopy for complex elbow pain.[6] These indications have been expanded to include débridement, drilling, and autograft replacement for osteochondritis dissecans; débridement and repair of lateral epicondylitis; and débridement of radiocapitellar arthritis, olecranon bursectomy, arthrofibrosis, and fractures of the radial head, capitellum, and distal humerus.[6,8,9,23]

Removal of loose bodies is perhaps the most common and rewarding arthroscopic procedure involving the elbow.[4,24,25] Arthroscopic identification and removal of such impediments to joint motion has significant advantages. Scar formation is limited by the small portal site incisions needed to fully evaluate and perform loose body removal. All compartments of the elbow are readily accessible for a thorough evaluation of intra-articular pathology with the arthroscope.

ANATOMY

The elbow is a complex joint that permits flexion and extension at the ulnohumeral articulation and pronation and supination at the radiocapitellar joint. Ligamentous stability is provided by the medial collateral ligament and lateral collateral ligament. An in-depth understanding of the neurovascular structures that traverse the elbow and their relation to bony landmarks enables the surgeon to perform arthroscopy of the elbow safely and effectively.

PATIENT EVALUATION

History and Physical Examination

A careful history, physical examination, and appropriate imaging are imperative before arthroscopic excision of loose bodies and osteophytes within the elbow joint. On presentation, patients with loose bodies often complain of pain, stiffness, catching, clicking, and locking of the elbow joint. Physical examination findings often include sometimes subtle losses of flexion, extension, and a small effusion that can be detected most often in the posterolateral gutter.[26]

When preparing for arthroscopic loose body excision, a detailed history of past surgical ulnar nerve neurolysis or transposition, along with physical examination for subluxation of the ulnar nerve, cannot be overemphasized. A subluxated or dislocated ulnar nerve can be found in 16% of the normal population.[26] Awareness of these variations in normal anatomy is essential to prevent iatrogenic neural injury.

Diagnostic Imaging

Anteroposterior and lateral radiographs of the elbow should be routinely obtained (Fig. 2-1). However, standard imaging fails to demonstrate almost 30% of loose bodies, and in such cases, further diagnostic testing, such as computed tomography or magnetic resonance imaging, may be warranted.[4,5,26,27] In most cases, loose bodies are found in the coronoid fossa, olecranon fossa, and posterior aspect of the lateral gutter. Although careful attention must be paid to these areas, loose bodies often migrate and may be difficult to see on imaging. In some cases, arthroscopic evaluation may prove to be the gold standard for demonstrating loose bodies when classic presentations are encountered.[26]

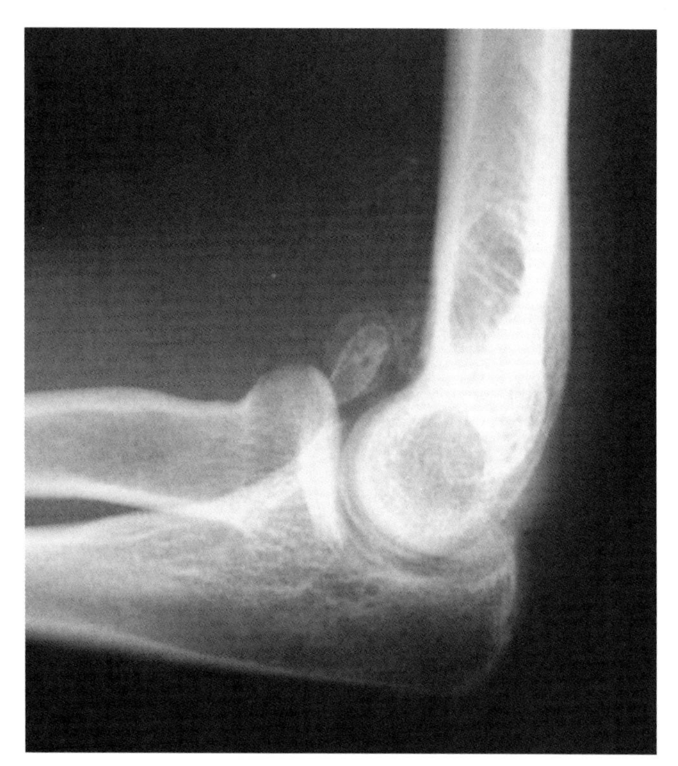

FIGURE 2-1 A large loose body in the anterior compartment of the elbow is seen on a lateral radiograph.

TREATMENT

Indications and Contraindications

Patients who have failed conservative management for loose bodies within the elbow are candidates for elbow arthroscopy and loose body removal. However, before surgical intervention is undertaken, the treating surgeon must ascertain the cause of these impediments to normal joint motion. Loose bodies may be the result of osteochondritis dissecans, degenerative arthritis, synovial chondromatosis, or trauma.[4,5,28] A carefully formulated plan to address the primary underlying pathology at the time of surgery can prevent the future formation of loose bodies.[28]

Absolute contraindications to elbow arthroscopy include any variation in the normal bony or soft tissue anatomy that precludes the safe insertion of the arthroscope into the elbow joint.[28] Other contraindications include an ankylosed elbow joint that would preclude joint distention and local soft tissue infection in the area of portal sites. Prior ulnar nerve transposition is a relative contraindication if it interferes with portal positioning.[28] However, elbow arthroscopy can be used if the ulnar nerve is identified with surgical dissection before portal creation.

Conservative Management

Loose bodies in the elbow often manifest with mechanical symptoms that obstruct normal joint motion and predispose the joint to premature osteoarthritic wear. As a result, the role of conservative management is limited to asymptomatic loose bodies.

Elbow Arthroscopy

Anesthesia

General anesthesia or regional blocks are the most common methods used in elbow arthroscopy. General anesthesia is more commonly used because of the flexibility it permits with respect to patient positioning and postoperative examination. The prone and lateral decubitus positions are poorly tolerated in awake patients, and these positioning methods are most amenable to general anesthesia.[12] Use of general anesthesia in the absence of a neurologic block enables immediate postoperative neurologic examination.

In patients who are unable to tolerate general anesthesia, interscalene, axillary, and regional intravenous (Bier) blocks can be used. Although these blocks can be used in combination with general anesthesia for postoperative pain management, their use as the primary means of anesthesia has several disadvantages, including limited tourniquet time, incomplete blockade of the surgical site, and pain from tourniquet constriction.

Patient Positioning

Supine Position. Supine positioning for elbow arthroscopy was first described in 1985.[9] After supine positioning of the patient on the operating table, the operative extremity is lateralized on the operating table so that the shoulder is placed at the edge of the bed. The patient is secured, and all pertinent prominences are appropriately padded. The operative extremity is placed in 90 degrees of shoulder abduction, 90 degrees of elbow flexion, and neutral forearm rotation, and a nonsterile arm tourniquet is applied (Fig. 2-2). Traction is facilitated with the use of a traction device.

The supine position offers several advantages to the elbow arthroscopist.[2] A three-dimensional understanding and application of elbow anatomy is facilitated by the anatomic and familiar position of the elbow. This also benefits the surgeon if open procedures follow. This position enables quick access to the patient's airway and the choice of multiple effective anesthetic regimens. Drawbacks of the supine position include the necessity of a traction setup, which makes manipulating the elbow cumbersome, and the inability to easily visualize and work in the posterior compartment.

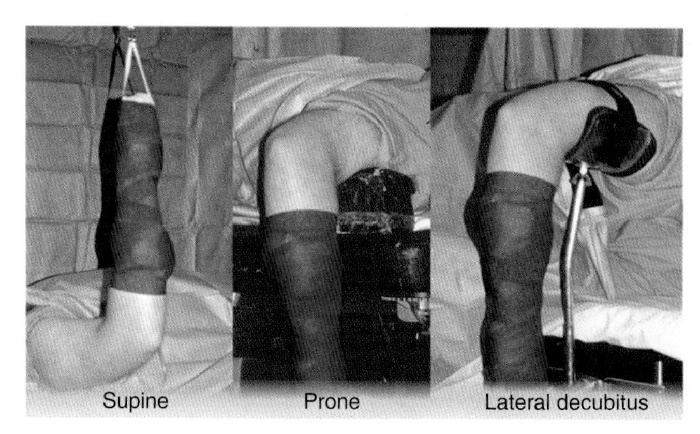

FIGURE 2-2 Each of three patient positions for elbow arthroscopy has inherent advantages and disadvantages with respect to anesthesia options, the need for positioning or traction devices, and the ease with which conversion to open procedures can be accomplished.

Prone Position. The prone position was first described in 1989 as an alternative method for positioning.[29] The aims of this method were to improve access to the posterior compartment of the elbow and eliminate the need for a traction device for intraoperative elbow manipulation.

The patient is initially intubated on a gurney and rolled to the prone position on the operating table. The face and chest are padded and supported by a foam airway and head positioner and by padded chest rolls. The nonoperative extremity is brought into 90 degrees of shoulder abduction and neutral rotation with the elbow in 90 degrees of flexion. The elbow and wrist are supported by a padded arm board. On the operative side, an arm board is placed parallel to the operating table centered at the shoulder level. A nonsterile arm tourniquet is applied, and the arm is placed in 90 degrees of shoulder abduction and neutral rotation. The arm is supported at the middle humeral level by a padded bolster attached the operating table or by a rolled towel bump that is positioned on top of the arm board, which suspends the elbow in 90 degrees of flexion (see Fig. 2-2).

The prone position has several advantages. With the arm freely hanging, the elbow is easily manipulated from flexion to full extension. This can be done without the use of a traction setup or arm positioner and without an assistant. The posterior compartment of the elbow is easily accessible. Flexion of the elbow allows the neurovascular structures to sag anteriorly, providing a greater margin of error when establishing anterior portal sites. As with the supine position, open procedures are easily conducted on the medial and lateral sides of the elbow if necessary.[30]

Disadvantages of the prone position primarily are related to patient positioning, ventilation, and anesthetic options. Care must be taken to support the head and face with foam padding to secure the airway. Chest rolls are needed to facilitate ventilation, and additional padding is needed to protect the patient from pressure sores at the knees and ulnar neuropathies at the elbow of the contralateral extremity. Regional anesthesia is poorly tolerated, and blocks may not provide adequate anesthesia, necessitating conversion to general anesthesia. In such cases, repositioning is necessary to establish an airway. Repositioning to a supine position also becomes necessary if an anterior, open procedure is undertaken.

Lateral Decubitus Position. The lateral decubitus position was described by O'Driscoll and Morrey in 1993.[30] The aim of this position was to exploit the benefits of the supine and prone positions while avoiding the major pitfalls inherent to each setup. The patient is initially placed in the lateral decubitus position with the aid of a bean bag or sand bag kidney rests and secure taping or strapping. An axillary roll is appropriately placed. The operative extremity is positioned over an arm holder or over a padded bolster, with the shoulder internally rotated and flexed to 90 degrees. The elbow is maintained in 90 degrees of flexion (see Fig. 2-2).

The elbow is essentially maintained in the prone position, affording the advantages of the prone position. Patient positioning is simplified with respect to prone positioning, and airway maintenance is easily monitored, with adequate exposure for conversion from regional to general anesthesia. Disadvantages include the need for a padded bolster and the inconvenience of repositioning if the need for an open procedure arises.

Arthroscopic Portals

Establishing arthroscopic portals about the elbow requires a thorough understanding of the underlying neurovascular, bony, and intra-articular anatomy. Surface landmarks and their relationship to the three-dimensional model of the elbow enable the surgeon to establish working portals that can be used for numerous arthroscopic procedures about the elbow. Ten common portal sites, dictated by bony, neurovascular, and musculotendinous anatomy, have been described in the literature. These portal sites can be used in various combinations to address pertinent pathology and surgical goals.

At the outset of any elbow arthroscopic procedure, various landmarks must be localized and marked. The ulnar nerve, radial head, olecranon, lateral epicondyle, and medial epicondyle should be traced with a marking pen. Palpating and outlining the course of the ulnar nerve cannot be overemphasized to ensure that it is not subluxated or subluxatable. An 18-gauge spinal needle is used to insufflate the elbow joint with approximately 20 to 30 mL of sterile saline. This can be accomplished through a posterior injection into the olecranon fossa or through the lateral soft spot portal site, which is bounded by the radial head, lateral epicondyle, and olecranon (Fig. 2-3). The intra-articular injection can be confirmed by resistance to further inflow and often by the slight extension of the elbow seen as fluid is introduced. Distention of the joint capsule further protects the anterior neurovascular structures by displacing them anteriorly and farther away from planned portal sites.[32,33]

Proximal Anteromedial Portal. The proximal anteromedial portal was first described in 1989 and has been recommended as the initial portal for elbow arthroscopy in the prone and lateral decubitus positions.[32,34] Initial creation of this portal is suggested because it provides the best view of intra-articular structures and is

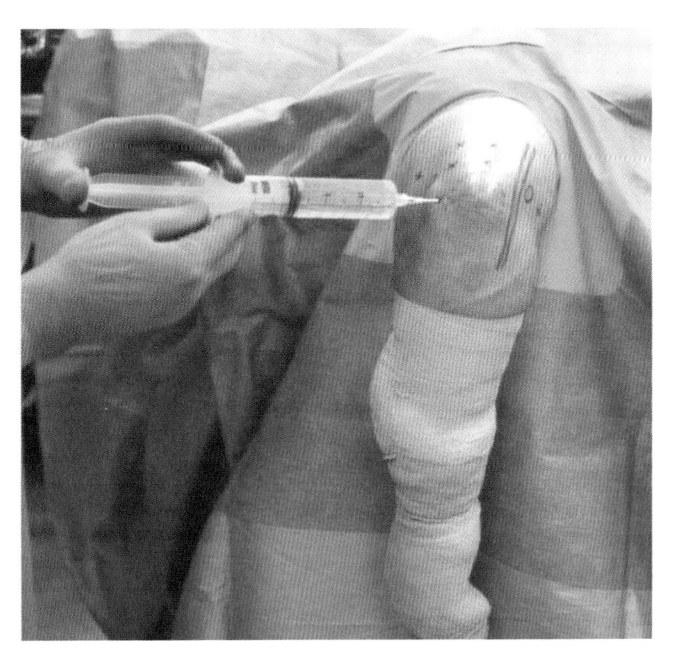

FIGURE 2-3 The patient is in the prone position, with outlining showing pertinent landmarks of the elbow, including the medial and lateral epicondyles *(circles)*, ulnar nerve *(parallel lines)*, and portal sites *(x marks)*. The joint before insufflation is seen through the lateral soft spot portal.

less likely than the anterolateral portal to be affected by extravasation.[32] This portal provides visualization of the anterior elbow joint structures, including the anterior capsule, coronoid process, trochlea, radial head, capitellum, and medial and lateral gutters.

The proximal anteromedial portal is made approximately 2 cm proximal to the medial epicondyle and just anterior to the intermuscular septum (Fig. 2-4). Placement anterior to the medial intermuscular septum avoids injury to the ulnar nerve, which courses posterior to this structure at this level. A blunt trocar is introduced through a nick in the skin (alternatively, a nick and spread technique can be employed with a small hemostat before trocar entry) and advanced distally along the anterior edge humerus toward the radiocapitellar joint. Maintaining contact with the humeral cortex during trocar advancement allows the brachialis muscle to serve as a partition between the trocar and anterior neurovascular structures. The trocar enters the elbow through the tendinous origin of the flexor-pronator group and medial capsule.[35]

Relative contraindications to creation of this portal include ulnar nerve subluxation or previous ulnar nerve transposition.[32,36,37] This portal can be used if care is taken to identify the course of the nerve with dissection before trocar placement. In the absence of ulnar nerve subluxation or a history of transposition, the ulnar nerve is located between 12 and 23.7 mm from the portal site, and it is not at risk as long as the trocar entry site is placed anterior to the intermuscular septum.[32,37]

The main structure at risk during creation of this portal site is the medial antebrachial cutaneous nerve as it courses approximately 2.3 mm from the entry site (see Fig. 2-4). The median nerve is at risk as the trocar is advanced distally between the humerus and brachialis muscle. The average distance from the trocar tip is 12.4 to 22 mm.[32,37]

Anteromedial Portal. The anteromedial portal, which is positioned 2 cm distal to and 2 cm anterior to the medial epicondyle, was originally described in 1985.[9] This portal can be established with an outside-in or inside-out technique.[32] The outside-in technique is accomplished by passing the blunt trocar toward the center of the joint while remaining in the plane between the humerus and brachialis muscle. The trocar tip is advanced through the flexor-pronator origin and into the joint at a position anterior to the medial collateral ligament.

The main structure at risk during creation of the anteromedial portal site is the medial antebrachial cutaneous nerve, which lies within 1 to 2 mm from the portal site.[37] The median nerve travels approximately 7 to 14 mm away from the portal site.[33,37] The safe distance between the trocar and nerve can be increased to 22 mm if the portal site is moved to 1 cm anterior to the medial epicondyle.[32]

Proximal Anterolateral Portal. The proximal anterolateral portal has been described by several surgeons[27,37,38] and is positioned approximately 2 cm proximal to and 2 cm anterior to the lateral epicondyle (Fig. 2-5). It can be established as the initial portal in elbow arthroscopy. As the trocar is advanced distally toward the elbow joint, the brachioradialis and brachialis muscle are pierced before entering the lateral joint capsule. With the arthroscope placed into the cannula, the anterior capsule, lateral gutter, radial head, capitellum, coronoid, and anterolateral aspect of the ulnohumeral articulation can be visualized.

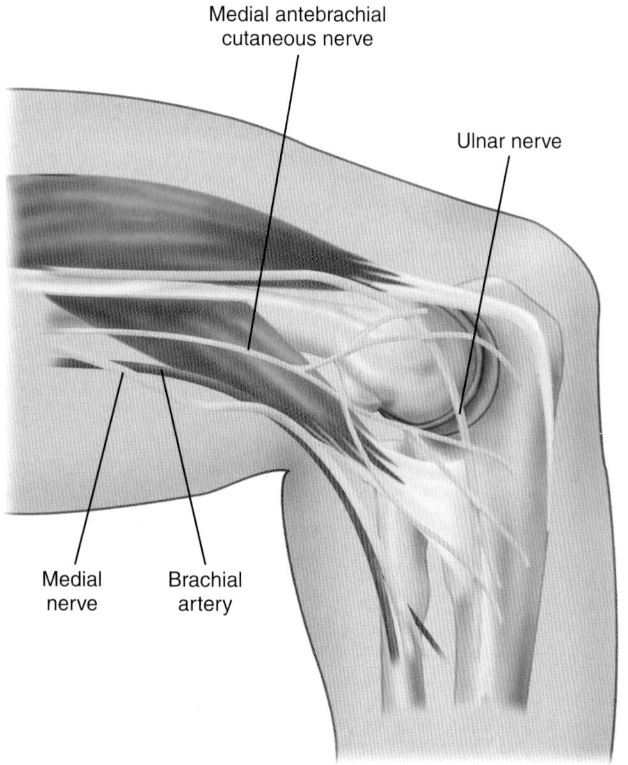

FIGURE 2-4 The proximal anteromedial portal is approximately 2 cm proximal and 2 cm anterior to the medial epicondyle. The medial antebrachial cutaneous nerve is placed at risk with the creation of this portal.

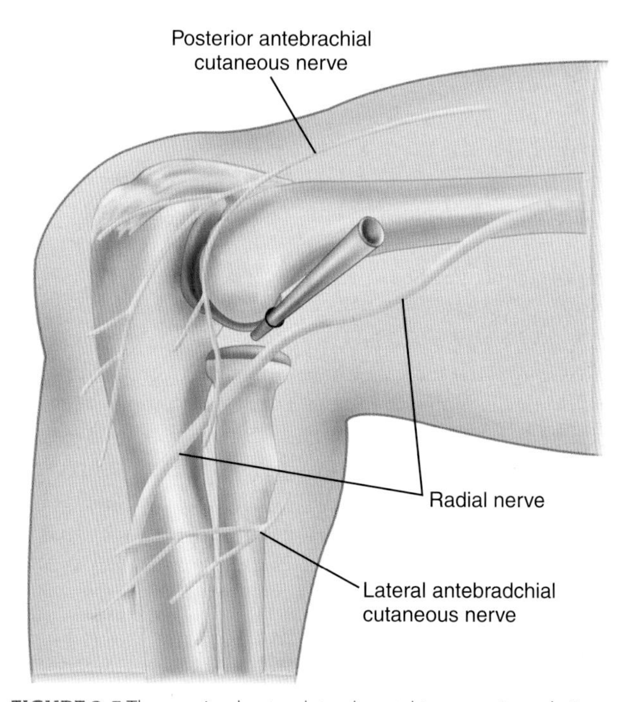

FIGURE 2-5 The proximal anterolateral portal is approximately 2 cm proximal and 2 cm anterior to the lateral epicondyle. The radial nerve is placed at risk with the creation of this portal.

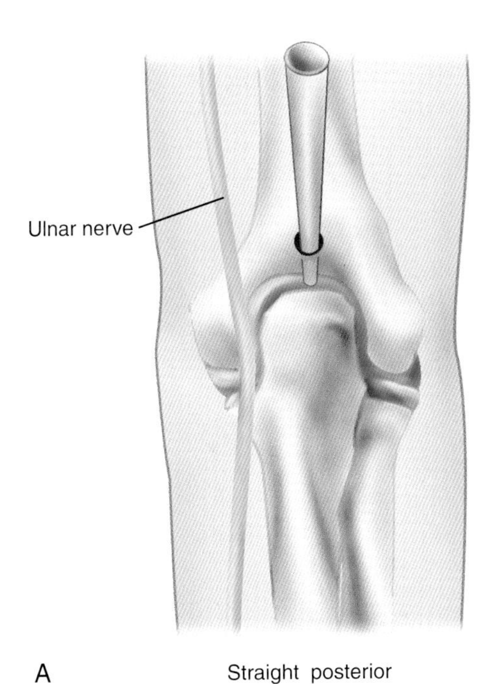

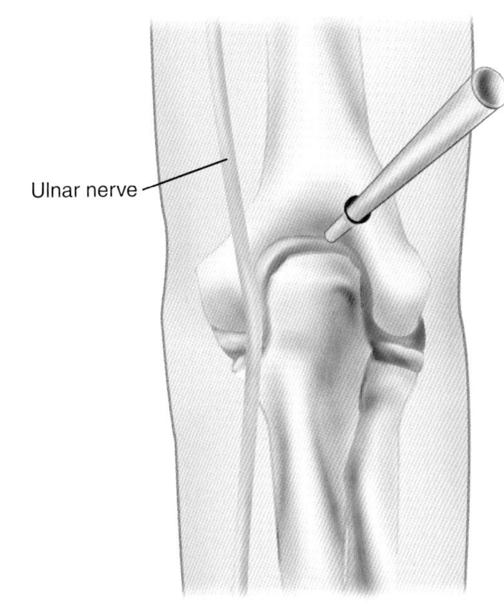

FIGURE 2-6 A, The straight posterior portal is established approximately 3 cm proximal to the olecranon tip. **B,** The posterolateral portal is made 3 cm proximal to the olecranon tip and immediately lateral to the triceps tendon. These portals can be used interchangeably for working in the posterior compartment.

Two neural structures are at risk with the creation of the proximal anterolateral portal. The development of the proximal anterolateral portal site was in response to the relative proximity of the radial nerve to the standard anterolateral portal (see Fig. 2-5). Anatomic studies with the elbow in 90 degrees of flexion and distended with fluid at the time of proximal anterolateral portal creation reveal a safe distance of 9.9 to 14.2 mm between the trocar and radial nerve.[37,38] This distance is markedly decreased to 4.9 to 9.1 mm when the standard anterolateral portal is created.[37,38] Cutaneous sensation in the forearm can likewise be disrupted if the posterior branch of the lateral antebrachial cutaneous nerve is injured. The pathway of this portal site is an average of 6.1 mm from this sensory nerve.[37]

Anterolateral Portal. The standard anterolateral portal, created 3 cm distal to and 1 cm anterior to the lateral epicondyle, was first described in 1985.[9] As the blunt trocar is introduced, it passes through the extensor carpi radialis brevis muscle before transversing the lateral joint capsule. This portal position is limited in its capabilities with respect to the lateral joint. However, it permits visualization of the anteromedial aspect of the joint, including the trochlea, coronoid fossa, coronoid process, and medial aspect of the radial head.[38] In conjunction with the proximal anterolateral portal, the standard anterolateral portal can be used for procedures involving the radial head and annular ligament.

As with the anteromedial portal, the anterolateral portal site can be established with an inside-out technique. This can be accomplished with the aid of a proximal anteromedial or anteromedial viewing portal. In either case, the arthroscope tip is advanced to the capsule lateral to the radial head and held in this position as the arthroscope is removed from the cannula. A blunt switching stick is then placed in the cannula and forced through the capsule. The overlying tented skin is incised, the rod is advanced, and a cannula is introduced in a retrograde fashion to create the anterolateral portal. Care must be taken to place the portal site lateral to the radial head, because moving anterior to this position puts the radial nerve in jeopardy of injury.[32,35,37]

The primary structures at risk with creation of the standard anterolateral portal include the posterior antebrachial cutaneous and radial nerves. The distance of the portal site to these vital structures is approximately 2 mm and between 4.9 and 9.1 mm, respectively.[33,37,38] A more proximal anterolateral portal site risks radial nerve injury.

Midlateral Portal. The midlateral portal is synonymously referred to as the direct lateral or soft spot portal in the literature. The surface landmarks used to locate this portal are the lateral epicondyle, olecranon process, and the radial head. An 18-gauge needle can be inserted in the center of this triangular area for joint insufflation with sterile saline as an alternative to the straight posterior portal. When establishing this portal, the trocar is advanced through the anconeus muscle, and entry to the lateral elbow joint is attained through the posterior elbow capsule. Visualization of the radioulnar joint and inferior aspect of the radial head and capitellum can be achieved through this portal site. This portal also provides a safe entry site for instrumentation of the radiocapitellar joint and lateral gutter.

The midlateral portal is relatively safe with respect to neurovascular structures, and the sole risk is injury to the posterior antebrachial cutaneous nerve, which courses approximately 7 mm away.[39] Caveats to creation of this portal center on the propensity for soft tissue fluid extravasation and the risk of iatrogenic articular cartilage damage due to the limited space available.[36,37,40]

Straight Posterior Portal. The straight posterior portal breeches the central midsubstance of the triceps tendon and is located 3 cm proximal to the tip of the olecranon in the midline (Fig. 2-6). In this position, the entire posterior compartment can be visualized in addition to the medial and lateral gutters.[35] As the blunt trocar is introduced through the triceps tendon and joint capsule, it is placed directly on the bone of the olecranon fossa. As the trocar is held in place, the cannula is advanced to the bone. The return of fluid with trocar removal confirms successful entry, and the arthroscope can then be introduced. This portal also provides an alternative site for insufflation of the joint with an 18-gauge spinal needle and sterile saline. Several common procedures can be performed through this portal site, including the removal of olecranon spurs and loose bodies and contouring or humeral fenestration of the olecranon fossa for ulnohumeral arthroplasty.[35,36]

Posterolateral Portal. The location of the posterolateral portal is 3 cm proximal to the olecranon tip and immediately lateral to the triceps tendon (see Fig. 2-6). Insertion of the trocar is directed toward the olecranon fossa, passing just lateral to the triceps tendon and through the posterolateral joint capsule. Visualization of the olecranon fossa and the medial and lateral gutters is afforded through this portal site.

The posterolateral portal can be used interchangeably with the straight posterior portal for viewing and instrumentation of the olecranon fossa and the medial and lateral gutters. Care must be taken to avoid injury to the ulnar nerve when instrumenting the medial gutter. The ulnar nerve is susceptible to injury posterior to the medial epicondyle, where it transverses obliquely and just superficial to the medial capsule of the elbow.[33]

Accessory Posterolateral Portal. The posterolateral aspect of the elbow consists of the radiocapitellar joint and the lateral olecranon process. This portal is useful for the excision of a posterolateral plica, excision of lateral olecranon spurs, and débridement of the radial side of the ulnohumeral articulation.[41] The placement of this portal can be accomplished in the area between the midlateral portal and the posterolateral portal, which is 3 cm proximal to the olecranon tip. Spinal needle localization under direct visualization is suggested for accurate portal placement to address pertinent pathology. There is limited risk to neurovascular structures. However, the triceps tendon and ulnohumeral articulation are at risk for iatrogenic damage with errant trocar or instrument placement.[27]

Surgical Technique

After the administration of general anesthesia, the patient is transferred to the operative table and placed in the prone position, with attention to all pertinent prominences and to securing the airway. The shoulder is placed in 90 degrees of abduction and neutral rotation, with the elbow suspended in 90 degrees of flexion (see Fig. 2-2). A nonsterile upper arm tourniquet is applied. An arm board, parallel to the operating table and centered under the shoulder, is used to support a rolled towel bump and the operative extremity. A DuraPrep solution is used to prepare the arm and forearm. An impervious, sterile stockinette is applied to the hand and covered with self-adherent Coban to seal the hand and forearm contents from the operative field. Standard sterile draping is followed by exsanguination of the limb with an Esmarch bandage. The tourniquet is inflated.

All pertinent landmarks are outlined, with emphasis on locating the ulnar nerve, olecranon process, and medial and lateral epicondyles (see Fig. 2-3). The course of the ulnar nerve is palpated, and it is evaluated for subluxation. An 18-guage spinal needle is introduced into the straight posterior portal site, and the joint is insufflated with 20 to 30 mL of sterile saline until resistance is felt (see Fig. 2-3). Intra-articular injection can be confirmed with the observation of slight elbow extension as the joint fills.

The proximal anteromedial portal site is established 2 cm proximal to the epicondyle and immediately anterior to the intermuscular septum (see Fig. 2-4). A blunt trocar and cannula for a 4.5-mm arthroscope are introduced through a nick made in the skin with a no. 11 blade knife and advanced distally toward the radiocapitellar joint. The trocar is advanced while in contact with the anterior aspect of the humerus, which ensures protection of the anterior neurovascular structures by the brachialis muscle. An egress of fluid with trocar removal confirms intra-articular placement. The 30-degree, 4.5-mm arthroscope is introduced, and diagnostic arthroscopy of the anterior compartment ensues.

The proximal anteromedial portal, if appropriately placed, permits a systematic evaluation of the lateral gutter, capitellum, radial head, anterior capsule, trochlea, coronoid process, and medial gutter. The radiocapitellar joint is assessed for instability and articular cartilage damage, with pronation and supination aiding the evaluation. The 30-degree arthroscope lens is rotated to facilitate evaluation of the anterior capsule and extensor carpi radialis brevis tendon insertion. The coronoid and trochlea are then evaluated by withdrawing the arthroscope and repositioning the lens of the arthroscope.

Loose bodies in the anterior compartment of the elbow are frequently found within the coronoid fossa (Fig. 2-7). Extraction of these osteochondral fragments is conducted after establishing a proximal anterolateral portal under direct spinal needle localization or by using and inside-out technique. The skin entry site for this portal is 2 cm proximal to the lateral epicondyle and 2 cm anteriorly. The spinal needle is removed, and a no. 11 blade knife is used to incise only the skin. A blunt trocar and cannula are in-

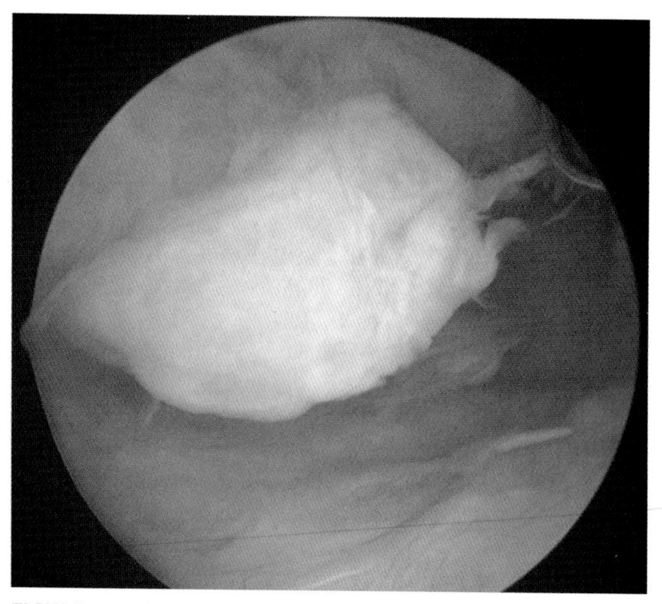

FIGURE 2-7 A large, loose osteochondral loose body is visualized in the anterior compartment of the elbow.

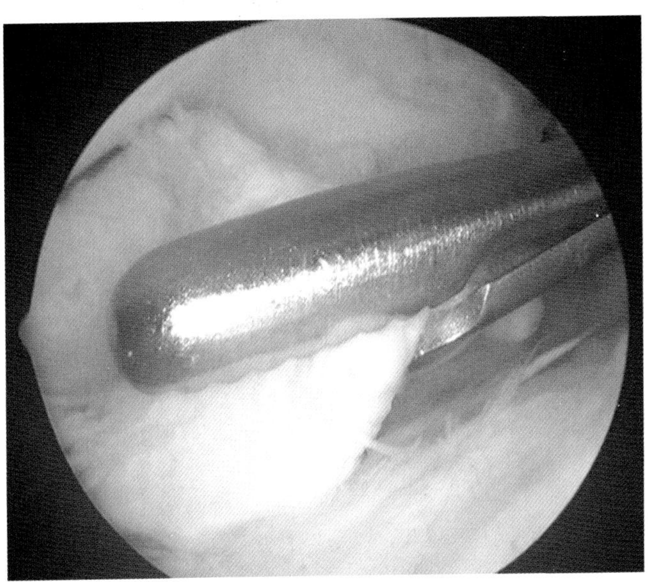

FIGURE 2-8 A grasper is used for the removal of a large loose body from the anterior compartment of the elbow.

serted into the elbow while maintaining constant contact with the anterior humeral cortex as the trocar is advanced. This minimizes the risk of damaging the radial nerve on transversing the soft tissue. A meniscal grasper is introduced through the proximal anterolateral portal and used to remove any loose bodies (Fig. 2-8). If the size of the osteochondral fragment exceeds that of the cannula, it may necessitate piecemeal removal or the use of a motorized shaver. In certain cases, the grasper can be used to pull the cannula and fragment together through the soft tissue and out of the body. This can be accomplished by rotating the grasper as it is removed from the soft tissues while maintaining firm grasp on the fragment. Alternatively, a spinal needle may be needed to skewer and stabilize the loose body for retrieval with a grasper (Fig. 2-9).

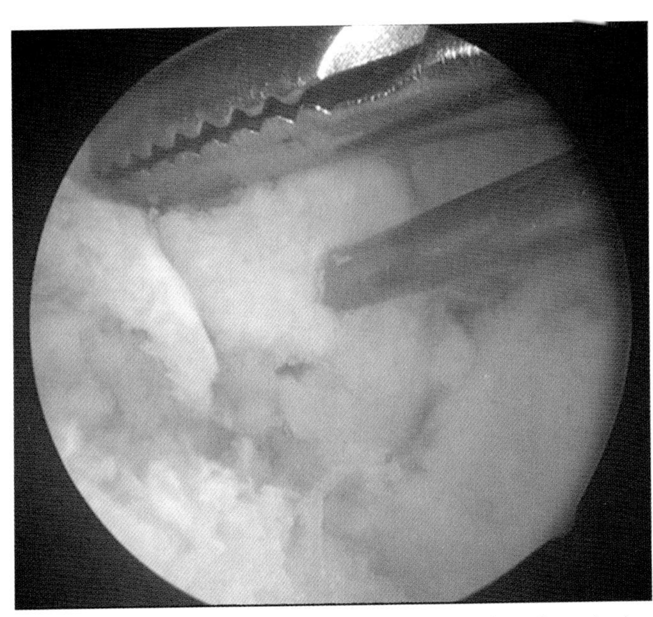

FIGURE 2-9 A spinal needle can be used to skewer a large loose body in the posterior compartment of the elbow to facilitate retrieval with a grasper.

After thorough evaluation of the anterior compartment and loose body removal, attention is focused on the posterior compartment. The water inflow is generally switched to the proximal anteromedial cannula.[26] The straight posterior portal is established using a no. 11 blade knife 3 cm proximal to the tip of the olecranon (see Fig. 2-6). After introducing the 30-degree, 4.5-mm arthroscope into the straight posterior portal, the posterolateral portal is created 3 cm proximal to the olecranon tip and just lateral to the triceps tendon under direct spinal needle localization (see Fig. 2-6). Commonly, a motorized shaver in the posterolateral portal is used to remove soft tissue obscuring the view to the olecranon fossa. The straight posterior portal and the posterolateral portal can be used interchangeably for removal of loose bodies. The olecranon fossa should be evaluated in its entirety because it is a common source of loose bodies.

The arthroscope is then introduced into the medial gutter from the straight posterior portal. A milking maneuver can be performed from a distal to proximal direction on the medial side of the elbow, which often propels loose bodies posteriorly.[26] In the lateral aspect of the elbow, entry through an accessory posterolateral portal or midlateral portal is needed for débridement. These portals are localized under direct visualization with a spinal needle. A cannula, trocar, and motorized shaver are introduced in succession through the established portal. Often, a soft tissue plica or synovial band may need to be removed with the shaver for adequate visualization. In this posterolateral location, loose bodies are often hidden, and it is imperative that a thorough evaluation be performed.

After arthroscopic examination and removal of all loose bodies in the anterior and posterior compartments, the arthroscopic equipment is removed, Steri-Strips are applied to the portal sites, and the lateral portal sites are sutured with an interrupted single nylon suture to help prevent fistula formation. A sterile dressing is applied, allowing the elbow to move freely in an arc of flexion-extension and pronation-supination.

PEARLS & PITFALLS

- Define and mark surface landmarks, especially the ulnar nerve.
- Palpate the ulnar nerve, and examine for dislocation or subluxation.
- Dissect out, identify, and protect the ulnar nerve if its location is in question.
- Insufflate before portal creation.
- Keep the elbow in 90 degrees of flexion to ensure that the distance between portal sites and neural structures is maximized.
- Avoid the anteromedial and anterolateral portals when possible.
- Do not use pressurized infusion pumps to avoid extravasation.
- Use only blunt trocars.
- Use sharp dissection to penetrate the skin only.
- Avoid using suction, which can cause capsular collapse and inadvertent neurovascular injury.

Postoperative Rehabilitation

The primary goal in the postoperative period is to attain a full range of motion. Surgeons should refrain from splinting the elbow and instead encourage use of the operative extremity immediately postoperatively. Dressings should not interfere with early flexion, extension, supination, and pronation. Institution of a home exercise program or physical therapy should be emphasized. Patients should return to the office within 1 week to check the wound and monitor the range of motion. Aggressive physical therapy should begin immediately if improvements in motion are not attained.

CONCLUSIONS

It is well documented in the literature that the success rates for arthroscopic loose body excision from the elbow approach 90%.[4,24,25] These findings have been supported by the work of O'Driscoll and colleagues, who reported 71 consecutive patients undergoing loose body removal.[6] All patients with isolated loose bodies reported clinical improvement after arthroscopic removal. However, failure to address the primary pathology responsible for loose body production (i.e., osteoarthritis) results in limited patient improvement over time.[6,14]

REFERENCES

1. Burman M. Arthroscopy of the elbow joint: a cadaver study. *J Bone Joint Surg*. 1932;14:349.
2. McKenzie PJ. Supine position. In :Savoie FH, Field LD, eds. *Arthroscopy of the Elbow*. New York NY: Churchill Livingstone; 1996:35-39.
3. Morrey BF. Arthroscopy of the elbow. *Instr Course Lect*. 1986;35:102-107.
4. O'Driscoll SW. Elbow arthroscopy for loose bodies. *Orthopaedics*. 1992;15:855-859.
5. O'Driscoll SW. Elbow arthroscopy: loose bodies. In: Morrey BF, ed. *The Elbow and Its Disorders*. 3rd ed. Philadelphia, PA: WB Saunders; 2000:510-514.
6. O'Driscoll SW, Morrey BF. Arthroscopy of the elbow: diagnostic and therapeutic benefits and hazards. *J Bone Joint Surg Am*. 1992;74:84-94.
7. Savoie FH. Arthroscopic management of loose bodies of the elbow. *Oper Tech Sports Med*. 2001;9:241-244.
8. Savoie FH. Guidelines to becoming an expert elbow arthroscopist. *J Arthrosc Relat Surg*. 2007;23:1237-1240.
9. Andrews JR, Baumgarten TE. Arthroscopic anatomy of the elbow. *Orthop Clin North Am*. 1995;26:671.
10. Wiesler ER, Poehling GG. Elbow arthroscopy: introduction, indications, complications, and results. In: McGinty JB, Burkhart SS, Jackson RW, et al, eds. *Operative Arthroscopy*. 3rd ed. Philadelphia, PA: Lippincott-Raven; 2003:661-664.
11. Byrd JW. Elbow arthroscopy for arthrofibrosis after type I radial head fractures. *Arthroscopy*. 1994;10:162-165.
12. Jones GS, Savoie FH. Arthroscopic capsular release of flexion contractures (arthrofibrosis) of the elbow. *Arthroscopy*. 1993;9:277-283.
13. O'Driscoll SW. Arthroscopic treatment for osteoarthritis of the elbow. *Orthop Clin North Am*. 1995;26:691-706.
14. Ogilvie-Harris DJ, Gordon R, MacKay M. Arthroscopic treatment for posterior impingement in degenerative arthritis of the elbow. *Arthroscopy*. 1995;11:437-443.
15. Baumgarten TE, Andrew JR, Satterwhite YE. The arthroscopic evaluation and treatment of osteochondritis dissecans of the capitellum. *Am J Sports Med*. 1998;26:520-523.
16. Ruch DS, Cory JW, Poehling GG. The arthroscopic management of osteochondritis dissecans of the adolescent elbow. *Arthroscopy*. 1998;14:797-803.
17. Savoie FH, Field LD. Basics of elbow arthroscopy. *Tech Orthop*. 2000;15:138-146.
18. Menth-Chiari WA, Ruch DS, Poehling GG. Arthroscopic excision of the radial head: clinical outcome in 12 patients with post-traumatic arthritis after fracture of the radial head or rheumatoid arthritis. *Arthroscopy*. 2001;17:918-923.
19. Andrews JR, Carson WG. Arthroscopy of the elbow. *Arthroscopy*. 1985;1:97-107.
20. Clarke R. Symptomatic lateral synovial fringe of the elbow joint. *Arthroscopy*. 1988;4:112-116.
21. Smith JP 3rd, Savoie FH, Field LD. Posterolateral rotatory instability of the elbow. *Clin Sports Med*. 2001;20:47-58.
22. Thomas MA, Fast A, Shapiro DL. Radial nerve damage as a complication of elbow arthroscopy. *Clin Orthop*. 1987;215:130-131.
23. Moskal JH, Savioe FH, Field LD. Elbow arthroscopy in trauma and reconstruction. *Orthop Clin North Am*. 1999;30:163-177.
24. Boe S. Arthroscopy of the elbow: diagnosis and extraction of loose bodies. *Acta Orthop Scand*. 1986;57:52-53.
25. McGinty J. Arthroscopic removal of loose bodies. *Orthop Clin North Am* 1982;13:313-328.
26. Savoie FH, Nunley PD, Field LD. Arthroscopic management of the arthritic elbow: indications, technique and results. *J Shoulder Elbow Surg*. 1999;8:214-219.
27. Savoie FH, Field LD. Anatomy. In: Savoie FH, Field LD, eds. *Arthroscopy of the Elbow*. New York, NY: Churchill Livingstone; 1996:3-24.
28. Baker CL, Jones GL. Arthroscopy of the elbow. *Am J Sports Med*. 1999;27:251-264.
29. Poehling GG, Ekman EF. Arthroscopy of the elbow. *Inst Course Lect*. 1995;44:217-228.
30. Rubin CJ. Prone or lateral decubitus position. In: Savoie FH, Field LD, eds. *Arthroscopy of the Elbow*. New York, NY: Churchill Livingstone; 1996:41-47.
31. O'Driscoll SW, Morrey BF. Arthroscopy of the elbow. In: Morrey BF, ed. *The Elbow and Its Disorders*. 2nd ed. Philadelphia, PA: WB Saunders; 1993:120-130.
32. Lindenfield TN. Medial approach in elbow arthroscopy. *Am J Sports Med* 1990;18:413-417.
33. Lynch GJ, Meyers JF, Whipple TL. Neurovascular anatomy and elbow arthroscopy: inherent risks. *Arthroscopy*. 1986;2:191-197.
34. Poehling GG, Whipple TL, Sisco L. Elbow arthroscopy: a new technique. *Arthroscopy*. 1989;5:222-224.
35. Lyons TR, Field LD, Savoie FH. Basics of elbow arthroscopy. In: Price CT, ed. *Instr Course Lect*. 2000;49:239-246.
36. Plancher KD, Peterson RK, Breezenoff L. Diagnostic arthroscopy of the elbow: set-up, portals, and technique. *Oper Tech Sports Med*. 1998;6:2-10.
37. Stothers K, Day B, Reagan WR. Arthroscopy of the elbow: anatomy, portal sites, and a description of the proximal lateral portal. *Arthroscopy*. 1995;11:449-457.
38. Field LD, Altchek DW, Warren RF. Arthroscopic anatomy of the lateral elbow: a comparison of three portals. *Arthroscopy*. 1994;10:602-607.
39. Aboud JA, Ricchetti ET, Tjoumakaris F, Ramsey ML. Elbow arthroscopy: basic setup and portal placement. *J Am Acad Orthop Surg*. 2006;14:312-318.
40. Poehling GG, Ekman EF, Ruch DS. Elbow arthroscopy: Introduction and overview. In: McGinty JB, Caspari RB, et al, eds. *Operative Arthroscopy*. 2nd ed. Philadelphia, PA: Lippincott-Raven; 1996:821-828.
41. McClung GA, Field LD, Savoie, FH. Diagnostic arthroscopy and loose body removal. *Surg Tech Sports Med*. 2007;22:211-219.
42. Kelly EW, Morrey BF, O'Driscoll SW. Complications in elbow arthroscopy. *J Bone Joint Surg Am*. 2001;83:25-34.
43. Papilion JD, Neff RS, Shall LM. Compression neuropathy of the radial nerve as a complication of elbow arthroscopy: a case report and review of the literature. *Arthroscopy*. 1988;4:284-286.
44. Rodeo SA, Forester RA, Weiland AJ. Neurologic complications due to arthroscopy. *J Bone Joint Surg Am*. 1993;75:917-926.
45. Ruch DS, Poehling GG. Anterior interosseous nerve injury following elbow arthroscopy. *Arthroscopy*. 1997;13:756-758.
46. Casscells SW. Neurovascular anatomy and elbow arthroscopy: inherent risks [editor's comment]. *Arthroscopy*. 1987;2:190.

SUGGESTED READINGS

Aldolfsson L. Arthroscopy of the elbow joint: a cadaveric study of portal placement. *J Shoulder Elbow Surg*. 1994;3:53-61.

Savoie FH, Field LD. Anatomy. In: Savoie FH, Field LD, eds. *Arthroscopy of the Elbow*. New York, NY: Churchill Livingstone; 1996:3-24.

CHAPTER

3

Lateral Epicondylitis: Débridement, Repair, and Associated Pathology

Champ L. Baker, Jr. • Champ L. Baker III

Lateral humeral epicondylitis was first described in the German literature by Runge in 1873.[1] Ten years later, Morris reported an association between lateral epicondylitis and lawn tennis, leading to its common designation as *tennis elbow*.[2] Since these original descriptions were published, multiple causes and various treatments for this condition have been proposed.

Despite advances in our understanding of the pathoanatomy of lateral epicondylitis, controversy remains regarding its optimal nonoperative and operative management. Most patients respond successfully to a variety of conservative methods. In the studies reported by Boyd and McLeod,[3] Coonrad and Hooper,[4] and Nirschl and Pettrone,[5] 4% to 11% of patients ultimately required operative intervention for recalcitrant symptoms. Many different operative procedures have been described in the orthopedic literature: percutaneous,[6-11] endoscopic,[12,13] and myriad open techniques, such as excision of abnormal degenerative tissue with simple suture repair[4,5,7,10,14-17] or formal repair of the extensor tendons back to the lateral epicondyle.[18-20] Clinical outcomes of arthroscopic treatment have been reported.[10,16,21-29] In one study, we found high rates of clinical success for our patients with lateral epicondylitis treated arthroscopically using the technique described in this chapter.[21,22]

ANATOMY

Nirschl and associates detailed the most commonly accepted theory of the pathogenesis of lateral epicondylitis.[5,30] Building on the previous findings of Cyriax,[31] Goldie,[32] and Coonrad and Hooper,[4] Nirschl observed that the basic underlying lesion was in the origin of the extensor carpi radialis brevis (ECRB) tendon. Repetitive overuse leads to microtears in the ECRB origin. Tendinous nonrepair and replacement with immature reparative tissue often follow. Histopathologic examination revealed an absence of inflammatory cells and the presence of a degenerative process, with tissue first characterized as angiofibroblastic hyperplasia and later modified to angiofibroblastic tendinosis.[5,30,33,34]

In a cadaveric study, Cohen and associates[35] characterized the ECRB origin as diamond shaped and as beginning just anterior to the most distal aspect of the lateral supracondylar ridge. The anatomic ECRB footprint is located between the most proximal aspect of the capitellum and the midline of the radiocapitellar joint (Fig. 3-1). The lateral collateral ligamentous complex, consisting of the radial collateral ligament, annular ligament, accessory collateral ligament, and lateral ulnar collateral ligament, lies

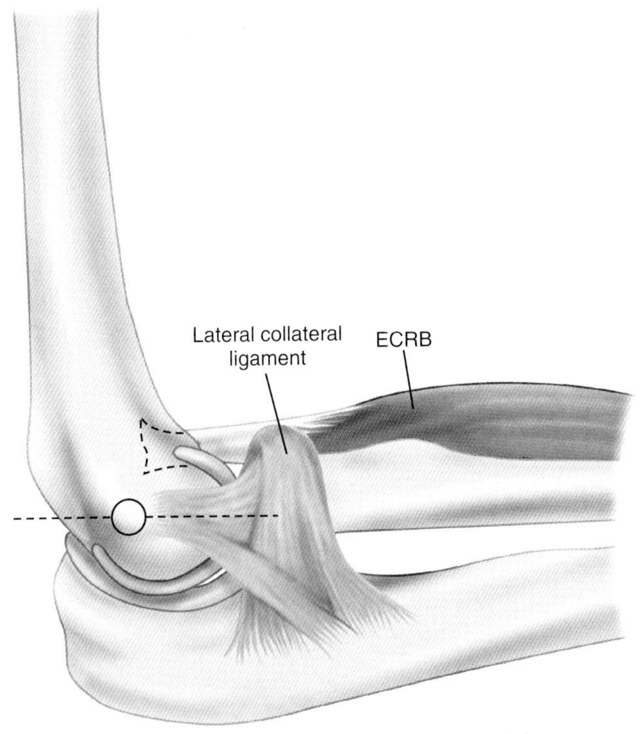

FIGURE 3-1 Anatomic origin of the extensor carpi radialis brevis tendon between the top of the capitellum and the midpoint of the radiocapitellar joint.

posterior to the ECRB origin. This lateral collateral ligamentous complex is not disrupted during arthroscopy as long as resection of the ECRB and elbow capsule is kept anterior to a line bisecting the radial head.[36]

PATIENT EVALUATION

History and Physical Examination

Typically, patients with lateral epicondylitis present with lateral elbow pain. The pain may extend proximally or distally into the dorsal forearm. Lifting or gripping movements encountered with activities of daily living often exacerbate the pain. During physical examination, the patient may wince or give submaximal effort with a handshake. Tenderness is typically localized to an area slightly anterior and distal to the lateral epicondyle. Provocative testing reveals pain localized to the lateral epicondyle with resisted wrist extension or passive wrist flexion with the elbow in full extension. Examination of the cervical spine should be performed to exclude cervical radiculopathy as a source of elbow pain.

Diagnostic Imaging

Lateral epicondylitis is a clinical diagnosis. We routinely obtain plain anteroposterior, lateral, and axial radiographic views of the elbow as part of the initial evaluation in the patient presenting with elbow pain. Although they are frequently normal, the radiographs may show radiocapitellar arthrosis, which should be included in the differential diagnosis. Plain radiographs may show soft tissue calcification adjacent to the lateral epicondyle in approximately 25% of patients, especially if the patient previously had steroid injections. Although unnecessary for the diagnosis, magnetic resonance imaging (MRI) can provide additional information regarding suspected intra-articular pathology, the integrity of the lateral collateral ligamentous complex, and the presence and extent of extensor tendon tearing.[37]

TREATMENT

Indications and Contraindications

Indications for surgical intervention for lateral epicondylitis include persistent, disabling symptoms despite an appropriate course of nonoperative management. Relative contraindications to the arthroscopic technique include previous medial elbow surgery with an ulnar nerve transposition or the presence of a subluxating ulnar nerve. In these instances, the ulnar nerve should be exposed and protected before the creation of the proximal medial portal to prevent iatrogenic injury. An absolute contraindication is the presence of an active infection.

Conservative Management

Many nonoperative treatments have been reported. A regimen that includes activity modification, physical therapy, nonsteroidal anti-inflammatory medications, counterforce bracing, and corticosteroid injections is usually successful in reducing symptoms and allowing a progressive return to unrestricted activities. Novel approaches include injections of buffered platelet-rich plasma[38] or botulinum toxin[39] and application of extracorporeal shock wave therapy.[40]

Arthroscopic Technique

For the arthroscopic procedure, the patient can be placed in the supine, lateral decubitus, or prone position. We prefer the prone position with the use of a general anesthesia to allow accurate postoperative neurovascular assessment. A well-padded tourniquet is applied to the upper arm, which is then placed into a commercially available arm holder (Fig. 3-2). The extremity is then prepared and draped in standard fashion. A compressive dressing is wrapped around the forearm to help prevent leakage of fluid into the distal soft tissues. Several bony anatomic landmarks and important structures are outlined with a marking pen to assist in proper portal creation: medial and lateral epicondyles, radial head, olecranon tip, and ulnar nerve (Fig. 3-3).

The limb is exsanguinated, and the tourniquet is inflated to 250 mm Hg. An 18-gauge spinal needle is introduced into

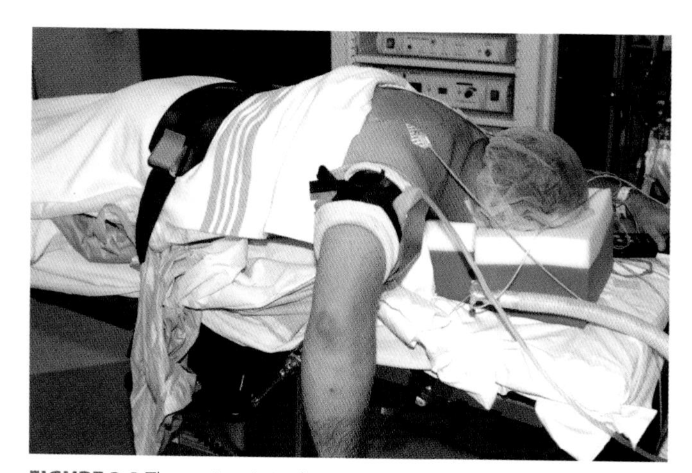

FIGURE 3-2 The patient is in the prone position with the right arm placed in an arm holder.

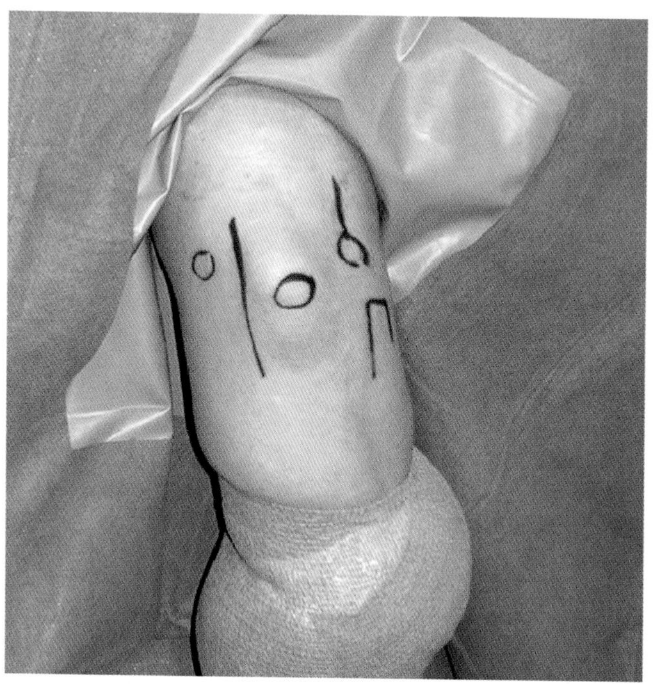

FIGURE 3-3 Landmarks outlined include the medial epicondyle, ulnar nerve, olecranon tip, lateral epicondyle, and radial head.

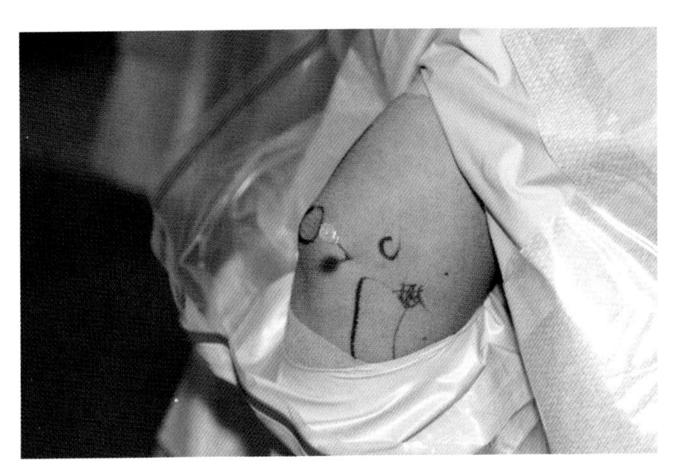

FIGURE 3-4 To distend the joint and displace the neurovascular structures anteriorly, the lateral soft spot is injected with 20 to 30 mL of saline.

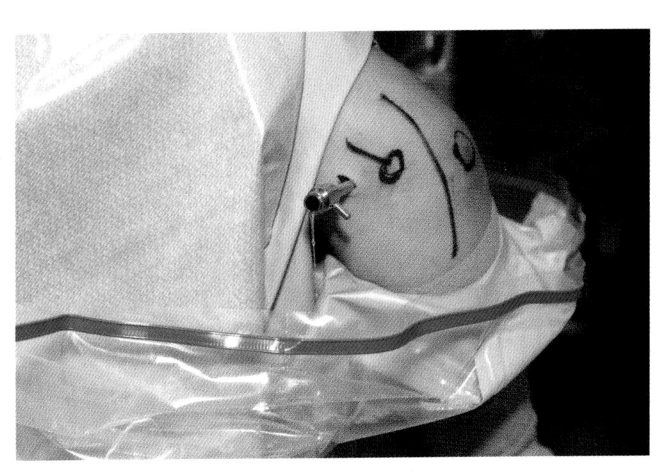

FIGURE 3-6 Leaking of fluid confirms joint entry.

the lateral soft spot, which can be found in the center of a triangle formed by the palpable radial head, lateral epicondyle, and olecranon. The joint is injected with approximately 20 to 30 mL of saline (Fig. 3-4). Joint distention pushes the neurovascular structures more anterior, thereby protecting them from iatrogenic injury.

The proximal medial portal is created approximately 2 cm proximal to the medial epicondyle and 1 cm anterior to the medial intermuscular septum (Fig. 3-5). To protect against injury to the sensory nerves, we use a nick and spread technique, in which only the skin is incised, and a hemostat is used to spread the subcutaneous tissues. Stothers and colleagues[41] found the proximal medial portal to be, on average, 2.3 mm away from the medial antebrachial cutaneous nerve, 7.6 mm away from the median nerve, and 18 mm away from the brachial artery with the elbow in flexion. The ulnar nerve is typically located 12 mm from this portal and lies anterior to and is protected by the medial intermuscular septum.

A blunt trocar is inserted through the portal. The surgeon should aim toward the center of the joint and maintain contact with the anterior surface of the humerus. Backflow of fluid through the cannula confirms entry into the joint (Fig. 3-6).

The 4-mm, 30-degree arthroscope is inserted into the joint. The lateral capsule and radiocapitellar articulation are easily inspected. According to Baker's classification system,[21] the condition of the capsule is classified as type 1 (i.e., intact capsule), type 2 (i.e., linear capsular tears), or type 3 (i.e., capsular rupture) (Fig. 3-7). Irregular extension of the annular ligament overlying the radial head, or synovial fringe, can be appreciated in some cases. We believe that this structure can be a source of lateral elbow symptoms that often mimic lateral epicondylitis and that it should be removed concomitant with the ECRB resection.[26]

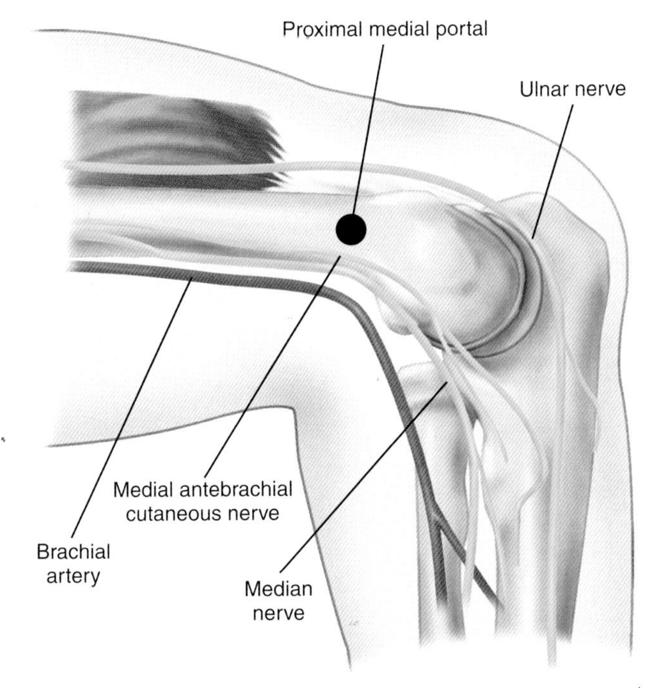

FIGURE 3-5 The proximal medial portal and surrounding neurovascular structures.

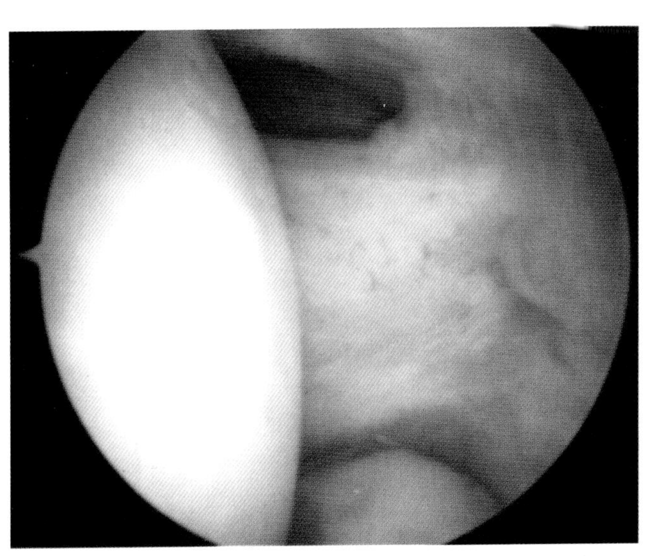

FIGURE 3-7 View from the proximal medial portal shows a complete Type III capsular tear.

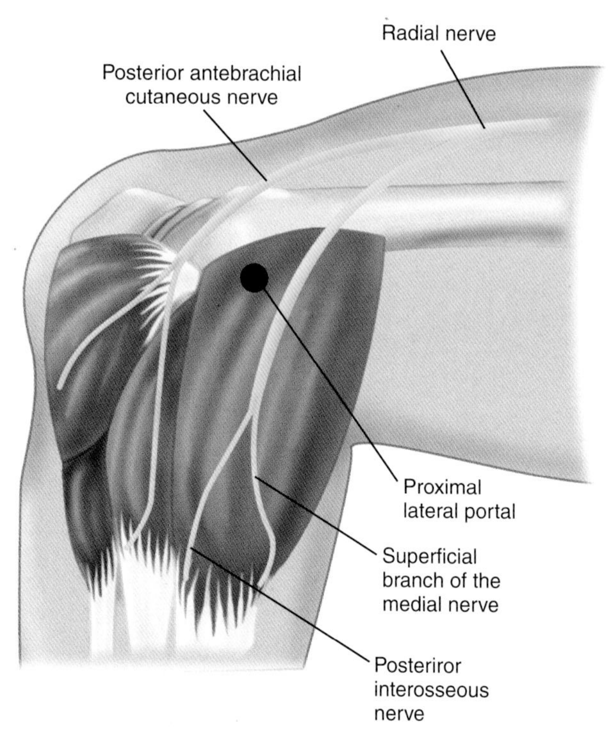

FIGURE 3-8 The proximal lateral portal and surrounding neurovascular structures.

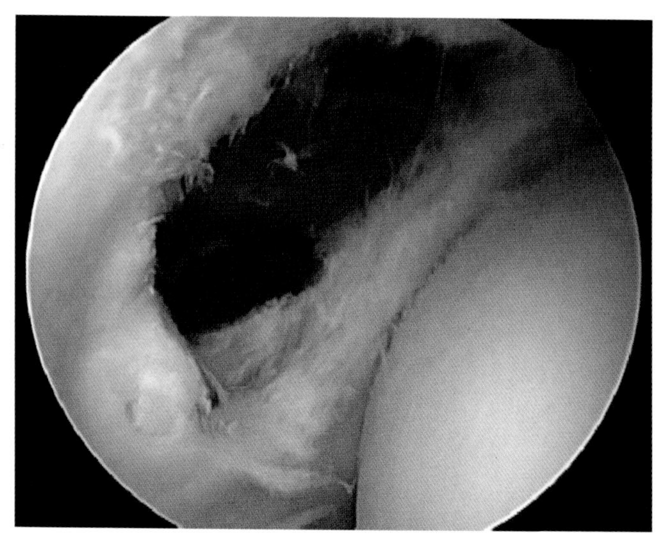

FIGURE 3-10 A portion of the lateral capsule is removed to reveal the underlying extensor carpi radialis brevis tendon.

The proximal lateral portal is typically located 1 to 2 cm proximal to the lateral epicondyle along the anterior humeral surface (Fig. 3-8). This portal is established after needle localization using an outside-in technique (Fig. 3-9). Stothers and coworkers[41] found the radial nerve to be 9.9 mm away from this portal and the posterior branch of the antebrachial cutaneous nerve to be an average of 6.6 mm away from the portal with the elbow flexed.

A blunt trocar is used to enter the joint, followed by a small, motorized shaver. A portion of the lateral capsule is resected to reveal the underlying common extensor origin (Fig. 3-10). The ECRB tendon lies between the common extensor origin and the removed capsule. The shaver is exchanged for a monopolar radiofrequency device (Fig. 3-11) The ECRB origin is then completely released from its insertion and the tendinosis tissue ablated (Fig. 3-12). To protect the lateral ligamentous structures, care is taken not to extend the release posterior to a line bisecting the radial head. Early in our experience, we decorticated the lateral epicondyle; however, several patients developed postoperative bony tenderness that was not present preoperatively. We no longer routinely decorticate the lateral epicondyle.

If the patient had preoperative concurrent posterior or posterolateral pain on terminal elbow extension, we inspect the posterior compartment through the posterior and direct lateral portals. If no such symptoms were present at the preoperative evaluation, we do not routinely examine the posterior compartment. The portal sites are closed with simple nylon sutures, and a sterile dressing is applied.

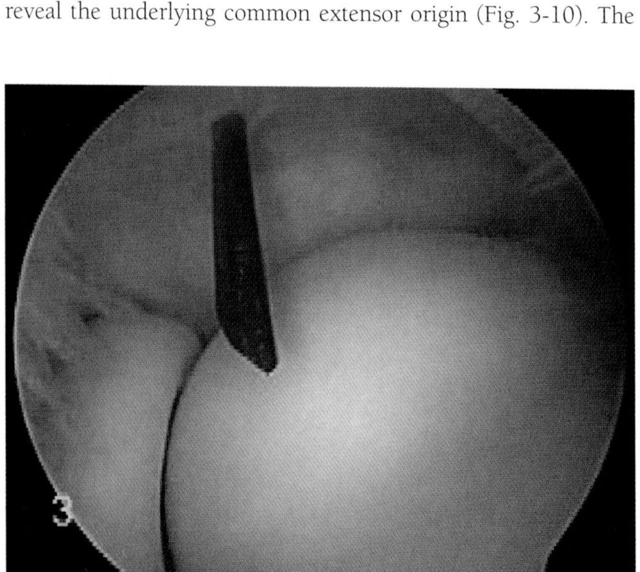

FIGURE 3-9 The proximal lateral portal is created with an outside-in technique for correct portal localization.

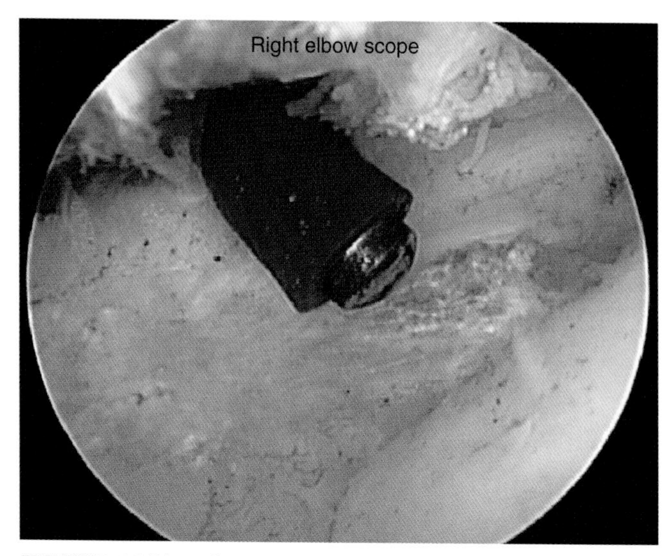

FIGURE 3-11 We prefer to use a radiofrequency device to resect the extensor carpi radialis brevis origin from its insertion.

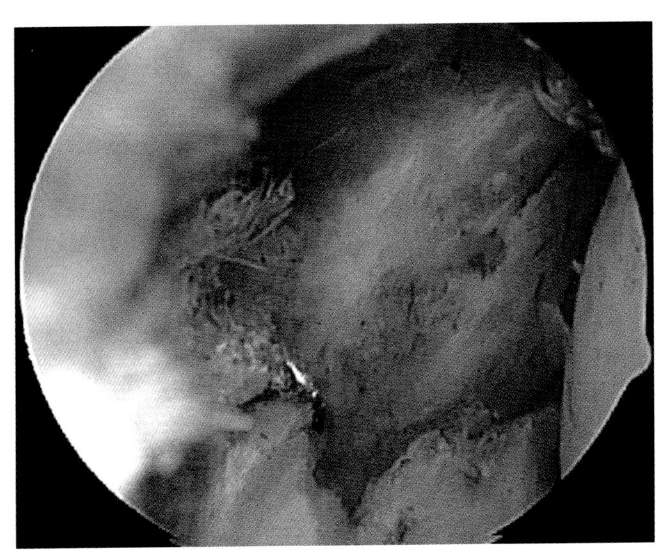

FIGURE 3-12 Completed resection.

PEARLS & PITFALLS

PEARLS

- If a concurrent open procedure is planned, a side board can be affixed to the table.
- The tourniquet and arm holder should be placed as far proximally as possible to allow easy joint access with instrumentation.
- The nick and spread technique decreases the likelihood of injury to the medial sensory nerves during the creation of the proximal medial portal.
- Annular ligament extension with synovial tissue can become entrapped between the radial head and capitellum, and it can be a source of lateral elbow pain. It should be excised concurrently with the tendinosis resection.

PITFALLS

- Before the procedure, the surgeon must identify a prior ulnar nerve transfer or subluxating ulnar nerve.
- Using cannulas with side ports allows fluid extravasation into the soft tissues. We use cannulas without side ports to decrease extravasation.
- If visualization becomes difficult, a second, more proximal lateral portal can be created to insert a retractor.
- To prevent iatrogenic posterolateral rotatory instability, resection should not extend posterior to a line bisecting the radial head with the elbow in 90 degrees of flexion.

Postoperative Rehabilitation

All procedures are performed on an outpatient basis. Initially, the arm is placed in a sling for comfort only. The patient is encouraged to begin immediate active and passive range-of-motion exercises of the elbow.

The first postoperative visit is scheduled within 7 days of surgery. Sutures are removed at that time. If potential motion loss is a concern or the patient has difficulty regaining full extension, formal physical therapy is prescribed. Home exercises, including simple stretching and strengthening, are initiated as the patient's symptoms allow. Patients typically return to light activities at 2 weeks after surgery and to sports at approximately 6 weeks postoperatively.

OUTCOMES

We reviewed the long-term outcomes of our initial series of patients who were treated with arthroscopic resection of the ECRB origin for recalcitrant lateral epicondylitis.[22] Thirty elbows in 30 patients were evaluated at a mean follow-up of 130 months. Patients were asked to rate their level of pain using a numeric scale from 0 (no pain) to 10 (severe pain). They were also asked to rate their elbows according to the 12-point functional portion of the Mayo Clinic Elbow Performance Index.

The mean pain score was 0 at rest, 1.0 for activities of daily living, and 1.9 of 10 for work or sports. The mean functional score was 11.7 of a possible 12 points. No patient required repeat injections or surgery. One patient did continue to wear a counterforce brace during heavy activities. When asked to rate their overall results, 87% of patients were satisfied, and 97% of patients stated they were "much better" or "better" at the final follow-up evaluation.

The high rate of success in Baker's initial series of patients was maintained at long-term follow-up. Other investigators also reported high rates of success with this technique in limited follow-up studies.[10,25,27-29]

CONCLUSIONS

Lateral epicondylitis is a common cause of lateral elbow pain. Although controversy exists regarding the optimal treatment for this condition, in our hands, arthroscopic release of the ECRB origin with resection of the pathologic tendinosis tissue provides reproducible pain relief and allows patients to return to unrestricted activities. Other surgeons have reported similar short-term success with this technique with minor modifications.[10,16,25,27-29] We have documented maintenance of successful outcomes at long-term follow up.[21,22]

Cadaveric studies have demonstrated the ability to resect the entire ECRB origin safely without violation of the important lateral ligamentous complex.[35,36,42] The arthroscopic technique enables identification and treatment of coexistent intra-articular pathology. Successful operative treatment of lateral epicondylitis primarily depends on proper patient selection, identification of pathology, and complete resection of the ECRB tendinosis.

REFERENCES

1. Runge F. Zur genese und behandlung des schreibekrampfes. *Berl Klin Wochenschr*. 1873;10:245-248.
2. Morris HP. Lawn-tennis elbow. *Br Med J*. 1883;2:557.
3. Boyd HB, McLeod AC Jr. Tennis elbow. *J Bone Joint Surg Am*. 1973;55:1177-1182.
4. Coonrad RW, Hooper WR. Tennis elbow: its course, natural history, conservative, and surgical management. *J Bone Joint Surg Am*. 1973;55:1183-1187.
5. Nirschl RP, Pettrone FA. Tennis elbow: the surgical treatment of lateral epicondylitis. *J Bone Joint Surg Am*. 1979;61:832-839.
6. Baumgard SH, Schwartz DR. Percutaneous release of the epicondylar muscles for humeral epicondylitis. *Am J Sports Med*. 1982;10:233-236.
7. Dunkow PD, Jatti M, Muddu BN. A comparison of open and percutaneous techniques in the surgical treatment of tennis elbow. *J Bone Joint Surg Br*. 2004;86:701-704.
8. Grundberg AB, Dobson JF. Percutaneous release of the common extensor origin for tennis elbow. *Clin Orthop Relat Res*. 2000;376:137-140.
9. Savoie FH 3rd. Management of lateral epicondylitis with percutaneous release. *Tech Shoulder Elbow Surg*. 2001;2:243-246.

10. Szabo SJ, Savoie FH 3rd, Field LD, et al. Tendinosis of the extensor carpi radialis brevis: an evaluation of three methods of operative treatment. *J Shoulder Elbow Surg*. 2006;15:721-727.
11. Yerger B, Turner T. Percutaneous extensor tenotomy for chronic tennis elbow: an office procedure. *Orthopaedics*. 1985;8:1261-1263.
12. Grifka J, Boenke S, Kramer J. Endoscopic therapy in epicondylitis radialis humeri. *Arthroscopy*. 1995;11:743-748.
13. Rubenthaler F, Wiese M, Senge A, et al. Long-term follow-up of open and endoscopic Hohmann procedures for lateral epicondylitis. *Arthroscopy*. 2005;21:684-690.
14. Dunn JH, Kim JJ, Davis L, Nirschl RP. Ten-to-14 year follow-up of the Nirschl surgical technique for lateral epicondylitis. *Am J Sports Med*. 2008; 36:261-266.
15. Khashaba A. Nirschl tennis elbow release with or without drilling. *Br J Sports Med*. 2001;35:200-201.
16. Peart RE, Strickler SS, Schweitzer KM Jr. Lateral epicondylitis: a comparative study of open and arthroscopic lateral release. *Am J Orthop*. 2004;33:565-567.
17. Zingg PO, Schneeberger AG. Debridement of extensors and drilling of the lateral epicondyle for tennis elbow: a retrospective study. *J Shoulder Elbow Surg*. 2006;15:347-350.
18. Jobe FW, Cicotti MG. Lateral and medial epicondylitis of the elbow. *J Am Acad Orthop Surg*. 1994;2:1-8.
19. Rosenberg N, Henerdon I. Surgical treatment of resistant lateral epicondylitis: follow-up study of 19 patients after excision, release and repair of proximal common extensor tendon origin. *Arch Orthop Trauma Surg*. 2002;122:514-517.
20. Thornton SJ, Rogers JR, Prickett WD, et al. Treatment of recalcitrant lateral epicondylitis with suture anchor repair. *Am J Sports Med*. 2005; 33:1558-1564.
21. Baker CL Jr, Murphy KP, Gottlob CA, Curd DT. Arthroscopic classification and treatment of lateral epicondylitis: two-year clinical results. *J Shoulder Elbow Surg*. 2000;9:475-482.
22. Baker CL Jr, Baker CL 3rd. Long-term follow-up of arthroscopic treatment of lateral epicondylitis. *Am J Sports Med*. 2008; 36:254-260
23. Brooks-Hill AL, Regan RD. Extra-articular arthroscopic lateral elbow release. *Arthroscopy*. 2008; 24:483-485.
24. Cummins CA. Lateral epicondylitis: in vivo assessment of arthroscopic debridement and correlation with patient outcomes. *Am J Sports Med*. 2006;34:1486-1491.
25. Jerosch J, Schunck J. Arthroscopic treatment of lateral epicondylitis: indications, technique and early results. *Knee Surg Sports Traumatol Arthrosc*. 2006;14:379-382.
26. Mullett H, Sprague M, Brown G, Hausman M. Arthroscopic treatment of lateral epicondylitis: clinical and cadaveric studies. *Clin Orthop Relat Res*. 2005;439:123-128.
27. Owens BD, Murphy KP, Kuklo TR. Arthroscopic release for lateral epicondylitis. *Arthroscopy* 2001;17:582-587.
28. Romeo AA, Fox JA. Arthroscopic treatment of lateral epicondylitis: the 4-step technique. *Orthop Tech Rev*. 2002;4:206.
29. Sennoune B, Costa V, Dumontier C. Arthroscopic treatment of tennis elbow: preliminary experience with 14 patients. *Rev Chir Orthop Reparatrice Appar Mot*. 2005;91:158-164.
30. Nirschl RP. Elbow tendinosis/tennis elbow. *Clin Sports Med*. 1992;11: 851-870.
31. Cyriax JH. The pathology and treatment of tennis elbow. *J Bone Joint Surg Am*. 1936;18:921-940.
32. Goldie I. Epicondylitis lateralis humeri (epicondylalgia or tennis elbow): a pathogenetical study. *Acta Chir Scand Suppl*. 1964;57:339.
33. Kraushaar BS, Nirschl RP. Tendinosis of the elbow (tennis elbow): clinical features and findings of histological, immunohistochemical, and electron microscopy studies. *J Bone Joint Surg Am*. 1999;81:259-278.
34. Regan W, Wold LE, Coonrad R, Morrey BF. Microscopic histopathology of chronic refractory lateral epicondylitis. *Am J Sports Med*. 1992;20: 746-749.
35. Cohen MS, Romeo AA, Hennigan SP, Gordon M. Lateral epicondylitis: anatomic relationships of the extensor tendon origins and implications for arthroscopic treatment. *J Shoulder Elbow Surg*. 2008;17:954-960.
36. Smith AM, Castle JA, Ruch DS. Arthroscopic resection of the common extensor origin: anatomic considerations. *J Shoulder Elbow Surg*. 2003; 12:375-379.
37. Calfee RP, Patel A, DaSilva MF, Akelman E. Management of lateral epicondylitis: current concepts. *J Am Acad Orthop Surg*. 2008;16:19-29.
38. Mishra A, Pavelko T. Treatment of chronic elbow tendinosis with buffered platelet-rich plasma. *Am J Sports Med*. 2006;34:1774-1778.
39. Placzek R, Drescher W, Deuretzbacher G, et al. Treatment of chronic radial epicondylitis with botulinum toxin A. A double-blind, placebo-controlled, randomized multicenter study. *J Bone Joint Surg Am*. 2007; 89:255-260.
40. Pettrone FA, McCall BR. Extracorporeal shock wave therapy without local anesthesia for chronic lateral epicondylitis. *J Bone Joint Surg Am*. 2005;87:1297-1304.
41. Stothers K, Day B, Regan WR. Arthroscopy of the elbow: anatomy, portal sites, and a description of the proximal lateral portal. *Arthroscopy*. 1995;11:449-457.
42. Kuklo TR, Taylor KF, Murphy KP, et al. Arthroscopic release for lateral epicondylitis: a cadaveric model. *Arthroscopy*. 1999;15:259-264.

CHAPTER

4

Plica Synovialis of the Elbow

Bernard F. Morrey • Scott P. Steinmann

Documentation of synovial plica as an anatomic structure began in 1912, when Testut described the "humeral radialis labrum."[1,2] Descriptions of this as a pathologic condition began in the 1950s.[3-5] Since then, the pathologic condition has been described as the lateral synovial fringe,[6] snapping plica,[7] and synovial fold of the humeral radial joint.[1] Identification of the plica as a pathologic condition can be traced to individual case reports within the past 30 years that described symptoms, clinical presentation, and treatment. The true significance has been dramatically enhanced with the advent of arthroscopy.

ANATOMY

Most of the early and recent anatomic descriptions of this structure come from the Japanese or French literature.[8-12] One of the most detailed accounts was provided by Isogai and colleagues.[10] Anterior and posterior folds have been documented in embryo and adult elbows, confirming these folds as normal anatomic structures (Fig. 4-1).[13] The so-called lateral fold has been identified only in adults.[10] This finding prompted the theory that a single event, repetitive trauma, or anatomic variant combined with activity may give rise to the development of the pathologic structure. This theory is enhanced by recognition that the histology of the normal anterior and posterior folds is that of fibrous fatty tissue; however, the lateral plica consists of hyaluronized bundles with fibrous tissue, making it histologically different from the anterior and posterior bands.[10] Others have recognized that histologically, normal plica reveals uninflamed fibrofatty synovial tissue with no evidence of necrosis.[1] However, a hard, fibrous type of tissue is characteristic of the lateral or circumferential variation of the plica.

Duparc and coworkers[1] performed careful dissections on 50 elbows and demonstrated some form of a synovial fold in 43 (86%). They described six orientations, including four (9%) that were circumferential. In 30, the structure was described as rigid, and in the remaining 13, it was soft and pliable. The relationship with degenerative changes of the radial head was also recognized. A later German investigation sought to define the accuracy of MRI detection of the plica. These investigators determined that MRI detected some form of a plica in 88 studies. Dividing the folds into small (31%), medium (57%), and large (12%), they also correlated degenerative changes with the larger plicae.[14]

PATIENT EVALUATION

Early recognition of the potential pathologic features of this tissue has been offered in case reports.[9] Circumferential synovial flow was found to roll over the radial head and then slide back over the radial neck with extension and flexion, respectively.[6] Duparc and collagues[1] also recognized that 4 of 43 folds were actually circumferential and seemed to blend with the annular ligament and the margin of the radial head. It is this particular variant that appears to be the pathologic lesion (see Fig. 4-1).

Clinical Presentation

In the early descriptions, the pain was confused with that of tennis elbow. It might have been confusion with this lesion that prompted the so-called Bosworth approach to tennis elbow.[15] In this procedure, arthrotomy and inspection of the joint was recommended because it was recognized that intra-articular changes correlated to lateral elbow pain. Numerous investigators have subsequently pointed out the difficulty of differentiating a pathologic plica from lateral epicondylitis when the characteristic snapping is absent.[1,6,16] The diagnosis becomes simplified when the clinical presentation is not so much lateral or posterolateral joint pain, but rather catching, snapping, and locking. The differential diagnosis may be tennis elbow or a loose body, depending on the presence or absence of the mechanical features.[6,7]

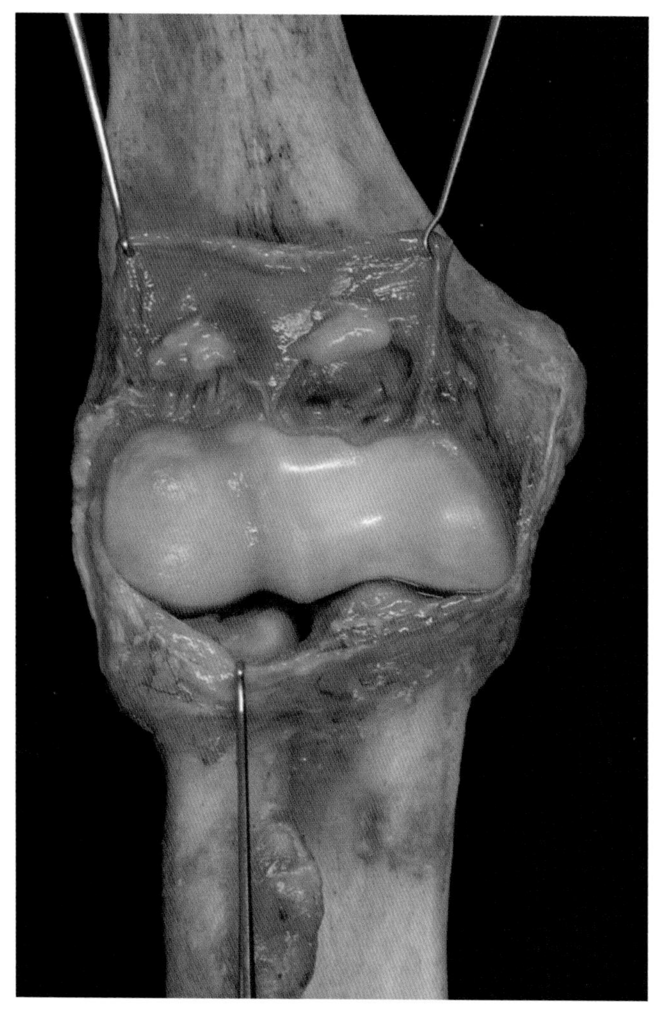

FIGURE 4-1 Anatomic dissection reveals the oblique anterior band emanating from the anterior capsule and annular ligament. Symptomatic plicae appear to be thickening of this structure. *(From Llusá Pérez M, Ballesteros Betancourt JR, Forcada Calvet P, Carrera Burgaya A.* Atlas de disccíón Anatomoquirúrgica del Codo. *Barcelona, Spain: Elsevier Masson; 2009.)*

Early descriptions found this entity to be sufficiently and interestingly uncommon to be the source of case reports.[3,6,8,9,12] They characterized the pathologic tissue as enveloping the radial head in extension. These early observations also recognized the coexistence of chondromalacia of the margin of the radial head. Isogai and coworkers[10] carefully assessed the size, shape, and location and correlated these observations with pathologic changes. The lateral or circumferential component of the complex is considered to be the pathologic anatomy that is associated with the clinical syndrome. The anterior and posterior bundles are considered to be normal variants. The gross anatomy of the pathologic version is that of a prominent intra-articular band that parallels the annual ligament: the intra-articular fold slips over the radial head in extension of less than 90 degrees and then slides over the radial neck with flexion beyond 90 to 100 degrees.[6,7] This translation results in a well-recognized chondromalacia of the margin of the radial head. Others[16] have speculated that there is an association of this lesion and subtle posterolateral rotatory instability.[10,16] However, this relationship is poorly understood.

Diagnosis

The patient typically presents with chronic, repetitive injury or a single traumatic episode. The most common and obvious presentation is snapping or catching of the elbow, which occurs at about 90 to 100 degrees of flexion and is exacerbated by pronation.[6,7,11] The patient may experience aching over the lateral epicondyle. This pattern is responsible for confusion with lateral epicondylitis. Because MRI can identify a fold in most patients, it is not very specific.[14] The diagnosis is usually made clinically and confirmed arthroscopically.

TREATMENT

Indications

Treatment of this lesion is straightforward. It is especially suited for arthroscopic intervention.

Technique

The patient is positioned according to the surgeon's preference. An anteromedial portal is commonly used (Fig. 4-2), although some prefer a midlateral observation portal. The plica is usually readily seen around the head when the elbow is extended past 60 degrees and slides over the head and around the neck with flexion beyond 90 to 100 degrees. Observing the altered position of the plica with flexion and extension provides absolute confirmation of the diagnosis.

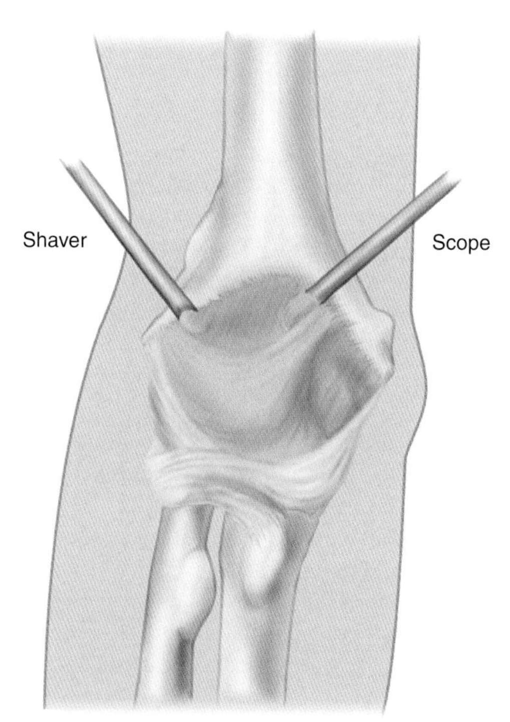

FIGURE 4-2 Most surgeons initially prefer an anterior medial viewing portal and an anterior lateral working portal. *(Courtesy of the Mayo Foundation for Medical Education and Research, Rochester, MN.)*

Resection occurs through an anterolateral portal but may be somewhat difficult because the hardened fibrous tissue may require a sharp incision into the plica to provide an edge against which the powered shaver can be effective. A second midlateral and posterolateral or distal lateral portal is needed for completion of resection of the posterolateral portions of the plica.

Removing the plica is all that is required to relieve the symptoms, and additional lateral portals may be used (Fig. 4-3). Davis and coworkers[17] described the use and value of dual direct lateral portals and found they afforded excellent visualization for osteochondritis dissecans and lateral elbow plica.

Resection must remove, not just release, the plica. However, care should be taken not to continue the resection too far into the capsule because it is possible to violate the lateral collateral ligament complex if the resection proceeds posterior to the meridian of the radial head.

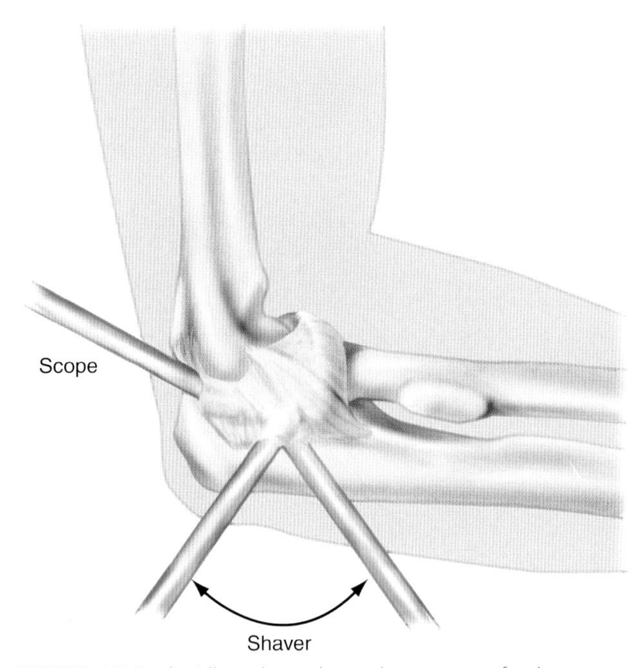

FIGURE 4-3 Dual midlateral portals may be necessary for the scope and shaver to adequately reseat the plica. *(Courtesy of the Mayo Foundation for Medical Education and Research, Rochester, MN.)*

PEARLS & PITFALLS

PEARLS

- Recognize that plica can simulate epicondylitis, but snapping may not be present.
- The plica tends to snap over the radial head at about 60 degrees.
- Flexion engages the plica.
- In extension, the plica slips off the radial head and neck.
- MRI is accurate in defining the presence of a plica if diagnostic questions exist.
- If secondary arthrosis develops, some aching discomfort may persist over the lateral joint after plica resection.

PITFALLS

- Complete resection may not be possible from a single portal.
- Be prepared to employ several lateral portals to adequately visualize and resect the plica.
- A midlateral portal in the soft spot may be the most effective for diagnosing and visualizing the resection.
- Inaccurate portal placement may result in a lack of appreciation of the extent of the pathology.

OUTCOMES

Several studies have had relatively large sample sizes of 10 to 14 patients.[7,11,16] These investigators universally demonstrated a high likelihood of success with arthroscopic resection; more than 90% of patients were free of all symptoms within a short postoperative surveillance period. There was minimal postoperative morbidity. However, Antuna and O'Driscoll did observe that 2 (15%) of 14 patients had some residual discomfort, and 1 patient developed recurrence of the snapping several months after resolution of symptoms postoperatively. The articular changes that frequently occur at the radial head may become symptomatic in the future (Fig. 4-4).

COMPLICATIONS

The most likely complication is development of instability from an aggressive capsular release of the plica that violates the lateral ulnar collateral ligament. This situation causes posterior lateral rotatory instability.

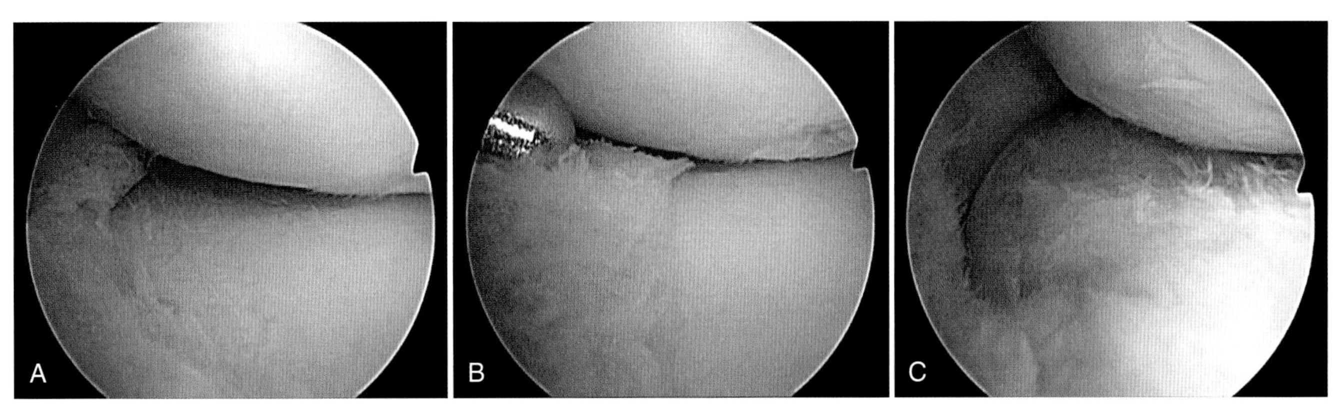

FIGURE 4-4 A, In extension, the plica slips over the margin of the radial head. **B,** With flexion, the plica envelops the lateral and anterior portion of the radial head. **C,** After resection, chondromalacial changes are observed on the radial head.

REFERENCES

1. Duparc F, Putz R, Michot C, Muller JM. The synovial fold of the humeroradial joint: anatomical and histological features, and clinical relevance in lateral epicondylalgia of the elbow. *Surg Radiol Anat*. 2002; 24:302-307.
2. Testut L. *Traite' d'Anatomie Humaine*. Paris, France: Doin, 1928.
3. Miyazaki K, Murakami H. Report of a case of snapping elbow. *J Jpn Orthop Assoc*. 1958;32:250-254.
4. Paturet G. *Membres Superieur et Inferieur*. Vol. II. *Traite d'Anatomic Humaine*. Paris, France: Masson; 1951.
5. Wightman JAK. Clicking elbow from a torn annular ligament: report of a case. *J Bone Joint Surg Br*. 1963;45B:380-381.
6. Clarke RP. Symptomatic, lateral synovial fringe (plica) of the elbow joint. *Arthroscopy*. 1988;4:112-116.
7. Antuna SA, O'Driscoll SW. Snapping plicae associated with radiocapitellar chondromalacia. *Arthroscopy*. 2001;17:491-495.
8. Akagi M, Nakamura T. Snapping elbow caused by the synovial fold in the radiohumeral joint. *J Shoulder Elbow Surg*. 1998;7:427-429.
9. Commandre FA, Taillan B, Benezis C, et al. Plica synovialis (synovial fold) of the elbow: report of one case. *J Sports Med Phys Fitness*. 1988; 28:209-210.
10. Isogai S, Murakami G, Wada T, Ishii S. Which morphologies of synovial folds result from degeneration and/or aging of the radiohumeral joint? An anatomic study with cadavers and embryos. *J Shoulder Elbow Surg*. 2001;10:169-181.
11. Kim DH, Gambardella RA, Elattrache NS, et al. Arthroscopic treatment of posterolateral elbow impingement from lateral synovial plicae in throwing athletes and golfers. *Am J Sports Med*. 2006;34:438-444.
12. Kurosawa H, Koide S, Yaoita T, Nakajima H. Snapping elbow caused by the plica synovialis patellaris. *Rinsyo Seikei Geka*. 1976;11:231-237, 1976.
13. Llusá Pérez M, Ballesteros Betancourt JR, Forcada Calvet P, Carrera Burgaya A. *Atlas de disccíon Anatomoquirúrgica del Codo*. Barcelona, Spain: Elsevier Masson; 2009.
14. Vahlensieck M, Wiche U, Schmidt HM. Humeroradial plica: frequency and visualization on MRI. *Rofo*. 2004;176:959-964.
15. Bosworth D. The role of the orbicular ligament in tennis elbow. *J Bone Joint Surg Am*. 1955;37A:527.
16. Ruch DS, Papadonikolakis A, Campolattaro RM. The posterolateral plica: a cause of refractory lateral elbow pain. *J Shoulder Elbow Surg*. 2006;15:367-370.
17. Davis JT, Idjadi JA, Siskosky MJ, ElAttrache NS. Dual direct lateral portals for treatment of osteochondritis dissecans of the capitellum: an anatomic study. *Arthroscopy*. 2007;23:723-728.

CHAPTER

5

Arthroscopic Resection of the Olecranon Bursa

Darrell J. Ogilvie-Harris • Wayne S.O. Palmer

A prominent and painful olecranon bursa occurs as a result of inflammation. The cause is often repetitive trauma with thickening of the bursal wall, and there may be fibrinous loose bodies within the bursa. Other rheumatologic conditions, such as rheumatoid arthritis or gout, are often associated with olecranon bursitis.

PATIENT EVALUATION

History and Physical Examination

The bursa lies over the point of the olecranon. A general medical history and physical examination are carried out and followed by specific assessments. When the bursa wall is markedly thickened and especially when there are fibrinous loose bodies, it usually does not respond to conservative management. Resection of the bursa should be considered. Infection and other rheumatologic conditions should be excluded.

Diagnostic Imaging

Plain radiographs can rule out significant bony pathology underneath the bursa. They are useful in detecting arthritis in the joint. Other imaging modalities are probably not useful unless specifically indicated.

TREATMENT

Indications and Contraindications

The main indication for surgery is a bursa that has failed to respond to conservative management. A previously infected bursa with a thickened wall should be removed to prevent further episodes. When the bursa wall is markedly thickened and especially when there are fibrinous loose bodies, it usually does not respond to conservative management, and resection of the bursa should be considered.

Arthroscopic resection should not be carried out in the presence of infection. Infection in the bursa should first be eradicated with débridement and antibiotics. An acutely infected bursa should be drained. Initial drainage can be achieved with open or arthroscopic approaches (with limited débridement). After the infection has been eradicated, a formal arthroscopic bursal excision can be perfumed safely.

Before performing arthroscopic resection, significant rheumatologic conditions such as rheumatoid arthritis or gouty arthritis should be excluded. In this situation, the bursa pathology is likely to recur, and this represents a relative contraindication to resection.

Conservative Management

The initial management for olecranon bursitis is conservative. The patient should be given a trial of nonsteroidal anti-inflammatory drugs (NSAIDs). The bursa may be aspirated under sterile conditions, and cortisone can be injected into the bursa. In many cases, bursitis will resolve. Use of a compression wrap or sleeve helps to decrease the swelling. The use of topical NSAIDs has not been clearly defined.

Open Excision

The alternative to arthroscopic resection is open resection of the bursa. There have been no comparisons of open and arthroscopic treatment. However, open treatment does involve a relatively large incision, with the attendant risk of wound complications such as poor healing.[1] Patients may be left with residual hypersensitivity over the scar. However, it usually is considered a satisfactory alternative treatment in the absence of the necessary arthroscopic skills.

Control of Septic Bursitis

In a patient with septic bursitis, the sepsis should be controlled before carrying out an arthroscopic resection. The study from Stell[2] indicated that acute olecranon septic bursitis could be managed on a conservative basis in many cases. The principle is to determine the infective agent. An aspirate of the bursa should be carried out with cultures and sensitivity tests performed.

Appropriate intravenous antibiotics may be given in the emergency department, followed by oral antibiotics. The patient needs careful observation. If the infection fails to resolve, the area may require surgical drainage.

Stell[2] showed that most patients with acute septic bursitis could be managed conservatively without the need for surgical intervention. If intervention is required, we recommend drainage of the bursa and allowing it to heal.

After the infection has been eradicated, an arthroscopic bursectomy or open bursectomy can be carried out under intravenous antibiotic coverage. We do not favor bursal resection in the presence of acute infection.

Arthroscopic Technique

The arthroscopic procedure is carried out under general anesthesia. A tourniquet is used. Although we have favored using a general anesthesia, there is no contraindication to using a regional technique. The procedure is done in the following steps:

1. Bursal distention. A needle is introduced into the bursa, and saline is injected to distend it. This may not be necessary if there is marked fluid in the bursa already. Distention of the bursa helps significantly in entering with the arthroscope.
2. Portals. The arthroscopic portals are proximal to the bursa (Fig. 5-1). Direct entry into the bursa lets the bursa collapse around the arthroscope and makes resection difficult. The portals therefore are started approximately 2 cm proximal to the margin of the bursa. The arthroscope is then introduced subcutaneously with a sharp obturator into the bursal sac (Fig. 5-2). Low pressure is used to prevent overdistention of the bursa (Fig. 5-3). A second portal is used to introduce a 4.5-mm, full-radius resector (Fig. 5-4). We favor using a curved resector to get around all areas of the bursal sac.

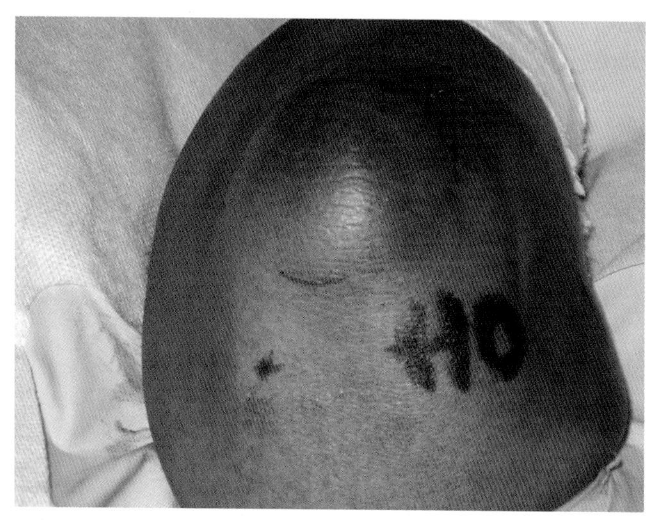

FIGURE 5-1 The positions of the portals are marked. They are 2 cm proximal to the bursal sac medially and laterally. The elbow is flexed slightly to gain access. The patient is supine with the arm across the chest. Notice that the surgeon's initials are used to identify the side to be scoped in keeping with the World Health Organization's recommendations.

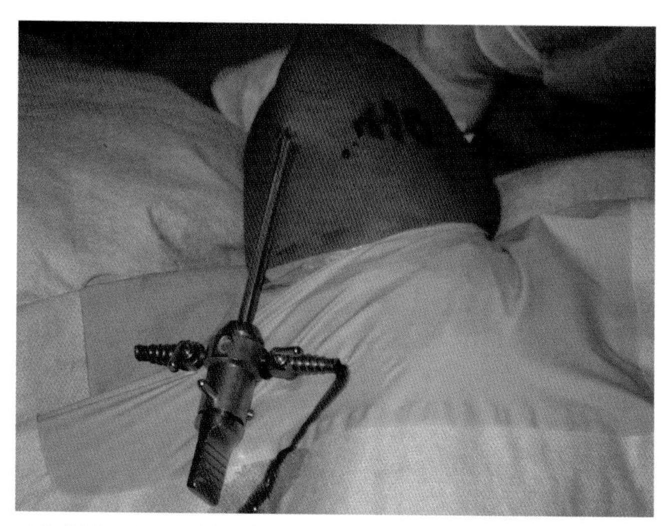

FIGURE 5-2 Bursal fluid drains as the scope enters a distended bursa.

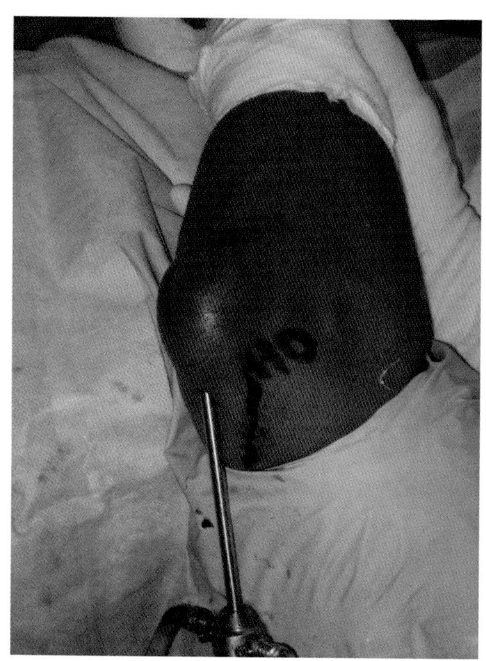

FIGURE 5-3 The arthroscope is introduced into the bursa with transillumination. Low pressure is used to prevent overdistention of the bursa.

3. Removal of the bursal sac. We progressively remove the thickened bursal sac (Figs. 5-5 and 5-6). We start off on the olecranon surface and remove the sac until we can see the fibers of the triceps tendon (Fig. 5-7). We then progressively remove the bursal sac from the peripheral rim and then remove the bursal sac from the subcutaneous area. Care is taken not to perforate the skin in this area (Fig. 5-8).

After completely removing the bursa, we remove the arthroscope but leave the shaver in situ. The tourniquet is then released. We ensure there is minimal or no residual blood in the resected area by sucking through the shaver tip.

The portals are then closed with nylon. Marcaine is injected locally into the portals, and a compressive soft tissue dressing is applied over the olecranon.

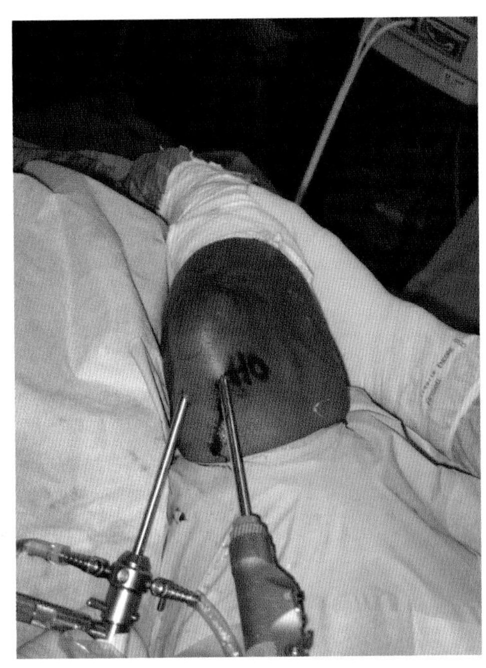

FIGURE 5-4 A second portal is used to introduce the arthroscope and shaver into the bursal sac.

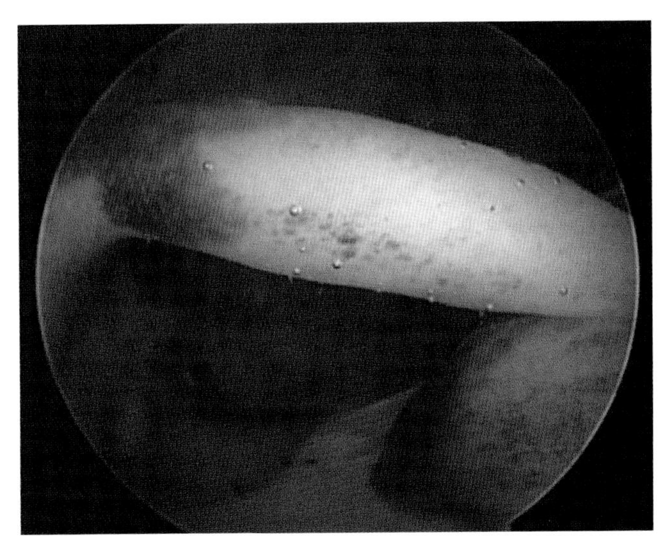

FIGURE 5-5 The view inside the olecranon bursa shows a thickened bursal sac with villous hyperplasia.

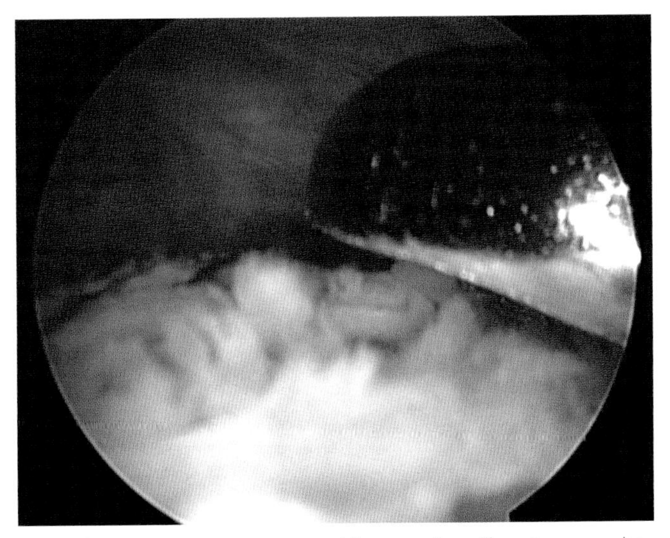

FIGURE 5-6 A 4.5-mm resector used for removing villous tissue can be seen at the 1-o'clock position.

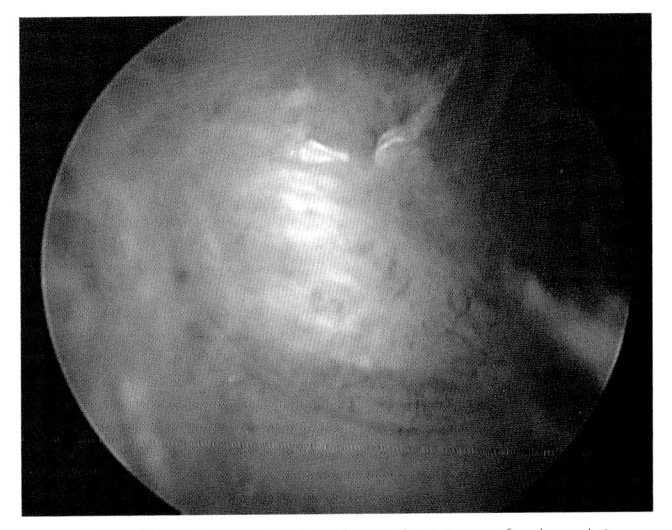

FIGURE 5-7 The arthroscopic view shows the triceps after bursal tissue has been removed. Notice the shiny fibers of the triceps tendon after stripping the bursal sac.

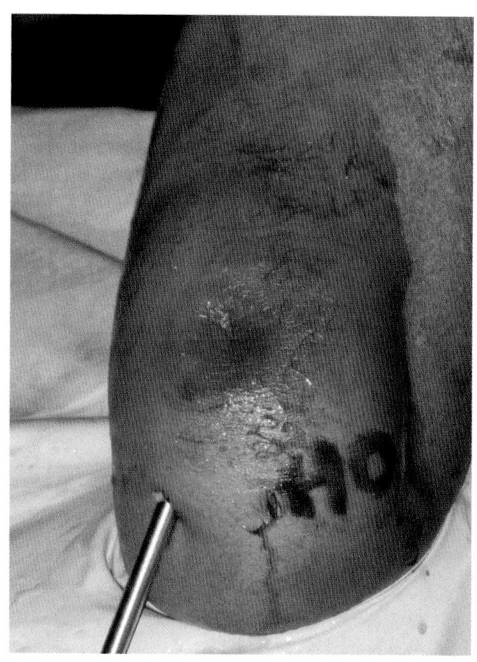

FIGURE 5-8 The bursal tissue has been resected, and the thin skin overlying the bursa is intact. Surgeons must take care not to penetrate the skin.

PEARLS & PITFALLS

- The major problem is achieving insufflation of the bursa, and the key is to inject saline into the bursa before inserting the arthroscope, which is introduced sharply to get it into the bursa.
- After the bursa has been penetrated by the arthroscope, low-pressure irrigation can keep the bursa patent for resection without overdistending the surrounding tissue.
- No one knows how much of the bursa must be resected to prevent disease recurrence. Avoid perforating the thin olecranon skin, because this can delay healing.
- Check the transillumination of the bursa and the arthroscopic view as you proceed.
- Resect the bursa until the shiny fivers of the triceps tendon are seen.
- Ensure patients do not have a rheumatologic disease, such as gout or rheumatoid arthritis, because they have a high recurrence rate.
- Avoid arthroscopic resection in the face of an infection. Treat the septic process first, and resect the bursa later.
- Avoid damage to the ulnar nerve. Carefully identify and mark the nerve preoperatively.

Postoperative Management

During the first 7 to 10 days, the patient wears an elastic compressive bandage. The bandage is taken off only for hygiene. It is important to keep some compression locally over the bursal area to prevent re-accumulation of blood and fluid.

At the end of 7 to 10 days, the sutures are removed. The patient is then allowed to mobilize the elbow. However, he or she should avoid direct contact on the point of the elbow for about 6 weeks to allow healing.

OUTCOMES AND CONCLUSIONS

There are only three reported arthroscopic series in the literature. In the report by Nussbaumer and colleagues,[3] nine patients had resection of the olecranon bursa. There were no complications. In the report by Kerr and Carpenter,[4] six patients had resection of the olecranon bursa, with complications occurring in two patients; one had gouty arthritis, and the other had CREST syndrome (calcinosis, Raynaud phenomenon, esophageal dysmotility, sclerodactyly, and telangiectasia), a limited form of scleroderma. In the report by Ogilvie-Harris,[5] there were 31 cases of olecranon bursitis. Eight-six percent of the patients had no residual pain. There was residual pain over the olecranon in the remaining patients. In an unpublished review, another 14 cases were done with no complications or recurrences. These results indicate that the arthroscopic resection of the olecranon bursa can be a highly successful procedure.

REFERENCES

1. Degreef I, De Smet L. Complications following resection of the olecranon bursa. *Acta Orthop Belg*. 2006;72:400-403.
2. Stell IM. Management of acute bursitis: outcome study of a structured approach. *J R Soc Med*. 1999;92:516-521.
3. Nussbaumer P, Candrian C, Hollinger A. [Endoscopic bursa shaving in acute bursitis.] *Swiss Surg*. 2001;7:121-125.
4. Kerr DR, Carpenter CW. Arthroscopic resection of olecranon and prepatellar bursae. *Arthroscopy*. 1990;6:86-88.
5. Ogilvie-Harris DJ, Gilbart M. Endoscopic bursal resection: the olecranon bursa and prepatellar bursa. *Arthroscopy*. 2000;16:249-253.

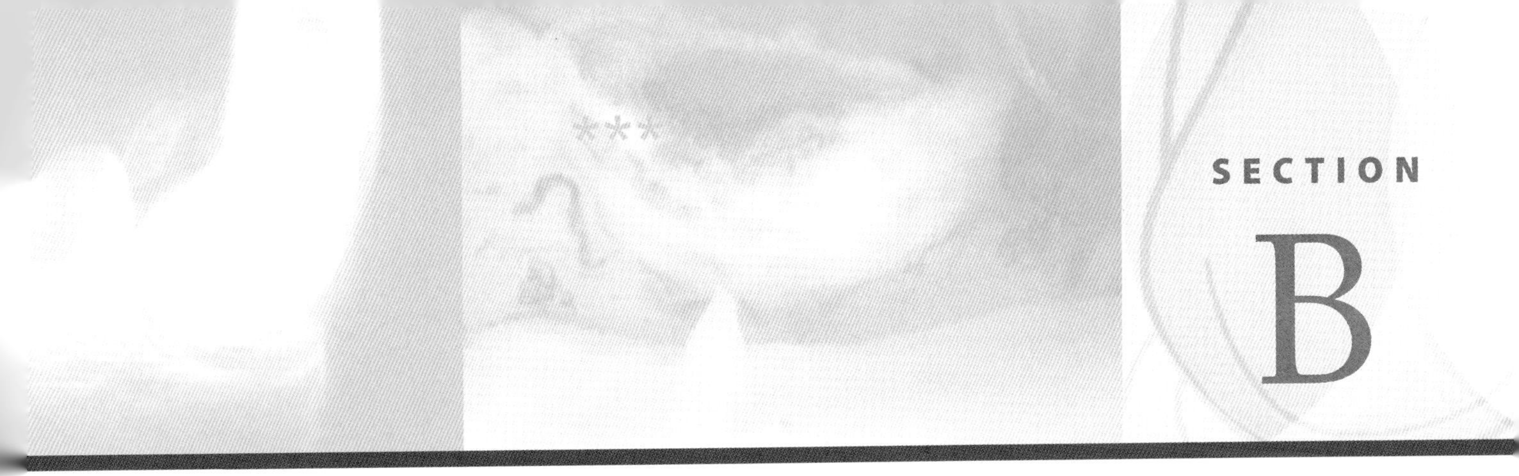

SECTION B

Advanced Procedures of the Elbow

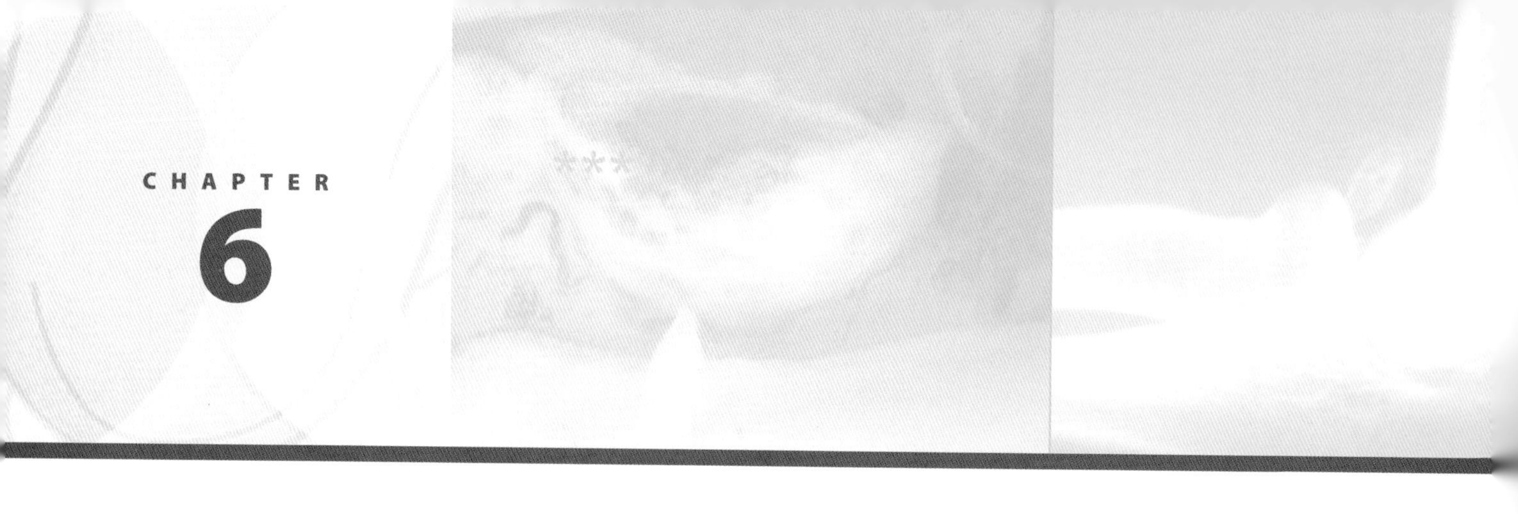

Osteochondritis Dissecans of the Elbow

Guillem Gonzalez-Lomas • Christopher S. Ahmad • Tony Wanich • Neal S. ElAttrache

Sport-specific injuries more frequently affect young athletes with earlier and more rigorous participation in sports. The radiocapitellar compartment of the young athlete's elbow is punished by significant stresses during repetitive throwing or during sports (e.g., gymnastics) that convert the elbow joint into a weight-bearing joint.[1] Lateral compartment compression can lead to Panner's disease (i.e., osteochondrosis) in the 6- to 10-year old patient or to various stages of capitellar osteochondritis dissecans (OCD) in the adolescent or young adult.[2-5] This chapter describes Panner's disease and OCD and outlines a treatment algorithm, including arthroscopic management using osteochondral grafting.

PANNER'S DISEASE

In 1927, Hans Jessen Panner published a description of osteochondrosis of the capitellum, likening it to Legg-Calvé-Perthes disease of the hip.[6] Like other ostochondroses, it consists of noninflammatory, disordered endochondral ossification. Its specific cause and relation to OCD remain debatable. It is known that abnormal radiocapitellar compressive forces during a period of vulnerability, typically while the physes are still open, predispose children to Panner's disease.[2,5,7] It may result from the combination of an avascular insult (likely related to the capitellum's predominantly end-artery supply) and repetitive microtrauma.[8]

Epidemiology

Panner's disease predominantly affects boys younger than age 10 years.[9] Young boys may be predisposed to it for two reasons. First, compared with girls, they have a delayed appearance and maturation of their secondary growth centers. Second, boys traditionally are more prone to trauma during the more aggressive early childhood activities they select.[7] This may change as more girls choose higher-risk athletic activities at younger ages. Although Panner's disease can be confused with OCD, and the age of onset may overlap, it is distinguished by three epidemiologic characteristics. Panner's disease does not share the strict association with repetitive throwing that OCD does, it is usually self-limited, and it resolves without any long-term sequelae.

Patient Evaluation

Panner's disease initially manifests as pain and stiffness in the elbow, which is relieved by rest. On physical examination, patients have poorly localized tenderness over the lateral elbow. Radiographs initially show fissuring, lucencies, fragmentation, and irregularity of the capitellum (Fig. 6-1), particularly near or at the chondral surface. Subsequent x-ray films, taken at 3 to 5 months, demonstrate larger radiolucent areas followed by reossification of the bony epiphysis, with a corresponding resolution of symptoms. In 1 to 2 years, the epiphysis regains its contour, usually without flattening.[4] As in Legg-Calvé-Perthes, radiographs often lag behind clinical symptoms. Magnetic resonance imaging (MRI) may be used effectively to document the extent of the lesion. Typically, edema is localized to the chondral surface and the bone adjacent to it, with less involvement of the deeper subchondral bone compared with the OCD (Fig. 6-2).

Treatment

Treatment involves rest and cessation of the aggravating activity and administering therapeutic modalities such as ice and anti-inflammatory medication. The elbow occasionally may need to be immobilized for 3 to 4 weeks to control symptoms. We favor a hinged elbow brace set at the pain-free motion to protect the area while allowing some motion and decreasing the risk of stiffness.

Symptoms usually resolve within 6 to 8 weeks, although they occasionally persist for months. Activities should be reinstituted progressively and as tolerated. The condition has an excellent long-term prognosis, although some patients may have a slight residual flexion contracture.

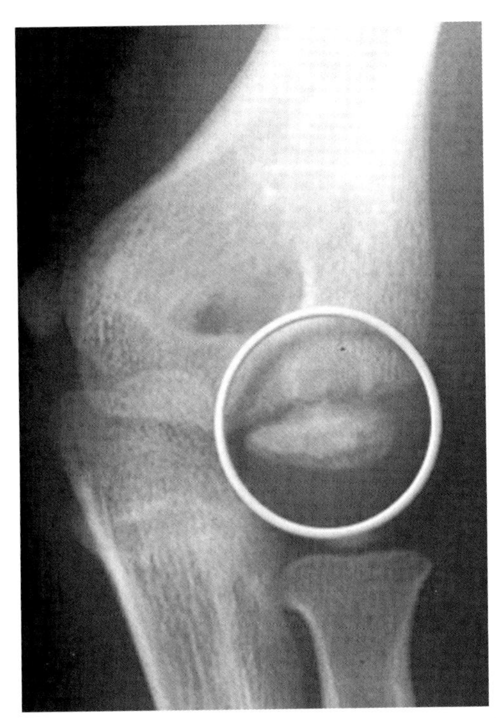

FIGURE 6-1 Panner's disease. An anteroposterior radiograph of the left elbow demonstrates fragmentation and lucency of the capitellum *(circle)* near the chondral surface. *(Courtesy of Neal S. ElAttrache, MD, Kerlan-Jobe Orthopaedic Clinic, Los Angeles, CA.)*

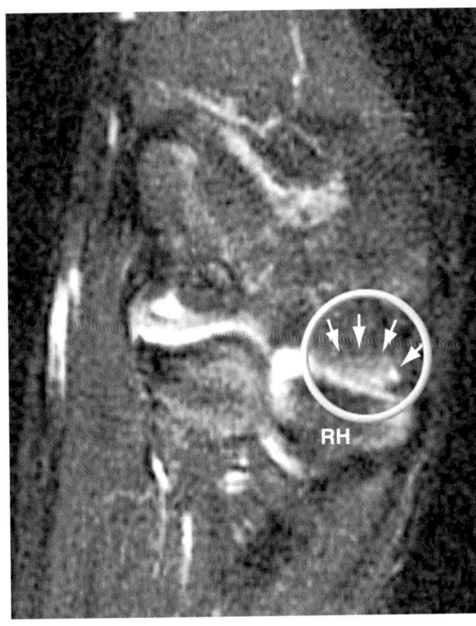

FIGURE 6-2 T2-weighted magnetic resonance imaging shows the effects of Panner's disease. A Panner's lesion *(circle)* is demarcated by *small arrows* opposite the radial head (RH). Notice the more typical finding of edema adjacent to the capitellar chondral surface, rather than deeper in the subchondral bone, as in osteochondritis dissecans. *(Courtesy of Neal S. ElAttrache, MD, Kerlan-Jobe Orthopaedic Clinic, Los Angeles, CA.)*

OSTEOCHONDRITIS DISSECANS

OCD of the capitellum is a non-inflammatory degeneration of subchondral bone occurring in the context of repetitive trauma to the lateral compartment of the elbow. Panner's disease and OCD may represent two different stages of the same disorder,[4] but they do have different characteristics: age of onset, cause, and natural history. Although Panner's disease affects children younger than 10 years, OCD victimizes older athletes, usually between the ages of 11 and 15 years.[10] Unlike Panner's disease, OCD is thought to be directly linked to repetitive trauma. OCD is not always a self-limited disease, and if left unaddressed, it results in profound destruction of the capitellum.[10]

Anatomy

The elbow's osseous anatomy and the capitellum's idiosyncratic blood supply may predispose young athletes to OCD. The elbow is a diarthrodial joint in which the distal humerus articulates with the proximal ulna and the radial head. Its unique bony configuration allows for −15 to 0 degrees° of extension to 150 degrees of flexion. Rotation of the radial head over the stationary ulna gives an arc of almost 180 degrees of forearm rotation.[11] The osseous and articular congruency of the humerus, ulna, and radial head accounts for the greater part of elbow stability, particularly at less than 20 degrees of extension or more than 120 degrees of elbow flexion.[12]

In young, skeletally immature athletes, the elbow possesses a greater degree of cartilaginous elasticity. Hyperextension, facilitated by this increased range of motion, can generate increased radiocapitellar compressive loads and tension of the medial capsule and ulnar collateral ligament (UCL). Overhead throwing athletes during the throwing motion and gymnasts during weight-bearing handstands in elbow hyperextension further exaggerate these stresses. Repetitive stress on this system can precipitate OCD. Medial-sided pathologies, such as medial apophysitis, UCL injury, and posteromedial impingement from the excess valgus stress, can occur concurrently.[13]

The tenuous end-artery vascular supply to the capitellum predisposes it to injury. In the young adult population, the capitellum is supplied by two end arteries coursing from posterior to anterior, which are branches of the radial recurrent and interosseous recurrent arteries (Fig. 6-3).[14] As a result of the longitudinal blood supply to the capitellar epiphyseal plate and minimal collateral circulation in the area, blood flow to the capitellum may be disrupted by repetitive microtrauma resulting in an avascular state and by a single traumatic event leading to post-traumatic subchondral bone bruises.[15,16]

Patient Evaluation

History

OCD arises from repetitive, excessive compressive forces generated by large valgus stresses on the elbow during throwing or racket swinging or by constant axial compressive loads on the elbow, such as those endured by gymnasts.[10,17,18] Specific risk factors predispose to the condition. In the case of baseball players, throwing sliders and breaking pitches, throwing more than 600 pitches per season, and increased age of the athlete increase the risk of developing OCD.[18] In female gymnasts, overtraining involving excessive handstand maneuvers has been linked to OCD.[19,20] There also may be a genetic predisposition to OCD.

Patients with OCD initially complain of pain and stiffness in the elbow that is relieved by rest. The onset is usually insidious, and a

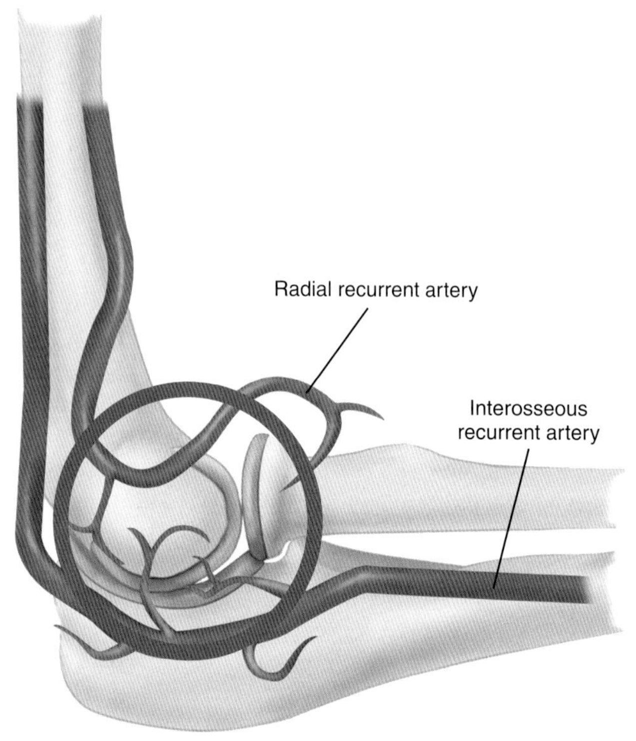

FIGURE 6-3 Capitellar blood supply. In young adults (<20 years), the radial recurrent and interosseous recurrent arteries give off branches that course from posterior to anterior and supply the capitellum *(circle)*. This end-artery blood supply makes the capitellum susceptible to an avascular insult. *(Modified from Mirzayan R, Itamura JM, Rockwood CA.* Shoulder and Elbow Trauma. *New York, NY: Thieme; 2004.)*

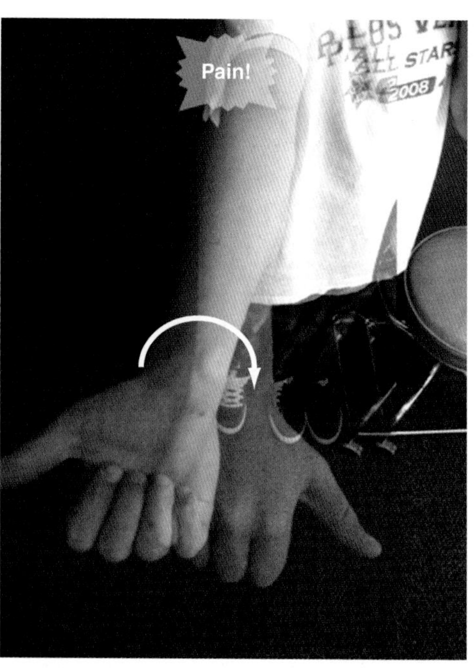

FIGURE 6-4 In the radiocapitellar compression test, pain in the lateral elbow is elicited when the extended arm is pronated and supinated. *(Courtesy of Neal S. ElAttrache, MD, Kerlan-Jobe Orthopaedic Clinic, Los Angeles, CA.)*

history of specific trauma is often absent. If left unaddressed, the symptoms may progress to locking or catching due to intra-articular loose bodies or an inflamed plica. Throwing athletes may present with painful posterolateral clicking or catching caused by a radiocapitellar plica. These symptoms can overlap with those from the OCD lesion, and the plica itself may be responsible for chondral wear in the radiocapitellar compartment.

Physical Examination

Because throwing athletes may have injured medial and lateral and posterior elbow structures, a full elbow examination is essential. We test UCL integrity by performing a valgus stress test at 30 degrees, the milking maneuver, and the moving valgus stress test. We screen for posteromedial impingement by performing a bounce test. A positive test result elicits pain posteromedially when the elbow undergoes forced hyperextension.

In athletes with OCD, physical examination findings tend to be remarkable for poorly localized lateral elbow tenderness over the radiocapitellar joint. Loss of range of motion with a 15- to 20-degree flexion contracture is common. Loss of extension is more common than loss of flexion. An effusion is often apparent and can be palpated by flexing the elbow and feeling the lateral portal area, triangulated by the radial head, olecranon, and lateral epicondyle. The provocative maneuver for the radiocapitellar joint we prefer is the active radiocapitellar compression test (Fig. 6-4). A positive test result elicits pain in the lateral compartment of the elbow when the patient pronates and supinates the forearm with the arm in extension. In patients with an associated symptomatic radiocapitellar plica, snapping typically occurs at greater than 90 degrees of elbow flexion with the forearm in pronation.

Diagnostic Imaging

Anteroposterior radiographs in full extension, anteroposterior radiographs in 45 degrees of flexion, and lateral views of the elbow should be obtained. Radiographic findings may be negative early in the disease process. As the condition progresses, flattening and sclerosis of the capitellum, typically on its anterolateral aspect, will become apparent. Irregular areas of lucency and intra-articular loose bodies also appear. The capitellar lesions of OCD and medial-sided epicondylar fragmentation are best seen on an anteroposterior radiograph at 45 degrees of elbow flexion (Fig. 6-5).

MRI should be used to assess suspected OCD. It can detect bone edema early in the disease process.[21] An MR arthrogram can further delineate the extent of the injury. Contrast can show separation of a detached or partially detached piece from subchondral bone (Fig. 6-6). This is important in determining whether to proceed with operative or nonoperative management. Peiss and colleagues[22] thought that fragment enhancement (Fig. 6-7B) (as opposed to the perifragment enhancement seen in Fig. 6-6) denoted viability and might be a reasonable indication for nonoperative treatment. They also suggested that enhancement of the fragment and subchondral bone interface was caused by vascular granulation tissue, indicating instability and requiring operative intervention.

Pseudolesions, which appear on the posteroinferior junction of the articular and nonarticular portions of the capitellum, must be differentiated from OCD, which almost always manifests on the anterolateral aspect. The examiner also should observe whether the capitellar physis is open or closed.

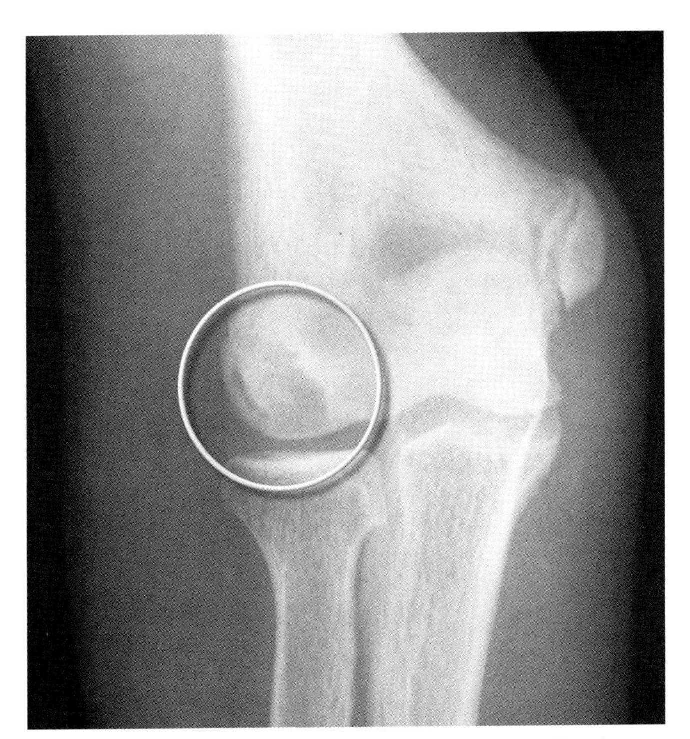

FIGURE 6-5 An anteroposterior radiograph shows the osteochondritis dissecans lesion *(circle)* more clearly with elbow flexed to 45 degrees. *(Courtesy of Neal S. ElAttrache, MD, Kerlan-Jobe Orthopaedic Clinic, Los Angeles, CA.)*

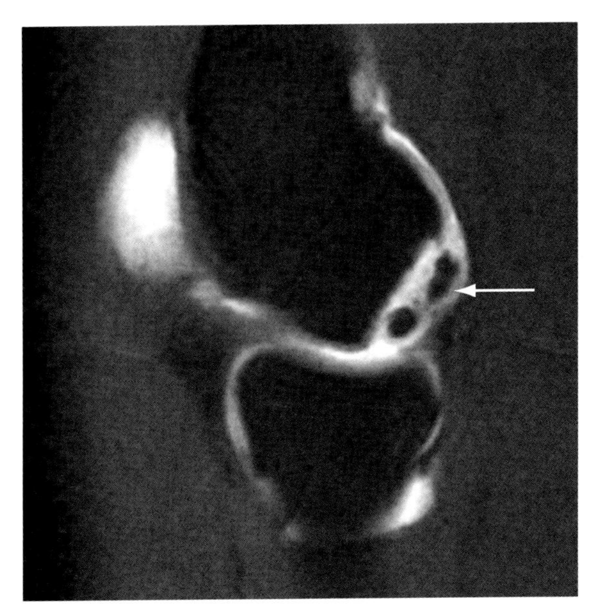

FIGURE 6-6 The MR arthrogram shows contrast surrounding an unstable osteochondritis dissecans fragment *(arrow)*. *(Courtesy of Neal S. ElAttrache, MD, Kerlan-Jobe Orthopaedic Clinic, Los Angeles, CA.)*

Treatment

Indications, Contraindications, and Classification

Management of OCD lesions is based primarily on the status and stability of the overlying cartilage. The size and location of the lesion and the patency of the capitellar growth plate also influence decision making.[23-25]

To guide treatment, detailed classification systems based on radiographic[26,27] and arthroscopic[23] findings have been delineated.[28,29] We have simplified these algorithms into a three-stage classification that provides a template for management. Table 6-1 shows the classification.

Stage 1. In stage 1, the osteochondral fragment is intact, stable, and not displaced. Radiographic findings are often negative. The MRI signal varies; it is typically abnormal on T1-weighted and normal on T2-weighted images, although the T2 signal may also be abnormal. Figure 6-7A and B shows a stage 1 lesion with coronal-slice signal that is abnormal on T1- and T2-weighted images. Arthroscopically, the articular cartilage is intact, with general preservation of subchondral stability.

This stage is best treated nonoperatively. All activity involving the affected arm should be stopped. The elbow should be rested in a hinged elbow brace for 3 to 6 weeks. Progressive physical therapy should ensue as symptoms abate. Return to sports usually can be expected at 3 to 6 months and should be governed by primarily by the patient's clinical response, because radiographic changes often lag behind the clinical symptoms by several months or years. Nevertheless, follow-up radiographs and MRI scans should be obtained at 2- to 3-month intervals to track progress. Figure 6-7C and D shows the same patient as in Figure 6-7A and B at the 6-month follow-up assessment after conservative treatment, with clear reconstitution of the subchondral bone.

If symptoms return, additional rest is mandated. With persistently refractory symptoms, pitchers may have to change positions, and gymnasts may have to change sports. Lesions that progress to stage 2 should be treated accordingly.

Stage 2. In stage 2, the osteochondral fragment is partially separated, as documented radiographically and arthroscopically. Radiographs demonstrate fissuring, lucencies, and fragmentation. On MRI, T1- and T2-weighted sequences show abnormal signal intensity and a margin around the fragment, denoting its instability (Fig. 6-8). Computed tomography (CT) may reveal the partially separated fragment. Arthroscopically, the cartilage is fractured, and the subchondral bone is unstable and partially displaced (Fig. 6-9).

When an unstable lesion is identified, conservative treatment should be bypassed. It warrants prompt surgical intervention to return the athlete to his or her sport or activities of daily living as soon as possible. In stage 2 lesions, the size and location of the lesion govern treatment. For smaller lesions, débridement is an option. Patients typically have immediate relief of symptoms, but the long-term natural history includes arthritis. Fragment fixation has been advocated by some for this stage, although questions linger concerning the long-term healing potential of fixed fragments and clinical results of the procedure.[26,27,30,31] Osteochondral autografts or synthetic grafts can address large, radial head–engaging defects involving the lateral buttress of the capitellum. If the decision rests between fixation and osteochondral restoration, we prefer osteochondral or synthetic plug grafting, because it has generated more reliable results.

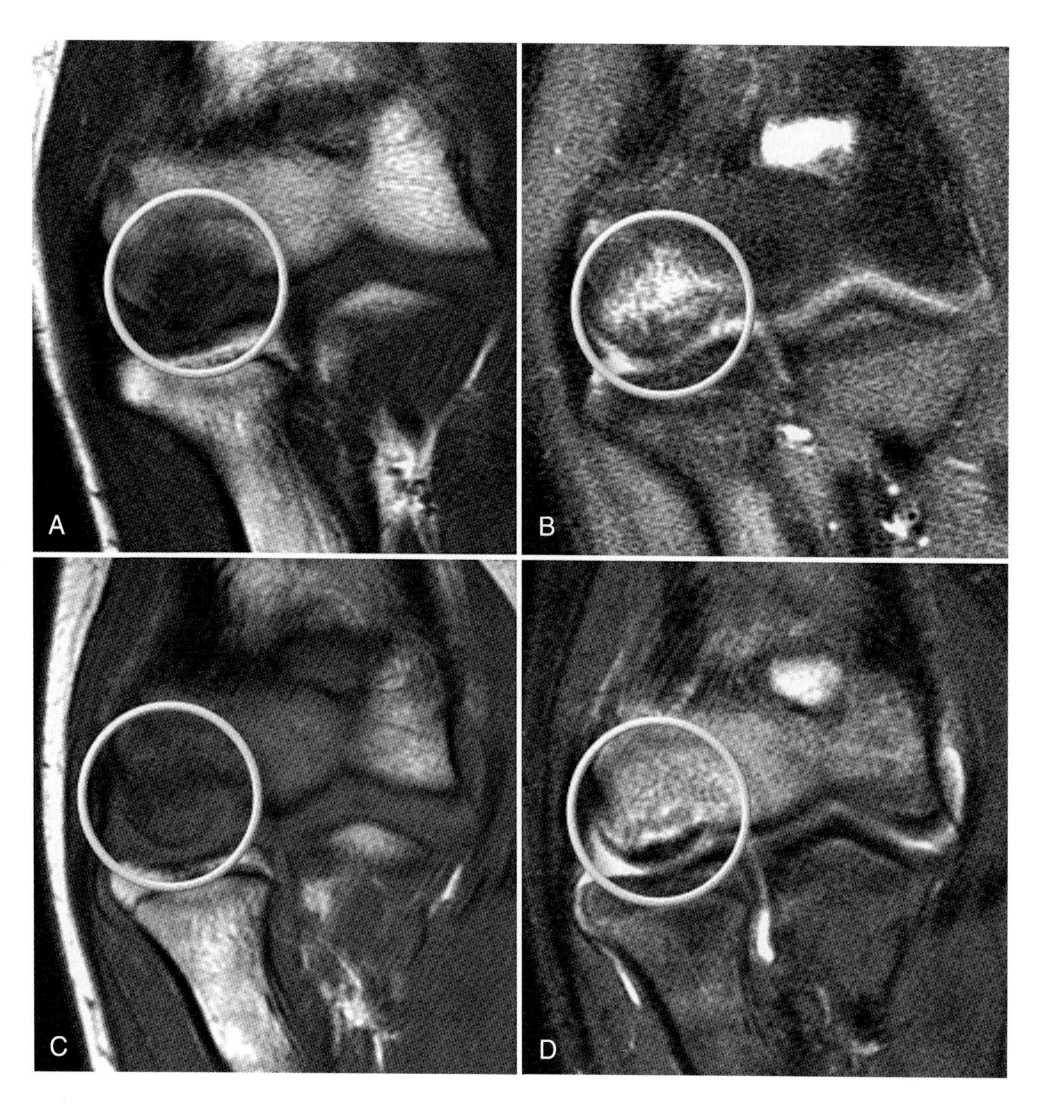

FIGURE 6-7 Progress of a stage 1 osteochondritis dissecans lesion is evaluated on magnetic resonance imaging (MRI). A stable, intact, nondisplaced fragment *(circles)* has abnormal signal intensity on coronal slices in T1-weighted (**A**) and T2-weighted (**B**) MRI sequences. After 6 months of conservative management, the T1-weighted (**C**) and T2-weighted (**D**) MRI sequences show reconstitution of subchondral bone in the area of the lesion. The patient was symptom free at the 6-month follow-up assessment. *(Courtesy of Neal S. ElAttrache, MD, Kerlan-Jobe Orthopaedic Clinic, Los Angeles, CA.)*

TABLE 6-1 Classification and Treatment of Capitellar Osteochondritis Dissecans Lesions

Stability	Stage	MRI Findings	Arthroscopic Findings	Treatment
Stable	1	Normal radiograph T1 abnormal T2 normal	Intact articular cartilage Subchondral bone edema but structurally sound	1. Hinged elbow brace for 3-6 wk 2. Physical therapy 3. NSAIDs 4. Follow-up radiograph and/or MRI at 3-6 mo
Unstable	2	Abnormal radiograph T1, T2 abnormal Contrast shows margin around lesion	Partially detached fragment Cartilage fracture Subchondral bone collapse Lateral buttress involved with a poorer prognosis	1. Acute: consider fragment fixation, but higher success treating as chronic condition 2. Chronic: a. <6-7 mm lateral buttress involved, radial head does not engage: fragment removal, microfracture drilling b. >6-7 mm lateral buttress involved, head engages: removal, osteochondral autograft, synthetic graft
Unstable	3	Loose bodies Associated radial head OCD	Completely detached Loose bodies Any of the above	1. Loose body removal 2. Treat as stage 2 lesion 1. <30% radial head involvement: treat as stage 2 lesion 2. >30% radial head involvement: no osteochondral grafting; microfracture drilling okay

MRI, magnetic resonance imaging; NSAIDs, nonsteroidal anti-inflammatory drugs; OCD, osteochondritis dissecans; T1, T1-weighted MRI; T2, T2-weighted MRI.

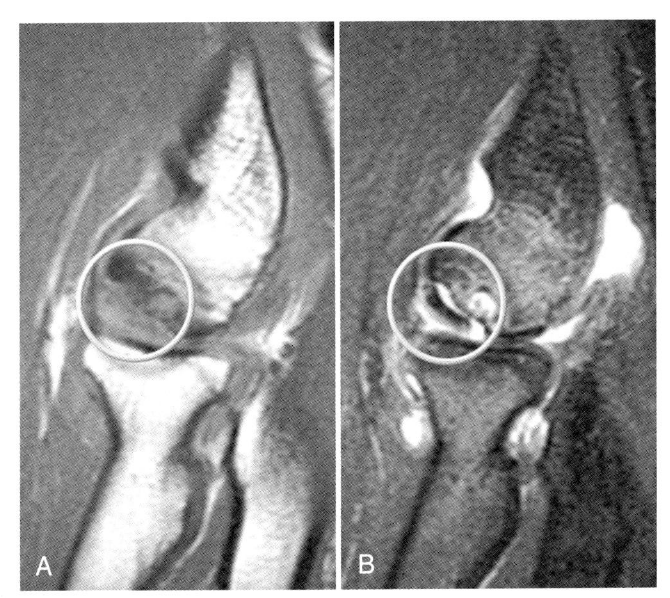

FIGURE 6-8 A stage 2 osteochondritis dissecans lesion is assessed by magnetic resonance imaging (MRI). T1-weighted (**A**) and T2-weighted (**B**) MRI sequences show a margin around the fragment *(circles)*, denoting its instability. *(Courtesy of Neal S. ElAttrache, MD, Kerlan-Jobe Orthopaedic Clinic, Los Angeles, CA.)*

Size. Takahara and coworkers[32] differentiated among small (<5% of the capitellum on an anteroposterior radiograph of the elbow, <60-degree angle formed by lines drawn along the borders of the lesion on a lateral radiograph), moderate (5% to 70%), and large (>70%, >90 degrees) lesions. They concluded that large lesions should be addressed operatively. Shimada and associates[33] suggested that smaller lesions (<1 cm^2) could be treated with débridement, chondroplasty, and possibly microfracture or drilling as described by Bradley and Dandy.[34] Larger lesions (>1 cm^2) should be treated with osteochondral autografts.

Location. We think the location of the lesion may be more important in guiding treatment than some other factors. Extension of the lesion into the lateral margin of the capitellum, as described by Chappell and ElAttrache[35] and by Ruch and colleagues,[36] is associated with a potentially poorer prognosis. The lateral column of the capitellum supports large compressive forces when the elbow is stressed in valgus or with axial loading. When the lateral column is intact, a defect treated with microfracture alone is relatively protected, and fibrocartilage healing may occur. Lesions that do not involve a significant portion of the lateral buttress of the capitellum and do not engage the radial head during arthroscopic observation (i.e., pronation and supination with the elbow in extension) have been successfully treated with microfracture or retrograde or antegrade subchondral drilling. Figure 6-10 shows an OCD lesion with a predominantly intact lateral column.

Lateral column involvement of more than about 6 to 7 mm cannot be dealt with acceptably by microfracture. The absence of a lateral buttress forestalls fibrocartilage healing by subjecting the defect to increased radiocapitellar forces. Engagement of the radial head in the defect also compromises healing and may lead to accelerated radiocapitellar arthrosis. For these larger, engaging defects or those that extend substantially into the lateral buttress (>6 to 7 mm) (Fig. 6-11), we recommend removal of the loose fragment and osteochondral restoration by means of mosaicplasty or osteochondral autograft transfer system (OATS).

For early, partially detached fragments, the detached portion (usually central) should be débrided from central to lateral aspects. After stable osteochondral borders have been obtained, the lesion is carefully evaluated arthroscopically to ascertain how much of the lateral column is involved and if the radial head engages with the defect. Chappell and ElAttrache[35] reported that lesions larger than 1 cm^2 (average, 1.32 cm^2) and no lateral column involvement were treated successfully with microfracture,

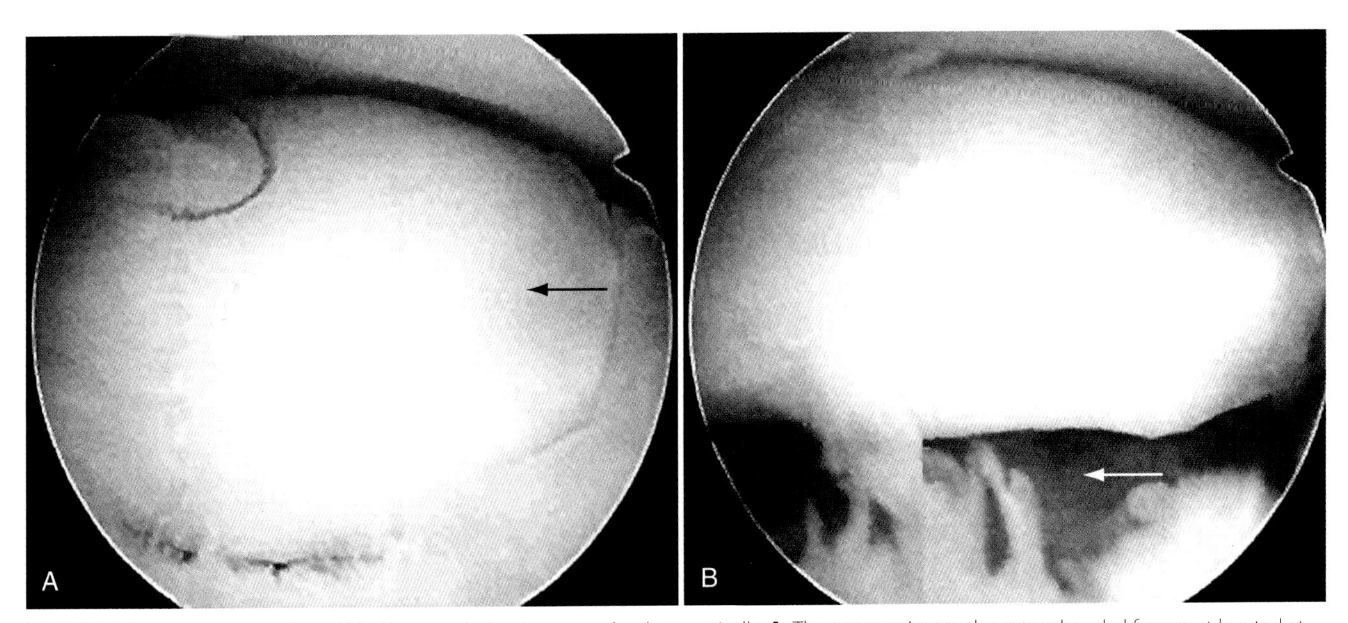

FIGURE 6-9 A stage 2 osteochondritis dissecans lesion is assessed arthroscopically. **A,** The *arrow* points to the osteochondral fragment located at its donor site. **B,** The arrow points to the space between the osteochondral fragment and bone, denoting fractured cartilage and instability. *(Courtesy of Neal S. ElAttrache, MD, Kerlan-Jobe Orthopaedic Clinic, Los Angeles, CA.)*

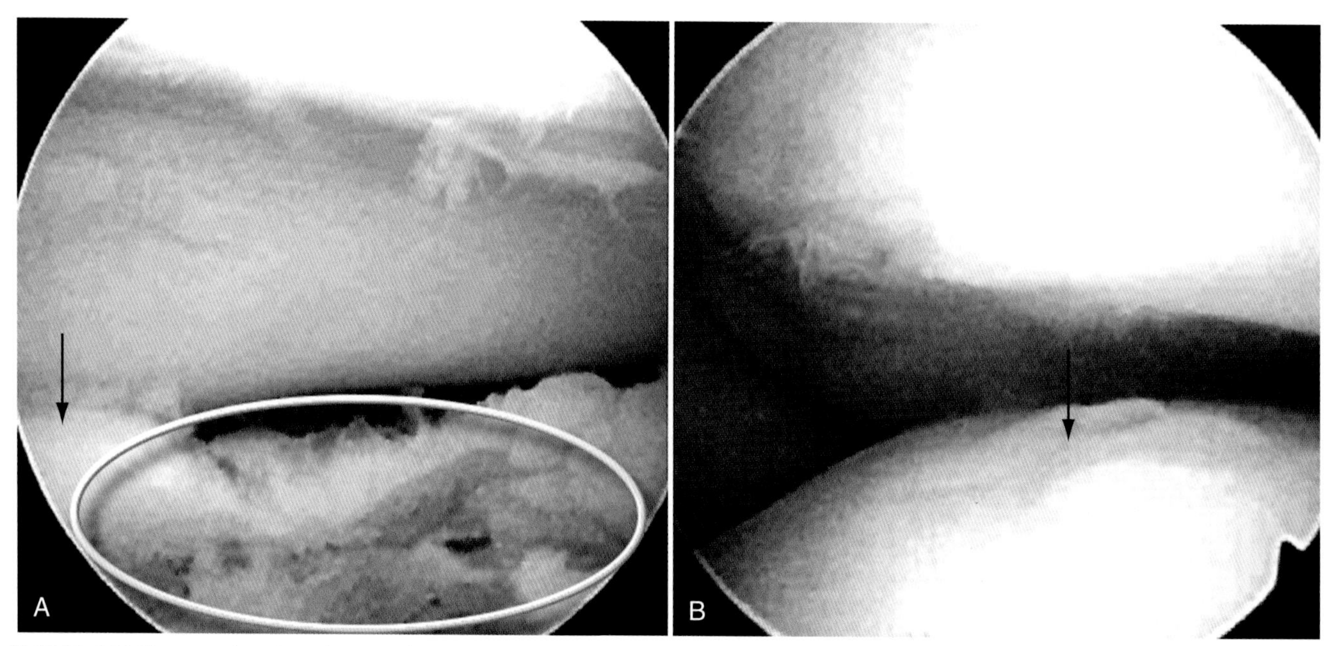

FIGURE 6-10 The osteochondritis dissecans lesion with an intact lateral column. **A,** The lesion *(oval)* is adjacent to a significant portion of the intact lateral column *(arrow)*. **B,** The lateral column *(arrow)* supports the radial head and does not permit engagement with the defect. *(Courtesy of Neal S. ElAttrache, MD, Kerlan-Jobe Orthopaedic Clinic, Los Angeles, CA.)*

whereas those involving the lateral column did well with osteochondral grafting. Fragment fixation also is an option, but we have had superior and more consistent results with grafting.

Stage 3. In stage 3, the fragment is fully displaced and has become or is imminently becoming a loose body. Figure 6-12 shows an example of a stage 3 lesion seen on MRI and arthroscopically. Patients may present with mechanical symptoms related to loose bodies, such as locking.

In this stage, débridement, drilling, or osteochondral replacement is indicated. If the loose osteochondral piece is acutely displaced in a patient with previously documented OCD, the surgeon can attempt to fix it to its donor site. Results of fixation are, however, inconsistent. Chronically loose bodies (documented by serial

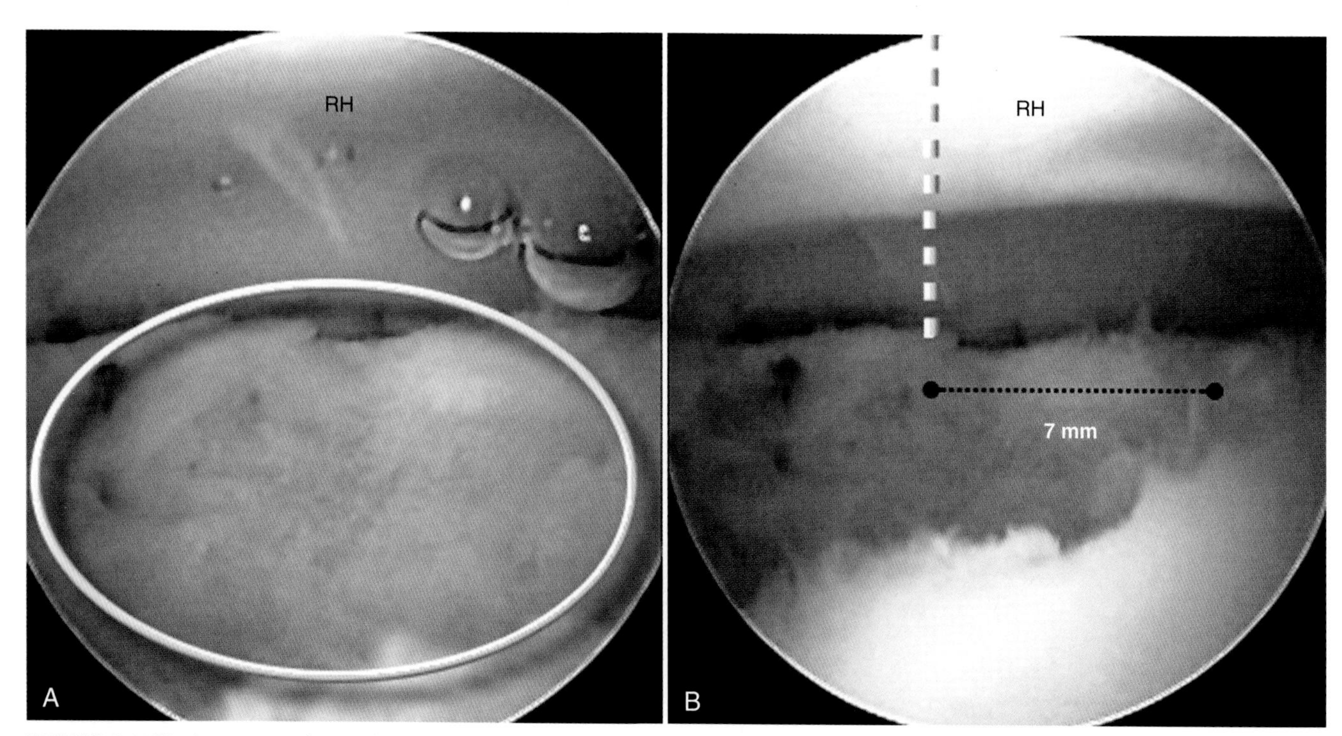

FIGURE 6-11 The lesion extends into the lateral column. **A,** The osteochondritis dissecans lesion *(circle)* can be seen. **B,** The *white dotted line* denotes the ulnar margin of the lateral column. The lesion extends 7 mm into the lateral column *(black dotted line)* and allows the radial head (RH) to engage. *(Courtesy of Neal S. ElAttrache, MD, Kerlan-Jobe Orthopaedic Clinic, Los Angeles, CA.)*

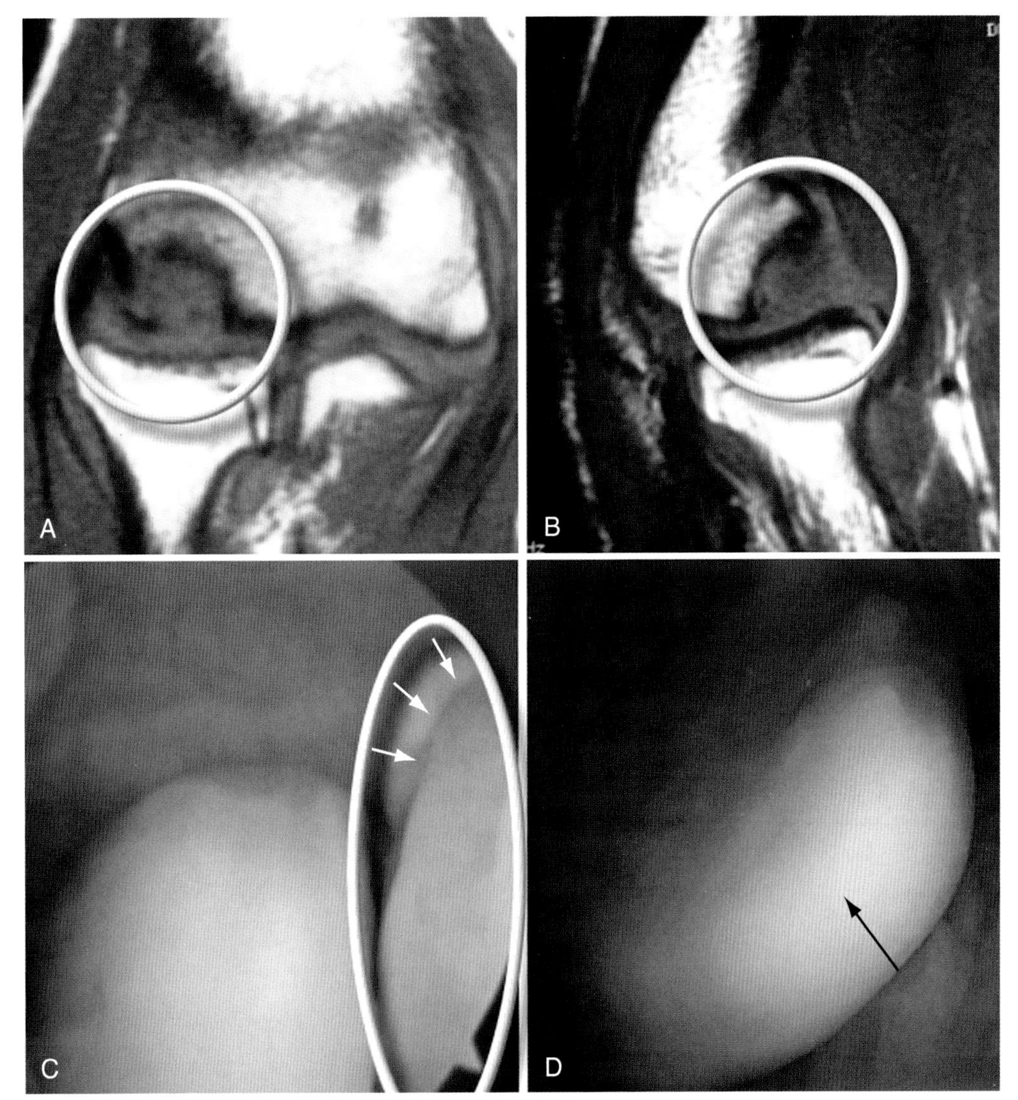

FIGURE 6-12 A stage 3 osteochondritis dissecans lesion is assessed by magnetic resonance imaging (MRI) and arthroscopy. T1-weighted, coronal MRI (**A**) and T1-weighted, sagittal MRI (**B**) show an unroofed lesion. **C,** Arthroscopy shows the lesion *(oval)* with no overlying cartilage. *Small arrows* demarcate edge of lesion. **D,** The loose body osteochondral fragment *(arrow)* is found in the joint. *(Courtesy of Neal S. ElAttrache, MD, Kerlan-Jobe Orthopaedic Clinic, Los Angeles, CA.)*

radiographs or MRI) should be removed and the donor bed débrided in preparation for one of the aforementioned treatment options, following the same algorithm. These patients often are unable to return to sports, and the long-term prognosis usually includes radiocapitellar arthrosis.

Radial Head Involvement. Radial head involvement, in addition to capitellar pathology, indicates advanced disease and usually does not occur in athletes. If the radial lesion is less than 30% of the radial head, treatment of the capitellar OCD should proceed as delineated earlier. For radial lesions that are greater than 30% of the radial head, treatment of the capitellar lesion should be limited to débridement, drilling, and microfracture.[9] Severe radiocapitellar degenerative arthritis is a relative contraindication to mosaicplasty.

Radiocapitellar Plica. A comorbid condition that may be found in throwing athletes at the time of arthroscopy for OCD is posterolateral elbow impingement caused by a thickened radiocapitellar plica. The plica can cause chondromalacic changes on the radial head and capitellum. Symptoms may include painful clicking or catching and effusions, and they can overlap with those from the OCD lesion. Snapping often occurs at more than 90 degrees of elbow flexion with the forearm in pronation. If found during arthroscopic inspection, the plica should be resected. Kim and colleagues[37] reported excellent results after plica débridement in throwing athletes and golfers.

Conservative Management

Nonoperative treatment is indicated for stage 1 OCD with a stable lesion and in patients with open capitellar growth plates. Takahara and coworkers[26,27] retrospectively reviewed 106 cases of capitellar OCD with an average 7-year follow-up. They found that stable lesions that healed completely with nonoperative treatment had three common characteristics at initial presentation: an open capitellar growth plate, localized flattening or radiolucency of the subchondral bone, and good elbow motion.

Nonoperative treatment mandates complete cessation of elbow use, including activities such as throwing, gymnastics, arm wrestling, push-ups, and weightlifting. The arm may be immobilized but not for more than 3 weeks.[29] Gentle range of motion should be instituted immediately after this period of immobilization if this therapeutic route is chosen. The patient is followed clinically at regular intervals (every 4 to 6 weeks) with serial radiographs. Gentle exercises are performed for the first 3 to 4 months, advancing to strengthening at 4 to 5 months. At that point, an interval throwing program can be initiated based on satisfactory clinical and radiographic findings. Return to sports should be governed by the patient's symptoms, because radiographic changes can persist for years.[38,39]

Rest. Takahara and associates[32,38] observed that repetitive forces on existing OCD lesions led to an increase in lesion size. Cessation of repetitive stress on the elbow should be emphasized to the athlete's parents, trainers, and coaches. They must be reminded that this is a potentially sport-ending injury, with degenerative arthritis as a possible outcome. The incidence of residual capitellar deformity in high-level pitchers is very low,[40] and this suggests that athletes who develop a degenerative elbow from failed OCD treatment do not go on to play high-level baseball. The athletes may be able to do active controlled rest by offloading with a brace and by continuing only those activities that are pain free.

Stage and Management. Because early-stage OCD responds better to nonoperative treatment than advanced stage lesions, identifying the disease promptly can have a significant impact on prognosis. Matsuura and colleagues[41] found that 91% of early-stage OCD but only 53% of advanced-stage OCD improved after nonoperative treatment.

Stability. Stability of the fragment also affects the final outcome. Mitsunaga and coworkers[42] showed that less than 50% of stable fragments went on to become unstable in the long term. However, Takahara and associates[26] demonstrated that fragments that did become unstable had a low rate of healing.

Patient Age and Growth Plate Status. Age has not been correlated with the likelihood of healing.[37,38] However, Mihara and colleagues[25] found a significant correlation between open capitellar growth plates and healing. In their study, 94% of patients with early-stage lesions and with open growth plates healed, whereas the rate for those with closed growth plates was only 71%.

Operative Treatment

Failure of conservative treatment for early-stage, stable lesions (i.e., about 6 weeks of no improvement or 4 to 6 months of persistent symptoms) or diagnosis of an advanced-stage, unstable lesion is an indication for pursuing operative treatment. The ultimate goals of surgery are to eliminate mechanical symptoms and stimulate a healing response. Takahara and coworkers[27] found that patients with unstable lesions that did well with surgery compared with elbow rest had the following common findings at presentation: a closed capitellar growth plate, radiographic fragmentation, and restriction of elbow motion of more than 20 degrees. Patients with closed capitellar physes did significantly better with surgery than with elbow rest. Larger lesions had better results with reconstruction of the articular surface than with simple fragment fixation.

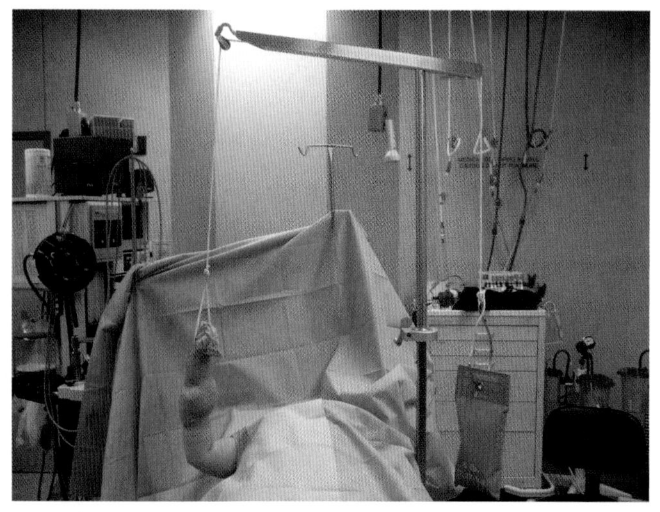

FIGURE 6-13 The patient is positioned supine with the arm held at 90 degrees of shoulder abduction, 90 degrees of elbow flexion, and in neutral rotation by a pulley system (i.e., 5 pounds of traction). *(Courtesy of Neal S. ElAttrache, MD, Kerlan-Jobe Orthopaedic Clinic, Los Angeles, CA.)*

Arthroscopic Positioning. Elbow arthroscopy can proceed with the patient supine, prone, or in the lateral decubitus position. We use the supine position because it facilitates general anesthesia and enables an easy conversion to an open procedure if needed (Fig. 6-13). Structures also may lie in a more anatomic orientation in this position. In the supine position, the elbow is positioned at 90 degrees of elbow flexion and 90 degrees of shoulder abduction with the hand suspended from a pulley and using 5 pounds of traction. The lateral position gives improved posterior compartment access. The prone position also gives good posterior compartment access and does not require traction. General anesthesia provides complete muscle relaxation and obviates the need for a regional block that may prevent diagnosing a postoperative neurologic problem. A tourniquet can be used at the surgeon's discretion.

Arthroscopic Technique. Available instruments include 2.9- and 4.0-mm, 30-degree arthroscopes, burrs, and shavers. The elbow is distended with 30 to 50 mL of saline through the direct lateral portal. Standard arthroscopic portals are created. Diagnostic arthroscopy is performed to look for loose bodies, osteophytes, and chondral damage. The arthroscope usually is in the anteromedial portal, and working instrumentation is in the anterolateral portal. In throwers, a valgus stress test with the elbow flexed to 70 degrees can be performed during the diagnostic portion of the procedure. A 1- to 2-mm opening of the ulnohumeral joint denotes laxity of the UCL, although clinical correlation is mandatory.

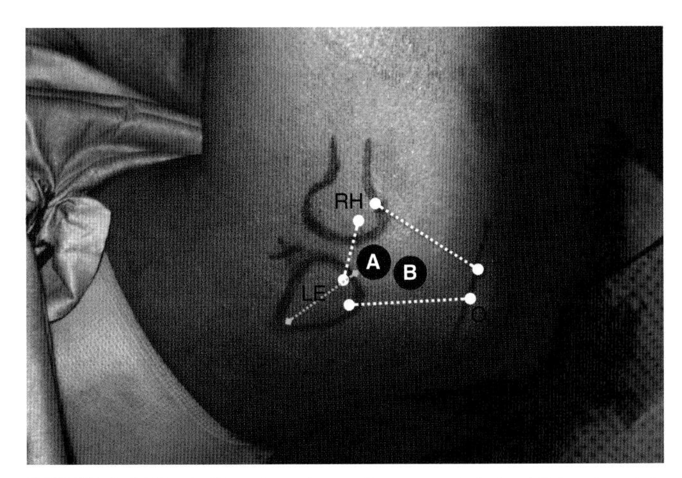

FIGURE 6-14 Dual, direct lateral portals are created. A midlateral portal (A) is created first by triangulating its location using the radial head (RH), lateral epicondyle (LE), and the lateral aspect of the olecranon (O). A working midlateral portal (B) is created adjacent and slightly lateral to the first portal. *(Courtesy of Neal S. ElAttrache, MD, Kerlan-Jobe Orthopaedic Clinic, Los Angeles, CA.)*

After the initial arthroscopic examination is complete, a midlateral portal (i.e., lateral soft spot) is created in line with the lateral epicondylar ridge and entered with the arthroscope. The radial head, capitellum, trochlear notch, and trochlear ridge are best seen through this portal. Care should be taken to avoid the posterior antebrachial cutaneous nerve, which is at risk near this portal. A working portal is created adjacent to and slightly ulnar to the midlateral portal (Fig. 6-14). Carefully placed dual direct lateral portals do not damage lateral ligamentous structures and provide superior exposure to the capitellum.[43] Patients with OCD and lateral compartment symptoms occasionally also have a thickened radiocapitellar plica (Fig. 6-15). If found, the plica should be resected.

The OCD lesion is evaluated and graded. If unstable and loose, the lesion is prepared by removing any loose fragments, shaving loose fragments of cartilage down to subchondral bone and establishing healthy cartilage borders (Fig. 6-16). The size of the lesions is determined by a calibrated probe. If osteochondral grafting is planned, the portals must allow access for the required 4- to 6-mm instruments. At this point, depending on the indication, one of the following procedures can be performed: abrasion chondroplasty, drilling, microfracture, fixation of large fragments, and osteochondral autograft transfer (i.e., OATS or mosaicplasty).

PEARLS & PITFALLS

PEARLS

- An accessory midlateral portal, placed adjacent and slightly ulnar to the standard midlateral portal, can facilitate access to the lesion.
- Resect a thickened radiocapitellar plica if present.
- Determine the size of the lesion after débriding damaged cartilage.
- Lesions involving more than 6 to 7 mm of the lateral column of the capitellum should be treated with osteochondral grafting.
- Microfracture can be used for smaller lesions or for a residual lesion after osteochondral grafting.

PITFALLS

- The size of 6 to 7 mm refers to the amount of lateral buttress involved, not the total diameter of the lesion.
- Any lesion that engages with the radial head in supination or pronation should be treated with osteochondral grafting. Microfracture alone will likely fail in these cases.
- Access to the lesion must be as perpendicular as possible for osteochondral grafting. Use a spinal needle to find the most direct angle.
- Articular step-off after grafting should be less than 1 mm.

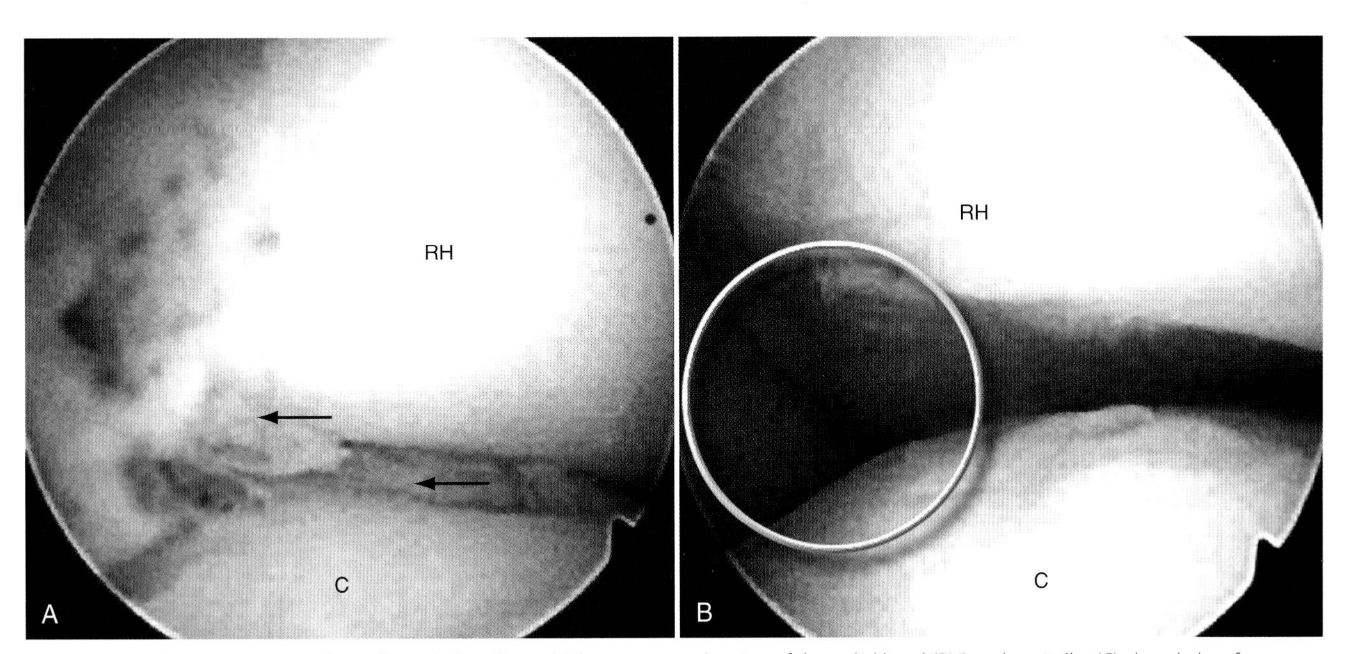

FIGURE 6-15 A, *Arrows* point to the radiocapitellar plica, which may cause abrasion of the radial head (RH) and capitellar (C) chondral surfaces. **B,** The *circle* demarcates the region formerly occupied by plica, which has been resected. *(Courtesy of Neal S. ElAttrache, MD, Kerlan-Jobe Orthopaedic Clinic, Los Angeles, CA.)*

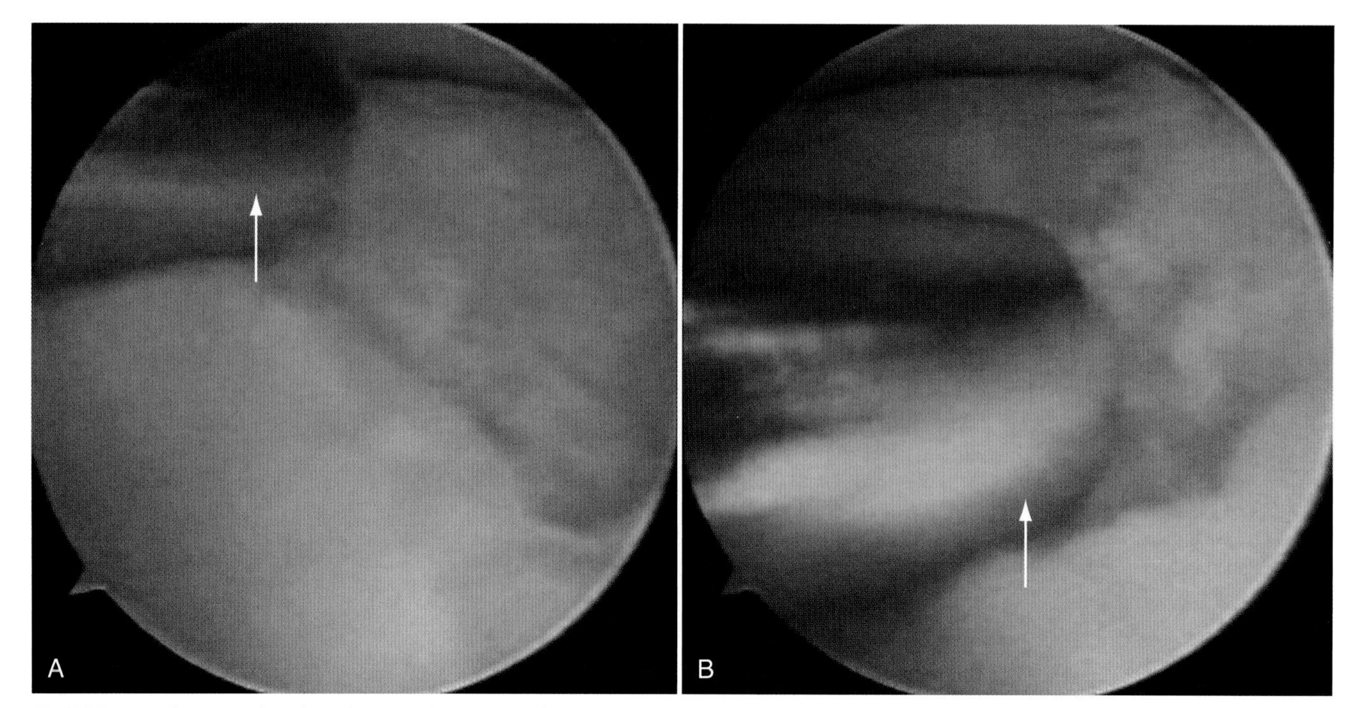

FIGURE 6-16 The osteochondritis dissecans lesion (**A**) is débrided with a shaver *(arrow)* to stable borders (**B**). *(Courtesy of Neal S. ElAttrache, MD, Kerlan-Jobe Orthopaedic Clinic, Los Angeles, CA.)*

Microfracture and Subchondral Drilling. The indications for microfracture or subchondral drilling are similar: early-stage lesions with cartilage fibrillation and fissuring and small, stage 2 lesions with exposed bone that do not significantly involve the lateral column of the capitellum. The lesion bed is prepared as described earlier (see Fig. 6-16). Detached fragments or loose bodies are removed. With the arthroscope in the direct lateral portal, a 0.062-inch Kirschner wire is inserted through the accessory lateral portal and used to perforate the lesion (Fig. 6-17A). Multiple holes are made in the lesion (see Fig. 6-17B). Marrow elements released from the holes induce a fibrocartilage healing response.

If microfracture is elected, a similar approach can be employed using microfracture awls instead of pins. Bojanic and as-

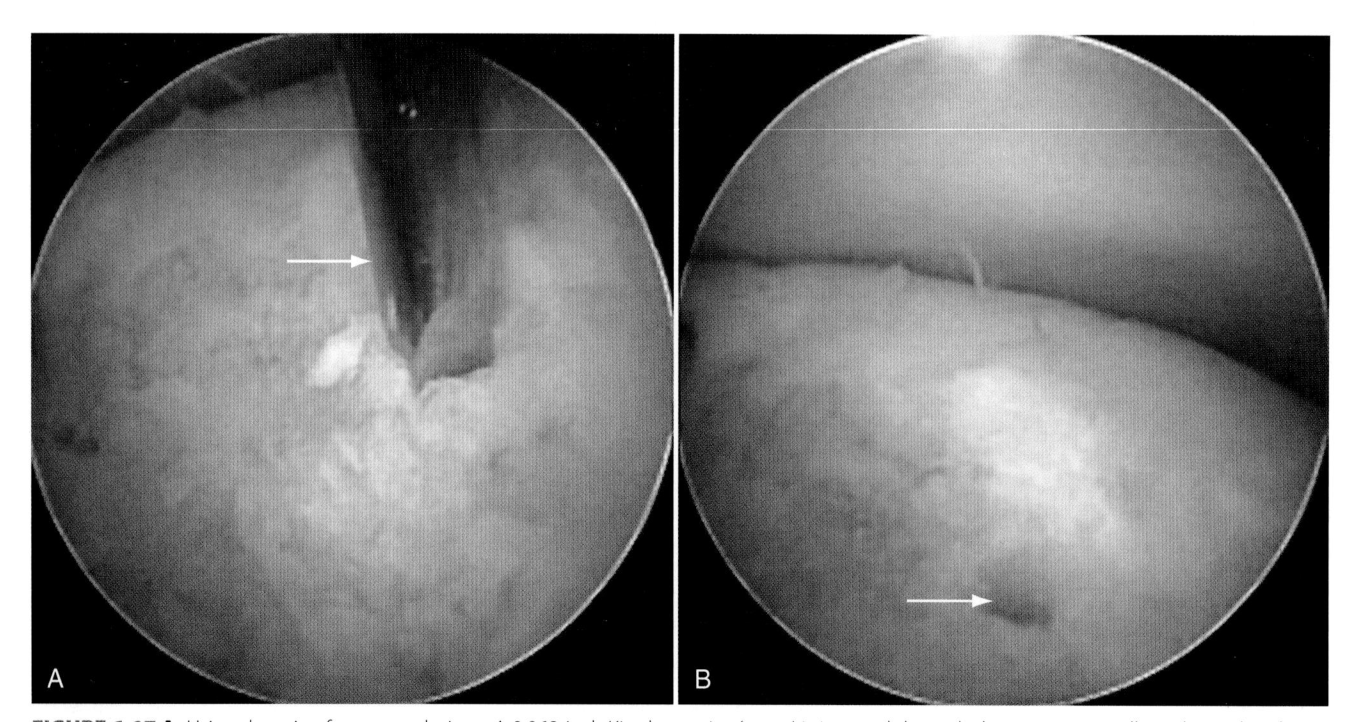

FIGURE 6-17 A, Using the microfracture technique, A 0.062-inch Kirschner wire *(arrow)* is inserted through the accessory midlateral portal and used to perforate the lesion. **B,** Holes *(arrow)* in the lesion allow marrow elements to induce a fibrocartilage healing response. *(Courtesy of Neal S. ElAttrache, MD, Kerlan-Jobe Orthopaedic Clinic, Los Angeles, CA.)*

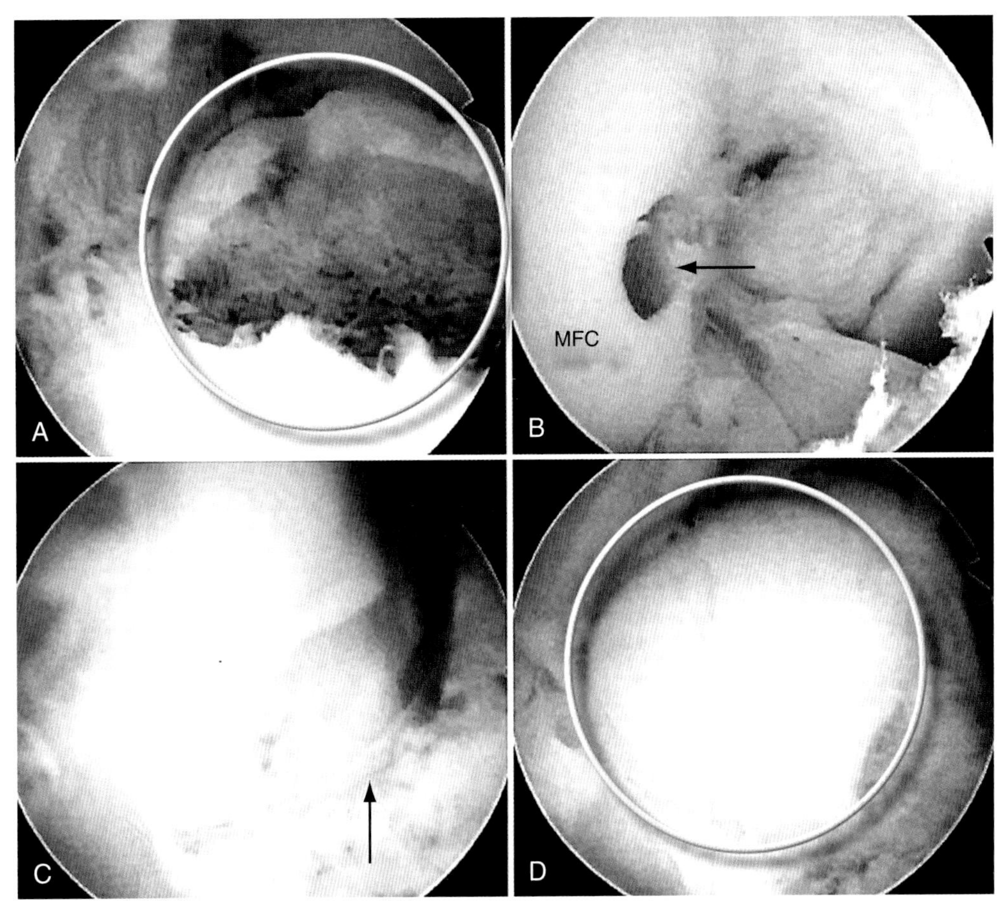

FIGURE 6-18 Osteochondral plug reconstruction is used for a capitellar osteochondritis dissecans defect that extends into the lateral column. **A,** The defect extends into the lateral column of the capitellum *(circle)*. **B,** The *arrow* points to the donor site for an osteochondral plug (i.e., 6 mm in diameter and 1 cm deep), which is harvested from the medial trochlea of the knee on the lateral aspect of the medial femoral condyle (MFC). **C,** The *arrow* points to implantation of an osteochondral plug using an inserter. **D,** The *circle* demarcates the osteochondral plug after implantation. *(Courtesy of Neal S. ElAttrache, MD, Kerlan-Jobe Orthopaedic Clinic, Los Angeles, CA.)*

sociates[44] reported symptom resolution in three adolescent (13- to 15-year-old) gymnasts 5 months after arthroscopic débridement and microfracture of lesions that were about stage 2. They remained symptom free 1 year postoperatively. Using microfracture in 11 athletes with an average age of 15 years, Chappell and ElAttrache[36] obtained excellent results at the 3-year follow-up, with a return to the previous level of activity by all 11. The size of the OCD lesions ranged from 7 × 6 mm to 17 × 15 mm.

Mosaicplasty. Mosaicplasty has been applied in the context of elbow OCD lesions. In this procedure, small, cylindrical osteochondral grafts are obtained from the lateral periphery or trochlear edge of the femoral condyles and transplanted to prepared osteochondral defects.[45] Mosaicplasty is indicated when a large capitellar lesion engages the radial head, as observed while rotating the extended arm during arthroscopy, or when there is significant (>6 to 7 mm) lateral column involvement (Fig. 6-18A). Radial head degeneration and severe deformities of the capitellum are relative contraindications.

A midlateral working portal is used to establish healthy, stable cartilage borders. In the case of a partially detached fragment, the detached area is first evaluated. Often, the detached region is located centrally. In this situation, ElAttrache recommends débriding the partially detached portion by beginning centrally and proceeding laterally toward the lateral column. Débridement proceeds until an area of bony integrity, consisting of an osseous connection between the fragment and the subchondral bone, is encountered, if one is present. The extent of posterolateral column involvement is then determined (see Fig. 6-18A), and an arthroscopic evaluation (i.e., supination and pronation of the extended forearm) of radial head engagement in the defect is performed. If more than 6 to 7 mm of the lateral column is involved or the radial head engages in the defect, osteochondral grafting proceeds. The goal should be to restore a bony buttress to prevent radial head subluxation into the defect, not necessarily replace every millimeter of the lesion.

If osteochondral grafting is elected, the elbow is then flexed 90 to 100 degrees, and a spinal needle is introduced through the anconeus to gauge the feasibility of a perfectly perpendicular approach to the lesion (typically 3 to 4 cm distal to the midlateral portal).[46] The incision is widened to provide access for a 4- to 6-mm diameter plug, so that it is in line with the perpendicular path delineated by the needle. After bluntly spreading the soft tissue to avoid neurovascular structures, the recipient site is then

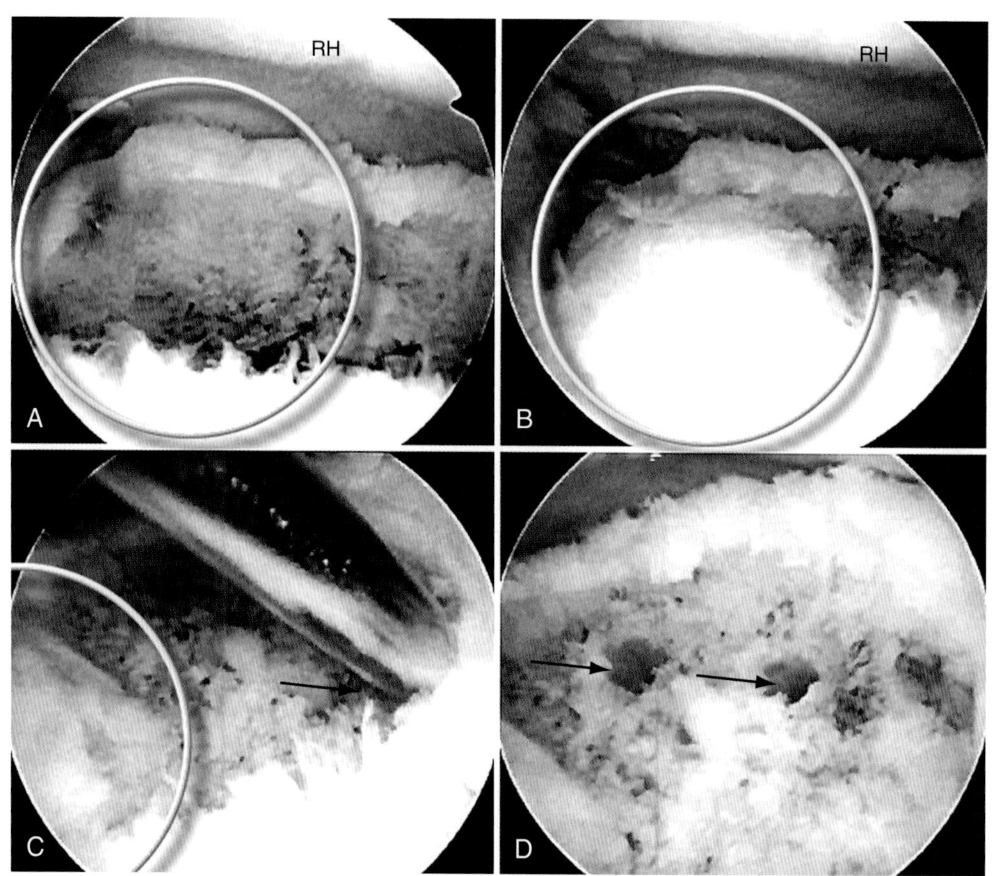

FIGURE 6-19 The lateral buttress of the capitellum is reconstructed with an osteochondral autograft. **A,** The osteochondritis dissecans lesion extends into the lateral column of the capitellum *(circle)*. During the arthroscopic examination (i.e., pronation and supination in extension), the radial head (RH) engages the defect. **B,** The osteochondral plug *(circle)* is placed in the lateral aspect of the capitellum, reconstituting the lateral buttress. The radial head no longer engages. **C,** The *circle* surrounds the osteochondral plug, and the *arrow* points to the remaining lesion, which is addressed with microfracture using a 0.0062-inch Kirschner wire. **D,** After microfracture, holes *(arrows)* allow release of the marrow elements. *(Courtesy of Neal S. ElAttrache, MD, Kerlan-Jobe Orthopaedic Clinic, Los Angeles, CA.)*

drilled as perpendicular to the chondral surface as possible, creating a tunnel of the necessary diameter.

At this point, the knee, which has been prepared, undergoes an arthroscopic harvest of an identically sized chondral plug from the intercondylar notch. The arthroscope is placed into an anterolateral portal. Instrumentation is inserted through an anteromedial portal. Using the harvesting instrumentation, a 6-mm-diameter, 1-cm-deep plug is harvested from the trochlear edge off the medial femoral condyle (see Fig. 6-18B). Usually, one plug is sufficient because of the small size of the capitellar lesions.

The plug is introduced into the recipient site and impacted flush with the surrounding cartilage (see Fig. 6-18C and D). The goal is to reconstitute the lateral buttress (Fig. 6-19A and B) so that the radial head does not subluxate into the defect. The process of osteochondral grafting is repeated until the lateral column integrity is adequately restored. If some corners of the lesion cannot be fully replaced, they are treated with drilling or microfracture (see Fig. 6-19C and D). If autograft is unavailable, allograft or synthetic scaffolding can be used.

With this method, Iwasaki and associates[45] obtained good or excellent results in 7 of 8 teenage baseball players with OCD. Yamamoto and colleagues[48] found that 6 of 9 adolescents with grade 3 and 8 of 9 with grade 4 OCD returned to competitive baseball after an OATS procedure. Chappell and ElAttrache[35] treated five baseball players with OCD using OATS. All five returned to competitive baseball and were still playing 5 years postoperatively. The investigators recommended the procedure, particularly when more than 6 to 7 mm of the lateral column is involved and when the radial head is seen to be engaging the lesion with a careful arthroscopic examination during supination and pronation and during flexion and extension of the forearm.

Fragment Fixation. Fragment fixation has been performed in patients with unstable, partially open OCD lesions.[30] Kuwahata and coworkers[31] described using cancellous bone grafts and a Herbert screw in an open technique. At 32 months of follow-up, they reported pain-free return to sports and an improvement in range of motion of 18 degrees in all seven patients who underwent the procedure. Takahara and colleagues[26,27] described using bone pegs harvested from the lateral olecranon to fix partially attached lesions. This was also done through an open approach. Newer bioabsorbable implants may allow fragment fixation to be performed routinely arthroscopically. Although these surgeons have reported encouraging results, data on fixation are still preliminary. Our recommendation remains excision and drilling or grafting for partially detached lesions.

Postoperative Rehabilitation

Postoperatively, all patients should be protected for 2 to 3 weeks with a long arm cast or hinged brace. Active motion should not be started until bony union is seen on radiographs. Gentle resistance exercises are initiated at 3 months, progressing to greater resistance at 4 months. For throwing athletes, a throwing program is started at 5 months. Full-effort return to sports is usually achieved 6 months after surgery. Athletes who have undergone simple débridement and drilling or microfracture can usually return 1 to 2 months sooner, depending on their rehabilitation progress.

Return to Sport. Return to sports has varied. Historically, gymnasts have had inferior outcomes compared with throwers, perhaps related to significantly increased axial loads borne by their elbows. Jackson and associates[3] treated 10 female gymnasts with removal of loose bodies and drilling after failure of nonoperative treatment. Only one returned to sport. Although surgery for lesions refractory to conservative treatment may improve symptoms, the investigators concluded that a return to gymnastics is unlikely.

Newer technical advancements and lesion-specific management may be improving these outcomes. Bojanic and colleagues[44] found that 3 of 3 female gymnasts successfully returned to their previous level after loose body removal and microfracture. Although Byrd and coworkers[47] suggested that arthroscopic surgery reliably improved symptoms but returned only 4 of 10 adolescent baseball players to competitive baseball, Yamamoto and associates[48] reported a return to competitive levels for 14 of 18 male baseball players with unstable fragments (in situ or displaced) after osteochondral autografting. Chappell and ElAttrache[36] had 8 of 8 male baseball players return to their sport and previous level at an average of 3 years of follow-up after microfracture or osteochondral autografting.

Prognosis. The prognosis for OCD of the capitellum is good when caught early at stage 1. Unfortunately, most cases are diagnosed at stage 2. Although surgery usually alleviates symptoms and allows a return to play, these patients have less favorable long-term outcomes. Longitudinal studies have documented that 50% of radiocapitellar OCD patients eventually develop osteoarthritis.[49] Nevertheless, newer techniques, including osteochondral grafting (mosaicplasty), may mitigate the onset of long-term degenerative joint disease.

Ultimately, prevention is the best treatment. For throwers, pitch counts should be monitored and kept under 600 per week. Players or gymnasts should never pitch or practice when in pain and should never be medicated to play.

CONCLUSIONS

Young throwers and gymnasts are at risk for Panner's disease and OCD as performance demands and expectations escalate. For Panner's disease and early OCD, nonoperative treatment, consisting primarily of strict activity cessation, is the mainstay of management. Advanced OCD lesions require operative intervention, if feasible arthroscopically. The size and location of the lesion and its functional relationship to the radial head help guide management. Prevention, by monitoring and limiting pitch counts and excessive training and by educating athletes, parents, and coaches on early warning signs, provides the most reproducible solution for these potentially sport-ending conditions.

REFERENCES

1. Brown R, Blazina ME, Kerlan RK, et al. Osteochondritis of the capitellum. *J Sports Med.* 1974;2:27-46.
2. Douglas G, Rang M. The role of trauma in the pathogenesis of the osteochondroses. *Clin Orthop Relat Res.* 1981;(158):28-32.
3. Jackson DW, Silvino N, Reiman P. Osteochondritis in the female gymnast's elbow. *Arthroscopy.* 1989;5:129-136.
4. Ruch DS, Poehling GG. Arthroscopic treatment of Panner's disease. *Clin Sports Med.* 1991;10:629-636.
5. Singer KM, Roy SP. Osteochondrosis of the humeral capitellum. *Am J Sports Med.* 1984;12:351-360.
6. Panner H. An affection of the capitulum humeri resembling Calvé-Perthes disease of the hip. *Acta Radiol.* 1927;8:617-618.
7. Duthie RB, Houghton GR. Constitutional aspects of the osteochondroses. *Clin Orthop Relat Res.* 1981;(158):19-27.
8. Yamaguchi K, Sweet FA, Bindra R, et al. The extraosseous and intraosseous arterial anatomy of the adult elbow. *J Bone Joint Surg Am.* 1997;79:1653-1662.
9. Kobayashi K, Burton KJ, Rodner C, et al. Lateral compression injuries in the pediatric elbow: Panner's disease and osteochondritis dissecans of the capitellum. *J Am Acad Orthop Surg.* 2004;12:246-254.
10. Voloshin I, Schena A. Elbow injuries. In: Schepsis AA, Busconi BD, eds. *Sports Medicine.* Philadelphia, PA: Lippincott Williams & Wilkins; 2006.
11. Do T, Herrera-Soto J. Elbow Injuries in children. *Curr Opin Pediatr.* 2003;15:68-73.
12. Morrey BF, Tanaka S, An KN. Valgus stability of the elbow. A definition of primary and secondary constraints. *Clin Orthop Relat Res.* 1991(265):187-195.
13. Kocher MS, Waters PM, Micheli LJ. Upper extremity injuries in the paediatric athlete. *Sports Med.* 2000;30:117-135.
14. Haraldsson S. On osteochondrosis deformas juvenilis capituli humeri including investigation of intra-osseous vasculature in distal humerus. *Acta Orthop Scand Suppl.* 1959;38:1-232.
15. Fa K, E B, U H. Are bone bruises a possible cause of osteochondritis dissecans of the capitellum? A case report and review of the literature. *Arch Orthop Trauma Surg.* 2005;125:545-549.
16. Yang Z, Wang Y, Gilula LA, Yamaguchi K. Microcirculation of the distal humeral epiphyseal cartilage: implications for post-traumatic growth deformities. *J Hand Surg Am.* 1998;23:165-172.
17. Lord J, Winell JJ. Overuse injuries in pediatric athletes. *Curr Opin Pediatr.* 2004;16:47-50.
18. Lyman S, Fleisig GS, Waterbor JW, et al. Longitudinal study of elbow and shoulder pain in youth baseball pitchers. *Med Sci Sports Exerc.* 2001;33:1803-1810.
19. Caine D, Howe W, Ross W, Bergman G. Does repetitive physical loading inhibit radial growth in female gymnasts? *Clin J Sport Med.* 1997;7:302-308.
20. Caine DJ, Nassar L. Gymnastics injuries. *Med Sport Sci.* 2005;48:18-58.
21. Griffith JF, Roebuck DJ, Cheng JC, et al. Acute elbow trauma in children: spectrum of injury revealed by MR imaging not apparent on radiographs. *AJR Am J Roentgenol.* 2001;176:53-60.
22. Peiss J, Adam G, Casser R, et al. Gadopentetate-dimeglumine-enhanced MR imaging of osteonecrosis and osteochondritis dissecans of the elbow: initial experience. *Skeletal Radiol.* 1995;24:17-20.
23. Baumgarten TE, Andrews JR, Satterwhite TE. The arthroscopic classification and treatment of osteochondritis dissecans of the capitellum. *Am J Sports Med.* 1998;26:520-523.
24. DiFelice GS, Meunier M, Paletta GJ. Elbow injury in the adolescent athlete. In: Altchek AJ, ed. *The Athlete's Elbow.* Philadelphia, PA: Lippincott Williams & Wilkins; 2001:231-248.
25. Mihara K, Tsutsui H, Nishinaka N, Yamaguchi K. Nonoperative treatment for osteochondritis dissecans of the capitellum. *Am J Sports Med.* 2009;37:298-304.

26. Takahara M, Mura N, Sasaki J, et al. Classification, treatment, and outcome of osteochondritis dissecans of the humeral capitellum. *J Bone Joint Surg Am.* 2007;89:1205-1214.
27. Takahara M, Mura N, Sasaki J, et al. Classification, treatment, and outcome of osteochondritis dissecans of the humeral capitellum. Surgical technique. *J Bone Joint Surg Am.* 2008;90(suppl 2, pt 1):47-62.
28. Petrie R, Bradley JP. Osteochondritis dissecans of the humeral capitellum. In: De Lee J, Drez D, Miller M, eds. *Orthopaedic Sports Medicine: Principles and Practice.* Philadelphia, PA: WB Saunders; 2003.
29. Bradley JP, Petrie RS. Osteochondritis dissecans of the humeral capitellum. Diagnosis and treatment. *Clin Sports Med.* 2001;20:565-590.
30. Larsen MW, Pietrzak WS, DeLee JC. Fixation of osteochondritis dissecans lesions using poly(l-lactic acid)/poly(glycolic acid) copolymer bioabsorbable screws. Am *J Sports Med.* 2005;33:68-76.
31. Kuwahata Y, Inoue G. Osteochondritis dissecans of the elbow managed by Herbert screw fixation. *Orthopedics.* 1998;21:449-451.
32. Takahara M, Ogino T, Fukushima S, et al. Nonoperative treatment of osteochondritis dissecans of the humeral capitellum. *Am J Sports Med.* 1999;27:728-732.
33. Shimada K, Yoshida T, Nakata K, et al. Reconstruction with an osteochondral autograft for advanced osteochondritis dissecans of the elbow. *Clin Orthop Relat Res.* 2005;(435):140-147.
34. Bradley J, Dandy DJ. Results of drilling osteochondritis dissecans before skeletal maturity. *J Bone Joint Surg Br.* 1989;71:642-644.
35. Chappell JD, ElAttrache NS. Clinical outcome of arthroscopic treatment of OCD lesions of the capitellum. Presented at the meeting of the American Orthopaedic Society for Sports Medicine, 2008; Orlando, FL.
36. Ruch DS, Cory JW, Poehling GG. The arthroscopic management of osteochondritis dissecans of the adolescent elbow. *Arthroscopy.* 1998; 14:797-803.
37. Kim DH, Gambardella RA, ElAttrache NS, et al. Arthroscopic treatment of posterolateral elbow impingement from lateral synovial plicae in throwing athletes and golfers. *Am J Sports Med.* 2006;34:438-444.
38. Takahara M, Ogino T, Sasaki I, et al. Long term outcome of osteochondritis dissecans of the humeral capitellum. *Clin Orthop Relat Res.* 1999;(363):108-115.
39. Takahara M, Shundo M, Kondo M, et al. Early detection of osteochondritis dissecans of the capitellum in young baseball players. Report of three cases. *J Bone Joint Surg Am.* 1998;80:892-897.
40. Mihara K. Osteoarthritic elbow caused by sports [in Japanese]. *Rinsho Seikei Geka.* 2000;35:1243-1249.
41. Matsuura T, Kashiwaguchi S, Iwase T, et al. Conservative treatment for osteochondrosis of the humeral capitellum. *Am J Sports Med.* 2008; 36:868-872.
42. Mitsunaga MM, Adishian DA, Bianco AJ Jr. Osteochondritis dissecans of the capitellum. *J Trauma.* 1982;22:53-55.
43. Davis JT, Idjadi JA, Siskosky MJ, et al. Dual direct lateral portals for treatment of osteochondritis dissecans of the capitellum: an anatomic study. *Arthroscopy.* 2007;23:723-728.
44. Bojanic I, Ivkovic A, Boric I. Arthroscopy and microfracture technique in the treatment of osteochondritis dissecans of the humeral capitellum: report of three adolescent gymnasts. *Knee Surg Sports Traumatol Arthrosc.* 2006;14:491-496.
45. Iwasaki N, Kato H, Ishikawa J, et al. Autologous osteochondral mosaicplasty for capitellar osteochondritis dissecans in teenaged patients. *Am J Sports Med.* 2006;34:1233-1239.
46. Ahmad CS, ElAttrache NS. Treatment of capitellar osteochondritis dissecans. *Tech Shoulder Elbow Surg.* 2006;7:169-174.
47. Byrd JW, Jones KS. Arthroscopic surgery for isolated capitellar osteochondritis dissecans in adolescent baseball players: minimum three-year follow-up. *Am J Sports Med.* 2002;30:474-478.
48. Yamamoto Y, Ishibashi Y, Tsuda E, et al. Osteochondral autograft transplantation for osteochondritis dissecans of the elbow in juvenile baseball players: minimum 2-year follow-up. *Am J Sports Med.* 2006; 34:714-720.
49. Bauer M, Jonsson K, Josefsson PO, Lindén B. Osteochondritis dissecans of the elbow. A long-term follow-up study. *Clin Orthop Relat Res.* 1992;(284):156-160.

CHAPTER

7

The Stiff Elbow: Arthrofibrosis

Mark S. Cohen

The elbow is particularly prone to stiffness following trauma. This propensity has been attributed to several factors, including the congruous nature of the joint, the presence of three articulations within a synovium-lined cavity, and the close relationship of the joint capsule to the intracapsular ligaments and surrounding muscles.[1] Because of these factors, post-traumatic loss of motion is the most common complication after injury to the elbow joint. Arthroscopic techniques can improve motion and function in selected cases that fail conservative measures.

ANATOMY

The capsule of the elbow is normally thin and transparent and has a high degree of elasticity (Fig. 7-1). However, after even relatively minor trauma, the capsule can undergo structural and biochemical alterations, leading to thickening, decreased compliance, and loss of motion.[2] Prolonged immobilization after trauma may be a separate risk factor for the development of stiffness. In addition to capsular changes, the concavities of the humerus above the trochlea—the olecranon and coronoid fossae—can become filled with scar and fibrous tissue after injury. These fossae must be clear to accept the coronoid and olecranon processes at terminal elbow flexion and extension, respectively. In longstanding cases, secondary contracture of the brachialis and triceps muscles can limit motion.

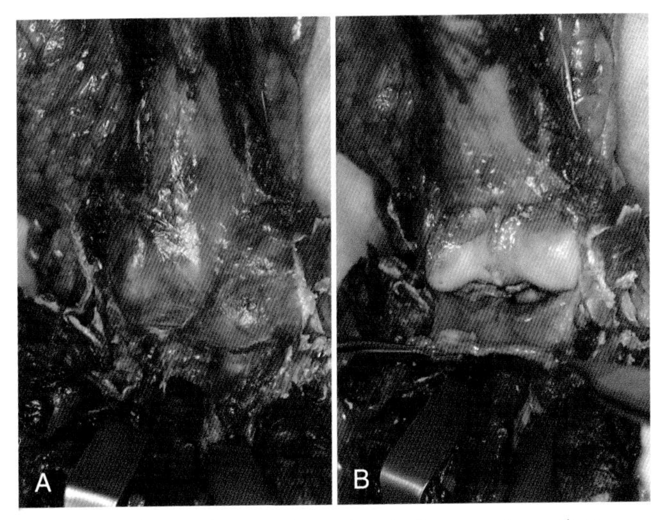

FIGURE 7-1 A, Anterior view of a cadaveric elbow specimen shows that the anterior muscles have been removed, revealing the elbow capsule. Notice that the normal capsule is thin and partially transparent. **B,** The capsule has been released and reflected distally, exposing the articular surfaces. The capsule originates well proximal to the trochlear cartilage along the anterior humerus. After trauma, this thin membrane can become thick and contracted, limiting joint mobility.

PATIENT EVALUATION

History and Physical Examination

Patients with post-traumatic stiffness typically present with limitation of motion. Important aspects of the history include the mechanism of trauma, the initial treatment, and whether they have plateaued in their motion during rehabilitation. Loss of elbow extension is more common than loss of flexion. The examination must include observation of the upper extremity, looking specifically for deformity, swelling, atrophy, and other diagnostic characteristics.

Range-of-motion evaluation should include the hand, wrist, forearm, and elbow. Motion should be compared with the contralateral, uninjured side. Motor and sensory testing is required to evaluate nerve function. In patients with elbow stiffness, it is important to evaluate the ulnar nerve in the cubital tunnel. The nerve lies along the medial elbow joint capsule, and it can become scarred and adherent to the surrounding soft tissues along the medial joint line after trauma. Although some patients may report tingling and numbness in their ulnar digits (especially with elbow flexion), traction neuritis can manifest as medial elbow pain alone. It may even be a factor contributing to elbow stiffness. It is important to document ulnar nerve sensitivity to percussion (i.e., Tinel's sign) and any medial joint pain or neurologic symptoms that occur at maximum elbow flexion.

Diagnostic Imaging

Plain radiographs of the elbow should include frontal, lateral, and oblique projections. In some cases, such as after fracture, advanced imaging can help to define joint congruity. A requirement for elbow release surgery includes a congruous joint with an adequate ulnohumeral joint space, at least centrally. This can typically be determined by plain radiographs. Occasionally, computed tomography is required to document joint congruency, especially in the post-traumatic setting. It also can document that there is no bony impingement or overgrowth in the olecranon and coronoid fossae.

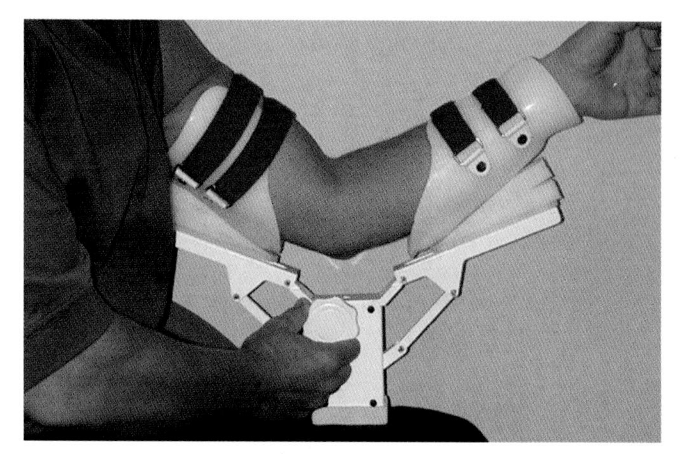

FIGURE 7-2 A patient-adjusted elbow brace is used to improve elbow motion. This device uses the principles of passive, progressive stretch. It is much more effective than dynamic braces and better tolerated, because it requires only short periods of use.

TREATMENT

Indications and Contraindications

Patients are candidates for contracture release if they have restricted elbow motion, with a flexion contracture of at least 25 to 30 degrees or less than 110 to 115 degrees of flexion, or both. Patients typically should have failed a course of supervised therapy, including proper splinting. A congruous ulnohumeral joint is required, as is adequate soft tissue coverage of the operative site. An interval from injury to operation of at least 3 to 4 months allows for resolution of post-traumatic inflammation.

Relative contraindications to arthroscopic elbow release include severe elbow contractures with minimal joint motion, prior ulnar nerve transposition surgery, and the presence of significant heterotopic bone. Surgical release of a contracted elbow is also contraindicated if a patient is deemed unable or unwilling to comply with the extensive program of postoperative therapy. Operative results depend on participation in a structured rehabilitation program. This is especially true for adolescents, who may not be dedicated to improving their elbow motion. If the ulnohumeral joint is incongruous, a simple release of the joint may not lead to improved motion and may worsen pain. Although pain at the extremes is common, patients who are candidates for elbow release surgery typically are pain free within their allowable arc of motion. If advanced post-traumatic arthritis exists in the ulnohumeral articulation, salvage-type procedures are required if surgery is undertaken.[3]

Conservative Management

Patients who are candidates for elbow release surgery should undergo a course of structured rehabilitation. This ensures compliance and helps document that they have reached a plateau in their motion and function. In the past, dynamic splints that apply a constant tension to the soft tissues over long periods (e.g., 23 hours per day) were popular. However, patient-adjusted static braces are more effective for the elbow (Fig. 7-2). These braces use the principle of passive progressive stretch, allowing for stress relaxation of the soft tissues. They are applied for much shorter periods and are better tolerated by patients. Only when conservative measures fail and there remains a significant loss of mobility is surgical intervention considered.

Arthroscopic Technique

Arthroscopic release of a post-traumatic elbow is much more difficult and complicated than arthroscopy for simpler conditions, such as loose bodies. The technique requires experience and knowledge of elbow stiffness surgery and demands advanced skills in elbow arthroscopy. Multiple portals are required, fluid management is essential, and arthroscopic joint retractors are helpful to aid in visualization. This is especially true after capsulectomy, when joint distention is more difficult.

Specialized instruments can be helpful, such as cannulas that do not have any holes near the tip (Fig. 7-3). Because the elbow

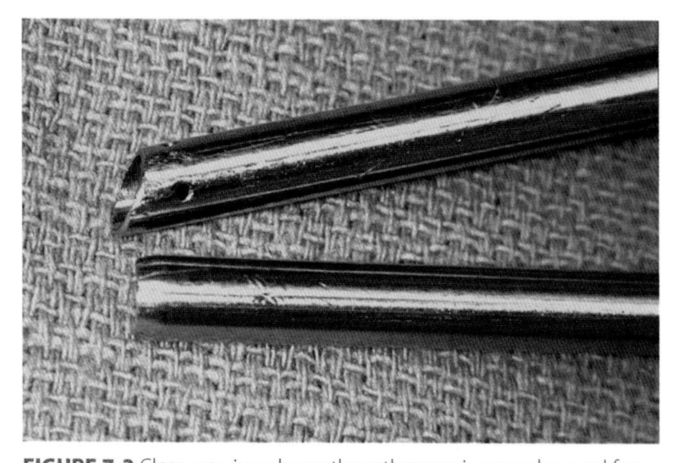

FIGURE 7-3 Close-up view shows the arthroscopic cannulas used for the elbow. Traditional cannulas *(top)* for larger joints commonly have an oblique end with holes near the tip to facilitate flow. Specialized cannulas *(bottom)* for the elbow do not have outflow holes. This is important because the distance between the cannula tip and the joint capsule can be quite small in the elbow, allowing fluid to extravasate inadvertently into the soft tissues. Fluid management is important when performing an elbow release arthroscopically.

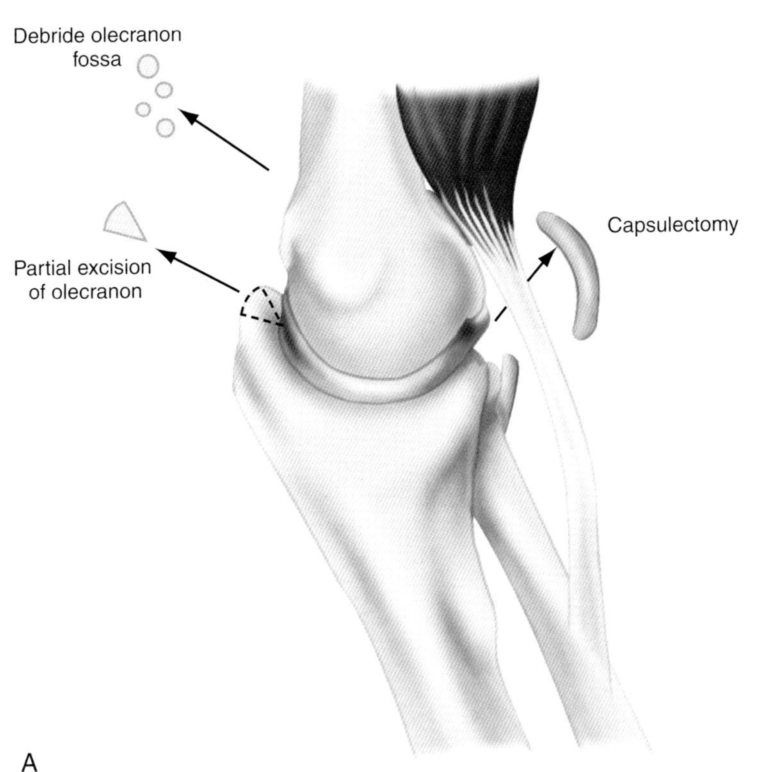

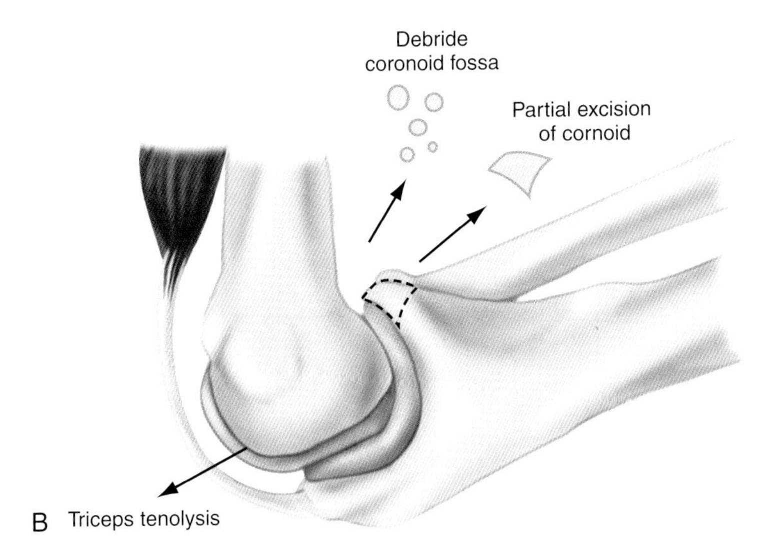

FIGURE 7-4 A, Improving elbow extension in stiff joints requires removal of posterior bony impingement and release of the anterior joint capsule. **B,** Improvement of flexion requires posterior soft tissue release and removal of any soft tissue or bony impingement anteriorly. *(Courtesy of Hill Hastings II, MD, The Indiana Hand Center, Indianapolis, IN.)*

is smaller than, for example, the knee, and has less intra-articular space, standard cannulas can lead to fluid inadvertently entering the soft tissues while visualizing the joint.

In very experienced hands, the procedure appears equivalent to more traditional open methods. However, there is clearly a learning curve, and potential complications must be appreciated. They include nerve injury, excessive fluid extravasation, and iatrogenic chondral damage.[4-9] If there is a question regarding visualization or safely, the surgeon must be prepared to convert the procedure to an open approach.[10-13]

From a purely mechanical standpoint, to improve elbow extension, posterior impingement must be removed between the olecranon tip and the olecranon fossa. Anteriorly, tethering soft tissues, such as the anterior joint capsule and any adhesions between the brachialis and the humerus, must be released (Fig. 7-4). Similarly, to improve elbow flexion, the surgeon must release any soft tissue structures posteriorly that may be tethering the joint. They include the posterior joint capsule and the triceps muscle, which can become adherent to the humerus. The surgeon must remove any bony or soft tissue impingement anteriorly, including any soft tissue overgrowth in the coronoid and radial fossae (see Fig. 7-4). There must be a concavity above the humeral trochlea and capitellum to accept the coronoid centrally and the radial head laterally for full flexion to occur.

Elbow release surgery is typically performed under regional anesthesia with a long-acting block that allows postoperative muscular relaxation and pain control. An indwelling axillary catheter also can be effective. We prefer the prone position for

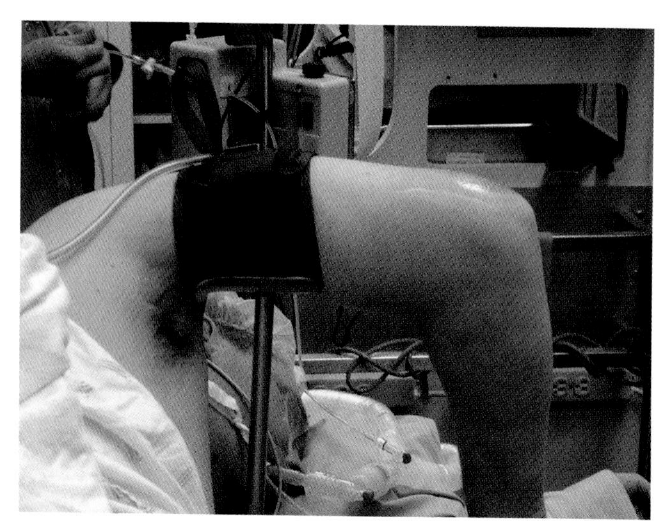

FIGURE 7-5 The patient is in the lateral decubitus position for elbow arthroscopy. Notice the specialized arm holder required to free the joint and allow maximum access in which to work.

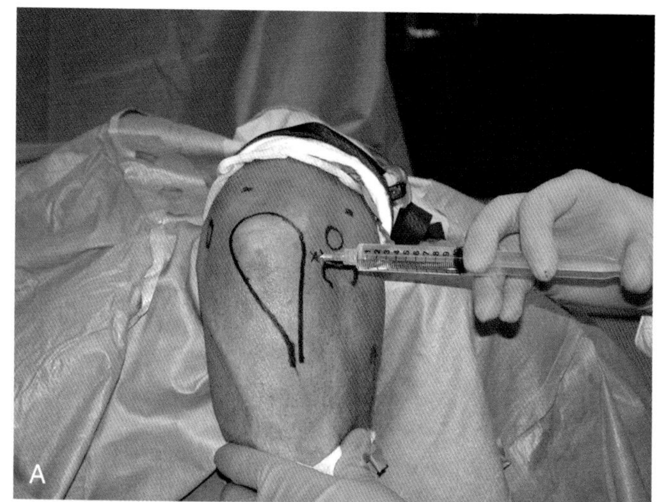

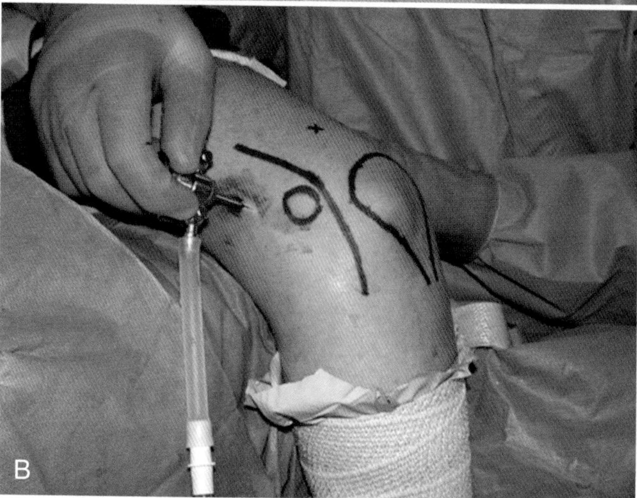

FIGURE 7-6 A, In the intra-operative photograph of elbow arthroscopy, notice how the bony landmarks and portals have been defined. The joint is being insufflated through the soft spot (i.e., direct midlateral portal). **B,** The medial portal has been established for viewing. It is started several centimeters proximal and anterior to the medial epicondyle. Notice how the path of the ulnar nerve has been documented.

elbow arthroscopy. The lateral decubitus position may also be used. It is facilitated by arthroscopic arm-holding devices (Fig. 7-5). The prone position is more complicated from an anesthesia perspective, but it does completely free the shoulder and makes conversion to an open approach easier if required.

Bony landmarks and portals are drawn. It is imperative to document the path of the ulnar nerve through the cubital tunnel. It lies posterior to the palpable intermuscular septum, which separates the triceps from the anterior musculature in the distal arm. Wrapping the hand and forearm in Coban tape helps with fluid extravasation in the dependent position.

The elbow is insufflated with saline introduced through the soft spot (direct midlateral) portal (Fig. 7-6). The anteromedial portal is established by placing a blunt trocar or switching stick along the anterior humerus, aiming toward the radial head laterally. This is started several centimeters proximal and anterior to the medial epicondyle (see Fig. 7-6). In cases of post-traumatic stiffness with a contracted capsule, it can be difficult to enter the joint. Care must be taken to hug the anterior humeral cortex because the capsule can be quite adherent, pushing the instrument into an extra-articular plane. Beneath the capsule and in the joint, the trocar or switching stick can be used to lever anteriorly to help strip the capsule and develop a space in which to work. The anterolateral portal is established using an inside-out technique. It is most effectively placed just anterior to the radiocapitellar articulation (Fig. 7-7).

The anterior joint is cleared of any synovitis or adhesions that are present. Mechanical instruments are typically used, although thermal devices can be quite effective at removing soft tissue. Care is taken to temporarily increase the inflow while using a thermal device to decrease heat generation within the joint. The coronoid fossa is cleared and deepened, removing any fibrous tissue down to the bony floor. This is also true of the radial fossa just above the capitellum. The radial fossa must be free to accept the radial head during elbow flexion. The arthroscope and the working instruments must be switched rapidly and effectively from medial to lateral positions during this work (see Fig. 7-7).

After the fossae are cleared and any necessary bony work is completed, the anterior capsule is addressed. It is first well defined and then partially or completely resected. The radial (posterior interosseous) nerve lives just anterior to the joint capsule and near the midline of the radiocapitellar joint. Removing the capsule proximal to the trochlea is much safer than distal excision. Any capsule work done at the level of the joint line must be done with great care. Retractors can be helpful to aid visualization. They can obviate the need for increased fluid pressure to distend the joint for visualization and are helpful for fluid management. After part of the capsule is released, fluid distention is less effective, and fluid extravasation into the periarticular soft tissues more readily occurs. This must be limited, because it is much more difficult to work within the elbow after a significant amount of fluid has extravasated. The capsule must be released all the way out to the supracondylar ridges to achieve a complete release (see Fig. 7-7).

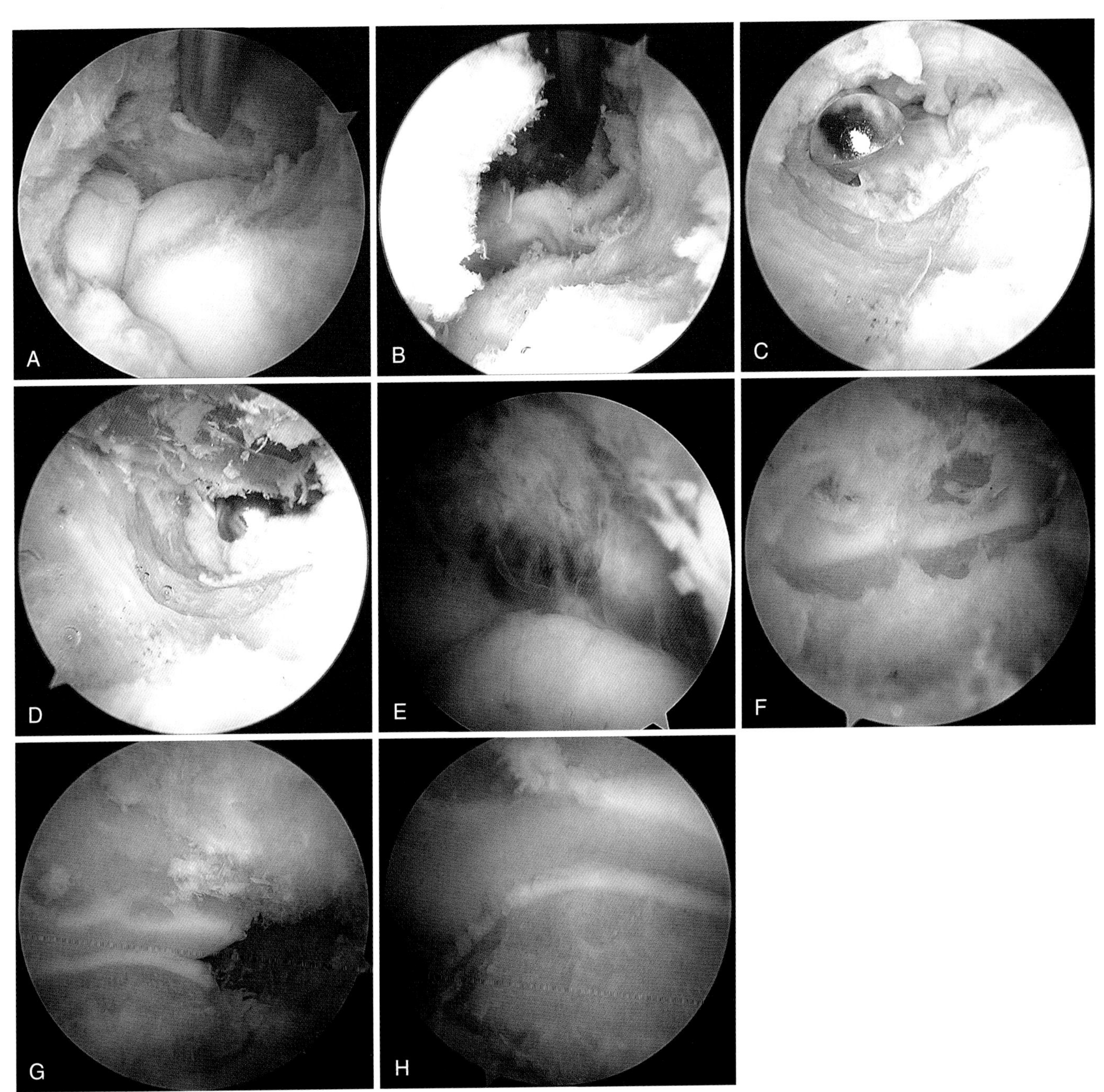

FIGURE 7-7 A, The initial intraoperative view of the anterior elbow joint in a patient with a post-traumatic joint contracture is seen from the anteromedial portal. The anterolateral portal has been established using an inside-out technique. It is positioned just anterior to the radiocapitellar joint. **B,** The coronoid and radial fossa have been débrided above the articular surface, creating a concavity. This removes anything that would cause impingement in flexion. **C,** The anterior concavity above the trochlea is viewed from the lateral side. **D,** The anterior capsule has been resected, revealing the undersurface of the brachialis muscle. Notice how the capsular release has been done at the level of the humerus above the joint line. The radial nerve is located just anterior to the capsule at the level of the radiocapitellar joint. Capsular removal more distally places this structure at risk. **E,** In the initial view of the posterior joint, the tip of the olecranon is seen, and the olecranon fossa is filled with fibrous tissue and scar. **F,** After posterior débridement, the olecranon fossa is clear, and the olecranon tip has been débrided to remove any posterior impingement that might limit extension. Lateral (**G**) and medial (**H**) views of the olecranon and gutters show the shaping of the olecranon tip to remove any impinging osteophytes.

After the anterior joint work is completed, attention is focused posteriorly. We typically leave a cannula in the anterior joint while working in the back. This helps to maintain outflow during the procedure. With the elbow extended maximally to protect the posterior trochlea, a blunt elevator is used to blindly strip and clear the olecranon fossa and elevate the posterior joint capsule. Identification of the concavity of the fossa should be possible using tactile feedback. The arthroscope is introduced into the posterior or the posterolateral portal. The latter is started approximately 1 cm proximal to the midpoint between a line drawn from the olecranon tip to the lateral epicondyle. The posterior portal is established

3 to 4 cm above the olecranon tip in the midline. The camera is then turned to look in a distal direction. In cases of post-traumatic stiffness, soft tissue often must be débrided in the olecranon fossa to allow for full visualization of the articular surfaces (see Fig. 7-7). Proximal retractors are also very helpful in the posterior joint. The posterior capsule is freed from the humerus proximally, and it can be partially resected. Typically, this capsule is less hypertrophic than the anterior capsule. Establishing a soft spot portal (direct midlateral) may facilitate visualization and help to free the posterolateral gutter. Any soft tissue or bony overgrowth at the tip of the olecranon is removed, including the medial and lateral corners (see Fig. 7-7).

The ulnar nerve requires special mention. It lies along the medial joint capsule in the cubital tunnel, and it can become adherent to the surrounding soft tissues after trauma. We recommend that the ulnar nerve be released in all cases when nerve symptoms are present or when nerve tension signs exist (i.e., positive Tinel's sign or positive elbow flexion test). This is also recommended when significant elbow extension contracture exists, for which acute improvement in joint flexion may precipitate ulnar nerve symptoms. Although the exact degree of flexion loss has not been determined, it is recommended that ulnar nerve release be considered when preoperative elbow flexion is limited below 90 to 110 degrees.

Because of the location of the ulnar nerve relative to the capsule, any mechanical or thermal instruments used along the medial ulnohumeral joint and medial gutter can place the nerve at risk. Suction makes the mechanical burrs and shavers more dangerous. Even when releasing the elbow joint arthroscopically, we prefer to address the ulnar nerve through a limited open approach. When there is significant loss of elbow flexion, the posteromedial capsule (which lies beneath the nerve in the cubital tunnel) may also need to be released. The nerve is approached through a limited incision centered on the cubital tunnel. After it is decompressed and isolated, the posteromedial joint capsule can be safely addressed. Release of this capsule can be done arthroscopically in experienced hands, but it can place the nerve at risk. If a limited open approach is chosen for the nerve, it is much easier to perform before the arthroscopic joint release. Swelling of the soft tissues can obliterate tissue planes, making nerve dissection more difficult. In post-traumatic cases with significant loss of flexion, we routinely dissect out the ulnar nerve before starting the arthroscopic procedure.

After the joint release is completed, care is taken to document recovery of elbow motion intra-operatively. Although soft tissue swelling can make this difficult, it is important to achieve terminal flexion and extension before leaving the operating room. If the ulnar nerve was decompressed, it can be left in the cubital tunnel (i.e., in situ decompression) or formally transposed anteriorly, depending on the surgeon's preference. A drain can be placed if significant bleeding is anticipated. The elbow is wrapped in a soft, compressive dressing. Cutting out some of the dressing anteriorly (in the antecubital fossa) allows greater mobility postoperatively.

PEARLS & PITFALLS

1. Nerve injury must be avoided. Know where nerves reside, and avoid suction near nerves. The radial nerve is most vulnerable deep to the capsule at the midline of the radiocapitellar joint. The ulnar nerve is at risk in the posteromedial gutter. Avoid penetrating the brachialis.
2. Arthroscopic elbow release requires experience and knowledge of elbow stiffness surgery and advanced skills in elbow arthroscopy. This is especially true for more complex contractures.
3. In post-traumatic contracture, the anterior joint capsule can become thick and adherent, limiting the ability to enter the joint and obtain visualization. Inside the joint, the capsule can be manually torn and released to facilitate the arthroscopic procedure.
4. Fluid management is key when releasing a stiff elbow arthroscopically. High-pressure inflow to distend the joint should be avoided, and retractors can aid in visualization, particularly after the capsule has been resected. Soft tissue swelling must be monitored throughout the operation.
5. If visualization of intra-articular structures becomes compromised, most commonly due to fluid extravasation, the surgeon must be prepared to convert the procedure to an open approach. Knowledge about the open approach for elbow release is required when performing these procedures arthroscopically.
6. The ulnar nerve can become adherent to surrounding soft tissues aft er trauma. Nerve tension can contribute to elbow contracture, specifically the loss of elbow flexion. Ulnar nerve tension can complicate rehabilitation after elbow joint release surgery (i.e., tardy ulnar nerve palsy), especially in individuals who lack significant flexion preoperatively.

Postoperative Rehabilitation

Several rehabilitation programs may be effective after elbow release surgery. We typically use continuous passive motion that is begun immediately in the recovery room (Fig. 7-8). It is used the next morning to help maintain the motion gained at surgery. Formal

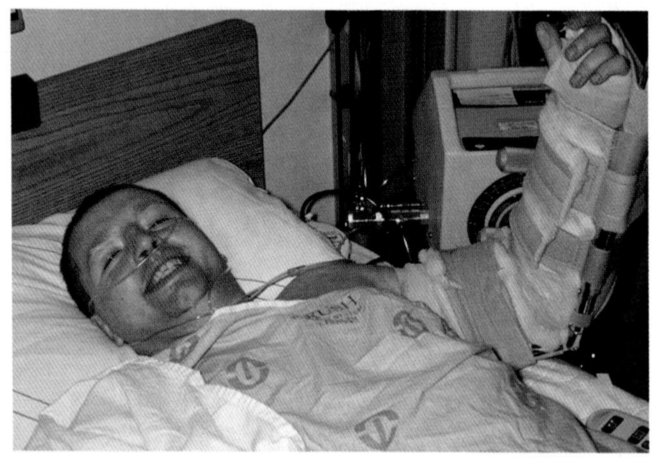

FIGURE 7-8 The patient is in a continuous passive motion machine after arthroscopic elbow release. At our institution, we use a long-acting regional block that allows immediate use of this modality.

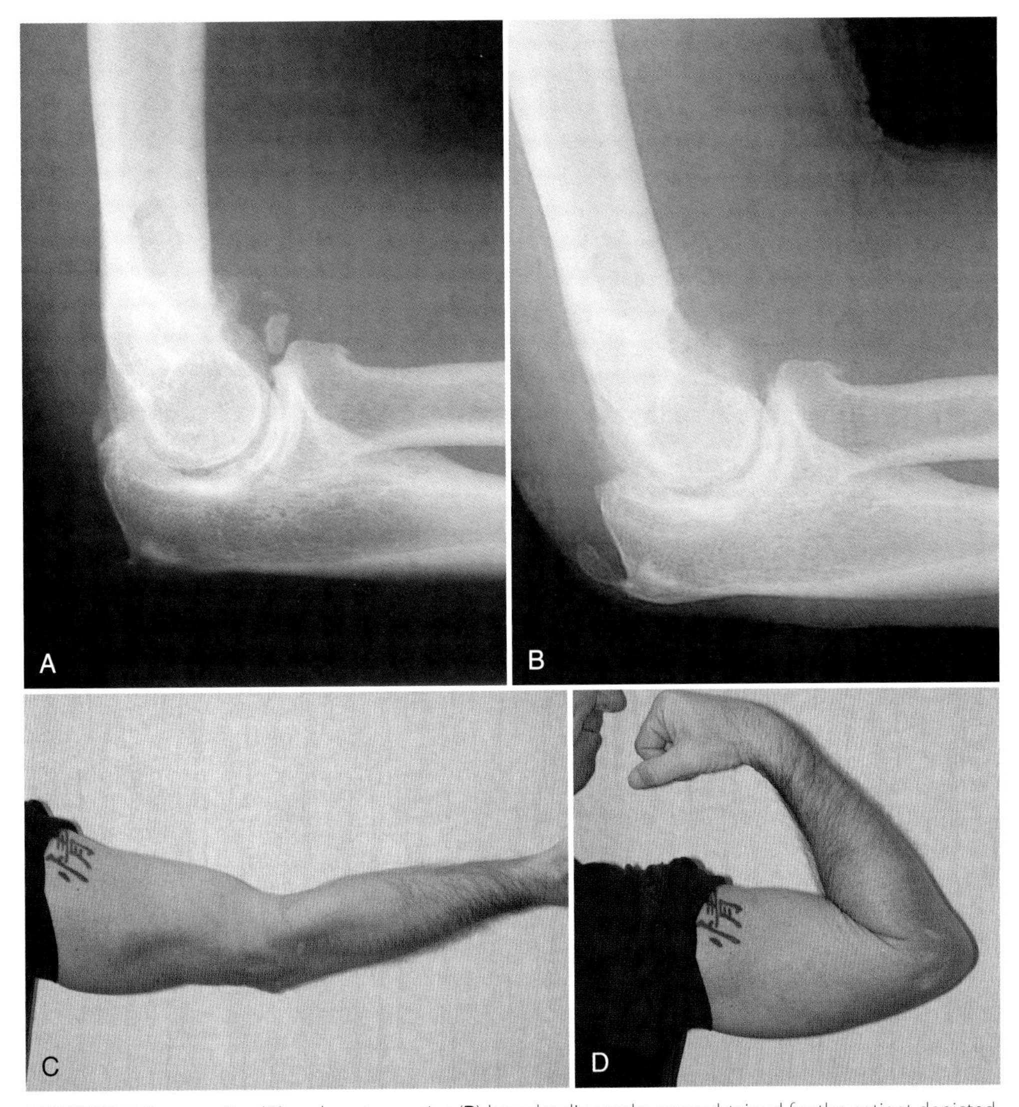

FIGURE 7-9 Preoperative (**A**) and postoperative (**B**) lateral radiographs were obtained for the patient depicted in Figure 7-7. He developed a post-traumatic elbow contracture, with preoperative motion measuring approximately 45 to 105 degrees. Notice the deepening of the anterior fossa above the trochlea and capitellum and removal of the posterior olecranon spur. Clinical photographs taken 1 week after arthroscopic elbow release show early improvement in elbow extension (**C**) and flexion (**D**).

therapy is commonly begun on postoperative day 1. The dressing is removed, and edema-control modalities (e.g., edema sleeve, Ace wrap) are used to limit swelling. Active and gentle passive elbow motion is combined with intermittent continuous passive motion. Static progressive elbow bracing is begun early in the postoperative period. Flexion and extension are alternated based on the preoperative deficit and the early progress of the elbow.

A nonsteroidal anti-inflammatory agent (e.g., Indocin) is commonly prescribed as a prophylaxis against heterotopic ossification for several weeks postoperatively. This also helps to limit inflammation of the joint and soft tissues during rehabilitation. The physician must follow these patients closely. Although most ultimate elbow motion is gained during the first 6 to 8 weeks, patients can continue to make gains in terminal flexion and extension for several months postoperatively. With proper patient selection, results can be gratifying, with predictable recovery of a functional arc of elbow motion and pain relief (Fig. 7-9).[14-18]

CONCLUSIONS

Arthroscopic release of the stiff elbow requires a high degree of surgical skill and knowledge of the bony and soft tissue anatomy of the elbow. In properly selected patient, this procedure can have gratifying results that are similar to those of traditional open procedures. Care must be taken to ensure proper visualization, management of fluid extravasation, and protection of important neurovascular structures. If any doubt exists, the surgeon must be prepared to convert to an open procedure.

REFERENCES

1. Modabber MR, Jupiter JB. Current concepts review: reconstruction for post-traumatic conditions of the elbow joint. *J Bone Joint Surg Am*. 1995;77A:1431-1446.
2. Cohen MS, Schimel DR, Masuda K, et al. Structural and biochemical evaluation of the elbow capsule following trauma. *J Shoulder Elbow Surg*. 2007;16:484-490.
3. Jupiter JB, O'Driscoll SW, Cohen MS. The assessment and management of the stiff elbow. *Instr Course Lect*. 2003;52:93-112.
4. Haapaniemi T, Berggren M, Adolfsson L. Complete transection of the median and radial nerves during arthroscopic release of post-traumatic elbow contracture. *Arthroscopy*. 1999;15:784-787.
5. Kelberine F, Landreau P, Cazal J. Arthroscopic management of the stiff elbow. *Chir Main*. 2006;25(suppl 1):S108-S113.
6. Kelly EW, Morrey BF, O'Driscoll SW. Complications of elbow arthroscopy. *J Bone Joint Surg Am*. 2001;83A:25-34.
7. Lynch GJ, Meyers JF, Whipple TL, Caspari RB. Neurovascular anatomy and elbow arthroscopy: inherent risks. *Arthroscopy*. 1986;2:190-197.
8. Park JY, Cho CH, Choi JH, et al. Radial nerve palsy after arthroscopic anterior capsular release for degenerative elbow contracture. *Arthroscopy*. 2007;23:1360.e1-1360.e3.
9. Ruch DS, Poehling GG. Anterior interosseus injury following elbow arthroscopy. *Arthroscopy*. 1997;13:756-758.
10. Cohen MS. Open capsular release for soft-tissue contracture of the elbow. In: Yamaguchi K, King GJW, McKee MD, O'Driscoll SW, eds. *Advanced Reconstruction: Elbow*. Rosemont, IL: American Academy of Orthopaedic Surgeons; 2007:195-204.
11. Cohen MS, Hastings H. Capsular release for contracture of the elbow: operative technique and functional results, *Orthop Clin North Am*. 1999; 30:133-139.
12. Cohen MS, Hastings H. Post-traumatic contracture of the elbow: operative release using a lateral collateral sparing approach. *J Bone Joint Surg Br*. 1998;80B:805-812.
13. Mansat P, Morrey BF. The column procedure: a limited lateral approach for extrinsic contracture of the elbow. *J Bone Joint Surg Am*. 1998; 80A:1603-1615.
14. Ball CM, Meunier M, Galatz LM, et al. Arthroscopic treatment of post-traumatic elbow contracture. *J Shoulder Elbow Surg*. 2002;11:624-629.
15. Kelly EW, Bryce R, Coghlan J, Bell W. Arthroscopic debridement without radial head excision of the osteoarthritis elbow. *Arthroscopy*. 2007; 23:151-156.
16. Nguyen D, Proper SI, MacDermid JC, et al. Functional outcomes of arthroscopic capsular release of the elbow. *Arthroscopy*. 2006;22:842-849.
17. Salini V, Palmieri D, Colucci C, et al. Arthroscopic treatment of post-traumatic elbow stiffness. *J Sports Med Phys Fitness*. 2006;46:99-103.
18. Savoie FH, Nunley PD, Field LD, Savoie FH. Arthroscopic management of the arthritic elbow: indications, technique, and results. *J Shoulder Elbow Surg*. 1999;8:214-219.

CHAPTER

8

The Stiff Elbow: Degenerative Joint Disease

Julie E. Adams • Scott P. Steinmann

Degenerative arthritis of the elbow remains uncommon, but when symptomatic, it can cause substantial disability.[1-4] Post-traumatic arthritis and osteoarthritis of the elbow have been treated with nonoperative means or open procedures. However, arthroscopic series have documented outcomes similar to those of open procedures and with acceptable complication rates.[5-9]

ANATOMY

Pathologic processes include the loss of cartilage and fragmentation with reactive bone formation in the form of osteophytes and loose bodies, which contribute to impingement and joint contracture as the capsule becomes abnormally thickened and fibrotic.[3,11] Bony osteophytes commonly occur on the tip of the olecranon and coronoid process. Significant osteophytes also can occur along the medial aspect of the coronoid and may not be obvious on standard plain radiographs. Similarly, osteophytes may be found at the radial head fossa and the posterior aspect of the capitellum. The osteophytes in this area are difficult to visualize at time of surgery but can be seen while viewing from the posterolateral gutter when performing the posterior portion of the procedure, and they can be removed through a working portal at the soft spot. These bony spurs contribute to the loss of extension, and osteophytes at the radial head fossa contribute to a lack of flexion by impingement.

PATIENT EVALUATION

History and Physical Examination

Primary osteoarthritis of the elbow is uncommon, but when it occurs, it tends to manifest in manual laborers, athletes, or crutch and wheelchair ambulators.[1-4,10] Post-traumatic stiffness and arthrosis can be problematic after fractures or dislocations of the elbow.

Symptoms include loss of motion, mechanical catching and locking, and pain.[4,10] Pain often is felt at the end arc of motion, and it is more likely to be improved by arthroscopic means than pain experienced throughout the arc of motion, which typically indicates severe joint changes.

Patients frequently have signs and symptoms of ulnar nerve compression at the elbow, and they should be examined for and queried about dysesthesias or paresthesias and weakness in the ulnar nerve distribution.[4,12] Electrical studies can document the severity of cubital tunnel compression, but they may not be necessary. Nerve compression occurs after progressive contracture of the elbow and scarring at the cubital tunnel. Postoperatively, if a large restoration of motion is achieved but the ulnar nerve is not addressed, symptomatic ulnar neuritis or neuropathy can occur as the nerve is stretched further.

Diagnostic Imaging

Plain radiographs should be obtained, and they typically demonstrate hypertrophic bony spurs and loose bodies (Fig. 8-1). The bone usually is sclerotic rather than osteopenic, as seen in rheumatoid arthritis. Computed tomography (CT) is useful, particularly with three-dimensional reconstructions, to map areas of interest that will require recontouring (Fig. 8-2). Using three-dimensional CT as a preoperative planning tool allows the surgeon to gain an increased appreciation of the osteophytic areas that require attention to improve range of motion. During the procedure, these areas may be overlooked without this three-dimensional map of normal and abnormal anatomy.

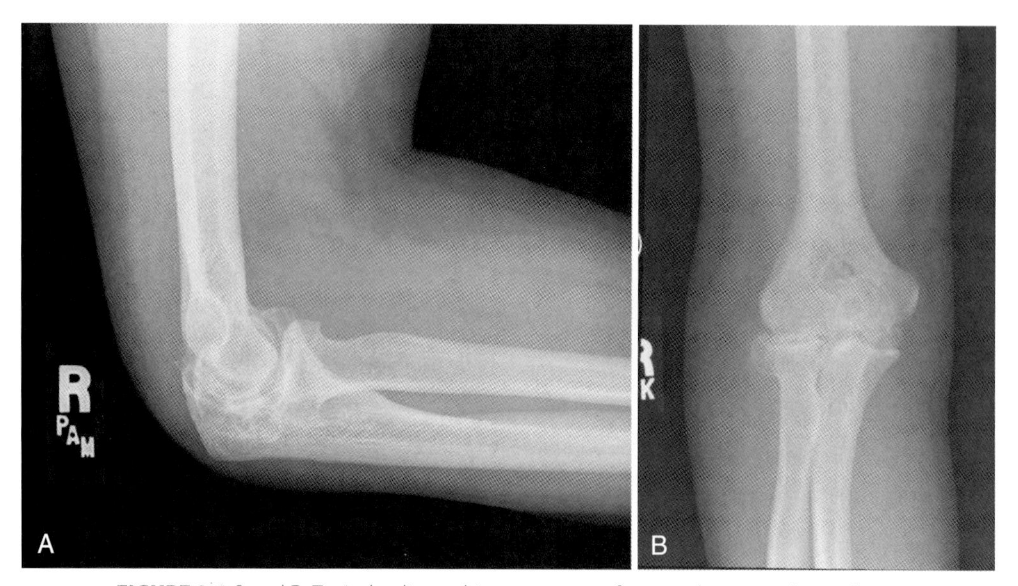

FIGURE 8-1 A and **B,** Typical radiographic appearance of a severely osteoarthritic elbow.

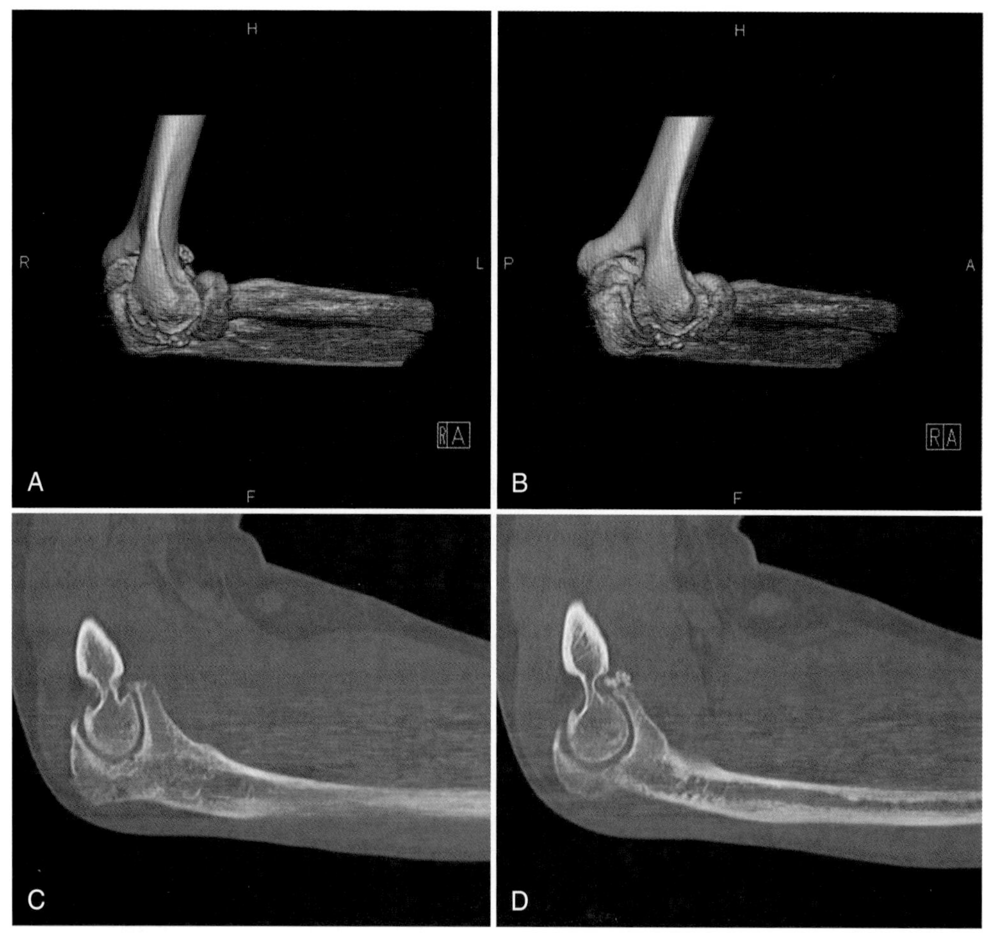

FIGURE 8-2 A–D, Computed tomography can provide a three-dimensional view of the pathology.

TREATMENT

Indications and Contraindications

Pain at the end arc of motion, symptomatic loose bodies with mechanical symptoms, and joint contracture that limits activity are indications for arthroscopic débridement or capsular release, or both. Pain in the middle arc range of motion may indicate severe joint changes and fail to respond to arthroscopic treatment. A subluxating ulnar nerve or a prior subcutaneous ulnar nerve transposition is not necessarily a contraindication to arthroscopy of the elbow; however, an intermuscular or submuscular transposition is often considered a relative contraindication unless the precise course of the nerve can be ascertained by visual inspection, palpation, or ultrasonography.

Conservative Management and Alternatives to Arthroscopy

Nonoperative treatment options such as nonsteroidal anti-inflammatory medications, corticosteroid injections, and activity modifications should be exhausted before considering surgery.[13]

Alternatives to arthroscopic procedures include open procedures such as resection arthroplasty of the ulnohumeral joint and open débridement such as the Outerbridge-Kashiwagi procedure. The medial "over-the-top" contracture release and the lateral column procedures allow access to the joint for excision of the thickened and abnormal capsule, with débridement of bony osteophytes.[14,15] Total elbow arthroplasty reliably relieves pain and motion, but early aseptic loosening is an unsolved problem, especially in young and active patients. Joint fusion can relieve pain, but it has dramatic implications on function and is sometimes difficult to achieve.[7]

Multiple open débridement procedures have been used with success and an acceptable complication rate, but open procedures remain the gold standard by which arthroscopic procedures are assessed.[3,4,10,12,15-21] Arthroscopic débridement and capsular release is an evolving technique that addresses underlying pathologic processes and provides outcomes similar to those of open procedures, and it is associated with an acceptable complication rate.[5,9,13,22-26]

Arthroscopic Technique

The arthroscopic technique and setup have been described previously.[1,19,20] General endotracheal anesthesia is induced, and the patient is placed in the lateral decubitus position. Various positions have been described for elbow arthroscopy, but we prefer the lateral decubitus position as described here.

A conforming bean bag is useful to position and secure the patient. The operative arm is secured in a dedicated arm holder with the elbow higher than the shoulder and the forearm hanging freely. This allows unrestricted access to the elbow. A nonsterile tourniquet may be applied, or a sterile one is used after the arm is prepared and draped in the usual fashion (Fig. 8-3).

The standard equipment used for elbow arthroscopy includes the 4-mm, 30-degree arthroscope; arthroscopic cannulas; retractors; and graspers. Retractors such a Howarth elevator and large, blunt Steinmann pins can improve the visual field. Special-use retractors have become available from various manufacturers. The standard arthroscopic shaver and burr are used. The suction tubing is placed to gravity only, because active suction by vacuum can injure structures that may be pulled inadvertently into the shaver.

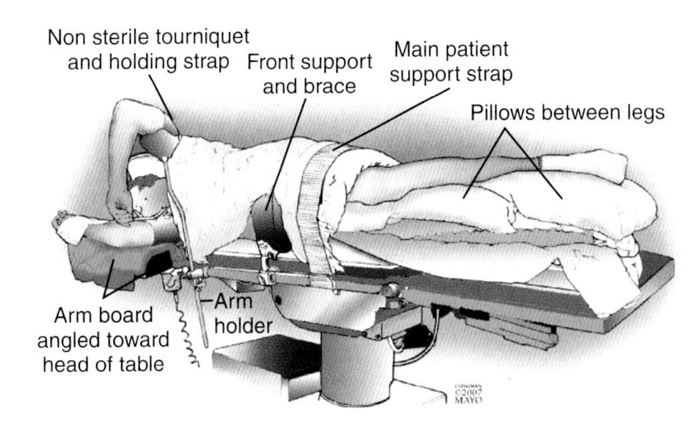

FIGURE 8-3 Operative setup.

Before insufflation, portal sites and landmarks should be marked, because after the operation proceeds, bony landmarks may become difficult to palpate because of soft tissue fluid extravasation. The radial head, medial and lateral epicondyles, capitellum, and olecranon are marked, as is the location of the ulnar nerve (Fig. 8-4).

It is essential to determine the position of the ulnar nerve and to rule out a subluxating ulnar nerve before starting the procedure. If there is any question about the nerve's location, ultrasonography in the operating room can confirm the location. Alternatively, a small incision may be made to identify and protect the nerve.

The joint is distended with 20 to 30 mL of saline introduced by means of an 18-gauge needle through the soft spot, which is the center of a triangle formed by the olecranon process, lateral epicondyle, and radial head. Fluid distention makes portal establishment easier and safer.

Portal sites are made by incising only the skin with the blade. Blunt dissection with a hemostat allows access to the capsule and joint. Capsular entry and joint location are confirmed by a sudden egress of fluid. The blunt trocar and sleeve are placed into the joint, and the arthroscope is then placed into the sleeve.

The order in which portal sites are established depends on surgeon's preference and comfort level. We prefer the sequence as described subsequently. The technique and order of the procedure depend on the indications. If the patient lacks flexion, the posterior joint must be addressed. If extension is limited, the anterior joint must be released and débrided.

Anterior Portals

The proximal anterolateral and proximal anteromedial portals typically are used first and are considered safer than the distal anterolateral and anteromedial portals. The anterolateral (see Fig. 8-4A) portal is established first, with care taken to avoid and protect the radial nerve. This portal is established just anterior and distal to the radiocapitellar joint.

The anteromedial portal (see Fig. 8-4B) can be established using an inside-out technique with direct visualization from the anterolateral portal. The arthroscope is withdrawn from the anterolateral portal while the canula is kept in place. The blunt trocar is replaced in the canula and then pushed directly across the joint until it tents the skin overlying the medial side of the elbow. The skin is then incised over this region, and the trocar is pushed through the remaining soft tissue. A cannula may be

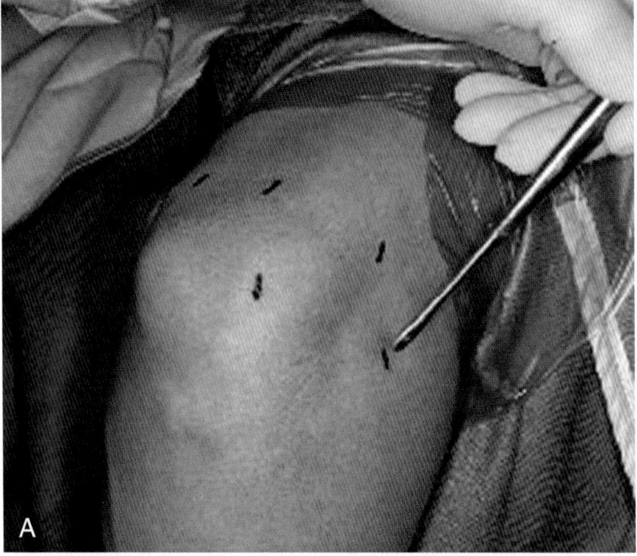

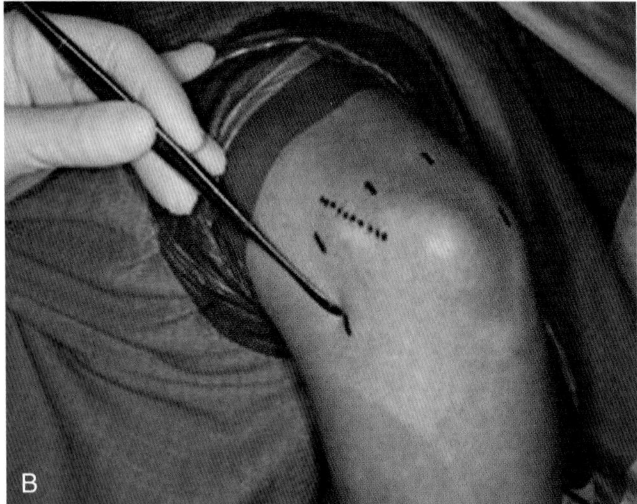

FIGURE 8-4 Portals sites and landmarks are marked before starting the procedure. **A,** On the lateral side, the elevator marks the anterolateral portal. **B,** On the medial side, the elevator marks the anteromedial portal.

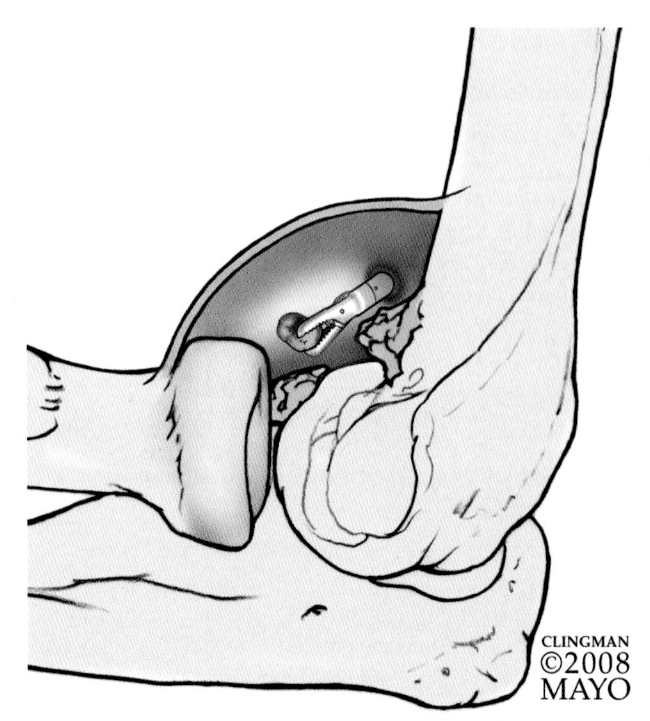

FIGURE 8-5 Loose bodies are removed as they are visualized.

placed over the trocar on the medial side, and the trocar is pulled back into the joint and out the lateral side.

A proximal anterolateral retraction portal may be established 2 cm proximal to the lateral epicondyle. It can be used as a retraction portal.

Anterior Capsulectomy and Débridement

A 4.8-mm arthroscopic shaver is introduced through the anteromedial portal. Retraction through a proximal anterolateral portal is useful as arthroscopy proceeds. The shaver is used initially to débride soft tissue and to improve visualization. Loose bodies may be removed as they are visualized (Fig. 8-5) with arthroscopic graspers or a narrow jaw needle driver through an enlarged portal. Alternatively, large loose bodies may be burred down to a size small enough to be extracted.

After visualization is adequate, bony work can proceed. A burr can be used to recontour the joint and remove osteophytes from the coronoid and radial head fossae (Fig. 8-6). Bony work should be near complete before addressing soft tissue contracture with capsular release, because after the capsulotomy is performed, fluid extravasation limits the duration of arthroscopy that may be safely performed.

For capsular release, the anteromedial capsule is first stripped off the humerus with an elevator (Fig. 8-7). Large Steinmann pins or Howarth elevators may be used for retraction.

The arthroscope is placed in the lateral portal, and an arthroscopic biter is used on the anterior capsule, working from medial to lateral aspects (Fig. 8-8). The appearance of the fat stripe anterior to the radial head marks the safe limit of resection. The shaver is then introduced to completely resect the anterior capsule (Fig. 8-9). The arthroscope is then placed in the medial portal site, and working from the lateral side, the capsulectomy and bony débridement are completed.

Radial head excision is not needed in many patients with primary osteoarthritis of the elbow, because they often have preservation of much of the cartilage on the capitellum and radial head. In patients with complete loss of cartilage at the radiocapitellar articulation, significant crepitus, or loss of pronosupination, radial head excision may be beneficial. Many of these patients also have osteophytes on the posterior aspect of the capitellum and the radial head fossa, which should be resected. Occasionally, significant osteophytes limit pronosupination. They can be resected with a burr without excising the radial head itself. Radial head excision may be performed while viewing from the medial side. The anterolateral portal provides a good working portal for resection of the anterior aspect of the radial head with a burr and shaver. With progressive supination and pronation, resection of a large portion of the radial head can be achieved. Complete resection may be facilitated while viewing posterolaterally and bringing in the burr through the soft spot portal as a working portal. A detailed description of this procedure is provided in Chapter 11.

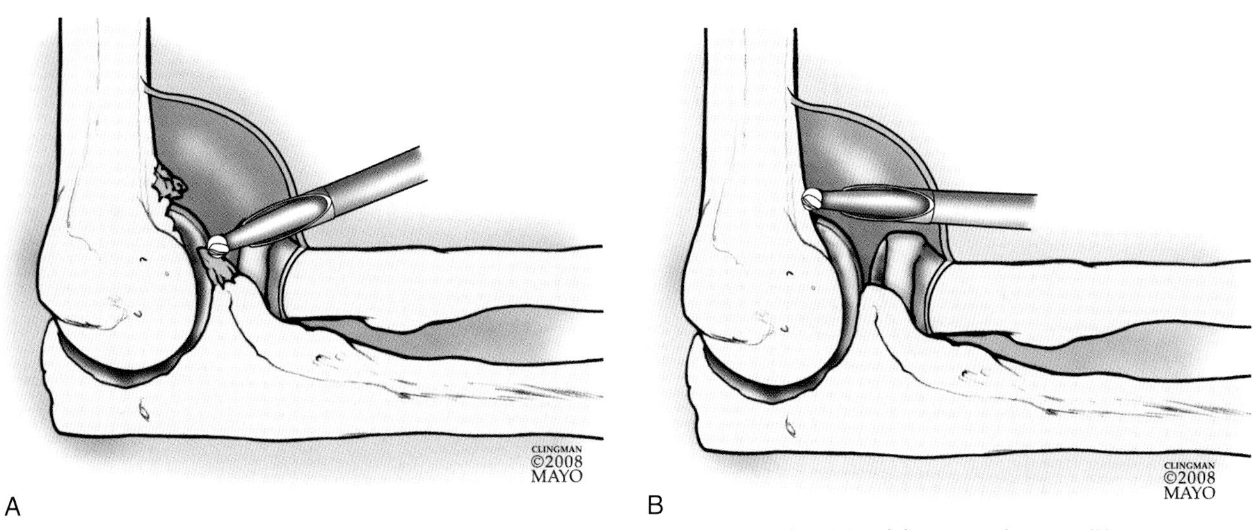

FIGURE 8-6 Osteophytes are removed from the radial head and coronoid tip (**A**) and the anterior humerus (**B**).

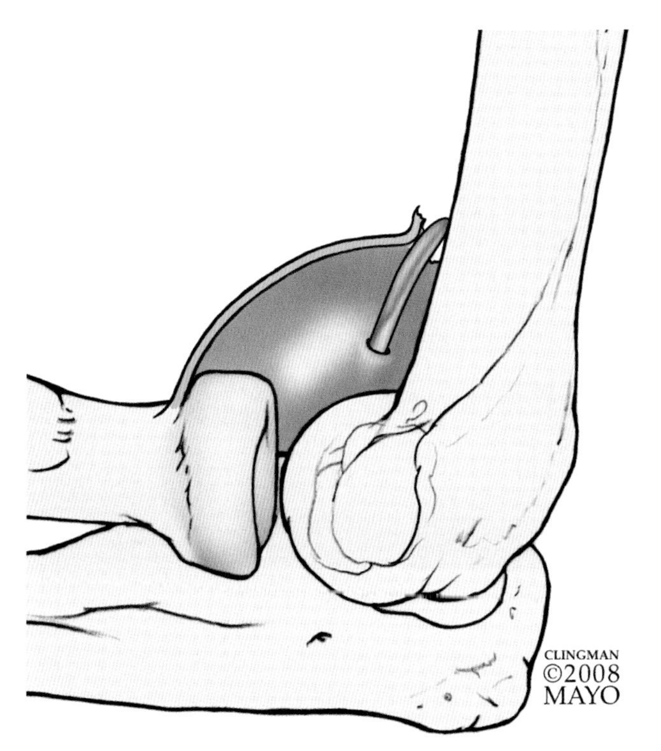

FIGURE 8-7 An elevator is used to lift the capsule off the anterior humerus.

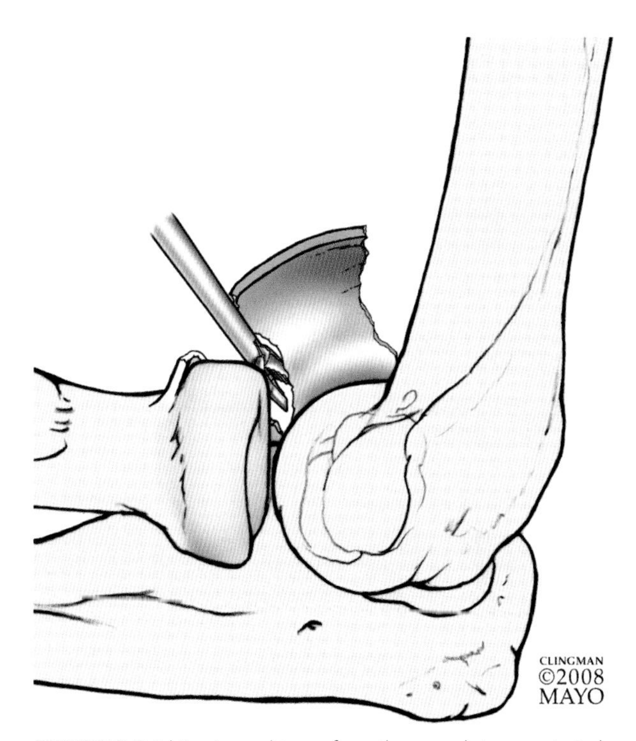

FIGURE 8-8 A biter is used to perform the capsulotomy anteriorly.

Posterior Portal Placement

After the anterior work is completed, the posterior aspect of the joint is addressed. The ulnar nerve, which was previously marked, should be confirmed at this point to prevent injury.

The posterolateral portal is the viewing portal and is made with the elbow at 90 degrees of flexion. The portal site is placed at the lateral joint line at a level with the tip of the olecranon. The direct posterior portal is the working portal, and it is made 2 to 3 cm proximal to the tip of the olecranon. It penetrates the triceps muscle, and a knife should be used to establish this portal, cutting through the thick triceps muscle all the way down to bone. Optional posterior retraction portals can be made 2 cm proximal to the direct posterior portal, situated slightly medially or laterally.

Posterior Capsular Débridement

After a posterolateral viewing portal and a direct posterior working portal are created, the shaver is placed in the direct posterior portal, and the view is improved by débridement of soft tissue. This is a potential space, and débridement is required to create a view. Subsequently, osteophytes are removed from the tip and sides of the olecranon and from the rim of the olecranon fossa (Fig. 8-10).

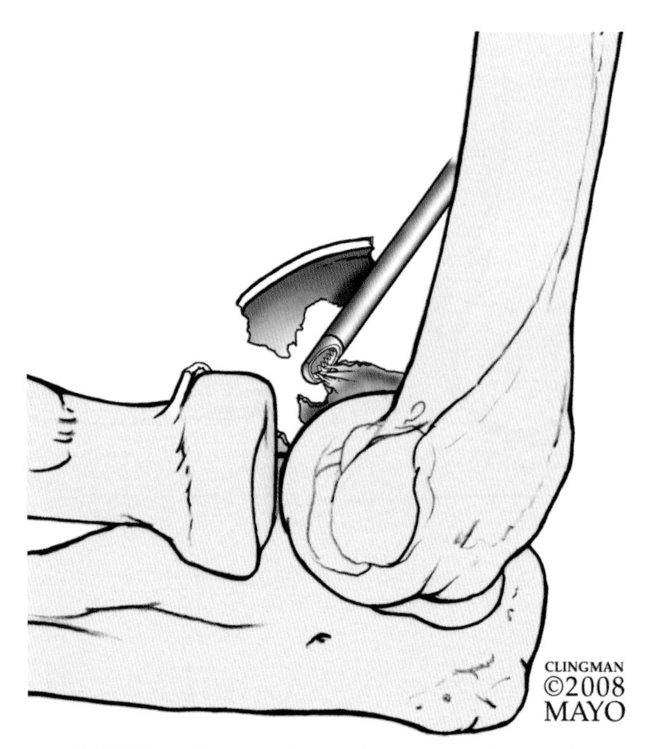

FIGURE 8-9 The shaver is brought in to resect the capsule.

An arthroscopic Outerbridge-Kashiwagi procedure can be performed using a burr or a large drill bit to remove the thickened bony bridge between the coronoid fossa and the olecranon fossa. The size of this fenestration should be limited to just the area of the olecranon fossa. In most individuals, this is a very thin portion of bone, measuring less than 3 to 4 mm. However, in throwing athletes with medial osteophytes, who may have instability, the osteophyte alone should be removed. Opposing osteophytes are often present on the medial aspect of the olecranon fossa. Resection should include only the osteophyte rather than additional native bone. If too much resection is performed in throwing athletes, additional strain will be placed upon the medial collateral ligament , potentially leading to instability.

Patients who lack flexion preoperatively should also undergo posterolateral and posteromedial capsular releases. When addressing the posteromedial capsule, care should be exercised to identify and protect the ulnar nerve (Fig. 8-11).

Management of the Ulnar Nerve

If a large restoration of motion is anticipated after the procedure, if preoperative ulnar nerve symptoms exist, or if preoperative flexion measures less than 90 degrees, ulnar nerve decompression or transposition should be considered. This may be done with arthroscopic decompression (see Fig. 8-11) if the surgeon possesses the requisite skill or with an open subcutaneous transposition or in situ decompression.

PEARLS & PITFALLS

1. Palpable landmarks and the intended portal sites must be marked before insufflation of the joint, which may obscure landmarks.
2. During the course of the procedure, suction tubing should be placed to gravity only to prevent accidently shaving objects that may be sucked into the shaver. Retractors, such as a Howarth elevator or a large, blunt Steinmann pin, make the procedure easier and safer by enhancing visualization and retracting structures out of harm's way.
3. Fluid management is important during the procedure. A low-flow, low-pressure system for inflow is useful, and early attention to providing outflow limits fluid extravasation and limb swelling.
4. The order of establishing portals is based on the surgeon's preference and experience and on the region where most work will be done. Portals may be started first anterolaterally or medially or can be started posteriorly.

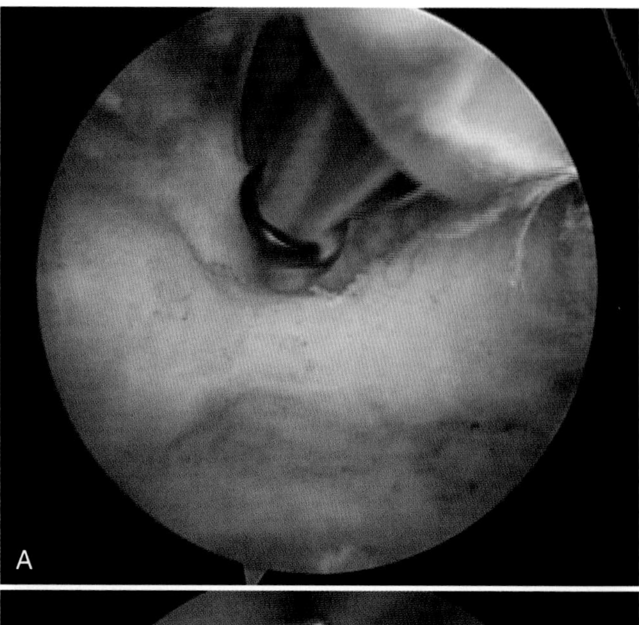

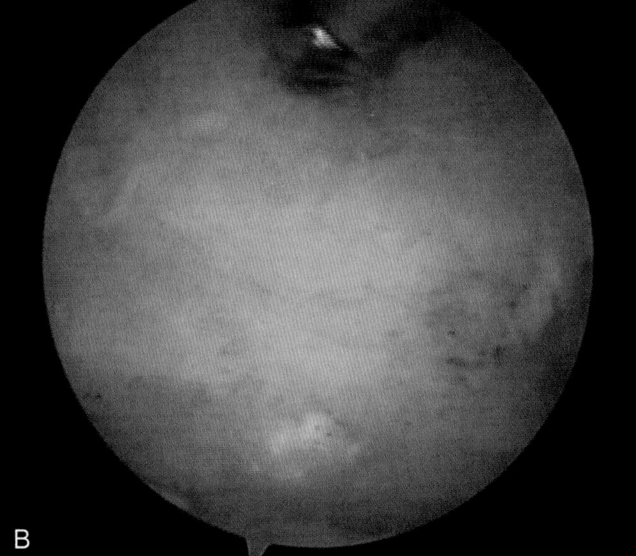

FIGURE 8-10 Posteriorly, osteophytes are seen at the olecranon fossa (**A**), and they are removed with the burr to improve motion (**B**).

Postoperative Rehabilitation

After completion of the procedure, motion is assessed in the operating room to ensure adequate release. Portals are closed

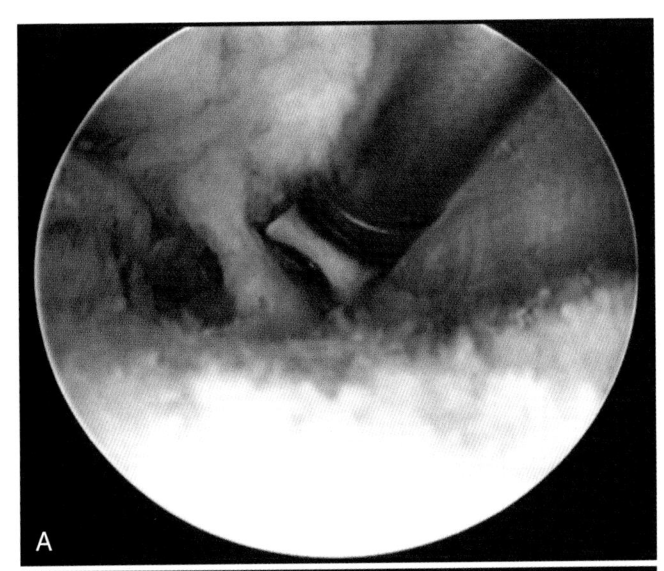

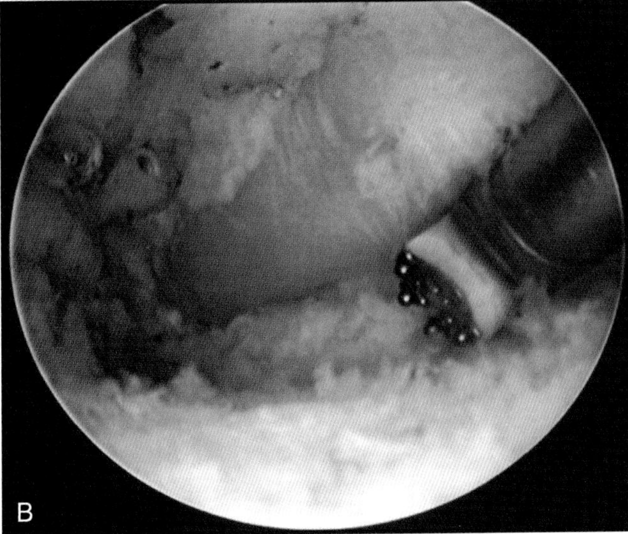

FIGURE 8-11 When performing a posteromedial capsulectomy (**A**), care is taken to identify and protect the ulnar nerve (**B**).

in the standard fashion with 3-0 nylon or Prolene sutures, and a sterile compressive dressing is applied. A posterior slab of plaster is used to splint the operative extremity in full extension, and the arm is elevated in the Statue of Liberty position overnight.

On the first postoperative day, the splint is removed, and the neurovascular status is evaluated with particular attention to the radial, median, and ulnar nerves. Full active range of motion is then initiated. No limitations are placed on use of the arm.

Heterotopic ossification prophylaxis, consisting of 75 mg of indomethacin three times daily for 6 weeks, is initiated. In selected patients who have had documented significant heterotopic ossification after an elbow procedure, radiation therapy is an option. A single dose of 700 cGy can be initiated within 72 hours of the procedure. We have found that this is rarely indicated for patients undergoing arthroscopic débridement of an arthritic elbow.

Splinting protocols, such as splints that may be adjusted from full extension to full flexion, are useful in many cases. The patient usually alternates hourly between the extremes of motion achieved at the time of surgery. In our experience, patients respond best to static progressive (turnbuckle) splints.

Continuous passive motion may be initiated using a continuous passive motion device with or without a nerve block, but in our experience, it is usually not necessary. In patients who are unable to move the elbow on their own or in those with severe contractures, it may beneficial, although a consensus regarding the indications and need for continuous passive motion is lacking.

CONCLUSIONS

Arthroscopic débridement and capsulectomy is an emerging technique for the treatment of elbow osteoarthritis. As more data become available, it appears that the results and complications are similar to those of open procedures. Although the theoretical benefits of early mobilization and recovery and decreased scar and pain may be associated with arthroscopic procedures, superiority over open releases has not been established. The surgeon must possess the requisite arthroscopic skills to perform the procedure safely and effectively.

REFERENCES

1. Stanley D. Prevalence and etiology of symptomatic elbow osteoarthritis. *J Shoulder Elbow Surg*. 1994;3:386-389.
2. Redden JF, Stanley D. Arthroscopic fenestration of the olecranon fossa in the treatment of osteoarthritis of the elbow. *Arthroscopy*. 1993;9:14-16.
3. Tsuge K, Mizuseki T. Debridement arthroplasty for advanced primary osteoarthritis of the elbow. Results of a new technique used for 29 elbows. *J Bone Joint Surg Br*. 1994;76:641-646.
4. Antuna SA, Morrey BF, Adams RA, O'Driscoll SW. Ulnohumeral arthroplasty for primary degenerative arthritis of the elbow: long-term outcome and complications. *J Bone Joint Surg Am*. 2002;84A:2168-2173.
5. Adams JE, Wolff LH 3rd, Merten SM, Steinmann SP. Osteoarthritis of the elbow: results of arthroscopic osteophyte resection and capsulectomy. *J Shoulder Elbow Surg*. 2008;17:126-131.
6. Ball CM, Meunier M, Galatz LM, et al. Arthroscopic treatment of post-traumatic elbow contracture. *J Shoulder Elbow Surg*. 2002;11:624-629.
7. Clasper JC, Carr AJ. Arthroscopy of the elbow for loose bodies. *Ann R Coll Surg Engl*. 2001;83:34-36.
8. Cohen AP, Redden JF, Stanley D. Treatment of osteoarthritis of the elbow: a comparison of open and arthroscopic debridement. *Arthroscopy*. 2000; 16:701-706.
9. O'Driscoll SW. Arthroscopic treatment for osteoarthritis of the elbow. *Orthop Clin North Am*. 1995;26:691-706.
10. Morrey BF. Primary degenerative arthritis of the elbow. Treatment by ulnohumeral arthroplasty. *J Bone Joint Surg Br*. 1992;74:409-413.
11. Suvarna SK, Stanley D. The histologic changes of the olecranon fossa membrane in primary osteoarthritis of the elbow. *J Shoulder Elbow Surg*. 2004;13:555-557.
12. Oka Y, Ohta K, Saitoh I. Debridement arthroplasty for osteoarthritis of the elbow. *Clin Orthop Relat Res*. 1998;(351):127-134.
13. Savoie FH 3rd, Nunley PD, Field LD. Arthroscopic management of the arthritic elbow: indications, technique, and results. *J Shoulder Elbow Surg*. 1999;8:214-219.
14. Tan V, Daluiski A, Simic P, Hotchkiss RN. Outcome of open release for post-traumatic elbow stiffness. *J Trauma*. 2006;61:673-678.
15. Mansat P, Morrey BF. The column procedure: a limited lateral approach for extrinsic contracture of the elbow. *J Bone Joint Surg Am*. 1998;80: 1603-1615.
16. Sarris I, Riano FA, Goebel F, et al. Ulnohumeral arthroplasty: results in primary degenerative arthritis of the elbow. *Clin Orthop Relat Res*. 2004; (420):190-193.

17. Phillips NJ, Ali A, Stanley D. Treatment of primary degenerative arthritis of the elbow by ulnohumeral arthroplasty. A long-term follow-up. *J Bone Joint Surg Br*. 2003;85:347-350.
18. Allen DM, Devries JP, Nunley JA. Ulnohumeral arthroplasty. *Iowa Orthop J*. 2004;24:49-52.
19. Vingerhoeds B, Degreef I, De Smet L. Debridement arthroplasty for osteoarthritis of the elbow (Outerbridge-Kashiwagi procedure). *Acta Orthop Belg*. 2004;70:306-310.
20. Kashigawi D, ed. *Osteoarthritis of the Elbow Joint*. Amersterdam, Netherlands: Elsevier Science; 1986:177-188.
21. Wada T, Isogai S, Ishii S, Yamashita T. Debridement arthroplasty for primary osteoarthritis of the elbow. *J Bone Joint Surg Am*. 2004;86A:233-241.
22. O'Driscoll SW. Operative treatment of elbow arthritis. *Curr Opin Rheumatol*. 1995;7:103-106.
23. Ogilvie-Harris DJ, Gordon R, MacKay M. Arthroscopic treatment for posterior impingement in degenerative arthritis of the elbow. *Arthroscopy*. 1995;11:437-443.
24. Steinmann SP, King GJ, Savoie FH 3rd. Arthroscopic treatment of the arthritic elbow. *J Bone Joint Surg Am*. 2005;87:2114-2121.
25. Gramstad GD, Galatz LM. Management of elbow osteoarthritis. *J Bone Joint Surg Am*. 2006;88:421-430.
26. Steinmann SP, King GJ, Savoie FH 3rd. Arthroscopic treatment of the arthritic elbow. *Instr Course Lect*. 2006;55:109-117.

CHAPTER 9

Osteocapsular Arthroplasty of the Elbow

Shawn W. O'Driscoll

Arthroscopic osteocapsular arthroplasty is a procedure involving three-dimensional reshaping of the bones (i.e., removal of osteophytes), removal of any loose bodies, and capsulectomy to restore motion and function and to eliminate pain.[1]

Arthroscopic release is effective for soft tissue contractures of the elbow.[2-5] When arthritic changes are present, bone work is also necessary.[1,6-12]

ANATOMY

Osteophytes build up in typical locations along the margins of the joint and in the fossae. Although the patient may have osteophytes on the posteromedial olecranon, osteophytes alone do not always cause impingement pain. The relationship between bony osteophytes and impingement pain poses an apparent dilemma. It is not unusual to see osteophytes that impinge at the limit of motion in patients who have no pain. The question is why some osteophytes are painful and others are not. Based on experience and unpublished research in progress, I think the usual cause for impingement pain in such circumstances is a fractured olecranon osteophyte that has typically progressed to nonunion by the time of referral to the orthopedic surgeon.[13] Nonunion fractures are best visualized (Fig. 9-1) on sagittal and coronal computed tomography (CT) reconstructions. The loose fragment is easily missed during arthroscopy because it is very small or covered with cartilage and not obviously loose. In some patients, the loose fragment is removed during osteophyte excision without ever being recognized. Other causes for the pain include loose bodies or buildup of inflamed soft tissue posteriorly.

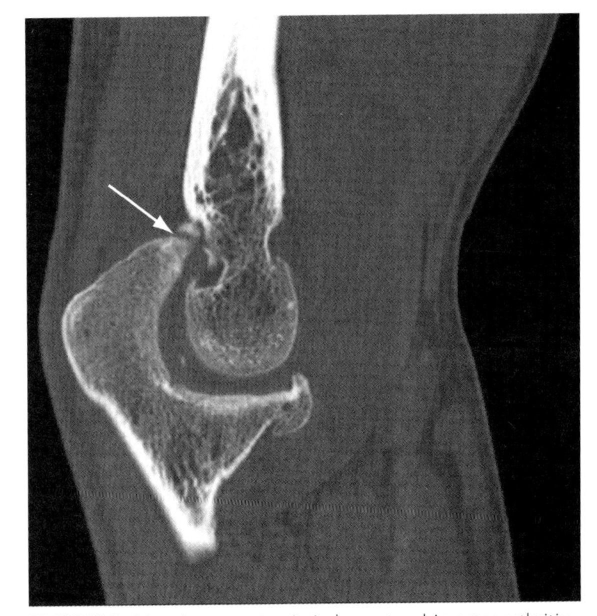

FIGURE 9-1 Impingement pain in hypertrophic osteoarthritis usually is caused by a painful nonunion of a fractured osteophyte, most commonly on the tip of the olecranon *(arrow)*.

PATIENT EVALUATION

History and Physical Examination

The patient reports posterior pain at the end point of extension. An associated contracture of some degree is almost invariably present.

I have found that the diagnosis of posterior impingement due to fractured nonunited osteophytes can be confirmed with confidence on physical examination using the extension impingement test and the arm bar test.[13] The extension impingement test is performed by starting with elbow near full extension and then quickly (but gently to prevent injury) snapping it into terminal extension. This maneuver reproduces the posterior or posteromedial pain experienced during provocative activities such as throwing. A simultaneous valgus load normally enhances the pain if the pathology is primarily posteromedial.

A similar test is the arm bar test, which is a variation of a martial arts maneuver. With the patient's shoulder in full internal rotation, the examiner extends the elbow to its full limit and then (gently at first) hyperextends it. This is reproducibly performed with the patient's shoulder in full internal rotation and 90 degrees of forward elevation. The patient's hand is placed on the shoulder of the examiner, and the examiner pulls down on the olecranon, leveraging the elbow into extension. Reproduction of the patient's pain is expected if impingement is present. I have found this test to be more sensitive than the extension impingement test if the patient's symptoms are relatively minor or have diminished just before consultation.

Diagnostic Imaging

CT with three-dimensional surface rendering provides excellent imaging of the bony pathology (Fig. 9-2A). The individual bones can be isolated from each other and spun around in three dimensions, demonstrating the location and structure of each osteophyte and loose body. Two-dimensional sagittal and coronal reconstructions are also necessary, because they reveal the fine details not available in the three-dimensional images (see Fig. 9-2B), including nonunited fractures, the original floors of the

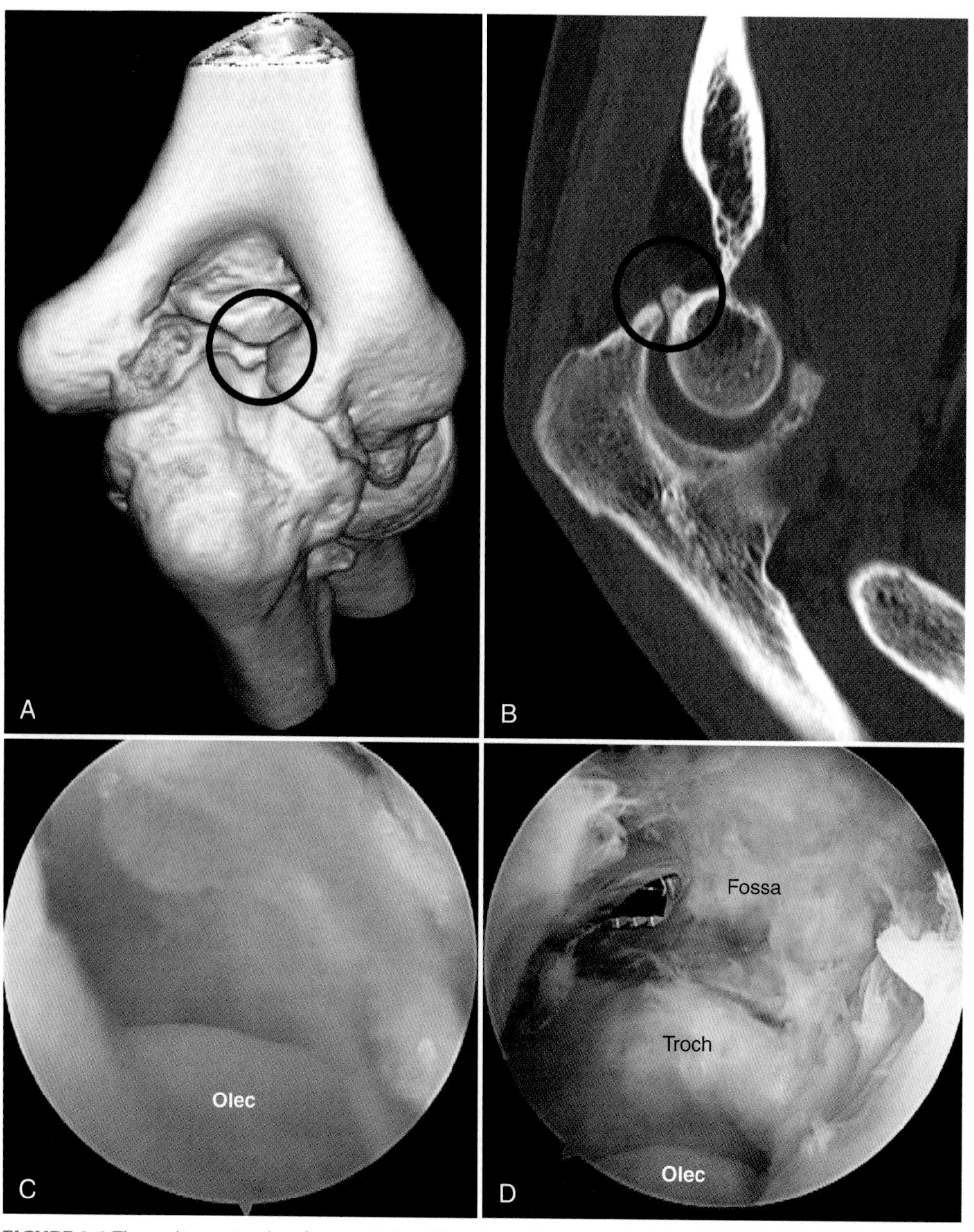

FIGURE 9-2 Three-dimensional surface rendering (**A**) and two-dimensional sagittal (**B**) computed tomographic reconstructions of the posterior compartment show osteophytes on the olecranon and in the olecranon fossa. The *circles* in **A** and **B** represent the arthroscopic fields of view in **C** and **D,** respectively. **C,** Step 1 is to get in and establish a view. The arthroscopic view is indicated by the *circles,* revealing the tip of the olecranon (Olec), which is just barely detectable within the surrounding scar tissue. **D,** Step 2 is to create a space in which to work by removing scar tissue, stripping the scar tissue and capsule off the bone, and inserting a retractor to elevate the soft tissues. A much larger view is then possible in which the olecranon (Olec) can be seen impinging on the marginal osteophyte on the trochlea (Troch). Above that area is scar tissue covering the floor of the olecranon fossa (Fossa). *(Courtesy of Shawn W. O'Driscoll, PhD, MD, Mayo Clinic, Rochester, MN.)*

fossae, and small loose bodies embedded in the cartilage surfaces. Axial two-dimensional reconstructions complete the imaging protocol.

TREATMENT

Indications and Contraindications

Arthroscopic osteocapsular arthroplasty is ideally indicated for symptomatic primary hypertrophic osteoarthritis of the elbow (with contracture and pain at the end range of motion) and for osteoarthritis resulting from osteochondritis dissecans. Relative indications include arthritis and contracture due to trauma or burned-out rheumatoid arthritis.

The main contraindication is questionable or inadequate expertise of the operating surgeon. The anterior capsulectomy portion of an arthroscopic osteocapsular arthroplasty may be relatively contraindicated in a patient with prior submuscular transposition of the ulnar nerve. Lying on the anterior capsule, to which it may be scarred, the nerve is theoretically at increased at risk for injury during anterior capsulectomy.

Relative contraindications include post-traumatic arthritis with severe joint surface irregularities and painful crepitus or nonhypertrophic osteoarthritis in the patients older than approximately 65 years.

Conservative Management

Nonsurgical treatment of hypertrophic arthritis with contracture is limited to symptomatic relief of pain by rest, activity modification, and nonsteroidal anti-inflammatory medications. Neither physical therapy nor splints have proved effective for established contractures.

Alternative Surgical Treatments

Alternatives to arthroscopic osteocapsular arthroplasty include arthroscopic or open Outerbridge-Kashiwagi, open column, and open Tsuge procedures.[6,8,12] In my experience, drilling a hole through the olecranon fossa does not adequately decompresses the coronoid fossa or the olecranon fossa, and it fails to address osteophytes in the radial fossa. It also eliminates the bony landmarks used to determine just how much bone should be removed from the fossa. The open column procedure does not permit as accurate and complete removal of osteophytes or contracted capsule (e.g., medial gutter) as the arthroscopic procedure. The Tsuge procedure has a high morbidity rate with no apparent advantages over arthroscopic osteocapsular arthroplasty.

Arthroscopic Technique

Patient positioning is critical for this procedure. With the patient in the lateral (preferred) or prone positions, it is necessary to have the shoulder forward flexed at least 90 degrees and abducted slightly (i.e., elbow higher than the shoulder). Failure to do so will result in the shaver handle hitting the chest of the patient and preventing access to the coronoid fossa. I do not recommend using the supine position for this procedure. A tourniquet is used.

Arthroscopic osteocapsular arthroplasty is a complex procedure requiring a high level of experience in elbow arthroscopy for its safe and effective performance. I have learned by experience that it is best performed in a stepwise sequence, starting posteriorly and completing the work in the gutters before going anteriorly (Box 9-1).

Box 9-1 Sequence for Elbow Arthroplasty

1. Get in and establish a view
2. Create a space in which to work
3. Bone removal
4. Capsulectomy

I perform a limited open decompression of the ulnar nerve through a 1.5- to 2-cm skin incision at the beginning of the procedure. This step was added to lessen the risk of developing a delayed-onset ulnar neuropathy postoperatively.

Posterior Joint Compartment

Three standard portals are used routinely, and one or two accessory portals may be added. The three standard portals are the posterolateral, posterior, and direct midlateral (i.e., soft spot). Accessory portals (i.e., proximal posterolateral and proximal posterior) can be used for retraction.

Step 1: Get In and Establish a View. The first step is to get in and establish a view. Place the scope in the posterolateral portal and the shaver in the posterior portal. Confirm by visualizing identifiable articular structures that you are inside the joint and that you have the correct anatomic orientation (see Fig. 9-2C). Touch the tips of the shaver and scope together by triangulation, and visualize the shaver blade. By using surface anatomic landmarks, it should be possible to verify the shaver is within the olecranon fossa. This can be confirmed by tactile feedback as the shaver is moved up and down the sides of the fossa and around its rim.

Step 2: Create a Space in Which to Work. Creating a space in which to work is the most important step in osteocapsular arthroplasty. If a surgeon can predictably create a space in which to work, he or she has most of the skills necessary to do the rest of the operation. More important, this makes the surgery safer and easier to perform.

Creating a space in which to work involves synovectomy and removal of debris, scar tissue, and loose bodies so that the surgeon can see clearly (see Fig. 9-2D). The surgeon strips the capsule off the humerus proximally and removes remaining loose bodies. Adding a retractor through the proximal posterolateral or proximal posterior portal increases the space, just as retraction does with open surgery. Slight elbow extension helps.

A radiofrequency device can be used to remove scar and adhesions from the olecranon and fossa so that they do not wrap up in the burr used to trim the bone. However, the surgeon must not to allow the irrigation fluid to heat up and cause thermal necrosis of cartilage.

Step 3: Bone Removal. Bone removal is performed before capsulectomy (Figs. 9-3 and 9-4). It is helpful to use a retractor to hold the triceps away from the burr. In re-creating the olecranon fossa, the key is to find the original floor of the fossa. The

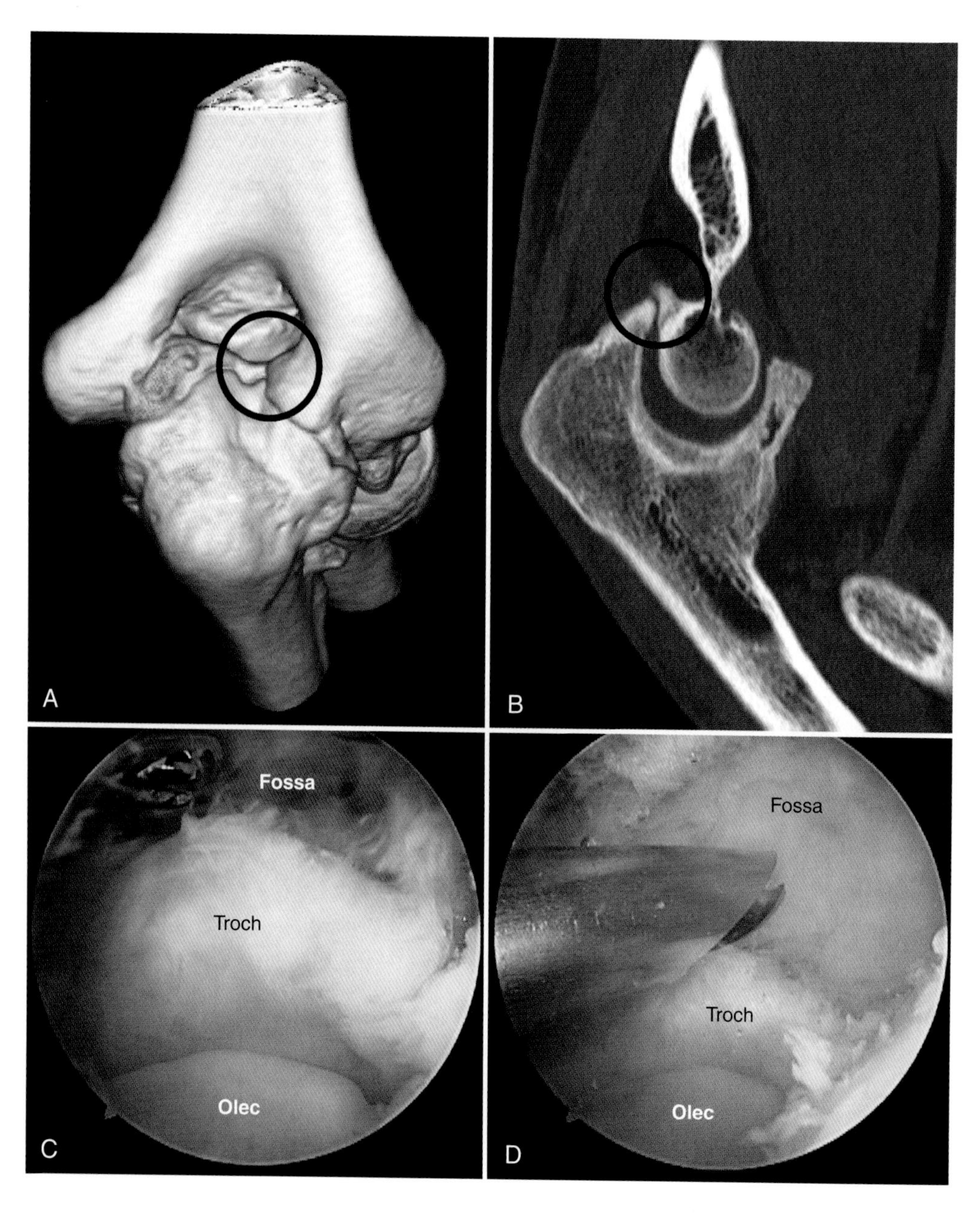

FIGURE 9-3 The three-dimensional surface rendering (**A**) and two-dimensional sagittal CT (**B**) reconstructions of the elbow show bony osteophytes on the olecranon (Olec) and around the olecranon fossa (Fossa). The *circles* in **A** and **B** represent the arthroscopic fields of view in **C** and **D,** respectively. **C** and **D,** Step 3 is bone removal. After an adequate space is created, the osteophytes must be removed. The marginal osteophyte is being resected from the top of the trochlea (Troch) at the bottom of the olecranon fossa (Fossa).

preoperative CT scans are used to determine whether the original floor of the fossa is preserved and where it is. Except in the most advanced cases, it is usually partially preserved under the osteophytes.

When trimming the olecranon, avoid removing normal olecranon bone (i.e., take off only the osteophytes) in an overhead athlete to prevent increased strain in the medial collateral ligament during valgus stress. I usually do avoid using a burr on the medial corner of the olecranon, because it can wrap up the soft tissues and injure the ulnar nerve. I try to prevent this by changing to a shaver blade (4.8-mm Gator), which cuts rather than wraps or pulls tissue, after I pass the corner of the olecranon (Fig. 9-5). Fortunately, exposed trabecular bone (from having already cut into it posteriorly) is relatively easy to cut with a shaver blade.

Step 4: Capsulectomy. After bone removal is complete, a posterior capsulectomy is performed with a 4.8-mm Gator blade or equivalent. I use a large shaver for three reasons. It can remove tissue more effectively; fluid outflow is more effective through a large-bore shaver (and swelling is less likely); and I sometimes use the device as a periosteal elevator to strip soft tissue off bone before resecting it, and the device needs to be physically strong.

Medial Gutter

The work in the medial gutter is performed with the arthroscope in the posterolateral portal and the shaver or working instrument in the posterior portal. Retractors can be placed through the proximal posterolateral or the proximal posterior portals (see Fig. 9-5D).

Step 1: Get In and Establish a View. The key landmarks to identify are the medial edge of the ulnohumeral articulation and the posterior bundle of the medial collateral ligament, which appears

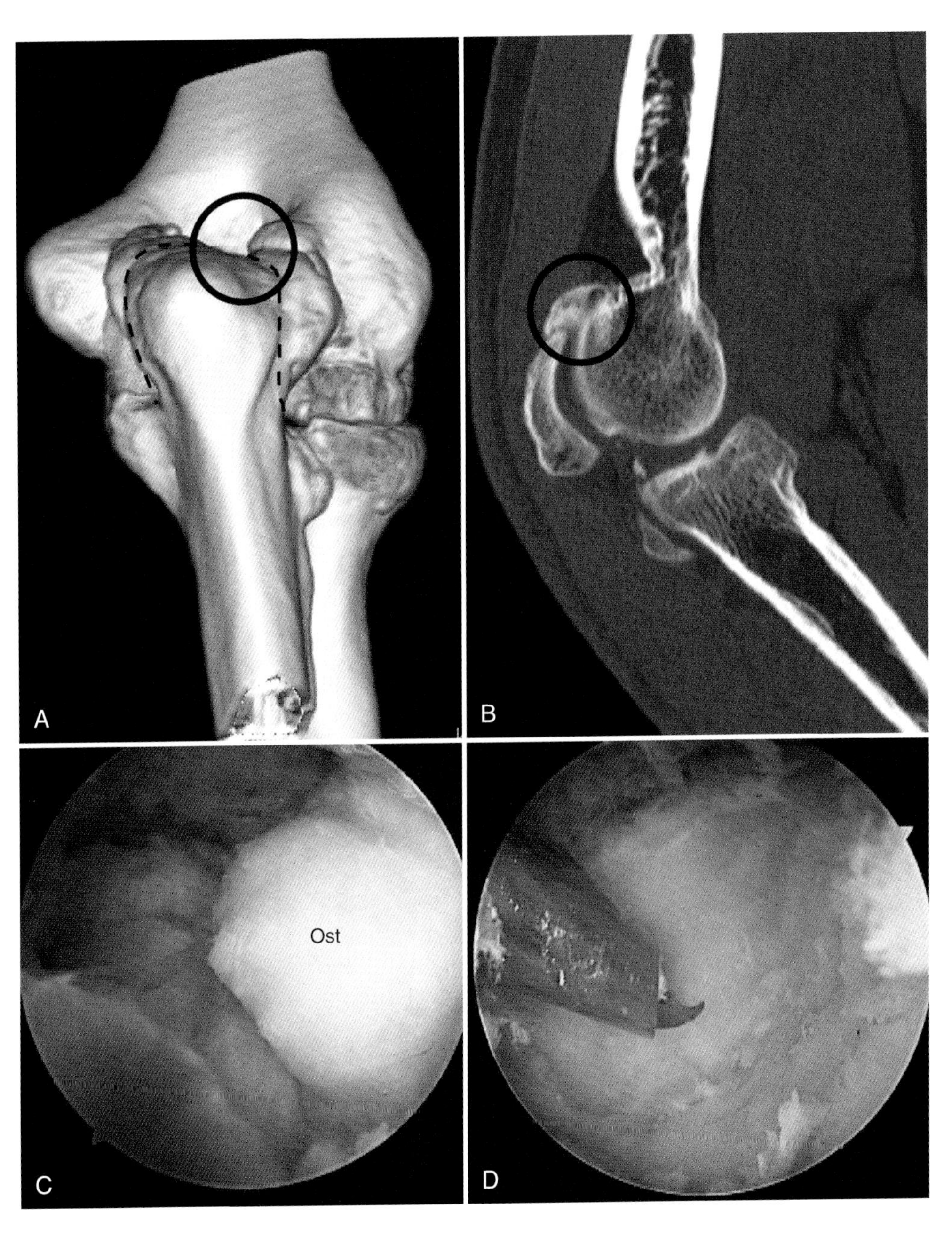

FIGURE 9-4 A-D, Step 4 is bone removal. Bone removal from the lateral side of the olecranon fossa continues. A large osteophyte (*circles* in **A** and **B,** Ost in **C**) encroaches on the olecranon fossa and abuts the posterolateral olecranon. The olecranon fossa is narrowed, and the olecranon is widened by these osteophytes (*dotted lines* in **A**), which must be removed. The posteromedial and posterolateral osteophytes on the olecranon give the typical appearance of Mickey Mouse ears (*dotted lines*).

as a series of corrugations or vertical bands within the posterior medial capsule.

Step 2: Create a Space in Which to Work. Before removing osteophytes from the medial gutter or releasing the posterior medial capsule, it is necessary to remove any synovitis. Disconnect the shaver from suction and turn the blade away from the capsule to minimize the chance of injuring the ulnar nerve. A retractor allows the surgeon to create a space in which to work and can be used to retract the ulnar nerve.

Step 3: Bone Removal. Extreme caution is necessary when using motorized instruments medial to the posteromedial corner of the olecranon. Beyond the posteromedial corner of the olecranon, I usually change from a burr to shaver blade, which avoids the risk of drawing tissues into the burr due to Bernoulli-Venturi effects (see Fig. 9-5B).

Step 4: Capsulectomy. The posteromedial capsule must be released to restore flexion in elbows that lack flexion preoperatively. It can be released through a small incision over the cubital tunnel, which permits concurrent ulnar nerve decompression. Alternatively, the posteromedial capsule can be released arthroscopically if the surgeon has the skill and is fully knowledgeable of the three-dimensional location of the nerve in this area (see Fig. 9-5C and D).

Lateral Gutter

Work in the lateral gutter begins by switching the instruments so that the arthroscope is in the posterior portal and the shaver is in

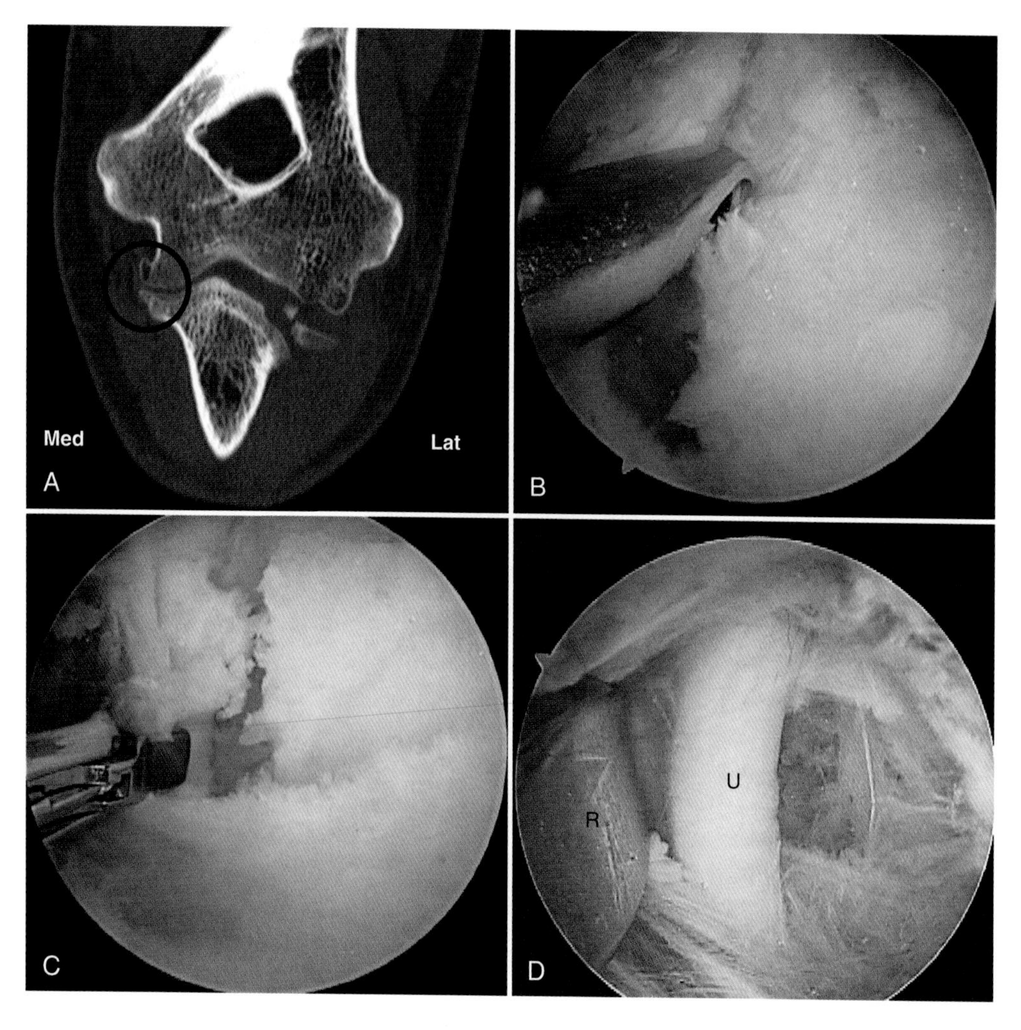

FIGURE 9-5 When removing the osteophytes from the medial gutter (**A,** *circle*), it is safer to change from a burr to a cutting shaver blade (**B**). **C,** The posteromedial capsule must be released by open or arthroscopic techniques to restore flexion. A wide duckbill is used to resect the posteromedial capsule. **D,** Immediately behind the posteromedial capsule lies the ulnar nerve (U), which can be seen by retracting the medial edge of the triceps with a retractor (R).

the posterolateral portal. It is helpful, but not always necessary, to use a retractor in the proximal posterolateral portal to retract the soft tissues at the posterolateral corner away from the olecranon and to open up the lateral gutter.

Step 1: Get In and Establish a View. Access to the lateral gutter can be obstructed by large osteophytes on the posterolateral corner of the olecranon, the lateral trochlea, or the posterior aspect of the capitellum. A switching stick is brought in through the posterolateral portal under direct vision down into the lateral gutter. The arthroscope is removed from the posterior portal and reinserted through posterolateral portal down into the lateral gutter over the switching stick. A spinal needle is then brought in through the direct midlateral (soft spot) portal, after which a knife blade is used to create the portal and the shaver brought in through the direct midlateral portal.

Step 2: Create a Space in Which to Work. Before removing osteophytes, it is necessary to remove or ablate soft tissue around the posterolateral corner and to perform a general débridement and synovectomy in the lateral gutter. A radiofrequency device is especially useful in this area. At this stage, any abnormal thickening of the annular ligament in the form of a plica is also trimmed.

Step 3: Bone Removal. Osteophytes are removed from the posterior capitellum (sometimes extending well out laterally) and the lateral ridges of the trochlea and olecranon. The osteophyte behind the capitellum is best appreciated on the two-dimensional, sagittal or three-dimensional, surface rendering CT reconstructions. The entire lateral compartment should be carefully inspected for loose bodies, because this is a typical location in which loose bodies may be nestled.

Step 4: Capsulectomy. If the patient lacks flexion, the posterolateral capsule must be released. The extent of the posterolateral capsular release depends on the severity of the loss of flexion. In extreme cases, the release should be continued down to the annular ligament but not through it. For less severe contractures, it is often necessary to release only around the corner of the olecranon to the proximal portion of the lateral gutter.

Anterior Joint Compartment

Three portals are routinely used for osteocapsular arthroplasty involving the anterior joint, and occasionally, a fourth is used. The anterolateral and proximal anteromedial portals are used for the arthroscope and working instruments, respectively, and the proximal anterolateral portal is used for a retractor. Occasionally,

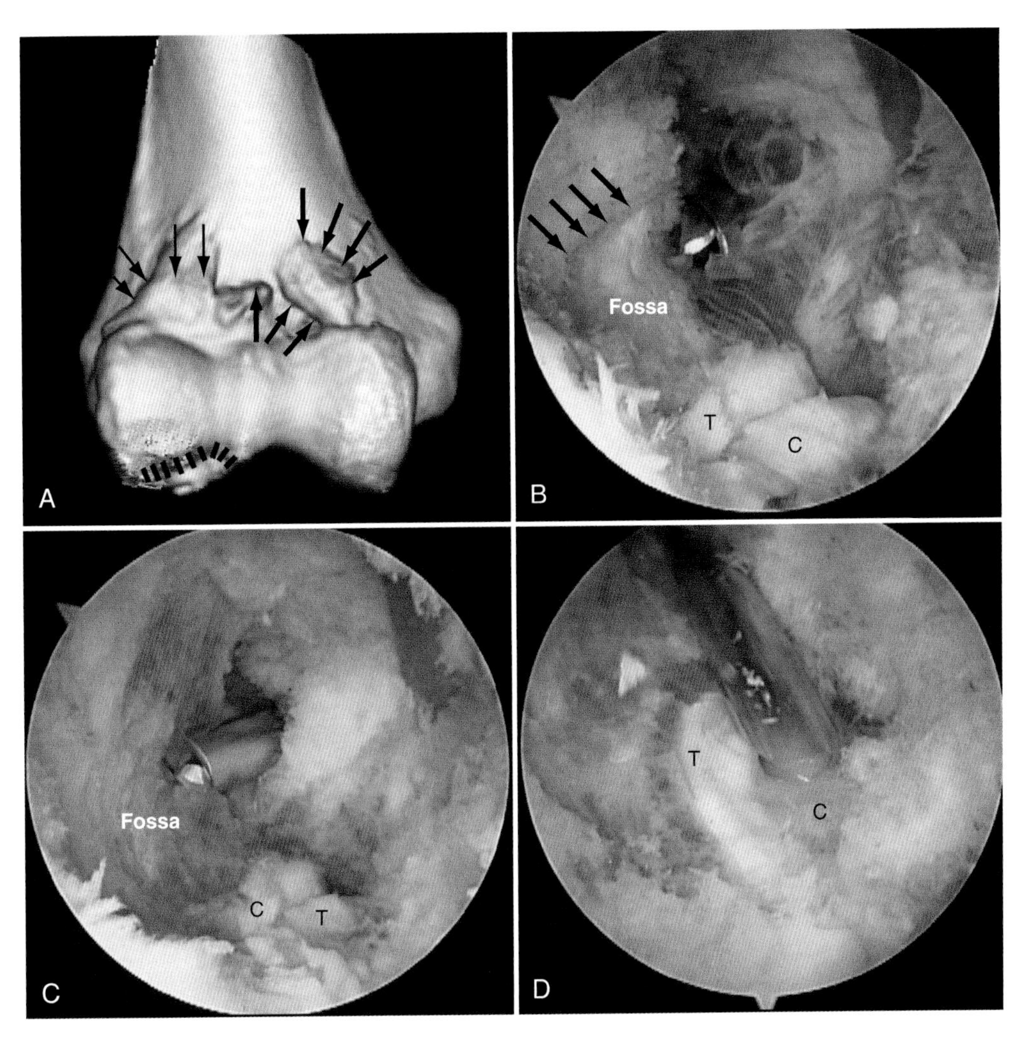

FIGURE 9-6 Step 3 is bony work in the anterior elbow compartment. **A,** Osteophytes anteriorly encroach on the radial fossa *(small arrows)* and the coronoid fossa *(large arrows)*, and they must be removed by recontouring the distal humerus. Osteophytes typically extend off the tip of the coronoid, as seen in Figures 9-2B and 9-3B, and they must be removed. By subtracting the radius and ulna, the osteophyte at the posterior margin of the capitellum can be seen *(arrows)*. **B,** A burr in the coronoid fossa (Fossa) is used to remove the osteophyte *(arrows)*. The coronoid (C) and the top of the trochlea (T) are seen at the bottom of the image. **C,** The coronoid fossa (Fossa) is restored. **D,** With hyperflexion, the osteophytes can be removed from the coronoid (C) flush with the top of the trochlea (T).

a second retractor is used, and it is placed in the anteromedial portal.

Step 1: Get In and Establish a View. In some elbows with contracture and arthritis, getting in and establishing a view is the most difficult and intimidating step. Contracted elbows are tight, with minimal or no space between the capsule and the cartilage surface. Entry into the joint should be performed with a pointed switching stick, which is pointed enough to penetrate dense scare tissue and the capsule but blunt enough to avoid injuring the cartilage. After the switching stick is in place, the sheath is inserted into the joint over the switching stick, and the scope is then inserted inside the sheath. Identify articular anatomy before proceeding further.

Step 2: Create a Space in Which to Work. This critical step in osteocapsular arthroplasty can be time consuming, but it is a major factor in making the bone removal and capsulectomy safer and more predictable. Mastery of this step requires most of the skills necessary to do the rest of the operation.

After establishing a view in step 1, it is time to create a space in which to work. This involves synovectomy and removal of debris, scar tissue, and loose bodies so that the surgeon can see clearly.

The capsule is stripped off the humerus proximally, and any loose soft tissue is removed. If not already done, a retractor is placed through the proximal anterolateral portal to retract the capsule anteriorly.

The capsular attachments are released along the medial and lateral supracondylar ridges if that has not already been done. This step allows the entire soft tissue mass (i.e., capsule, muscle, scar, and neurovascular structures) to be retracted further anteriorly away from the shaver or burr.

Step 3: Bone Removal. In re-creating the coronoid and radial fossae, the key is to find the floor of the fossa, which is usually at least partially preserved under the osteophytes (Fig. 9-6). Removing the periosteal soft tissue layer under the osteophytes exposes smooth cortical bone, which is readily distinguished from the overlying trabecular bone in the osteophytes. Bone debris is removed using the shaver, because it will not wash off the surface of exposed muscle with irrigation alone.

Step 4: Capsulectomy. Anterior capsulectomy is performed by first releasing the capsule along the supracondylar ridges if this was not done during the stage of creating a space in which to work. The

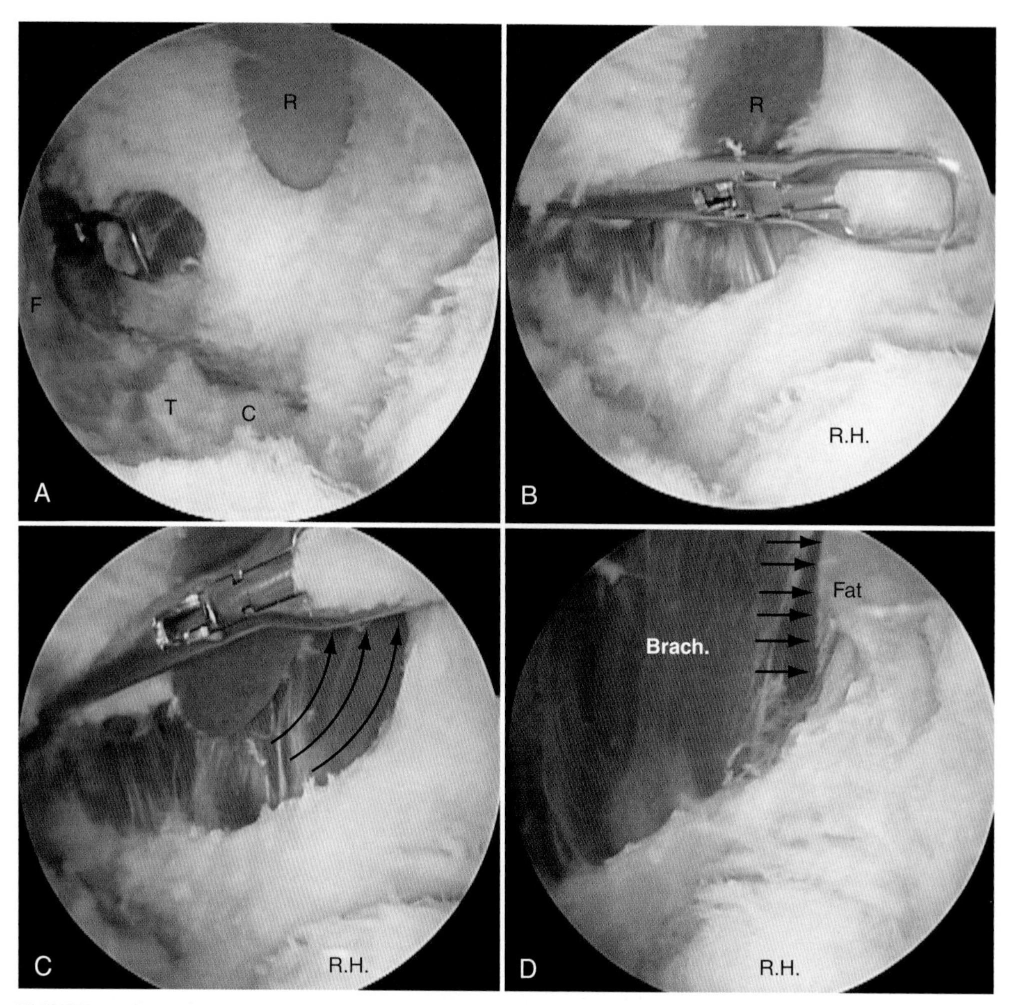

FIGURE 9-7 Step 4 is an anterior capsulectomy, which is best performed by starting with a capsulotomy from medial to lateral aspects. **A,** View from anterolateral portal showing trochlea (T), coronoid (C), coronoid fossa (F), and retractor (R). A wide duckbill is used to take a bite out of the anterior capsule, starting at the medial side of the elbow, where the interval between the capsule and the brachialis is well defined. A retractor (R) is used to position and tension the capsule. **B** and **C,** The bite and peel action *(curved arrows)* involves biting the capsule with the duckbill and then peeling it off the brachialis proximally to create a wide strip, exposing the brachialis. **D,** When the lateral edge *(small arrows)* of the brachialis (Brach.) is reached at the midpoint of the radial head (R.H.), a strip of fat (Fat) that encloses the radial nerve can be seen. This is a consistent anatomic landmark and the point at which the capsulotomy is stopped until the instruments are switched around.

capsule is cut from medial to lateral aspects with a wide duckbill (i.e., duckling or punch biopsy) (Fig. 9-7). Release proceeds laterally to the lateral edge of the brachialis, indicated by a strip of fatty tissue surrounding the radial nerve (see Fig. 9-7D). The capsule is excised proximally on the medial side and centrally with the shaver disconnected from suction (see Fig. 9-7E and F). The remaining lateral capsule is divided with a fine, pointed scissors or other suitable instrument, and the proximal portion is excised (see Fig. 9-7G and H). I prefer to make the capsulotomy distally, where the interval between brachioradialis and extensor carpi radialis longus is readily identifiable, and I then excise the whole capsule. Some surgeons wisely recommend cutting the capsule more proximally, where the radial nerve is farther away. In either case, a small triangle of capsule may be left intact over the interval between the brachioradialis and extensor carpi radialis longus to protect the radial nerve. The capsular release must go right down to the collateral ligaments on each side for complete release.

PEARLS & PITFALLS

- Major concerns are related to the possibility of nerve injury during arthroscopy.
- To avoid nerve injury, elbow arthroscopists must work within the scope of their technical abilities and experience; need to have intricate knowledge of the three-dimensional anatomy of the nerves; and should use retractors to maintain a working space and keep the nerves away from power instruments.
- Major restoration of motion in these elbows may cause delayed-onset ulnar neuropathy. In most cases, this problem manifests as partial loss of the restored motion, because the ulnar neuritis is too painful to permit continued rehabilitation with full motion.
- Resulting neuropathy can be severe, but prophylactic decompression of the ulnar nerve at the cubital tunnel can prevent this problem.

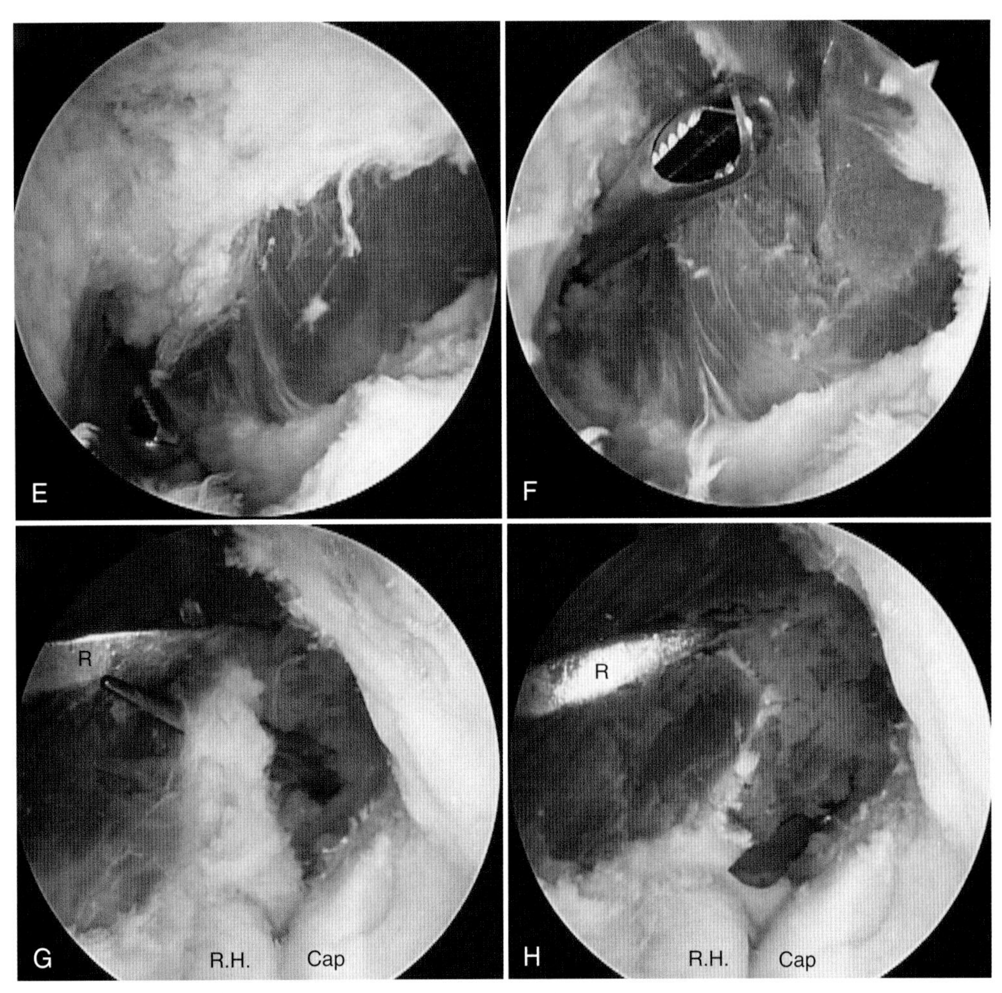

FIGURE 9-7, cont'd **E** and **F,** The capsulectomy is performed using a shaver facing into the joint and working from distal to proximal aspects. **G,** With the scope in the anteromedial portal, all that is left to see of the capsule is a small triangle of tissue in front of the radial head (R.H.) and capitellum (Cap). This can be left in place to protect the radial nerve, or it can be dissected away from the overlying tissues with fine dissecting scissors. A retractor (R) maintains the space and retracts the brachialis and the anterior neurovascular structures. **H,** A knife blade is used to release the capsule down to the level of the collateral ligaments, because this is difficult to perform with the shaver. A retractable blade can be brought in through the anterolateral portal to perform this.

Postoperative Rehabilitation

After the patient is confirmed to have normal neurologic function, an indwelling axillary catheter is placed for continuous infusion of a long-acting local anesthetic for pain control. Continuous passive motion (CPM) is commenced through a full range of motion, with the patient instructed in end-range stretching. The arm is removed from the CPM device each hour for 5 minutes to prevent pressure sores or nerve palsies. This program continues for 3 days in the hospital, after which the block is removed, and the patient commences a CPM program at home for 3.5 more weeks. Intervals out of the CPM machine are increased progressively to wean the patient, as tolerated without loss of motion.

OUTCOMES

There are no published series of results for arthroscopic osteocapsular arthroplasty. The lack of studies reflects the fact that the safety of the procedure had not been proved for several years, and it is only recently being performed in many centers.

My experience has been that for the proper indications, the results are among the most reliable and gratifying for the patient and physician of any shoulder or elbow operation performed. Data should be available in the peer-review literature in the future.

REFERENCES

1. O'Driscoll SW. Arthroscopic osteocapsular arthroplasty. In: Yamaguchi K, King G, McKee M, O'Driscoll S, eds. *Advanced Reconstruction Elbow*. 1st ed. Rosemont, IL: American Academy of Orthopedic Surgeons; 2007:59-68.
2. O'Driscoll S. The arthroscopic treatment of the stiff elbow. In: Celli A, ed. *Treatment of the Elbow Lesions: New Aspects in Diagnosis and Surgical Techniques*. New York, NY: Springer; 2008:211-219.
3. O'Driscoll SW, Savoie FH 3rd. Arthroscopy of the elbow. In: Morrey BF, editor. *Master Techniques in Orthopedic Surgery: The Elbow*. 2 ed. Philadelphia, PA: Lippincott Williams & Wilkins; 2002:27-45.
4. Jones GS, Savoie FH III. Arthroscopic capsular release of flexion contractures (arthrofibrosis) of the elbow. *Arthroscopy*. 1993;9:277-283.
5. Ward WG, Anderson TE. Elbow arthroscopy in a mostly athletic population. *J Hand Surg Am*. 1993;18A:220-224.
6. Redden JF, Stanley D. Arthroscopic fenestration of the olecranon fossa in the treatment of osteoarthritis of the elbow. *Arthroscopy*. 1993;9:14-16.

7. O'Driscoll SW. Arthroscopic treatment for osteoarthritis of the elbow. *Orthop Clin North Am*. 1995;26:691-706.
8. Ogilvie-Harris DJ, Gordon R, MacKay M. Arthroscopic treatment for posterior impingement in degenerative arthritis of the elbow. *Arthroscopy*. 1995;11:437-443.
9. Savoie FH 3rd, Nunley PD, Field LD. Arthroscopic management of the arthritic elbow: indications, technique, and results. *J Shoulder Elbow Surg*. 1999;8:214-219.
10. Cohen AP, Redden JF, Stanley D. Treatment of osteoarthritis of the elbow: a comparison of open and arthroscopic debridement. *Arthroscopy*. 2000;16:701-706.
11. Krishnan S, Pennington S, Burkhead W. Arthroscopic ulnohumeral arthroplasty for degenerative arthritis of the elbow in patients under the age of 50. *Tech Shoulder Elbow Surg*. 2005;6:208-213.
12. Adams JE, Wolff LH 3rd, Merten SM, Steinmann SP. Osteoarthritis of the elbow: results of arthroscopic osteophyte resection and capsulectomy. *J Shoulder Elbow Surg*. 2008;17:126-131.
13. O'Driscoll S. Valgus extension overload and plica. In: Levine WN, ed. *Athlete's Elbow*. Rosemont, IL: American Academy of Orthopaedic Surgeons; 2008:71-83.
14. Miller C, Jobe C, Wright M. Neuroanatomy in elbow arthroscopy. *J Shoulder Elbow Surg*. 1995;4:168-174.
15. Gallay SH, Richards RR, O'Driscoll SW. Intraarticular capacity and compliance of stiff and normal elbows. *Arthroscopy*. 1993;9:9-13.

CHAPTER

10

Arthroscopic Radial Head Resection

Darryl K. Young • Graham J.W. King

Radial head resection is a useful treatment alternative for symptomatic radiocapitellar or proximal radioulnar joint pathology. Radial head excision may improve forearm rotation and reduce impingement between the radial head and the capitellum or proximal ulna. Most reports in the literature involve open radial head resection.[1] Arthroscopic radial head resection has been described only recently,[2] and reports of outcomes are limited.[3-5] However, as experience with arthroscopic radial head resection continues to increase, we expect more evidence to be forthcoming.

The primary theoretical advantages of arthroscopic compared with open resection include better intra-articular visualization, which allows the surgeon to address concomitant pathologies such as synovitis, capsular contracture, osteophytes, or loose bodies, and less soft tissue disruption, potentially reducing the severity and duration of postoperative pain and stiffness.

ANATOMY AND BIOMECHANICS

The radial head is an important stabilizer of the elbow. A number of biomechanical studies have investigated the effect of radial head resection on the kinematics and stability of the elbow. The radial head is particularly important as a stabilizer in the setting of valgus instability due to medial collateral ligament insufficiency.[6-9] It is also important in tensioning the lateral collateral ligament,[7] and posterolateral rotatory instability has been reported after radial head excision in vitro[7,10] and clinically.[11,12] The role of the radial head in axial stability of the forearm is evident by the common finding of proximal migration of the radius after radial head resection.[13-17]

Radial head excision results in increased loading of the remaining ulnohumeral articulation. This effect is caused by the altered elbow kinematics and the fact that the loads originally borne by the radiocapitellar articulation must be accepted by the ulnohumeral joint.[8] Although this increased ulnohumeral load has not been studied biomechanically, it is thought to explain the high incidence of ulnohumeral osteoarthritis reported in patients after acute radial head resection for radial head fractures.[14-17] Extensive biomechanical evidence supports the beneficial stabilizing effects of prosthetic replacement of the radial head.[7-9],[18,19] These findings suggest that, whenever possible, the radial head should be replaced after it is resected, particularly in cases of acute trauma, in which occult ligament injuries are common.

PATIENT EVALUATION

History and Physical Examination

Several considerations are important in deciding whether to perform an arthroscopic radial head resection. The assessment starts with a thorough history. Pain and stiffness are common complaints related to the radiocapitellar deformity, both of which may be more pronounced with pronosupination rather than flexion and extension. Mechanical symptoms, including clicking, catching, or locking, may be prominent. The examiner should elicit a history surrounding any underlying disease process (e.g., inflammatory arthritis, primary osteoarthritis, hemophilia) and prior treatment. A history of trauma and surgical procedures is important. Obtaining previous operative reports and imaging can be helpful.

A detailed physical examination should be performed. The carrying angle and bony contours of the elbow should be observed. Prior traumatic and surgical incisions should be documented. The range of motion of the elbow and forearm should be measured with the use of a goniometer. The examiner should confirm that the proximal radius articular deformity is the impediment to rotation. Motion can be lost as a result of soft tissue or osseous deformities. The synovial tissue in patients with hemophilic arthropathy is hypertrophic, highly vascular, and prone to impingement between the articular surfaces.[22] A soft end point suggests a soft tissue cause, whereas a firm end point suggests osseous impingement. The distal radioulnar joint may be contributing to the forearm rotational stiffness.

Physical examination and imaging of the wrist are important, especially in patients with prior traumatic injuries, congenital deformities, and rheumatoid arthritis, in which distal radioulnar joint pathology is common. A careful examination of elbow and forearm stability is critical because valgus, posterolateral rotational, and axial instability are contraindications to radial head resection. Joint laxity may be caused by loss of articular cartilage, ligament attenuation resulting from chronic inflammation, or prior traumatic injuries. The examination for valgus instability includes valgus stress testing,[26,27] the milking maneuver,[28] and the moving valgus stress test.[29] The examination for posterolateral rotatory instability includes the pivot shift test,[12] the posterolateral drawer test,[30] and the supine and seated push-up tests.[31,32] Longitudinal radioulnar instability is difficult to detect on clinical examination. These patients often have tenderness or dorsal prominence of the ulna at the distal radioulnar joint.

As for any planned arthroscopic procedure, the location and function of the ulnar nerve should be assessed. A previous ulnar nerve transposition makes percutaneous placement of medial portals risky, and open placement is advocated to prevent iatrogenic nerve injury.

Diagnostic Imaging

Imaging can confirm the presence of a proximal radius articular deformity or arthritis (Fig. 10-1). In addition to anteroposterior and lateral views, a radiocapitellar view can help to throw the radial head into profile. Bilateral radiographs of the wrists should be performed to assess for other contributions to the painful or limited rotation, such as radioulnar synostosis or distal radioulnar joint pathology, and to assess for longitudinal radioulnar dissociation. Stress views or a fluoroscopic examination should be considered to rule out valgus, varus, and axial instability if there is any concern resulting from the physical examination. Computed tomography (CT) with sagittal, coronal, and three-dimensional reconstructions can better define the bony anatomy (Fig. 10-2). CT may offer additional information about the ulnohumeral, radiocapitellar, and proximal radioulnar joint spaces and about articular congruity. Loose bodies and heterotopic ossification also may be better defined. Resecting the radial head without addressing these other osseous deformities may result in suboptimal results.

TREATMENT

Indications and Contraindications

The indication for arthroscopic radial head resection is proximal radius articular deformity or arthritis causing pain or impeding motion in the presence of competent medial and lateral collateral ligaments of the elbow and the interosseous membrane of the forearm. Limitation in rotation is particularly amenable to radial head resection. The radial head deformity can cause a mechanical block at the radiocapitellar or proximal radioulnar articulation, or both. The goal of this procedure is to remove the mechanical block, increase rotation, and decrease pain. If the capitellum is relatively intact and judged suitable for prosthetic replacement intraoperatively, radial head excision with prosthetic replacement may be preferred over radial head excision for the reasons previously discussed.

The most common conditions for which arthroscopic radial head resection has been described are rheumatoid arthritis[3-5,20,21] and post-traumatic arthritis (particularly radial head fractures).[2-5,20,21] Radial head resection is sometimes indicated for hemophilic arthropathy of the elbow. Chronic hemophilic synovitis of the elbow can lead to enlargement and irregularity of the radial head. The margins of this hypertrophic radial head impinge against the proximal ulnar facet, acting as a mechanical block to forearm rotation. Reports in the literature of radial head resection for hemophilic arthropathy are limited to open techniques.[22-25] Congenital and acquired radial head dislocations can also be treated by arthroscopic radial head resection in selected cases. Surgical intervention is typically reserved for symptoms refractory to nonoperative measures, such as activity modification and anti-inflammatory drugs. In the setting of rheumatoid arthritis, this includes an adequate trial of disease-modifying medications.

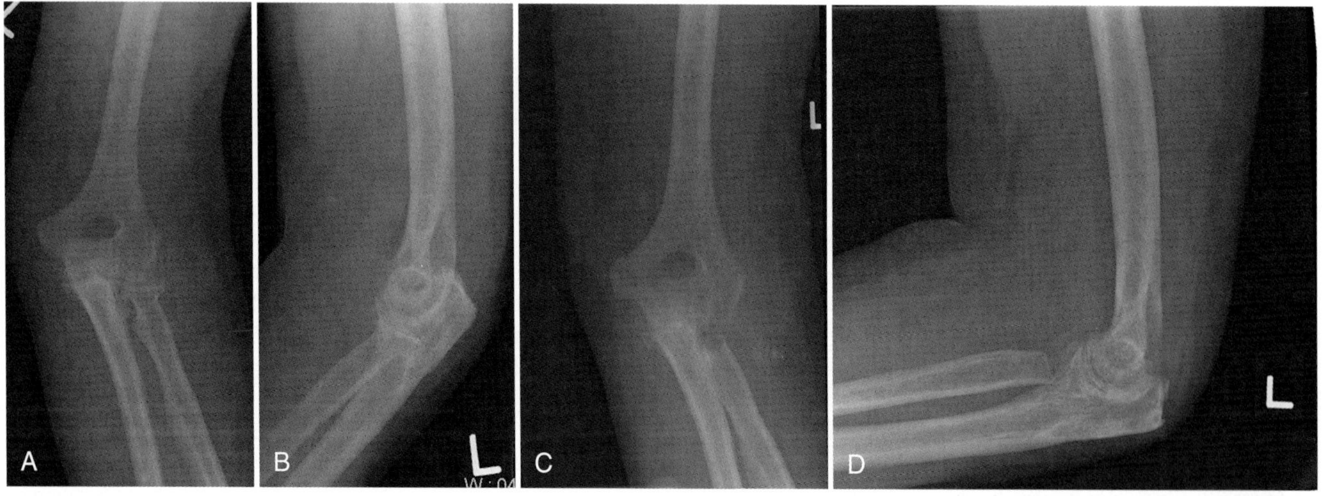

FIGURE 10-1 Imaging was performed for a 65-year-old woman with Mayo grade III rheumatoid arthritis of the left elbow associated with intractable synovitis, painful rotation, and significant radial head deformity. Preoperative flexion was 15 to 140 degrees, with 60 degrees of pronation and 60 degrees of supination. The difference is shown between the preoperative anteroposterior (**A**) and lateral (**B**) radiographs and the anteroposterior (**C**) and lateral (**D**) radiographs obtained after arthroscopic radial head resection.

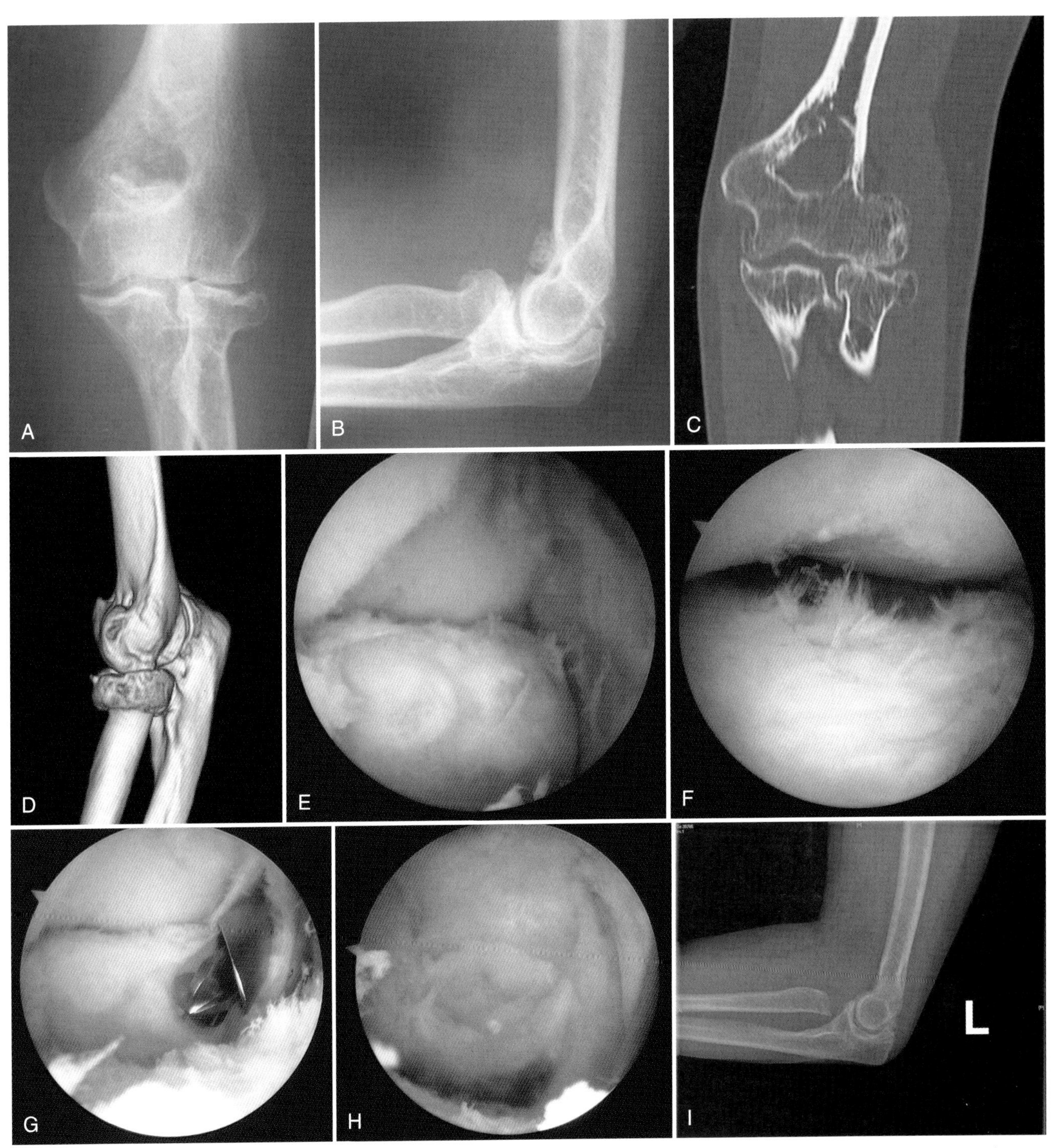

FIGURE 10-2 A 53-year-old woman has post-traumatic arthritis resulting from a remote elbow injury. She had undergone open débridement but presented with persistent posterior impingement and lateral elbow pain. Preoperative radiographs (**A** and **B**) and CT scans (**C** and **D**) reveal the radial head deformity. **E,** The radial head deformity is viewed from a proximal anteromedial portal. **F,** An arthroscopic view shows the associated full-thickness loss of capitellar articular cartilage. **G,** The burr is introduced from an anterolateral portal. **H,** An arthroscopic view shows the appearance after resection of the radial head. **I,** A lateral radiograph shows the joint postoperatively.

Radial head excision is contraindicated in patients with valgus, posterolateral rotatory, or axial instability. The loss of this secondary stabilizer can exacerbate preexisting instability. Advanced ulnohumeral arthritis is a relative contraindication because radial head excision alone cannot address symptoms originating from the ulnohumeral articulation. Radial head excision results in increased loading of the remaining ulnohumeral articulation, which may further exacerbate ulnohumeral joint pain.[8] Radial head replacement and radiocapitellar replacement can be considered when isolated radial head excision is contraindicated, such as in the setting of instability.[33] Older, lower-demand patients with advanced articular destruction and bony deformity may be better treated with a total elbow arthroplasty. Arthroscopic excision of the radial head usually is not recommended for acute radial head fractures because of the high incidence of concomitant ligament injuries.[34,35] The torn capsule in the acute fracture setting can result in significant extravasation of fluid, making it a higher-risk procedure and more technically challenging.

A surgeon's inexperience with arthroscopy of synovitic elbows can be considered a relative contraindication. Arthroscopy of synovitic elbows is technically demanding because synovial proliferation, stiffness, and deformity result in diminished capsular volume, reducing the available working room in the elbow.[36] An inexperienced surgeon may better manage these patients with open surgery because of the increased risk of nerve injuries in the setting of inflammatory arthritis.[37]

Alternative Treatments

Radial head resection is uncommonly indicated and should be avoided if other options are available. Alternative treatment options include open radial head resection, synovectomy alone with retention of the radial head, radial head débridement, radial head replacement, radiocapitellar arthroplasty, and total elbow arthroplasty. Because of the technical difficulty and theoretical increased risk of nerve injury associated with elbow arthroscopy, open radial head resection should be considered in the hands of surgeons who are not experienced with elbow arthroscopy.

Retention of the radial head should be considered in most patients undergoing synovectomy and débridement for rheumatoid and primary osteoarthritis unless there is severe deformity interfering with rotation or there are symptoms specifically referable to the radial head. Removing the stabilizing effect of the radial head can result in long-term overload of the medial collateral ligament, valgus instability, posterolateral rotatory instability, proximal migration of the radius, and progressive articular destruction due to increased ulnohumeral loading.[38,39] Although not well studied, radial head contouring has been used by some surgeons in the setting of rheumatoid arthritis with the aim of improved forearm rotation.[38]

If radial head resection is deemed necessary, radial head replacement can preserve the stabilizing effect of the radial head.[7-9,18,19] However, radial head replacement is not ideal if there is anticipated maltracking of a prosthetic radial head, as seen in the setting of chronic subluxation or dislocation of the proximal radioulnar joint. Likewise, a significantly deformed native capitellum may become a pain generator if it articulates with a radial head hemiarthroplasty, making excision without replacement more ideal in that setting. Radiocapitellar prostheses have recently become available but have not been extensively studied.

Total elbow arthroplasty remains the procedure of choice for patients with more advanced arthritis of the radiocapitellar and ulnohumeral joints.

Arthroscopic Technique

General anesthesia is typically employed. In patients with more severe stiffness and advanced articular damage, a continuous brachial plexus block is useful for postoperative pain control and early mobilization. Standard elbow arthroscopic positioning, equipment, and portals are used. We prefer a lateral decubitus position with the arm positioned over a well-padded bolster. Gravity inflow is used to maintain low pressures to avoid excessive joint swelling. A 4.0-mm arthroscope is used for visualization. The initial view after arthroscope insertion is often poor because of extensive synovitis. A full radius resector is used for synovectomy as needed for visualization (see Chapter 11). In addition to the radial head deformity, the entire elbow should be inspected for the presence of associated abnormalities, such as cartilage defects of the capitellum, synovitis, loose bodies, and capsular contracture.

Resection of the radial head is initiated with the arthroscope in the proximal anteromedial portal and a drainage cannula placed in the posterior central portal for outflow. After achieving an adequate view, a motorized burr is introduced through a cannula placed in the middle anterolateral portal, which is placed at the level of the radial head. To improve visualization and to protect the posterior interosseous nerve, a retractor can be placed in the proximal anterolateral portal.

The radial head is resected in a piecemeal fashion, starting anteriorly and working posteriorly. The cutting surface of the resector should be kept facing in a posterior direction to avoid injury to the posterior interosseous nerve, which lies closely adjacent to the anterior capsule at this level. Resection is continued to the radial neck, just past the level of the sigmoid notch of the ulna. Care should be taken to avoid resection of the annular ligament and the lateral ulnar collateral ligament, which contributes to varus and posterolateral rotatory stability of the elbow. The burr is transferred to a posterolateral (soft spot) portal to complete the posterior resection of the radial head while continuing to view from the proximal anteromedial portal. A full-radius resector and a pituitary rongeur are used to remove the remaining cartilage and bony debris from the joint. An image intensifier is used to confirm that an adequate amount of bone has been resected from the radial neck.

The goal is to resect the head just distal to the sigmoid notch of the ulna so there is no impingement with rotation. The elbow should be supinated and pronated under arthroscopic vision to ensure that there is no remaining mechanical impingement or block to rotation. A fluoroscopic examination of the elbow is performed to evaluate for valgus, varus, posterolateral, and axial instability after resection of the radial head.

The portal sites are sutured to prevent formation of synovial fistulas. A bulky soft compressive dressing is applied for comfort and to allow early elbow range of motion.

PEARLS & PITFALLS

PEARLS

- Radial head resection is uncommonly indicated and should be avoided if other options are available.
- Use brachial plexus block for postoperative pain control and to allow early mobilization.
- Place a retractor in the proximal anterolateral portal to improve visualization and to protect the posterior interosseous nerve while resecting the radial head.
- Rotate the forearm under arthroscopic vision to ensure that there is no remaining mechanical impingement or block to rotation.
- Use fluoroscopy to evaluate the adequacy of bone resection and to assess valgus, varus, posterolateral, and axial instability.

PITFALLS

- Arthroscopic radial head resection is technically demanding and should be performed only by experienced elbow arthroscopists.
- Radial head excision is contraindicated in patients with valgus, posterolateral, or axial instability, because it can exacerbate preexisting instability.
- Radial head excision cannot address symptoms originating from the ulnohumeral articulation.
- Avoid resection of the annular ligament and the lateral ulnar collateral ligament.

Postoperative Management

Postoperative management involves discharge from the hospital on the same day and immediate active range of motion as tolerated. If a concomitant contracture release is performed, the patient is admitted for a continuous regional block for the first few days, combined with immediate rehabilitation efforts with a continuous passive motion device. Indomethacin (25 mg three times daily for 3 weeks) should be considered to reduce the incidence of heterotopic ossification in patients who do not have a contraindication to this medication.[40]

OUTCOMES

Our understanding of the outcomes of arthroscopic radial head resection is based largely on our experience with open radial head resection. The available literature on arthroscopic resection is limited to very few cases with only short-term follow-up.[2-5] There are no published clinical trials comparing the outcomes of open versus arthroscopic radial head resection.

McLaughlin and colleagues[3] reported the largest published series of arthroscopic radial head resections. They reviewed 36 patients who underwent surgery for radiocapitellar joint arthritis at a mean age of 46 years and had a mean follow-up of 52 months. Radiocapitellar arthrosis was caused by post-traumatic radial head fracture in 17 patients, primary osteoarthritis beginning with the radiocapitellar joint in 10 patients, rheumatoid arthritis with radiocapitellar subluxation in 3 patients, arthrofibrosis in 2 patients, and osteonecrosis, psoriatic arthritis, post-radial head fracture synostosis, and acute radial head fracture in 1 patient each. Eight patients underwent arthroscopic radial head resection alone, and the remaining 26 patients underwent a concurrent arthroscopic modification of the Outerbridge-Kashiwagi procedure, which was added if there was concurrent ulnohumeral arthritis. Both groups had similar flexion-extension loss preoperatively. They found that isolated radial head excision resulted in an increased flexion-extension arc averaging 62 degrees, whereas the average was 46 degrees with the combined procedure. Similarly, patients who underwent radial head excision alone had a greater increase in functional scores. All of the eight patients who underwent radial head excision alone were satisfied with the procedure and reported significant pain relief. The study authors concluded that patients treated early in the disease process had greater success overall than those who chose to receive later treatment. Two patients required additional surgery. One required a flexion contracture release, and one underwent radial head replacement for continued pain after excision of the radial head associated with proximal migration of the radial shaft.

Menth-Chiari and coworkers[4] reported a series of 12 patients (10 with post-traumatic arthrosis secondary to radial head fractures and 2 with rheumatoid arthritis) who underwent arthroscopic radial head resections. The average age was 38.5 years, and the mean follow-up was 39 months. Their indication for surgery was chronic mechanical elbow pain with arthroscopic findings of radiocapitellar arthritis primarily involving the radial head. Limitation in range of motion was not a major indication in this series. Eleven of 12 patients were satisfied with the procedure and experienced improved pain, mechanical symptoms, and range of motion. One patient who underwent partial radial head resection suffered from radiocapitellar impingement. Range of motion improved in all patients. The flexion arc improved from a preoperative mean of 23 to 110 degrees to a postoperative mean of 9 to 136 degrees. Preoperatively, two patients had limited pronation (both lacking 5 degrees), and two had limited supination (lacking 15 degrees in one and 30 degrees the other). All patients had full rotation postoperatively. The only complications identified were a moderate loss of strength (that did not interfere with activities of daily living) in three patients and proximal radial migration of 2 and 3 mm in two patients. There was no objective or subjective evidence of elbow instability, cubitus valgus, heterotopic ossification, infection, nerve injury, or vascular injury.

Savoie and associates[5] reported on series of 24 patients treated with an arthroscopic modification of the open Outerbridge-Kashiwagi procedure. Their indication was a painful arthritic elbow with restricted motion refractory to nonoperative treatment. The primary diagnosis was post-traumatic arthritis in 15 patients, rheumatoid arthritis in 5 patients, and primary osteoarthritis in 4 patients. The average age was 59 years, and the mean follow-up was 32 months. The technique they described included arthroscopic synovectomy, débridement, osteophyte removal, olecranon fossa fenestration, and radial head resection when indicated. The radial head was excised arthroscopically in 18 of the 24 patients. They found an increase in range of motion and a significant relief of pain in all of their patients, with 23 of 24 patients being satisfied with their results. The flexion arc improved from a preoperative mean of 40 to 90 degrees to a postoperative mean of 8 to 139 degrees. The 13% complication rate included a superficial infection in one patient, heterotopic ossification in one patient, and recurrent effusions in two patients. There was no report of late instability. One patient who did not undergo radial head resection continued to have radiocapitellar symptoms and required a radial head resection later. Because this study reported the results of treatment of the entire arthritic elbow (i.e., radiocapitellar, proximal radioulnar, and ulnohumeral articulations), it is difficult to extrapolate how much of the improvements seen can be attributed to the radial head resection alone or to the extensive joint débridement and capsulectomy.

These three small series comprise the bulk of information available about the results of arthroscopic radial head resection. However, there are numerous studies documenting the beneficial effects of open radial head excision and synovectomy in early to moderate rheumatoid arthritis.[1,41-49] Improvement in rotation has been consistently reported in this setting.[1] The beneficial effect deteriorates with time, and the procedure seems to fail more quickly in patients with valgus instability after excision of the radial head.[21] Radial head excision unbalances the elbow, concentrating stress on the lateral portion of the ulnohumeral articulation and thereby potentially accelerating degenerative wear.

Gendi and colleagues[42] reported the largest series of open radial head resections for rheumatoid arthritis. Of 115 patients treated by open synovectomy, 113 had a concomitant radial head resection. The average age was 55 years, and the mean follow-up was 6.5 years. The investigators reported a 19% failure rate during the first year and a decline in survival averaging 2.6% per year. Forearm rotation improved by 50 degrees, whereas the flexion-extension range improved by only 10 degrees compared with the preoperative state. Preoperative forearm rotation of less than 50% of normal and preservation of preoperative flexion-extension range were predictors of success. Complications included instability in 18% and recurrent synovitis in 43%, both of which were associated with poor outcomes.

Arthroscopic radial head excision will likely have complications similar to those reported after open resection, including cubitus valgus, proximal radial migration, distal radioulnar joint symptoms, posterolateral rotatory instability, residual radiocapitellar or proximal radioulnar impingement due to inadequate resection, loss of strength, degenerative osteoarthritis, heterotopic ossification, and nerve injury.[11,38,39,50] Although neurovascular structures are at risk with arthroscopic and open procedures, joint distention, the use of retractors, and careful portal placement should reduce the proximity of these structures and thereby reduce the incidence of injury.

CONCLUSIONS

Radial head resection is uncommonly indicated. Surgeons should aim to preserve or replace the radial head when possible to maintain the stability of the elbow and prevent late complications. Elbow instability must be assessed preoperatively, and radial head resection should be avoided if present. Arthroscopic radial head resection may offer theoretical benefits over open resection, such as less injury to the lateral collateral and annular ligaments, an earlier return of function, and less stiffness due to the less invasive surgical approach. However, comparative evidence in the literature is lacking. Much of what we know about the outcomes of arthroscopic radial head resection is extrapolated from our knowledge of open resections. Although complications associated with radial head resection are well recognized, resection of the radial head in selected patients with painful, deformed, and arthritic joints can be rewarding.

REFERENCES

1. Lee BPH, Morrey BF. Synovectomy of the elbow. In: Morrey BF, ed. *The Elbow and Its Disorders*. 3rd ed. Philadelphia, PA: WB Saunders; 2000:708-717.
2. Lo IK, King GJ. Arthroscopic radial head excision. *Arthroscopy*. 1994; 10:689-692.
3. McLaughlin RE, Savoie FH 3rd, Field LD, Ramsey JR. Arthroscopic treatment of the arthritic elbow due to primary radiocapitellar arthritis. *Arthroscopy*. 2006;22:63-69.
4. Menth-Chiari WA, Ruch DS, Poehling GG. Arthroscopic excision of the radial head: clinical outcome in 12 patients with post-traumatic arthritis after fracture of the radial head or rheumatoid arthritis. *Arthroscopy*. 2001;17:918-923.
5. Savoie FH 3rd, Nunley PD, Field LD. Arthroscopic management of the arthritic elbow: indications, technique, and results. *J Shoulder Elbow Surg*. 1999;8:214-219.
6. Morrey BF, Tanaka S, An KN. Valgus stability of the elbow. A definition of primary and secondary constraints. *Clin Orthop*. 1991;(265):187-195.
7. Beingessner DM, Dunning CE, Gordon KE, et al. The effect of radial head excision and arthroplasty on elbow kinematics and stability. *J Bone Joint Surg Am*. 2004;86:1730-1739.
8. Johnson JA, Beingessner DM, Gordon KD, et al. Kinematics and stability of the fractured and implant-reconstructed radial head. *J Shoulder Elbow Surg*. 2005;14:195S-201S.
9. King GJ, Zarzour ZD, Rath DA, et al. Metallic radial head arthroplasty improves valgus stability of the elbow. *Clin Orthop Relat Res*. 1999;(368):114-125.
10. Jensen SL, Olsen BS, Søjbjerg JO. Elbow joint kinematics after excision of the radial head. *J Shoulder Elbow Surg*. 1999;8:238-241.
11. Hall JA, McKee MD. Posterolateral rotatory instability of the elbow following radial head resection. *J Bone Joint Surg Am*. 2005;87A:1571-1579.
12. O'Driscoll SW, Bell DF, Morrey BF. Posterolateral rotatory instability of the elbow. *J Bone Joint Surg Am*. 1991;73:440-446.
13. Morrey BF, Chao EY, Hui FC. Biomechanical study of the elbow following excision of the radial head. *J Bone Joint Surg Am*. 1979;61:63-68.
14. Ikeda M, Oka Y. Function after early radial head resection for fracture: a retrospective evaluation of 15 patients followed for 3-18 years. *Acta Orthop Scand*. 2000;71:191-194.
15. Janssen RP, Vegter J. Resection of the radial head after Mason type-III fractures of the elbow: follow-up at 16 to 30 years. *J Bone Joint Surg Br*. 1998;80:231-233.
16. Leppilahti J, Jalovaara P. Early excision of the radial head for fracture. *Int Orthop*. 2000;24:160-162.
17. Stephen IB. Excision of the radial head for closed fracture. *Acta Orthop Scand*. 1981;52:409-412.
18. Pomianowski S, Morrey BF, Neale PG, et al. Contribution of monoblock and bipolar radial head prostheses to valgus stability of the elbow. *J Bone Joint Surg Am*. 2001;83:1829-1834.
19. Schneeberger AG, Sadowski MM, Jacob HA. Coronoid process and radial head as posterolateral rotatory stabilizers of the elbow. *J Bone Joint Surg Am*. 2004;86A:975-982.
20. Menth-Chiari WA, Poehling GG, Ruch DS. Arthroscopic resection of the radial head. *Arthroscopy*. 1999;15:226-230.
21. Steinmann SP, King GJW, Savoie FH. Arthroscopic treatment of the arthritic elbow. *Instr Course Lect*. 2006;55:109-117.
22. Silva M, Luck JV. Radial head excision and synovectomy in patients with hemophilia. *J Bone Joint Surg Am*. 2007;89:2156-2162.
23. Luck JV Jr, Kasper CK. Surgical management of advanced hemophilic arthropathy. An overview of 20 years' experience. *Clin Orthop Relat Res*. 1989;(242):60-82.
24. Lofqvist T, Nilsson IM, Petersson C. Orthopaedic surgery in hemophilia: 20 years' experience in Sweden. *Clin Orthop Relat Res*. 1996; (332):232-41, 1996
25. Rodriguez-Merchan EC, Magallon M, Galindo E, Lopez-Cabarcos C. Hemophilic synovitis of the knee and the elbow. *Clin Orthop Relat Res*. 1997;(343):47-53.
26. Jobe FW, Stark H, Lombardo SJ. Reconstruction of the ulnar collateral ligament in athletes. *J Bone Joint Surg Am*. 1986;68:1158-1163.
27. Chen FS, Rokito AS, Jobe FW. Medial elbow problems in the overhead-throwing athlete. *J Am Acad Orthop Surg*. 2001;9:99-113.
28. Veltri DM, O'Brien SJ, Field LD, et al. The milking maneuver: a new test to evaluate the MCL of the elbow in the throwing athlete. In: Programs and Abstracts of the 10th Open Meeting of the American Shoulder and Elbow Surgeons. Rosemont, IL: American Academy of Orthopaedic Surgeons; 1994.
29. O'Driscoll SWM, Lawton RL, Smith AM. The "moving valgus stress test" for medial collateral ligament tears of the elbow. *Am J Sports Med*. 2005;33:231-239.
30. O'Driscoll SW. Classification and spectrum of elbow instability: recurrent instability. In: Morrey BF, ed. *The Elbow and its Disorders*. 2nd ed. Philadelphia, PA: WB Saunders; 1993:453-463.
31. Regan WD, Morrey BF. The physical examination of the elbow. In: Morrey BF, ed. *The Elbow and its Disorders*. 2nd ed. Philadelphia, PA: WB Saunders; 1993:73-85.
32. Regan W, Lapner PC. Prospective evaluation of two diagnostic apprehension signs for posterolateral instability of the elbow. *J Shoulder Elbow Surg*. 2006;15:344-346.

33. Shore BJ, Mozzon JB, MacDermid JC, et al. Chronic posttraumatic elbow disorders treated with metallic radial head arthroplasty. *J Bone Joint Surg Am*. 2008;90:271-280.
34. van Riet RP, Morrey BF. Documentation of associated injuries occurring with radial head fracture. *Clin Orthop Relat Res*. 2008;466:130-134.
35. Itamura J, Roidis N, Mirzayan R, et al. Radial head fractures: MRI evaluation of associated injuries. *J Shoulder Elbow Surg*. 2005;14:421-424.
36. Gallay SH, Richards RR, O'Driscoll SW. Intra-articular capacity and compliance of stiff and normal elbows. *Arthroscopy*. 1993;9:9-13.
37. Kelly EW, Morrey BF, O'Driscoll SW. Complications of elbow arthroscopy. *J Bone Joint Surg Am*. 2001;83A:25-34.
38. Kauffman JI, Chen AL, Stuchin S, Di Cesare PE. Surgical management of the rheumatoid elbow. *J Am Acad Orthop Surg*. 2003;11:100-108.
39. Morrey BF. Radial head fracture. In: Morrey BF, ed. *The Elbow and Its Disorders*. 3rd ed. Philadelphia, PA: WB Saunders; 2000:341-364.
40. Gofton WT, King GJ. Heterotopic ossification following elbow arthroscopy. *Arthroscopy*. 2001;17:E2.
41. Woods DA, Williams JR, Gendi NS, et al. Surgery for rheumatoid arthritis of the elbow: a comparison of radial-head excision and synovectomy with total elbow replacement. *J Shoulder Elbow Surg*. 1999;8:291-295.
42. Gendi NST, Azon JMC, Carr AJ, et al. Synovectomy of the elbow and radial head excision in rheumatoid arthritis. *J Bone Joint Surg Br*. 1997;79B:918-923.
43. Lonner JH, Stuchin SA. Synovectomy, radial head excision, and anterior capsular release in stage III inflammatory arthritis of the elbow. *J Hand Surg Am*. 1997;22A:279-285.
44. Ferlic DC, Patchett CE, Clayton ML, Freemand AC. Elbow synovectomy in rheumatoid arthritis. Long-term results. *Clin Orthop Relat Res*. 1987;(220):119-225.
45. Maenpaa HM, Kuusela PP, Kaarela K, et al. Reoperation rate after elbow synovectomy in rheumatoid arthritis. *J Shoulder Elbow Surg*. 2003;12:480-483.
46. Makai F, Chudacek J. Long-term results of synovectomy of the elbow with excision of the radial head in rheumatoid arthritis. In: Hamalainen M, Hagena FW, eds. *Rheumatoid Surgery of the Elbow*. Vol. 15. Basel, Switzerland: Karger; 1991:22-26.
47. Tulp NJ, Winia WP. Synovectomy of the elbow in rheumatoid arthritis: long-term results. *J Bone Joint Surg Br*. 1989;71:664-666.
48. Taylor AR, Mukerjea SK, Rana NA. Excision of the head of the radius in rheumatoid arthritis. *J Bone Joint Surg Br*. 1976;58:485.
49. Rymaszewski LA, Mackay I, Amis AA, Miller JH. Long-term effects of excision of the radial head in rheumatoid arthritis. *J Bone Joint Surg Br*. 1984;66:109-113.
50. Morrey BF, Schneeberger AG. Anconeus arthroplasty: a new technique for reconstruction of the radiocapitellar and/or proximal radioulnar joint. *J Bone Joint Surg Am*. 2002;84:1960-1969.

CHAPTER

11

Arthroscopic Synovectomy for Inflammatory Arthritis

Darryl K. Young • Graham J.W. King

Elbow synovectomy is a well-recognized and accepted form of treatment for the rheumatoid elbow. Although it has traditionally been performed through an open arthrotomy, arthroscopic synovectomy is gaining popularity. Compared with open synovectomy, arthroscopic synovectomy is less invasive, can be done as an outpatient procedure, allows more rapid recovery, and enables better visualization of intra-articular pathology. However, it is a technically demanding procedure in this patient population, and it is associated with a risk of nerve injury. Before performing arthroscopic synovectomy, the surgeon should be familiar with the indications, contraindications, and important technical considerations.

ANATOMY

The early stages of inflammatory arthritis of the elbow are characterized by painful synovitis without articular or bony deformity. If synovitis persists, secondary changes may occur. Progressive ligamentous, cartilaginous, and bony destruction may result in progressive instability and deformity. Proliferation of the synovium or distention of the joint capsule may result in compression of the ulnar or radial nerves. The end stage of disease is characterized by severe cartilage loss, damage to the subchondral bone, and elbow instability that result in a joint that is painful, weak, and unstable.

PATIENT EVALUATION

History and Physical Examination

A complete history and physical examination aid in operative planning. Pain and stiffness are common complaints of early synovitis, whereas instability is usually associated with more advanced disease. The examiner should elicit information to help identify the underlying disease process and prior treatment. Review of systems may reveal other joint involvement by rheumatoid arthritis, skin lesions in psoriatic arthritis, or sequelae of bleeding disorders such as hemophilia.

Physical examination often reveals a boggy swelling posterolaterally, which indicates synovitis or effusion (Fig. 11-1). The range of motion of the elbow and forearm should be documented with the use of a goniometer. If there is a loss of motion, a soft end point suggests a soft tissue cause, such as a tense effusion with synovitis or capsular contracture, whereas a firm end point suggests osseous deformity. For instance, the synovial tissue in patients with hemophilic arthropathy is hypertrophic, highly vascular, and prone to impingement between the articular surfaces. Synovectomy alone cannot address the loss of motion due to a bony abnormality. Limitation in rotation may be caused by radial head deformity and may need to be addressed by radial head resection at the time of the synovectomy (see Chapter 10). In the setting of rotational stiffness, examination and imaging of

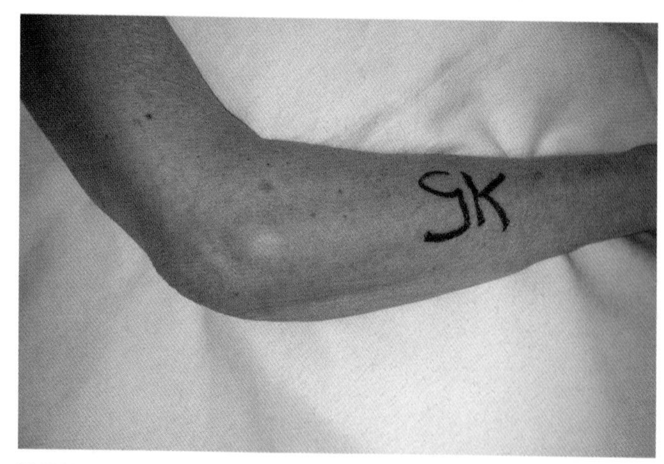

FIGURE 11-1 Lateral swelling is indicative of extensive synovitis in a 65-year-old woman with Mayo grade III rheumatoid arthritis of the right elbow.

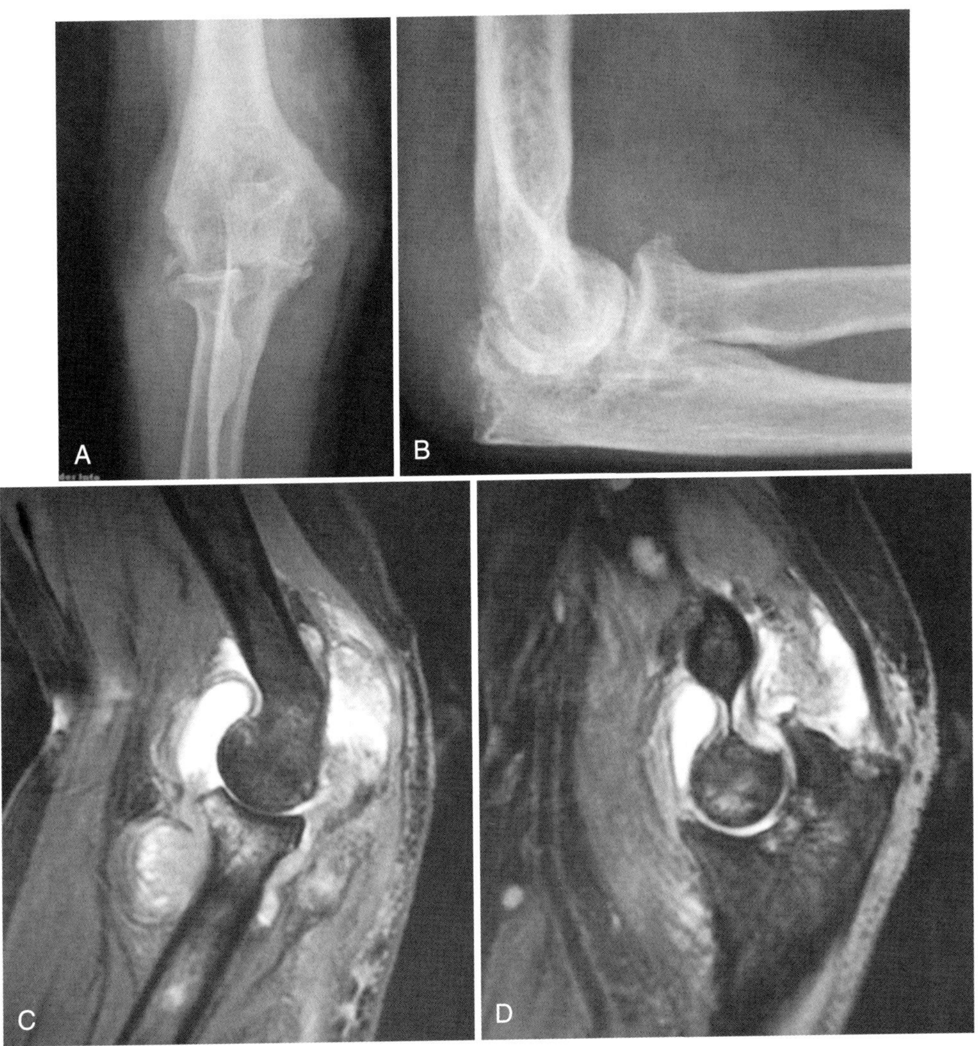

FIGURE 11-2 Preoperative anteroposterior (**A**) and lateral (**B**) radiographs were obtained for a 58-year-old woman with Mayo grade III rheumatoid arthritis with associated intractable synovitis. Preoperative sagittal magnetic resonance imaging shows the radiocapitellar (**C**) and ulnohumeral (**D**) joints.

the wrist are important to rule out pathology of the distal radioulnar joint as a cause, especially in patients with rheumatoid arthritis, in which involvement of this joint is common.

A routine neurovascular examination is important. The posterior interosseous and ulnar nerves may be compressed by synovitis of the elbow. The location of the ulnar nerve also should be assessed. Prior ulnar nerve transposition contraindicates percutaneous placement of medial portals. Preoperative ulnar nerve dysfunction is an indication for in situ release or transposition of the nerve at the time of arthroscopy.

Diagnostic Imaging

Plain radiographs of the elbow reveal the degree of joint destruction, which aids in estimating the expected efficacy of synovectomy in the rheumatoid elbow (Fig. 11-2A and B). The Mayo Clinic classification of rheumatoid elbows,[11] which grades the severity of disease based on the radiographic appearance, can be useful in guiding treatment. Grade I is primarily synovitis with no radiographic changes other than periarticular osteopenia or soft tissue swelling. In grade II, there is narrowing of the joint, but the architecture of the joint is intact. In grade III, there is alteration of the subchondral architecture of the joint, such as thinning of the olecranon or resorption of the trochlea or capitellum. In grade IV, there is gross destruction of the joint. Grade V is ankylosis.

Computed tomography (CT) can better define the osseous anatomy, including osteophytes and deformity of the radial head. Radial head deformities identified on imaging may need to be addressed by radial head resection at the time of the synovectomy (see Chapter 10). Magnetic resonance imaging (MRI) is useful for determining the extent of synovitis and nonossified loose bodies (see Fig. 11-2C and D).

Indications and Contraindications

Rheumatoid arthritis of the elbow is the most common indication for arthroscopic synovectomy in inflammatory arthritis.[1-4] Synovectomy for rheumatoid arthritis of the elbow is indicated in the setting of persistent, painful synovitis with associated loss of function despite an adequate trial of medical management. Although the best results are seen in patients with some preserved articular cartilage and only mild bony deformity, arthroscopic synovectomy also should be considered in patients with more advanced disease who are younger or have pauciarticular disease. Arthroscopic débridement and synovectomy is a reasonable option in this group given the concerns about the longevity of total elbow arthroplasty.

Arthroscopic synovectomy is used to treat patients with hemophilia who have recurrent elbow hemarthroses and synovitis.[5-7] Patients should have failed treatment with factor replacement for 3 to 6 months before being considered for synovectomy.[8] With improved factor replacement, the incidence hemophilic patients with persistent synovitis requiring surgery seems to be decreasing over time. Arthroscopic synovectomy is also indicated for psoriatic arthritis and acute septic arthritis.[9]

Inadequate expertise of the treating surgeon is a contraindication to arthroscopic synovectomy. Arthroscopy of the rheumatoid elbow is technically demanding and has been associated with an increased risk of nerve injury.[12] Patients with greater stiffness and deformity have diminished capsular volume, reducing the working room in the elbow.[13] Initial visualization is often poor, and the capsule is often very thin and friable, increasing the risk of inadvertent capsulectomy and nerve injury. Surgeons with less arthroscopic experience should manage these patients with open surgery or refer them to someone more skilled at advanced arthroscopic techniques of the elbow.

An inadequate trial of medical management is another contraindication to synovectomy for inflammatory arthritis. With improvements in nonsurgical management of rheumatoid arthritis, only patients who fail an adequate trial of disease-modifying agents, usually for a minimum of 6 months, should be considered for arthroscopic synovectomy.

Advanced articular destruction and bony deformity is a relative contraindication. The results of synovectomy are less favorable in this setting. Gross instability, often a result of severe joint destruction, is considered a contraindication, because synovectomy cannot address symptoms related to instability and may instead aggravate these symptoms.[14]

Treatment Alternatives

Alternative surgical treatment options include open synovectomy, combined synovectomy and radial head excision, interposition or excisional arthroplasty, and total elbow arthroplasty. Open synovectomy is a safer option in the hands of surgeons with less arthroscopic experience and is well supported by the literature for the treatment of rheumatoid synovitis in early stages of the disease.[15-30]

Conversion to an open procedure should be performed if there is an inadequate view to proceed safely or a slow progression of the arthroscopy due to technical challenges. Historically, most reports of open synovectomy for rheumatoid arthritis have included a radial head resection.[15-30] Currently, the decision to resect the radial head at the time of synovectomy is based on the degree of radial head deformity and how much it is thought to be contributing to the symptoms. The surgeon should retain the radial head if possible. An unstable elbow can be made worse by removing the stabilizing effect of the radial head (see Chapter 10). Even in a stable elbow, radial head excision increases loading on the ulnohumeral joint and may lead to more rapid progression of arthritis.

Interposition arthroplasty has fallen out of favor in treating inflammatory arthritis, because it tends to be unpredictable compared with total elbow arthroplasty.[31,32] Its use is currently limited to younger patients with polyarticular disease too advanced to benefit from synovectomy and débridement. Total elbow arthroplasty is the procedure of choice for most patients with advanced rheumatoid arthritis, particularly older patients with polyarticular disease.

Arthroscopic Technique

General anesthesia is typically employed. In patients with more severe stiffness, a continuous brachial plexus block is useful for postoperative pain control and to allow early mobilization. We prefer a lateral decubitus position with the arm positioned over a well-padded support. Standard elbow arthroscopic equipment and portals are used. Gravity inflow is used to maintain low inflow pressures to avoid excessive joint swelling. A 4.0-mm arthroscope is used for visualization and a 4.8-mm, full-radius resector is used for the synovectomy. Avoiding more aggressive shavers and opening the outflow to the floor rather than connecting to suction helps to preserve the integrity of the capsule and reduce the risk of nerve injury. Retractors can be used to retract the joint capsule or muscles if needed to improve visualization.

The extensive synovitis often makes the initial view very poor (Fig. 11-3). The full-radius resector should not be turned on until it is confirmed that the instruments are within the joint. The joint synovium is removed with the resector while preserving joint capsule. Visualization improves with the removal of synovium, and the surgeon should proceed cautiously until a good view is obtained. The capsule is typically very thin in rheumatoid elbows, making it easy to inadvertently penetrate or resect. Keeping the tip of the resector in view at all times and pointed away from the capsule can help to protect the capsule. Extra caution should be used when removing synovium anterior to the radial head in the region of the posterior interosseous nerve and in the posteromedial gutter near the ulnar nerve.

We prefer to start the synovectomy in the anterior compartment (Fig. 11-4A to D). The proximal anterolateral portal is the viewing portal, the proximal anteromedial portal is the working portal, and a direct posterior portal is used as an outflow portal with a drainage cannula. The viewing and working portals are exchanged using a switching stick to complete the anterior synovectomy. If the view is insufficient, a middle anterolateral or middle anteromedial portal can be established, and a retractor (e.g., Howarth elevator) is inserted to retract the capsule. The posterior synovectomy is performed next, starting with a direct posterior viewing portal and a middle posterolateral working portal. Care is taken in the area of the medial recess because of the risk of injury to the ulnar nerve. The lateral compartment can be addressed by viewing from the middle posterolateral portal and working through a distal posterolateral (i.e., soft spot) portal, and vice versa (see Fig. 11-4E and F).

Radial head excision should be reserved for patients with a stable elbow and a radial head deformity impeding rotation (see Chapter 10). Osteophyte débridement and capsulectomy may be indicated in some cases, and they can be performed arthroscopically with the synovectomy. Osteophytes that are impeding joint motion are removed with a burr if needed. An anterior or posterior capsulectomy is performed if there is significant restriction of el-

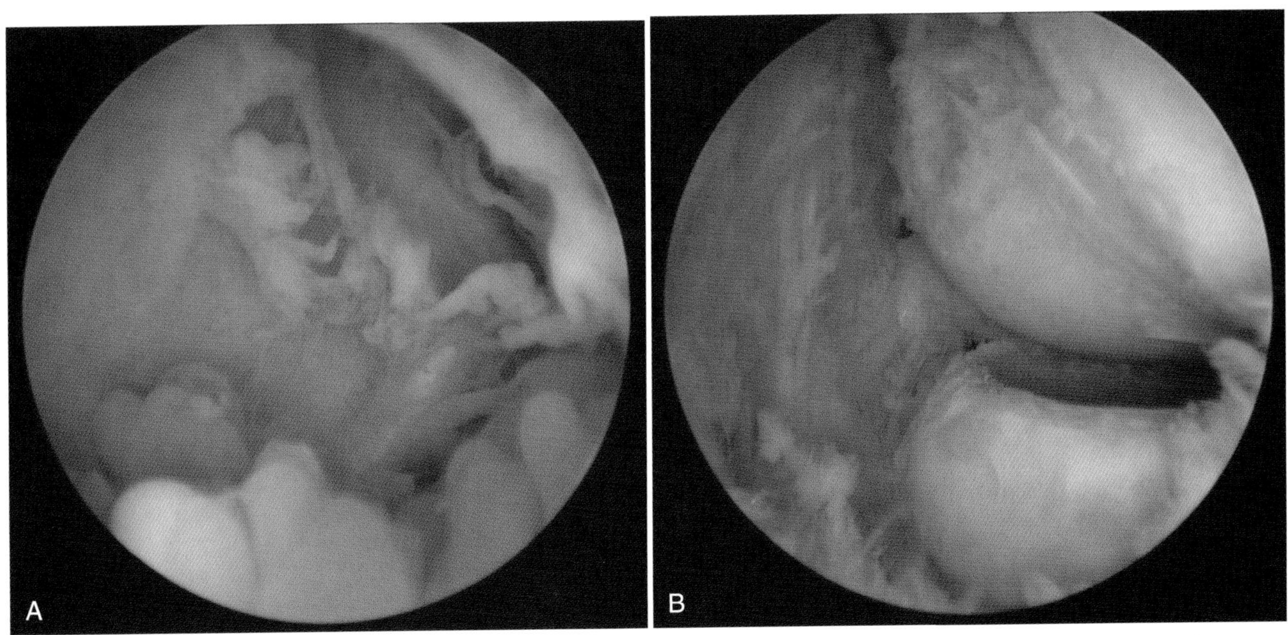

FIGURE 11-3 A, the arthroscopic view reveals the characteristic appearance of proliferative synovitis in patients with inflammatory arthritis. **B,** Improved visualization of the anterior radiocapitellar joint is achieved after synovectomy.

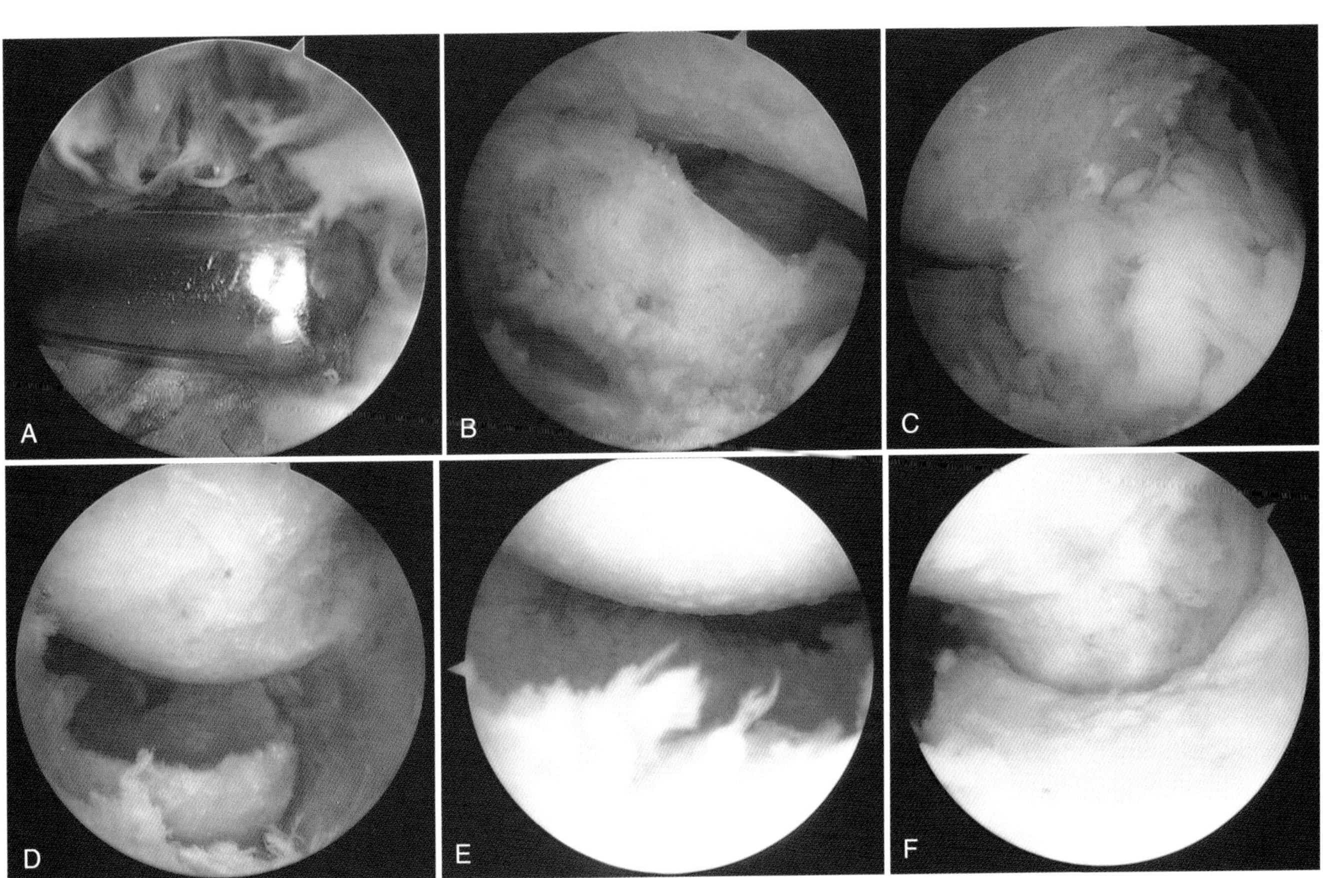

FIGURE 11-4 A 57-year-old woman had with Mayo Grade III rheumatoid arthritis of the left elbow with associated intractable synovitis. **A,** The initial view of the anterior joint from the proximal anterolateral portal reveals extensive synovitis. **B,** The arthroscopic view shows the coronoid after anterior synovectomy. **C,** Synovitis of the radiocapitellar joint is seen from the proximal anteromedial portal. **D,** The arthroscopic view shows the radiocapitellar joint after anterior synovectomy. **E** and **F,** The radiocapitellar and ulnohumeral joints are seen from the distal posterolateral portal after synovectomy.

bow flexion or extension and the patient desires improved motion. Caution should be exercised when removing the anterolateral capsule because of the proximity of the posterior interosseous nerve.

At the conclusion of the procedure, portal sites are sutured to prevent the formation of synovial fistulas. A bulky dressing is applied for comfort and to allow early elbow range of motion.

PEARLS & PITFALLS

PEARLS

- Review CT or MRI scans preoperatively to assess bone structure changes that may prevent normal portal access into the elbow, and change portals accordingly.
- Although visualization may be difficult, do not start shaving without confirming the position in the joint. Always keep the shaver under direct visualization.
- When shaving in the anterior compartment, always keep the shaver blade facing posteriorly; never point it toward the anterior area, where the neurovascular structures are present.
- Suture all portal sites.
- Start range-of-motion exercises early, and add continuous passive motion and physical therapy early if there is evidence of developing stiffness or slow return of motion.

PITFALLS

- Positioning the elbow such that there is inadequate portal access to the anterior compartment due to restrictions from the tourniquet or body.
- The transition from synovium to capsule to brachialis is often muddled in severe inflammatory synovitis, and failure to recognize and protect the brachialis can result in damage to the median nerve and brachial artery.
- Avoid aggressive débridement anterior to the radial neck because the posterior interosseous nerve is located adjacent to the capsule in this area.
- Failure to control swelling and begin motion early can result in postoperative stiffness.

Postoperative Management

Postoperative management depends on extent of the surgery. Synovectomy alone is usually an outpatient procedure managed postoperatively with early active range of motion. The bulky soft dressing is removed by the patient 48 hours postoperatively, and Band-Aids are applied to the portal sites. Sutures are removed at 10 days and physical therapy is initiated if motion recovery is slow. If the procedure is combined with a significant osseous débridement or capsulectomy, patients are admitted for 48 hours and placed on a continuous passive motion machine with a continuous brachial plexus block for postoperative analgesia. For these patients, we prefer to use a nighttime static progressive extension splint for 12 weeks to retain extension.

OUTCOMES

Open elbow synovectomy, with or without radial head excision, is an effective treatment for the rheumatoid elbow.[15-30] The best results are obtained in patients with some preserved articular cartilage and mild bony deformity (corresponding to grade I, II, and early III involvement).[14] Results vary, but studies indicate that 70% to 90% have satisfactory outcomes within the first 3 to 5 years, although these improvements deteriorate with time.[14] There is no evidence that open synovectomy arrests the progress of the disease process. Further studies are needed that employ more potent disease-modifying agents.

The literature provides limited information about the results of arthroscopic synovectomy for rheumatoid arthritis and even less information for other conditions (Table 11-1). Compared with open procedures, arthroscopic synovectomy offers theoretical advantages of being less invasive, which speeds recovery and limits postoperative pain, and allowing the surgeon to better visualize all areas of the elbow and address intra-articular pathology. Although there are no published randomized clinical trials comparing the relative efficacy and risks of open versus arthroscopic synovectomy, reports in the literature suggest that the outcomes of arthroscopic synovectomy are comparable to those of open synovectomy. As with open synovectomy, results deteriorate with time[1,2,4] and depend on the severity of arthritis, with better results expected for elbows without significant osseous destruction and with some preserved articular cartilage.[1,2]

In 1997, Lee and Morrey[1] initially reported good or excellent results for 93% of patients, but these results deteriorated to 57% by 42 months postoperatively. In 2001, Horiuchi and colleagues[2] reported good to excellent results for 71% of patients at 2 years, but the rate deteriorated to 43% by 8 years. However, if elbows with advanced cartilage loss and bony deformity were excluded, the results were 100% and 71% of patients with good or excellent results at 2 and 8 years, respectively. Patients maintained on disease-modifying agents had a lower incidence of recurrent synovitis and a better long-term outcome.

In 2006, Tanaka and coworkers[4] reported a prospective comparative study of arthroscopic versus open synovectomy with 23 elbows in each group. At a mean follow-up of 10 years, 48% of those treated arthroscopically and 70 % of those treated with open procedures had minimal or no pain. There were no significant differences found between the groups with respect to pain, function, or range of motion. Improvements in each of these outcomes deteriorated with time. A subgroup of patients with a preoperative flexion arc of less than 90 degrees had significantly better function when treated arthroscopically instead of with an open procedure.

Less is known about the results of arthroscopic synovectomy for hemophilic arthropathy of the elbow. Although studies are limited to very small numbers and they often combine results of synovectomy of other joints, there is evidence that arthroscopic synovectomy decreases the rate of recurrent hemarthrosis.[5-8]

Transient nerve paresthesias, recurrent synovitis, and persistent pain requiring repeated synovectomy or total elbow arthroplasty have been reported as complications of arthroscopic synovectomy.[1-4,12]

CONCLUSIONS

Although arthroscopic synovectomy is one of the most technically demanding arthroscopic elbow operations, early evidence supports its safety and efficacy. The outcomes and complications likely depend on the arthroscopic experience of the surgeon, the underlying disease severity of the patient, and the concomitant use of disease-modifying medications.

TABLE 11-1 Results of Synovectomy Studies

Study	No. of Elbows	Mean Age (Range)	Mean Follow-up (Range)	Results	Complications
Lee et al,[1] 1997	14	NA but patients < 65 yr	42 mo (24-84)	Pain and function (MEPS) improved, but improvement decreased over time Flexion and rotation improved slightly	One radial and one transient ulnar nerve paresthesia Four patients converted to total elbow arthroplasty
Horiuchi et al,[2] 2002	21	51 yr (19-71)	97 mo (42-160)	Pain and function (MEPS) improved, but improvement decreased over time Flexion improved, no change in rotation Joint arthritic damage increased over time; best results in patients with preserved joint space and those on disease-modifying antirheumatic drugs	Three transient ulnar nerve paresthesias Five with recurrent synovitis, two of which went on to total elbow arthroplasty
Nemoto et al,[3] 2004	11	54 yr (38-68)	37 mo (15-39)	Pain and function improved Flexion improved, no change in rotation Joint arthritic damage increased over time	One repeat synovectomy
Tanaka et al,[4] 2006	23	51 yr (31-64)	156 mo (120-216)	Pain and function improved, but improvement decreased over time Flexion and rotation improved Joint arthritic damage increased over time	Transient neuropraxia of the radial nerve in one and ulnar nerve in one Five with recurrent synovitis

MEPS, Mayo Elbow Performance Score; NA, not available.

REFERENCES

1. Lee BPH, Morrey BF. Arthroscopic synovectomy of the elbow for rheumatoid arthritis. *J Bone Joint Surg Br.* 1997;79B:770-772.
2. Horiuchi K, Momohara S, Tomatsu T, et al. Arthroscopic synovectomy of the elbow in rheumatoid arthritis. *J Bone Joint Surg Am.* 2002;84A:342-347.
3. Nemoto K, Arino H, Yoshihara Y, Fujikawa K. Arthroscopic synovectomy for the rheumatoid elbow: a short-term outcome. *J Shoulder Elbow Surg.* 2004;13:652-655.
4. Tanaka N, Sakahashi H, Hirose K, et al. Arthroscopic and open synovectomy of the elbow in rheumatoid arthritis. *J Bone Joint Surg Am.* 2006;88:521-525.
5. Dunn AL, Busch MT, Wyly JB, et al. Arthroscopic synovectomy for hemophilic joint disease in a pediatric population. *J Pediatr Orthop.* 2004;24:414-426.
6. Tamurian RM, Spencer EE, Wojtys EM. The role of arthroscopic synovectomy in the management of hemarthrosis in hemophilia patients: financial perspectives. *Arthroscopy.* 2002;18:789-794.
7. Journeycake JM, Miller KL, Anderson AM, et al. Arthroscopic synovectomy in children and adolescents with hemophilia. *J Pediatr Hematol Oncol.* 2003;9:726-731.
8. Verma N, Valentino LA, Chawla A. Arthroscopic synovectomy in haemophilia: indications, technique and results. *Haemophilia.* 2007; 13(suppl 3):38-44.
9. Jerosch J, Hoffstetter I, Schroder M, Castro W. Septic arthritis: arthroscopic management with local antibiotic treatment. *Acta Orthop Belg.* 1995;61:126-134.
10. Kamineni S, O'Driscoll S W, Morrey BF. Synovial osteochondromatosis of the elbow. *J Bone Joint Surg Br.* 2002;84B:961-966.
11. Morrey BF, Adams RA. Semiconstrained arthroplasty for the treatment of rheumatoid arthritis of the elbow. *J Bone Joint Surg Am.* 1992;74:479-490.
12. Kelly EW, Morrey BF, O'Driscoll SW. Complications of elbow arthroscopy. *J Bone Joint Surg Am.* 2001;83A:25-34.
13. Gallay SH, Richards RR, O'Driscoll SW. Intra-articular capacity and compliance of stiff and normal elbows. *Arthroscopy.* 1993;9:9-13.
14. Lee BPH, Morrey BF. Synovectomy of the elbow. In: Morrey BF, ed. *The Elbow and Its Disorders.* 3rd ed. Philadelphia, PA: WB Saunders; 2000: 708-717.
15. Woods DA, Williams JR, Gendi NS, et al. Surgery for rheumatoid arthritis of the elbow: a comparison of radial-head excision and synovectomy with total elbow replacement. *J Shoulder Elbow Surg.* 1999;8:291-295.
16. Gendi NST, Azon JMC, Carr AJ, et al. Synovectomy of the elbow and radial head excision in rheumatoid arthritis. *J Bone Joint Surg Br.* 1997; 79B:918-923.
17. Lonner JH, Stuchin SA. Synovectomy, radial head excision, and anterior capsular release in stage III inflammatory arthritis of the elbow: *J Hand Surg Am.* 1997;22A:279-285.
18. Ferlic DC, Patchett CE, Clayton ML, Freemand AC. Elbow synovectomy in rheumatoid arthritis. Long-term results. *Clin Orthop Relat Res.* 1987;(220):119-225.
19. Maenpaa HM, Kuusela PP, Kaarela K, et al. Reoperation rate after elbow synovectomy in rheumatoid arthritis. *J Shoulder Elbow Surg.* 2003; 12:480-483.
20. Makai F, Chudacek J. Long-term results of synovectomy of the elbow with excision of the radial head in rheumatoid arthritis. In: Hamalainen M, Hagena FW, eds. *Rheumatoid Surgery of the Elbow.* Vol. 15. Basel, Switzerland: Karger; 1991:22-26.
21. Tulp NJ, Winia WP. Synovectomy of the elbow in rheumatoid arthritis: long-term results. *J Bone Joint Surg Br.* 1989;71:664-666.
22. Taylor AR, Mukerjea SK, Rana NA. Excision of the head of the radius in rheumatoid arthritis. *J Bone Joint Surg Br.* 1986;58:485-487.
23. Rymaszewski LA, Mackay I, Amis AA, Miller JH. Long-term effects of excision of the radial head in rheumatoid arthritis. *J Bone Joint Surg Br.* 1984;66:109-113.
24. Wilson HDW, Arden GP, Ansell BM. Synovectomy of the elbow in rheumatoid arthritis. *J Bone Joint Surg Br.* 1973;55:106-111.
25. Eichenblat HM, Hass A, Kessler I. Synovectomy of the elbow in rheumatoid arthritis. *J Bone Joint Surg Am.* 1982;64:1074-1078.
26. Brumfield HRH, Resnick CT. Synovectomy of the elbow in rheumatoid arthritis. *J Bone Joint Surg Am.* 1985;67:16-20.
27. Herold N, Schrøder HA. Synovectomy and radial head excision in rheumatoid arthritis: 11 patients followed for 14 years. *Acta Orthop Scand.* 1995;66:252-254.
28. Rodríguez-Merchán EC, Magallón M, Galindo E, López-Cabarcos C. Hemophilic synovitis of the knee and the elbow. *Clin Orthop Relat Res.* 1997;(343):47-53.
29. Linclau LA, Winia WPCA, Korst JK. Synovectomy of the elbow in rheumatoid arthritis. *Acta Orthop Scand.* 1983;54:935-937.
30. Saito T, Koshino T, Okamoto R, Horiuchi S. Radical synovectomy with muscle release for the rheumatoid elbow. *Acta Orthop Scand.* 1986; 57:71-73.
31. Kauffman JI, Chen AL, Stuchin S, Di Cesare PE. Surgical management of the rheumatoid elbow. *J Am Acad Orthop Surg.* 2003;11:100-108.
32. Ljung P, Jonsson K, Larsson K, Rydholm U. Interposition arthroplasty of the elbow with rheumatoid arthritis. *J Shoulder Elbow Surg.* 1996; 5(pt 1):81-85.

CHAPTER

12

Arthroscopic and Open Radial Ulnohumeral Ligament Reconstruction for Posterolateral Rotatory Instability of the Elbow

Felix H. Savoie III • Larry D. Field • Daniel J. Gurley

Dysfunction of the lateral ligamentous complex of the elbow may produce considerable dysfunction in the activities of daily living.[1] Unlike the medial ulnar collateral ligament, whose injury results in disability during athletic activities, the radial ulnohumeral ligament (RUHL) complex is involved in even the simplest activities of the upper extremity. There has been a growing interest in the diagnosis and treatment of posterolateral rotatory instability (PLRI) of the elbow since the original description by O'Driscoll and colleagues in 1991.[1] Because the RUHL complex stabilizes the elbow during supination and extension activities, even mild injury to this area can cause difficulty in lifting and twisting activities, such as turning a key or opening a door.

ANATOMY

The RUHL complex as described by O'Driscoll and coworkers[1] is formed by three separate components that may have a variable expression. The radial collateral ligament is adjacent to the capsule and courses from the lateral epicondyle to the annular ligament and then down to the ulna. The RUHL begins at a variable point on the posterolateral aspect of the lateral epicondyle and courses distally to the crest of the ulna while sending fibers to the annular ligament and blending with the lateral collateral ligament (Fig. 12-1). The annular ligament originates and inserts on the ulna while following a course around the radial neck.

Anatomic studies have attempted to define the involved tissue. Dunning and colleagues[2] stated that the RUHL and the radial collateral ligament must be sectioned to achieve PLRI. They also found that they could not visually differentiate the two ligaments at their humeral origin. They could differentiate the RUHL from the radial collateral ligament only by identifying the distal extent of the RUHL at the supinator crest of the ulna.[2] Seki and associates[3] were able to show that sectioning just the anterior band of the lateral collateral complex induced instability. This suggests that an intact RUHL cannot stabilize

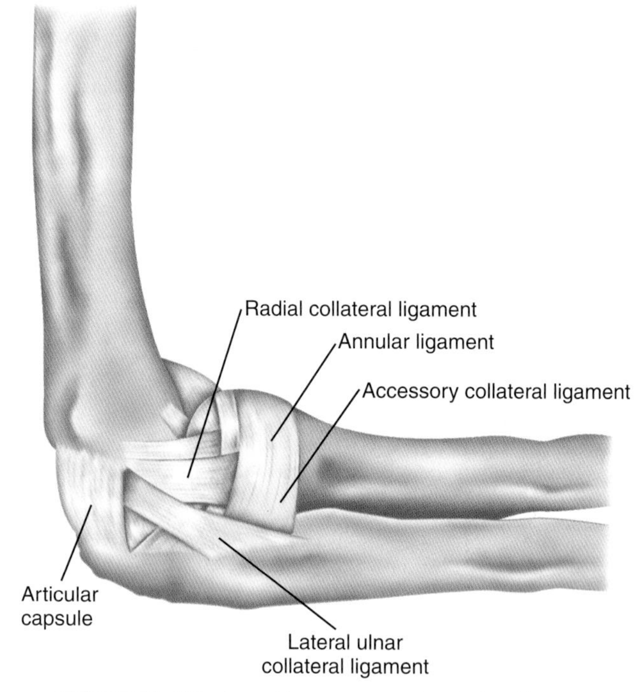

FIGURE 12-1 The lateral ligament complex of the elbow.

the elbow.[3] These data demonstrate that the cause of PLRI is a spectrum of injury. Although originally described as sequelae of an elbow dislocation, these anatomic studies and a report by Kalainov and Cohen[4] support our own experience that there is a continuum of injury between PLRI and frank elbow dislocation.[1,5]

Instability findings may coexist with the standard examination findings of lateral epicondylitis, radial tunnel, and posterolateral plica syndrome. Kalainov and Cohen[4] posit that PLRI may be a cause of these problems of the elbow. Twenty-five percent of patients in their study had previous surgery for chronic, recurrent lateral epicondylitis. We think that uncorrected posterolateral instability of the elbow may result in increased tension on the lateral musculature as it attempts to stabilize the elbow, thereby producing a secondary lateral epicondylitis. Other tertiary findings, such as an inflamed posterolateral plica and inflammation of the posterior interosseous nerve in or near the radial tunnel, may also occur with the instability. Physicians must look for the instability and fully evaluate the elbow of patients with all of these findings. The clinical examination recommended by O'Driscoll and colleagues[1] and by Regan and Lapner[6] can assist in the determination of a coexisting instability as a base cause of these problems in the elbow.

The data suggest that the proximity of the extensor carpi radialis brevis to the RUHL and lateral collateral ligament complex during lateral epicondylitis procedures may contribute to the iatrogenic development of PLRI. In performing a standard extensor carpi radialis brevis tendon release and repair for recalcitrant lateral epicondylitis, the surgeon must remain on the anterior aspect of the lateral epicondyle to avoid damage to the RUHL complex and resultant instability.

Smith and colleagues[5] initially described the role of arthroscopy in treating PLRI, and there have been various anecdotal reports since then.[7] In this chapter, we update and summarize the current information about the diagnosis and management of PLRI.

PATIENT EVALUATION

History and Physical Examination

A patient with PLRI often complains of a popping or catching of the elbow with activities. It is especially noticeable with certain routine daily activities, such as using the arms to help rise from a chair or in doing push-ups. Patients have histories of various injuries, with the spectrum ranging from an inconsequential fall to a frank elbow dislocation.

Instability is best demonstrated clinically with the pivot shift test of the elbow. As first described by O'Driscoll and colleagues,[1] this test with the patient in the supine position may elicit gross instability or pain and apprehension.[1] Two other clinical tests assess (1) pain when pushing up from an arm chair with the palms facing inward and (2) having the patient push up from a prone or wall-leaning position first with the forearms maximally pronated and then repeating the test with the forearms supinated, reproducing pain or instability, or both.[6,8]

We prefer to examine the elbow with the patient in the prone position and use the table as a base to stabilize the humerus. The elbow in this position mimics the examination of a flexed knee, and the findings seem to be more easily reproduced between examiners. We begin by manually trying to rotate the forearm from the humerus in 90 degrees of flexion, palpating the radiocapitellar joint and using the wrist to supinate and rotate the forearm to reproduce the radial column subluxation away from the humerus. The radial head movement on the capitellum is more easily seen and felt in this position, and the elbow can be flexed and extended while maintaining the subluxation force.

Diagnostic Imaging

Imaging studies for PLRI can be helpful. Radiographs may reveal an avulsion fragment from the posterior humeral lateral epicondyle in acute cases. However, radiographic findings often are normal. A stress radiograph or fluoroscopic scan while performing the pivot shift test may show the radial head and proximal ulna moving together in a subluxated and posterolaterally rotated position. Magnetic resonance imaging (MRI) of the elbow can identify a lesion in the RUHL.[9] It has been our experience that MRI is most helpful when contrast is added. This can be done for formal arthrography or, in the case of office MRI, an injection of 20 to 30 mL of sterile normal saline with or without gadolinium delivered into the olecranon fossa just before the scan can greatly enhance the effectiveness of the test.

TREATMENT

Indications and Contraindications

The indications for treatment of PLRI are the same as for any other injury: pain and functional impairment. Although much has been written about the pathologic anatomy and biomechanics of the lesion, little has been reported on the surgical treatment of these patients. Consequently, no level 1 studies comparing the effectiveness of operative or nonoperative management of this disorder have been published, nor are there any large published series describing the outcomes of the surgical treatment of PLRI. In the following sections, we review the outcomes of our experiences with arthroscopic repair, plication, and open grafting techniques.[5]

Nonoperative Treatment

In many patients, the functional disability produced by the milder versions of PLRI may be managed conservatively. Strengthening of the extensor wad of the elbow and tactile feedback of a simple elbow sleeve may allow the patient to control the subluxation events. Selective use of anti-inflammatory cream and gel compounds massaged directly into the posterolateral plica may help to reduce symptoms. When these simple feedback techniques fail to control the instability, surgical stabilization may be required.

Arthroscopic Technique

The surgical treatment of posterolateral instability may be divided into distinct subgroups based on cause: acute dislocations, recurrent dislocations, and PLRI. The procedures used may also be divided into subgroups based on available tissue at the time of reconstruction: repair of ligamentous avulsion, plication of the

RUHL complex with or without repair to bone, and tendon graft reconstruction.

Repair of Simple and Recurrent Dislocations

The anatomic injury pattern associated with simple and recurrent dislocation is avulsion of the humeral attachment of the RUHL complex. Most cases of simple dislocation respond to nonoperative management. The most common complication in the management of the acutely dislocated elbow is stiffness, not instability. However, several subsets may benefit from operative intervention: patients with a humeral avulsion fracture seen on radiographs, patents requiring a high level of function, those with damage to multiple areas of the joint, and those with recurrent instability after a satisfactory closed reduction or acute arthroscopic repair of the RUHL complex.

Arthroscopy of the acutely injured elbow demands efficiency and precision. A concrete preoperative plan must be formulated and followed, with adjustment made for arthroscopic findings. Patients with significant coronoid fracture, associated radial head fracture, or distal humerus fracture are not included in this chapter, but they may also be managed by arthroscopic means.

The procedure begins with establishment of a proximal anteromedial portal and diagnostic anterior compartment arthroscopy. In the acute setting, it may be necessary to establish a lateral portal to clean out the associated hematoma (Fig. 12-2). Tearing of the anterior capsule is readily apparent. In acute dislocations, the surgeon can often also see the damage to the brachialis muscle through the torn capsule (Fig. 12-3). The annular ligament should be surveyed for damage, and a suture is placed in it if necessary. The surgeon also can view around the corner of the proximal capitellum for damage to the collateral ligament part of the RUHL complex. In the acute setting, injuries to this ligament can tear the capsule in this area, and the musculature can be seen through the tear.

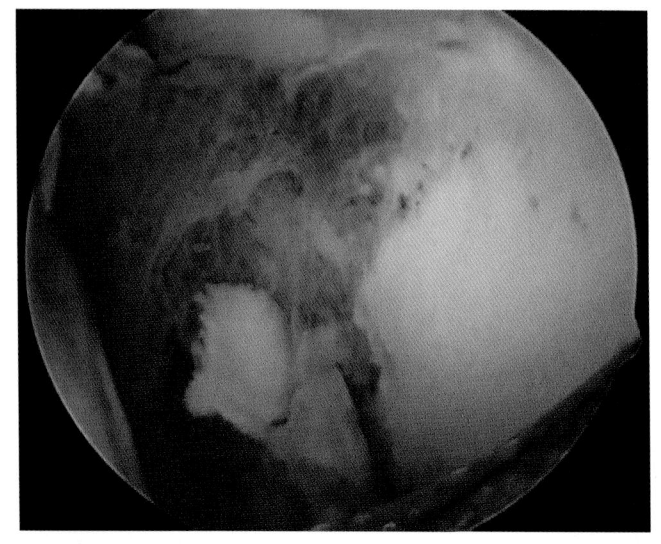

FIGURE 12-2 The anterior view from the proximal anteromedial portal of the elbow reveals an associated hematoma, which often is seen in an acute dislocation.

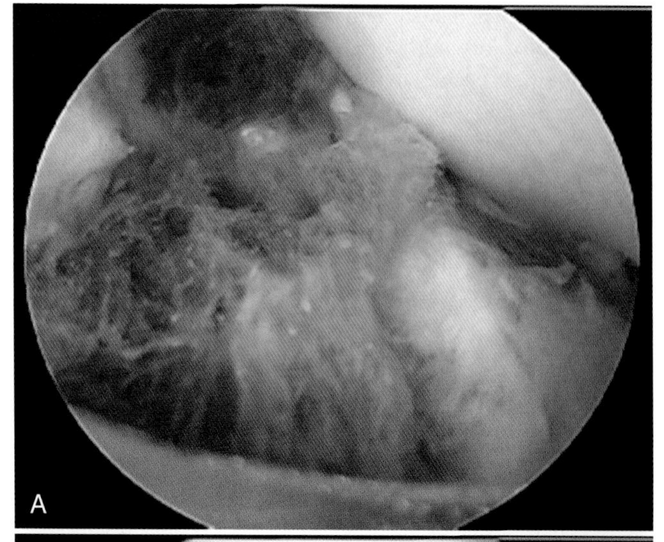

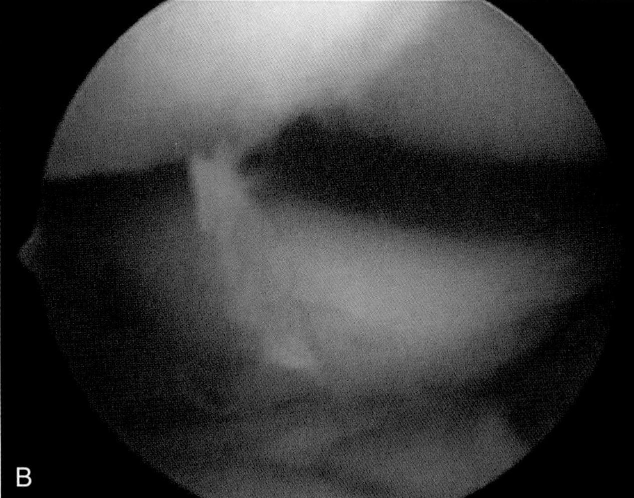

FIGURE 12-3 A, The arthroscopic view shows the damaged brachialis and torn anterior capsule that usually is the result of a traumatic dislocation. **B,** The laxity seen in the annular ligament and the displacement of the radial head from the capitellum in acute and chronic posterolateral rotatory instability are visualized from the proximal anteromedial portal.

The arthroscope is placed into the posterior central portal, and the hematoma in the back of the elbow compartment evacuated through a proximal posterior lateral portal. Both portals need to be relatively proximal, usually at least 3 cm above the olecranon tip, to allow the later repair of the ligament. A view of the medial gutter shows hemorrhage and sometimes shows tearing of the capsule near the posterior aspect of the medial epicondyle (Fig. 12-4).

The lateral gutter and capsule are evaluated. It is important to stay close to the ulna as the lateral gutter is evaluated and the hematoma débrided, because the avulsed ligament and bone fragments are displaced distally and may inadvertently be removed by the shaver (Fig. 12-5). The lateral aspect of the posterior humerus should be lightly débrided and the site of avulsion localized. It is usually directly lateral and slightly inferior to the center of the olecranon fossa, and it is easily seen after the hematoma has been removed.

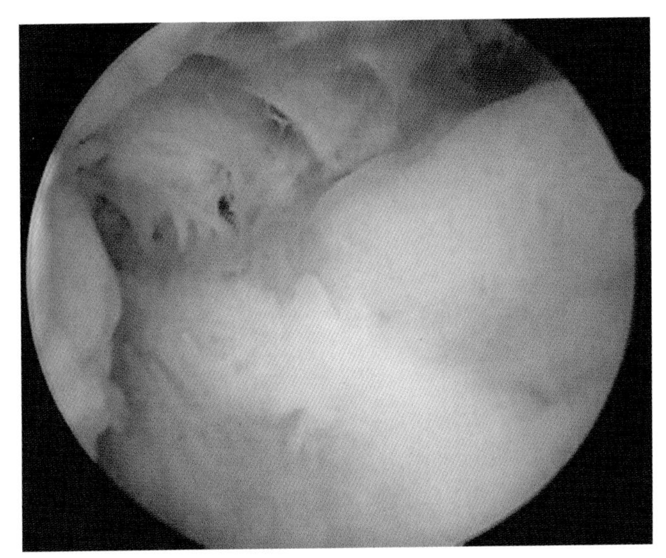

FIGURE 12-4 The posterior portals often reveal concomitant tearing of the capsule and the posterior band of the medial ulnar collateral ligament in acute instability cases.

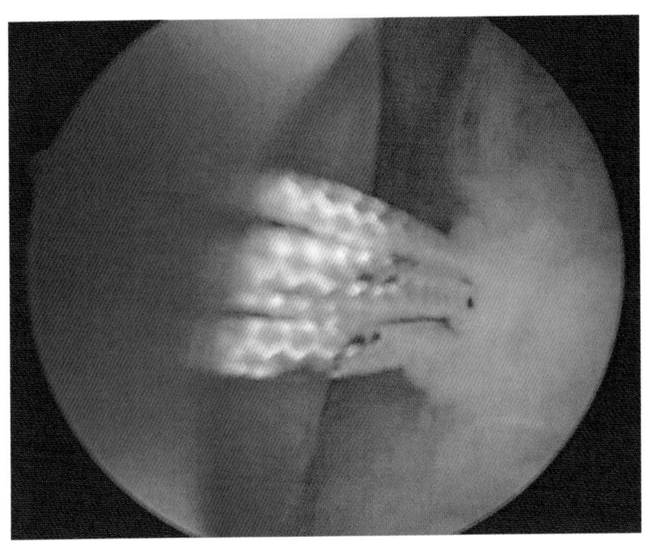

FIGURE 12-6 The site of anchor placement into the origin of the radial ulnohumeral ligament complex from the humerus is usually found lateral and slightly distal to the olecranon fossa of the humerus. This view is obtained from a straight posterior portal.

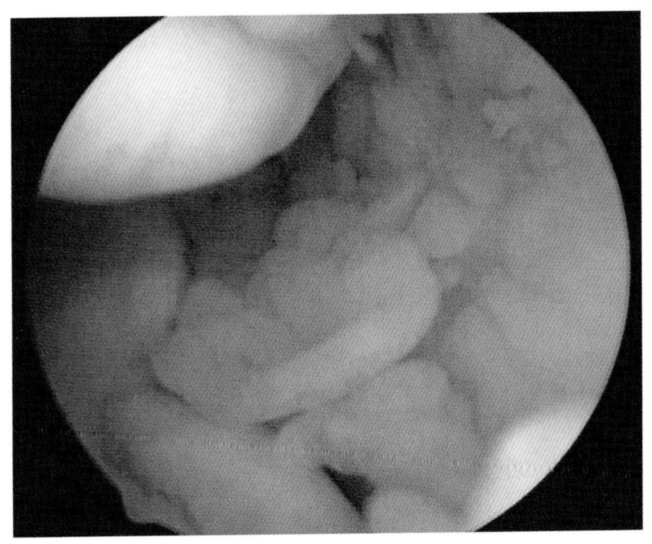

FIGURE 12-5 In acute and recurrent instability cases, the origin of the radial ulnohumeral ligament complex from the humerus and the distal displacement are revealed by the bone fragments and the ragged proximal edge of the ligament when the lateral gutter is evaluated.

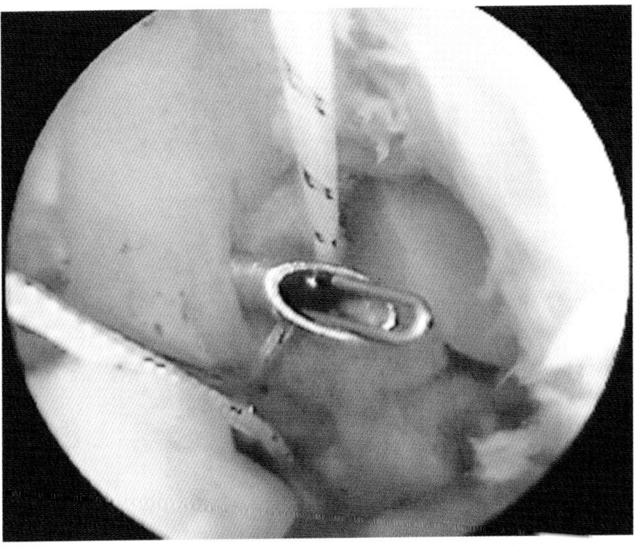

FIGURE 12-7 After anchor placement the attached multiple sutures are retrieved sequentially around the bone fragment and distal to the proximal end of the radial ulnohumeral ligament complex in preparation for repair.

After the area of damage has been defined, an arthroscopic anchor may be placed into the humerus at the origin of the RUHL (Fig. 12-6). The limbs of the suture are retrieved to place two horizontal mattress sutures through the noninjured part of the ligament. In the case of a bony avulsion, we place one set of sutures around the bone fragment and the other distal to the fragment (Fig. 12-7). The sutures are tensioned while viewing with the arthroscope, which should have the effect of pushing the arthroscope out of the lateral gutter. The elbow is then extended, and the sutures are tied beneath the anconeus muscle, tightening the ligament. Motion and stability are then evaluated with the arthroscope in the anterior compartment (Fig. 12-8). This ligament is lax in extension and tightens with flexion. We usually recommend placing the elbow in pronation and 45 to 60 degrees of flexion during tensioning to prevent overtightening and the resultant loss of flexion.

Arthroscopic Plication for Recurrent Posterolateral Rotatory Instability

The development of arthroscopic plication for recurrent or chronic PLRI was described by Smith and colleagues in 2001.[5] Chronic posterolateral instability is more readily seen during examination under anesthesia and by arthroscopic evaluation. While viewing from the proximal anteromedial portal, the ulna and radial head can be seen to subluxate posterolaterally during the performance of a pivot shift test. In most cases, the annular ligament is intact as the entire proximal radioulnar joint shifts on the humerus. A com-

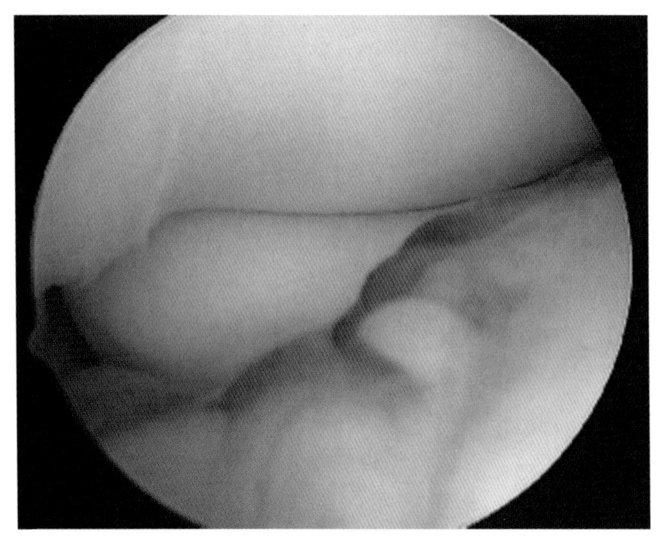

FIGURE 12-8 The sutures are tensioned while the elbow is ranged for stability. The ligament is then repaired back to the humerus with the elbow positioned between 45 and 90 degrees of flexion. The repaired ligament is visualized from the posterior portal.

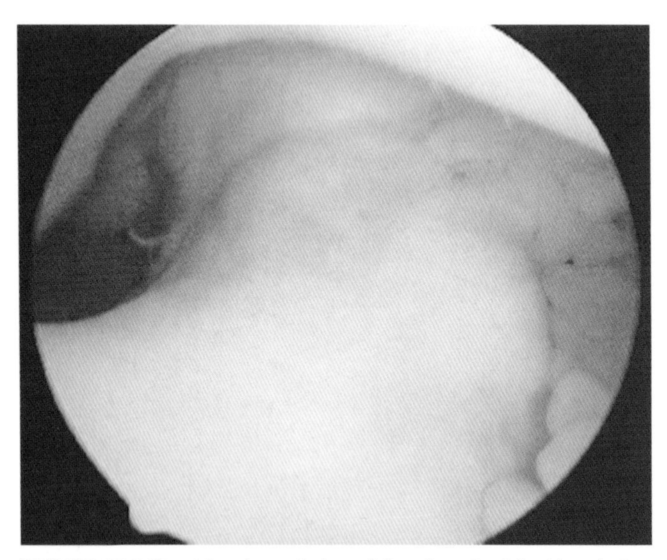

FIGURE 12-9 The drive-through sign of the elbow is elicited by placing the arthroscope into the lateral gutter and moving it straight across the ulnohumeral articulation into the medial gutter.

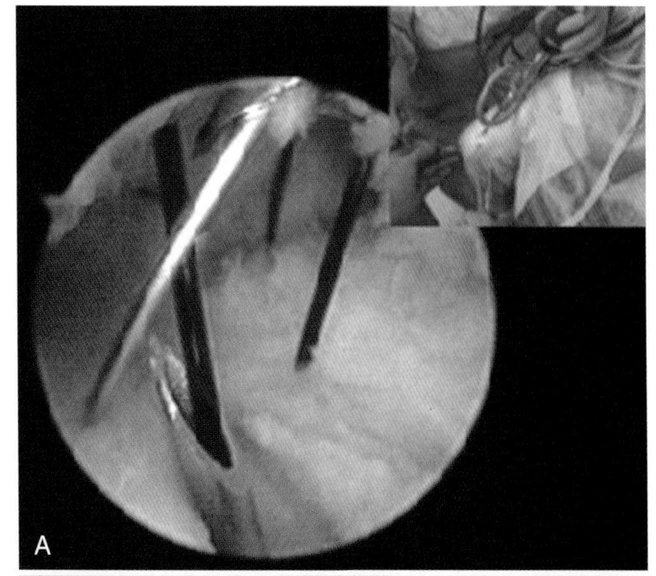

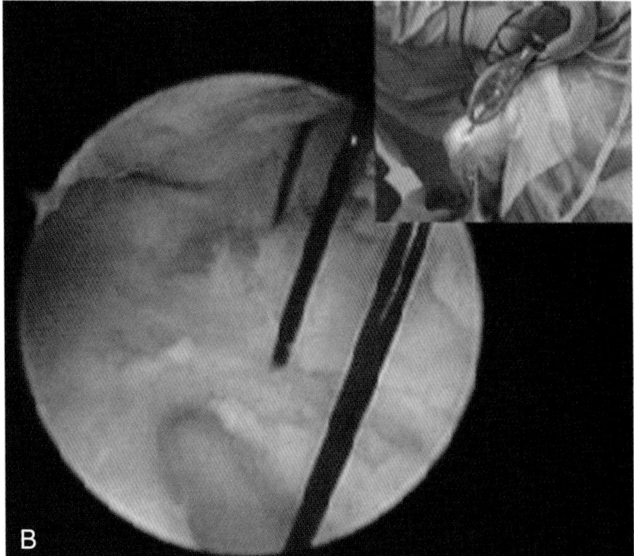

FIGURE 12-10 A, Multiple sutures are placed and retrieved using a retrograde retriever introduced along the posterior aspect of the lateral epicondyle and under the proximal end of the radial ulnohumeral ligament complex. **B,** As the sutures are tied sequentially, the view down the radial gutter is eliminated, as is the drive-through sign of the elbow.

mon finding is the ability to move an arthroscope placed down the posterolateral gutter from the posterior central portal straight across the ulnohumeral articulation into the medial gutter. This maneuver, called the ***drive-through sign***, is not possible in a stable elbow. It is somewhat analogous to the drive-through sign in shoulder instability (Fig. 12-9). Elimination of this drive-through sign is one of the key aspects of confirming an adequate arthroscopic reconstruction in patients with PLRI.

The arthroscopic technique for chronic instability has two key features: plication of the two major components of the complex and repair of the complex to the humerus. Both components can be managed with arthroscopic techniques if there is enough ligamentous and capsular tissue. This assessment is in part determined by the preoperative evaluation, including palpation of the structures in the area to be reconstructed, the amount of prior surgery, and the amount of tissue seen on MR arthrograms.

If adequate tissue is present, the tissue in the posterolateral gutter is assessed arthroscopically and prepared with a shaver or rasp. Four to seven absorbable sutures are placed in oblique fashion, beginning at the most distal extent of the RUHL complex attachment to the ulna. The sutures are placed into the lateral gutter with an 18-gauge spinal needle that slides along the radial border of the ulna. The first suture is delivered into the joint through the midportion of the annular ligament (Fig. 12-10A). Subsequent sutures are brought into the joint in a progressively more proximal position. Each suture is immediately retrieved with a retrograde suture retriever that passes into the joint from the posterolateral aspect of the lateral epicondyle (see Fig. 12-10B) using the curve of the retriever to hook under the radial collateral ligament. The retrograde retriever must come under the entire RUHL near its proximal attachment to the humerus. After all the sutures have been placed, they are retrieved one at a time percutaneously through the existing skin portals under or, in some cases, over the anconeus muscle and pulled to tension the sutures and evaluate the plication.

The surgeon can see the ulna move up to the humerus if the suture placement is correct. As the sutures are tied sequentially from distal to proximal, the arthroscope should be pushed out of the lateral joint. The examination under anesthesia is repeated with the arthroscope placed first in the posterior central portal and then in the proximal anteromedial portal while the PLRI pivot shift test is performed to evaluate the adequacy of the reconstruction. If laxity or subluxation remains after the sutures are pretensioned, an anchor can be placed at the isometric point of the lateral epicondyle, as in the acute repairs, and one limb of the suture can be passed under all of the loops of the plication sutures to a retriever and then retrieved back over the plicated sutures to pull the entire plicated complex back to the humerus. This is usually part of the preoperative planning and is accomplished before the plication sutures are tied.

PEARLS & PITFALLS

PEARLS

- Visualize the anatomy anteriorly from a proximal anteromedial portal.
- Always have the 70-degree arthroscope available to look down the lateral gutter and around the corner of the radial head.
- Use the prone or lateral decubitus position so that fluid runs downhill and out of the field.
- Wrap the forearm tightly so that fluid can egress at the end of the case and avoid a compartment syndrome.

PITFALLS

- Tightening the ligament or graft with the elbow fully extended can prevent the patient from regaining a full arc of motion unless the reconstruction fails.
- Do not spend time managing nonessential pathology; focus on the lesions that produce the problem.
- Maintain access by using cannulas and a low rate of flow.

Postoperative Management

In acute and chronic cases, the patients are placed in a splint or brace with the elbow in approximately 30 degrees of extension to relax tension on the repair. Fluoroscopy or radiography should be used to check the reduction after the splint is applied, because additional flexion may be necessary to tighten the reconstruction and keep the joint reduced. The first postoperative visit usually takes place within 3 to 5 days of the operation, and the patient is placed into a hinged elbow brace that allows comfortable movement, usually 0 to 45 degrees.

Shoulder, periscapular, wrist, and hand exercises are initiated and allowed as long as they do not produce pain in the elbow. The patient is seen at 2-week intervals, and motion is slowly increased as pain and swelling allows. After the repair begins to mature, usually between 5 and 8 weeks, physical therapy is increased to include more aggressive upper extremity and core exercises with the elbow brace in place. We expect normal motion of the elbow by 8 weeks postoperatively, if not earlier. Depending on individual progression, patients are allowed to start strengthening exercises out of the brace at 10 to 12 weeks. They must be able to perform all strengthening exercises in the brace without pain before progression to exercise out of the brace.

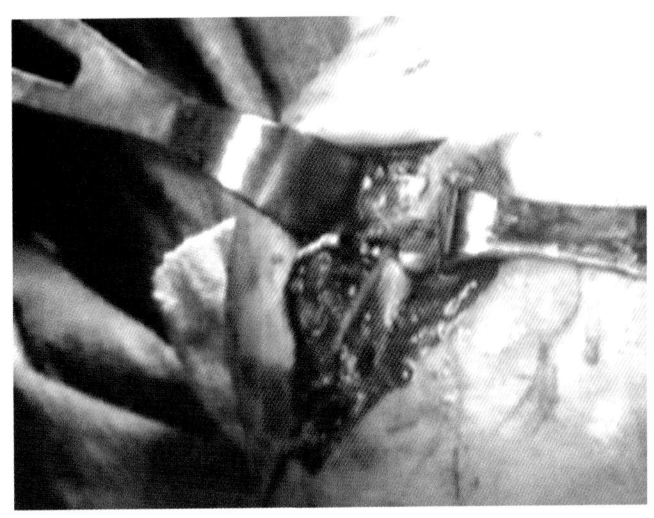

FIGURE 12-11 Anatomic picture of the graft reconstruction for posterolateral rotatory instability.

Open Technique

The open technique for plication and repair is similar to that described by O'Driscoll and colleagues.[1] After diagnostic arthroscopy confirms the instability and the absence of associated pathology, an extensile posterolateral approach is used, and the anconeus muscle is split or retracted anteriorly to access the RUHL complex. The ligaments are plicated and then repaired back to the humerus, as described for arthroscopic repair, if tissue is adequate to allow repair.

In patients undergoing revision surgery or in patients with inadequate tissue for repair, a palmaris longus or gracilis autograft may be used to reconstruct the joint. The supinator crest of the ulna just posterior to the radial neck is dissected free, and the insertion site is identified. A 4- to 6-mm tunnel is created in this spot. A Beath pin is drilled from this point out the ulnar side of the ulna and used to pull a passing suture out this side of the arm. The midportion of the graft is then pulled into the ulna and fixed using an interference screw technique. The two free graft limbs are then brought superiorly, pulling one under the annular ligament and one over the ligament, and they are attached to the isometric point on the posterior aspect of the lateral epicondyle. The graft should be slightly lax in extension and tighten with flexion (Fig. 12-11).

OUTCOMES

Savoie and associates published some of their data regarding the results of surgery for injuries to the lateral ligaments.[10] The results of the arthroscopic procedures were equal to those of open repair or grafting in their series. In the series, 54 patients had a PLRI repair, plication, or graft performed. Forty-one patients (20 arthroscopic, 21 open) had a combined plication and repair, 10 patients (6 open, 4 arthroscopic) had acute or subacute repairs for recurrent elbow instability, and 3 patients (all open) were reconstructed with a free tendon graft. Ten of the 20 arthroscopically treated and 11 of the 21 open plication or repair patients had the addition of an anchor to supplement the arthroscopic suture plication.

The average follow-up was 41 months (range, 12 to 103 months). Overall Andrews-Carson scores for all repairs improved from 145 to 180 ($P < .0001$).[7] Subjective scores improved from 57 to 85 ($P < .0001$), and objective scores improved from 88 to 95 ($P = .008$). Subdividing the technique yielded these overall results: arthroscopic repairs improved from 146 to 176 ($P = .0001$), and open repairs improved from 144 to 182 ($P < .001$). Acute repairs seemed to perform the best, with 9 of 10 patients returning to normal activities and 1 patient returning to near-normal activities. There was no statistical difference between the results of open and arthroscopic repairs.

CONCLUSIONS

The diagnosis of PLRI is made by a combination of positive clinical findings and radiologic confirmation, and it may be supplemented by arthroscopic confirmation of instability, including varus opening, the arthroscopic drive-through sign of the elbow, and abnormal movement of the radial head and proximal radioulnar joint on the humerus. The posterolateral pivot shift test described by O'Driscoll and colleagues[1] may be performed with the patient supine or prone, and combined with the internal rotation push-up and chair lift tests of Regan and Lapner,[6] it provides a clear clinical picture of instability.

Arthroscopic repair or plication is an effective method of managing PLRI. Although it is rarely necessary, surgeons should always be prepared to use a supplemental graft. We used a semitendinosus allograft with satisfactory results. We found the number of previous operations and the time from the initial injury to definitive treatment to be the best predictors of the need for a graft.

The four clinical tests for posterolateral instability are the supine pivot shift, prone pivot shift, internal rotation wall push-up, and chair push-up. MR arthrography provides the best assistance in evaluating the condition of the RUHL complex. In surgical cases, arthroscopic confirmation of the instability can be provided by the elbow drive-through sign from the posterior portal and by abnormal movement of the radial head and proximal radial ulnohumeral articulation on the humeral capitellum while viewing from the proximal anteromedial portal. Reconstructive techniques may be performed arthroscopically as a repair or a plication, or both, with a high rate of success.

REFERENCES

1. O'Driscoll SW, Bell DF, Morrey BF. Posterolateral rotatory instability of the elbow. *J Bone Joint Surg Am*. 1991;73:440-446.
2. Dunning CE, Zarzour ZD, Patterson SD, et al. Ligamentous stabilizers against posterolateral rotator instability of the elbow. *J Bone Joint Surg Am*. 2001;83A:1823-1828.
3. Seki A, Olsen BS, Jensen SL, et al. Functional anatomy of the lateral collateral ligament complex of the elbow: configuration of Y and its role. *J Shoulder Elbow Surg*. 2002;11:53-59.
4. Kalainov DM, Cohen MS. Posterolateral rotatory instability of the elbow in association with lateral epicondylitis. A report of three cases. *J Bone Joint Surg Am*. 2005;87:1120-1125.
5. Smith JP, Savoie FH, Field LD. Posterolateral rotatory instability of the elbow. *Clin Sports Med*. 2001;20:47-58.
6. Regan W, Lapner PC. Prospective evaluation of two diagnostic apprehension signs for posterolateral instability of the elbow. *J Shoulder Elbow Surg*. 2006;15:344-346.
7. Andrews JR, Carson WG. Arthroscopy of the elbow. *Arthroscopy*. 1985; 1:97-107.
8. Yadao MA, Savoie FH, Field LD. Posterolateral rotator instability of the elbow. *Inst Course Lect*. 2004;53:607-614.
9. Potter HG, Weiland AJ, Schatz JA, et al. Posterolateral rotator instability of the elbow: usefulness of MR imaging in diagnosis. *Radiology*. 1997; 204:185-189.
10. Savoie FH, Field LD, Gurley DJ. Arthroscopic and open radial ulnohumeral ligament reconstruction for posterolateral rotatory instability of the elbow. *Hand Clin*. 2009;25:323-329.

CHAPTER

13

Arthroscopy in the Throwing Athlete

Christopher C. Dodson • Robert L. Parisien • David W. Altchek

Excessive valgus and extension forces are generated during the throwing motion in several sports, especially baseball, tennis, football, and certain track and field events.[1] The repetition required to excel in these sports can ultimately lead to fatigue and even failure of key stabilizing structures in the elbow. The medial ulnar collateral ligament (MUCL) is the primary restraint to a valgus load during the throwing motion and is most susceptible to injury after repetitive throwing. MUCL insufficiency leads to valgus instability, a condition that is significant only in overhead athletes. Over time, chronic valgus instability can result in a unique constellation of elbow pathologies that are indicative of repetitive overhead throwing.

Several investigators have described the most common injuries seen in the elbow of the throwing athlete, including MUCL injuries, ulnar neuritis, posteromedial impingement with osteophyte formation, flexor-pronator strain, ulnar stress fractures, osteochondritis dissecans of the capitellum, and capsular contracture.[2-8] Although not all pathology in the thrower's elbow is amenable to arthroscopic management, clinicians who care for throwing athletes must be familiar with all pathologic conditions and comfortable with open and arthroscopic treatments.

During the past decade, clinicians have gained a better understanding of the complex interplay between the dynamic and static stabilizers of the elbow. The desire for minimally invasive treatment of these conditions has led to the development of advanced techniques and instrumentation for elbow arthroscopy. This discussion is limited to the arthroscopic treatment of common elbow injuries in throwing athletes, including those that can be managed entirely arthroscopically and in conjunction with a common open procedure for valgus instability (e.g., MUCL reconstruction).

ANATOMY

The elbow is a hinge joint with the bony ulnohumeral articulation that provides stability at the extremes of motion, from 0 to 20 degrees of flexion and beyond 120 degrees of flexion.[3] The intervening 100 degrees, which is the primary arc of motion used in overhead throwing, relies progressively on the static and dynamic soft tissue restraints to provide stability.

The MUCL is not a single ligament but is rather a complex consisting of an anterior bundle, a posterior bundle, and a transverse component (Fig. 13-1).[9] The anterior bundle is the most well-defined structure, and it originates on the medial epicondyle

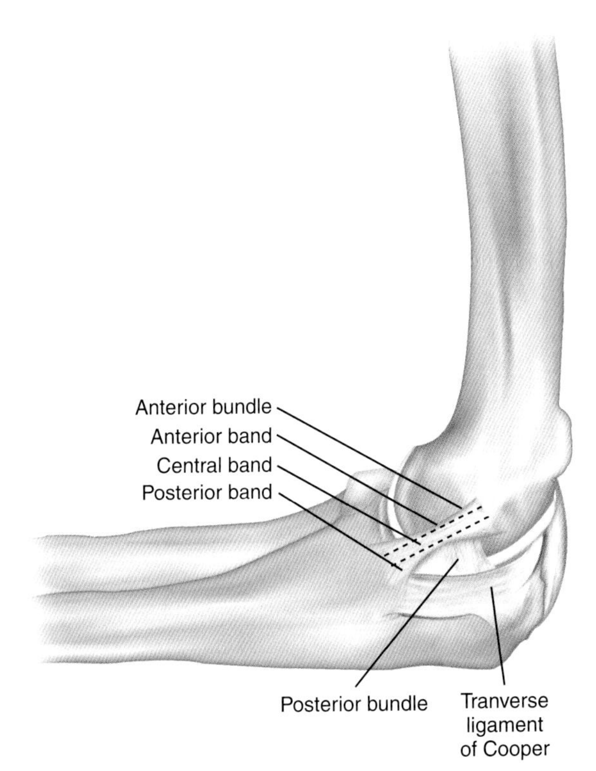

FIGURE 13-1 Schematic drawing of the medial collateral ligament complex. The anterior bundle is composed of three bands. The anterior band of the anterior bundle is the primary restraint to valgus stress.

and inserts on the sublime tubercle. The anterior bundle is subdivided into three components: an anterior band, a central band, and a posterior band. The anterior and posterior bands tighten in a reciprocal manner during flexion and extension, respectively. The posterior bundle is a less distinct fan-shaped structure. The transverse ligament is the least distinct anatomic structure and provides very little stability to the elbow because it does not cross the joint. Biomechanical studies have demonstrated that the anterior bundle is the primary constraint to valgus stress about the elbow.[10-12] Further studies have shown that the anterior band of the anterior bundle provides most of the stability from 30 to 90 degrees of flexion, whereas the posterior bundle becomes functionally significant between 60 degrees and maximum flexion.[13]

The mechanics of overhead throwing, particularly pitching, account for the various pathologies seen in overhead athletes. Valgus forces have been estimated to reach 64 N during the late cocking and early acceleration phases of throwing.[3,14] After the early and late cocking phases, the elbow goes from rapid flexion to extension, and the tangentially directed forces produce a valgus and extension moment, with resulting tensile forces across the medial side of the elbow, compressive forces across the lateral aspect of the joint, and shear forces in the posterior compartment.[3,4,15] The repetitive stress on the MUCL eventually leads to attenuation and ultimately rupture, resulting in an insufficient ligament complex, abnormal valgus rotation of the elbow, and instability. The term *valgus extension overload* describes this phenomenon.[2,16] As the athlete continues to throw with instability, the valgus overload is accentuated, and excessive valgus moments lead to stretch of other medial structures, resulting in ulnar neuritis, flexor-pronator tendinopathy, or medial epicondyle apophysitis in the skeletally immature patient.

Corresponding overload on the lateral side of the elbow may lead radiocapitellar chondromalacia, osteophyte formation, and loose bodies. During extension, posterior shear forces can produce olecranon osteophytes at the posteromedial tip with a corresponding kissing lesion on the posteromedial trochlea.[3] The clinician who treats throwing athletes must be familiar with these pathologies and be alert for underlying MUCL insufficiency as the cause of many of these disorders, because treating the pathology without ligament reconstruction often fails to relieve the athletes' symptoms and allow them to return to sport.

PATIENT EVALUATION

History

A comprehensive patient history is essential for developing a differential diagnosis for recalcitrant elbow pain and disability in the throwing athlete. The nature, mechanism, acuity of onset, and symptoms associated with the pain or injury are important factors. The phase of throwing and any change in accuracy, velocity, stamina, or strength can provide information about the specific diagnosis. Pain during the late cocking phase on the medial side of the elbow can indicate MUCL insufficiency. Young throwing athletes with osteochondritis dissecans lesions often report progressive lateral elbow pain during the late acceleration and follow-through phases, with loss of extension and episodes of locking. A history of mechanical symptoms, such as locking or catching, and of posterior pain exacerbated by forced extension is important, because these symptoms may be caused by loose bodies, chondral flaps, or posteromedial impingement.

The examiner must inquire about ulnar nerve symptoms, because they can be a source of elbow pain in the throwing athlete and because the nerve is vulnerable to arthroscopic injury. Sharp pain radiating down the medial portion of the forearm with paresthesias in the fifth digit and in the ulnar-innervated half of the fourth digit can indicate ulnar neuritis. When these symptoms are associated with a snapping or popping sensation, ulnar nerve subluxation may be the cause. Diagnosing a subluxating ulnar nerve is critical, because the nerve is at risk for injury when making and using medial portals during elbow arthroscopy.

Physical Examination

The physical examination of the elbow begins with the cervical spine and includes the ipsilateral shoulder and the contralateral elbow, followed by examination of the involved elbow. Neurovascular assessment of the involved extremity, including motor and sensory testing and reflexes, is equally important.

Inspection of the elbow begins with an assessment of the resting position of the elbow and its carrying angle. A normal carrying angle is approximately 11 degrees of valgus for men and 13 degrees of valgus for women.[3] An increase in the carrying angle of valgus may indicate an adaptation to the repetitive stress of valgus instability. Angles of greater than 15 degrees in professional pitchers have been documented in the literature.[17] The lateral, posterior, medial, and anterior regions of the involved elbow should be examined for swelling, obvious deformity, scars, or signs of previous trauma.

After careful inspection, the four regions of the elbow regions of the elbow should be palpated in an orderly fashion. The patients' history usually guides the examiner toward a specific location, but palpating all four anatomic regions ensures that concomitant pathology is not missed. The medial region of the elbow is often a focus when examining throwing athletes. Tenderness on the medial epicondyle and flexor-pronator mass can suggest an avulsion fracture (adolescents) or flexor-pronator tendinosis (adults). The patient with tendinosis typically exhibits local tenderness and pain with resisted flexion and forearm pronation. The MUCL can be palpated under the mass of the flexor-pronator origin when the elbow is flexed more than 90 degrees at its insertion at the sublime tubercle; tenderness to palpation at this location can indicate MUCL insufficiency.

In the posteromedial region of the elbow, the ulnar nerve is easily palpable in the groove, which is located between the medial epicondyle and the olecranon. The examiner should test for a Tinel sign and for hypermobility. This is done by palpating the nerve as the elbow is brought from extension to terminal flexion to determine whether the nerve subluxates or completely dislocates over the medial epicondyle. Palpation of the posteromedial region of the elbow should also focus on the olecranon, which can reveal osteophytes or swelling that occur in throwing athlete with valgus extension overload syndrome. The medial subcutaneous border of the olecranon should also be palpated for tenderness, which in the throwing athlete, can be caused by a stress fracture.[18]

Examination of the lateral region of the elbow begins with palpation of the lateral epicondyle. Tenderness directly over the epicondyle is consistent with lateral epicondylitis; tenderness directly over the anconeus soft spot can indicate a symptomatic lateral plica, a condition that is commonly found in throwing athletes. In one study, this was the most reproducible finding in a group of patients who were treated for this condition.[19]

Range of motion should be assessed for elbow flexion and extension and for forearm supination and pronation, as well as the nature of the extension and flexion end points. Cain and associates describe the "end feel" at the extremes of motion in the physical examination of the throwing athlete.[3] Normal extension terminates in the firm sensation of the posterior bony articulation making contact in the olecranon fossa, and normal flexion terminates in the abutment of the soft tissues of the distal humerus and the proximal forearm. Variations in the normal end points, particularly a bony end feel in extension, can indicate pathology such as posterior osteophytes. The examiner should focus on the end feel at extension and not necessarily on motion itself. Elbow flexion contractures have been detected in up to 50% of professional pitchers, and they do not necessarily indicate injury.

Evaluation of medial stability is the cornerstone of the assessment of the overhead athlete with valgus extension overload. Many techniques have been described in the literature for the optimal assessment of medial elbow stability. We typically find the valgus stress test and the moving valgus stress test to be the most specific, and we perform both provocative maneuvers when examining throwing athletes.

To perform the valgus stress test, the patient's distal forearm is placed under the examiner's axilla as a valgus load is applied to the elbow in 30 degrees of flexion (Fig. 13-2). The absence of a distinct end point combined with pain or tenderness indicates a positive test result and insufficiency of the anterior band of the anterior bundle of the medial collateral ligament (MCL).

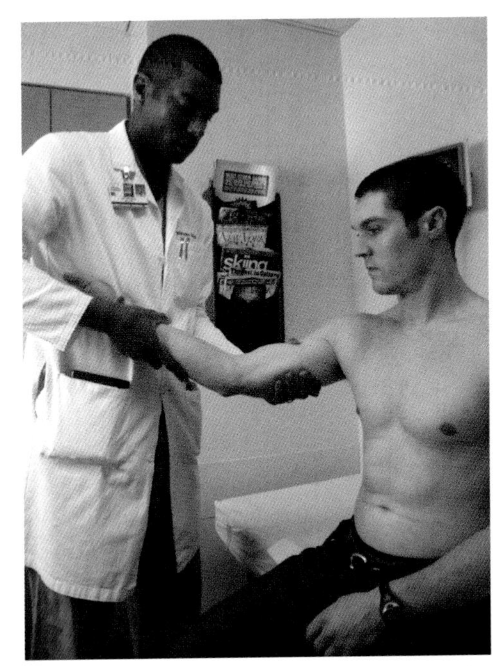

FIGURE 13-2 The valgus stress test is performed with the elbow at approximately 30 degrees. The distal forearm of the patient is placed under the axilla of the examiner to control rotation.

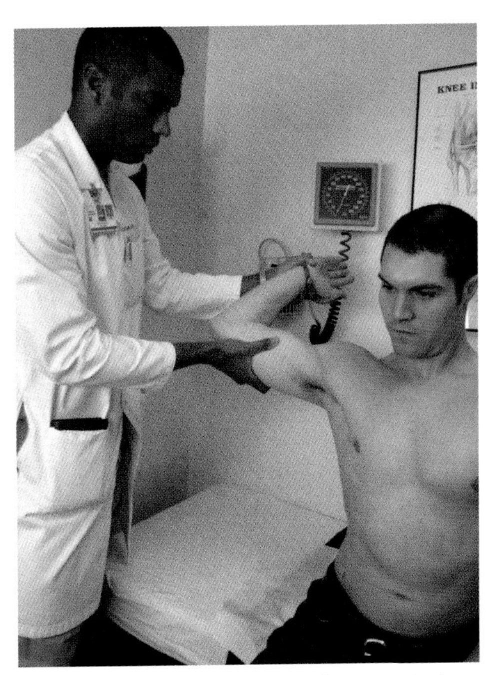

FIGURE 13-3 The moving valgus stress test begins with the arm in full flexion and the shoulder in maximal external rotation. The examiner applies a constant valgus force and quickly extends the elbow. The test result is positive test when the patient experiences pain, reproduction of symptoms, or apprehension from 120 degrees of flexion to 70 degrees of extension.

The moving valgus stress test, as described by O'Driscoll,[20] is performed with the patient in an upright position and the shoulder abducted 90 degrees (Fig. 13-3). Starting with the elbow in full flexion and the shoulder in maximal external rotation, the elbow is quickly extended while a constant valgus torque is maintained. For an examination result to be positive, the pain generated by the maneuver must reproduce the medial elbow pain that the patient has with activities, and the pain should be maximal between the position of late cocking (120 degrees) and early acceleration (70 degrees) as the elbow is extended.

Other relevant tests of the throwing athlete include the radiocapitellar compression test for osteochondritis dissecans of the radiocapitellar joint, the clunk test for posterior olecranon impingement, and the flexion-pronation test to detect a symptomatic snapping lateral plica. The radiocapitellar compression test is performed by placing the elbow in full extension and loading the joint with supination and pronation to produce mechanical symptoms. The clunk test for posterior olecranon impingement stabilizes the upper arm and brings the elbow into extension to produce posterior elbow pain (Fig. 13-4). The flexion pronation test is performed by placing the arm in maximum pronation and then passively flexing the elbow to approximately 90 degrees, which causes snapping in a positive test.[19]

We emphasize the importance of examining the ulnar nerve for subluxation. Many patients are unaware of this normal variant.

Diagnostic Imaging

The routine preoperative radiographic evaluation of the elbow includes anteroposterior, lateral, and oblique views. Stress views may be helpful in assessing ligamentous laxity, and olecranon

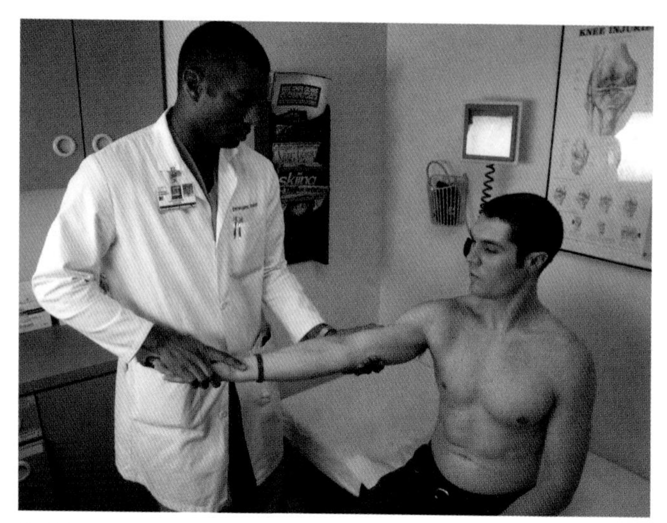

FIGURE 13-4 The clunk test for posterior olecranon impingement is performed by stabilizing the upper arm and bringing the elbow into extension to produce posterior elbow pain.

axial views at 110 degrees of flexion may reveal posteromedial osteophytes in valgus extension overload syndrome. However, it has been our experience that a true lateral view of the elbow in hyperflexion is adequate to diagnose posteromedial osteophytes. Contralateral comparison imaging studies of the elbow are helpful when evaluating elbow joint laxity and when trying to distinguish true growth disturbances from variant ossification centers in the pediatric population. Computed tomography can be helpful when trying to assess suspected bony pathology, including stress fractures and avulsion fractures.

Magnetic resonance imaging (MRI) remains the gold standard for evaluating pathology of the soft tissues about the elbow, including ligamentous injury, tendinopathy, and lesions of the articular cartilage. The accuracy of MRI in the evaluation of subtle MCL injuries and the role of arthrography and contrast remain controversial. At our institution, we use a noncontrast MRI with specially designed sequences (Fig. 13-5). Potter and colleagues demonstrated a high sensitivity and specificity for MRI in detecting ligamentous, soft tissue, and cartilaginous injuries.[21-23] This technique maintains the minimally invasive nature of the test and limits cost. A major additional advantage is excellent visualization of the articular cartilage in a highly specific and sensitive manner.[24]

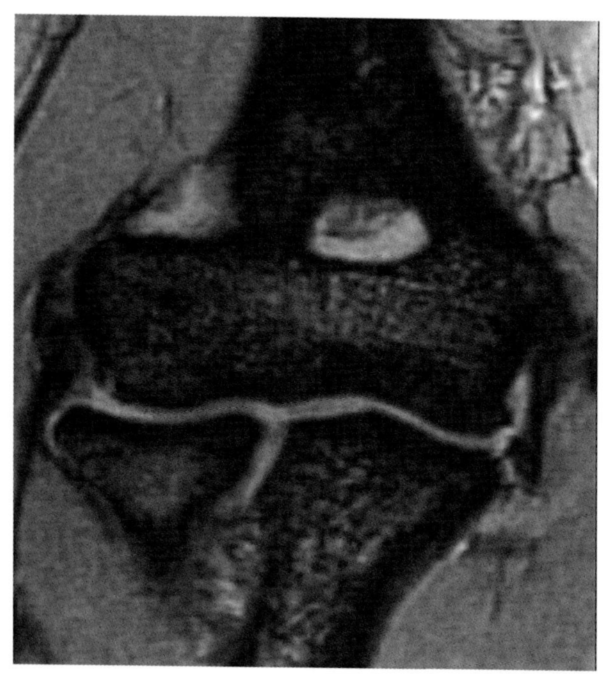

FIGURE 13-5 Coronal, fat-suppression MRI demonstrates a T sign, which indicates a complete tear of the medial collateral ligament complex at its humeral origin.

TREATMENT

Indications and Contraindications

Arthroscopy is an important method used for the diagnosis and treatment of valgus extension overload, with careful consideration given to choosing the appropriate indications. When valgus overload injury results in disabling symptoms for the athlete, surgical reconstruction of the anterior band of the ulnar collateral ligament may be indicated. Further indications for elbow arthroscopy in the throwing athlete include removal of loose bodies, excision of olecranon osteophytes, synovectomy, capsular release, capsular contracture, débridement of impinging osteophytes, articular cartilage lesions addressed, and the assessment and treatment of osteochondritis dissecans of the capitellum.[25-28]

The primary contraindication to elbow arthroscopy is any change in the normal bony or soft tissue anatomy that precludes safe entry of the arthroscope into the elbow joint.[29] We do not recommend performing arthroscopy when there has been a previous ulnar nerve transposition or when adequate distention of the joint cannot occur. Arthroscopy is contraindicated if there is soft tissue infection in the area of the portal sites.

The surgeon should have a comprehensive understanding of the surrounding anatomy and advanced technical experience of arthroscopic technique. Attention to detail is essential to prevent compromise of the surrounding neurovascular structures or damage to the delicate articular cartilage.[30]

Conservative Management

Initially, a nonoperative treatment regimen is initiated. It consists of a period of rest and anti-inflammatory medication to reduce pain and inflammation. Throwing athletes with partial MCL tears or those with overlapping symptoms resulting from medial epicondylitis or ulnar nerve symptoms are treated with activity modification and a shoulder and elbow-strengthening program. Cortisone injections should be avoided to prevent further tendon or ligament injury.

Athletes who fail conservative management are candidates for surgery. It is not uncommon for throwing athletes to have myriad pathologies that require arthroscopic treatment and open MCL reconstruction. In addition to our aforementioned criteria for arthroscopic management of valgus extension overload, we perform a MCL reconstruction concomitantly based on the following criteria: MRI evidence of MCL injury; a history of medial elbow pain in the region of the MCL that develops during the late cocking and early acceleration phase; and pain that is severe enough to prevent the athlete from an acceptable level of competition.

Arthroscopic Technique

Anesthesia

Regional or general anesthesia may be used for elbow arthroscopy. Regional anesthesia, with or without intravenous sedation, includes interscalene block, axillary block, and Bier block. In general, the advantage of regional anesthesia is that it optimizes postoperative pain control, minimizes postoperative nausea associated with general anesthesia, and facilitates positioning in cooperation with the patient. Disadvantages to regional anesthesia include limitations in the patient's tolerance of certain positions and the inability to perform a thorough postoperative neurologic examination of the involved extremity to determine whether nerve injury has occurred.

In our work with experienced regional anesthesiologist, we have not had any cases of nerve damage after regional anesthesia; therefore, we typically use axillary block anesthesia with intravenous sedation because we find it maximizes the patient's tolerance and allows supine positioning while maximizing postoperative comfort.

The advantages of general anesthesia include more options for patient positioning (prone and lateral decubitus positions) as well as total muscle relaxation. Disadvantages include postoperative pain tolerance and the potential for a longer postanesthesia recovery.

Patient Positioning

Patient positions routinely used for arthroscopic evaluation of the elbow include the prone position, lateral decubitus position, standard supine position, and supine-suspended position.

The prone position, first described by Poehling and coworkers,[31] places the patient prone on chest rolls with the arm stabilized by an arm holder and allowed to hang off the table. The shoulder is abducted to 90 degrees, and the elbow is flexed to 90 degrees. Some surgeons prefer this position because it eliminates the need for traction, places the elbow in a more stable position, and allows easier access to the posterior aspect of the joint.[26,31] If necessary, this position allows conversion from arthroscopy to an open surgical procedure, but we have found this to be very difficult.[31] Disadvantages of the prone position include general anesthesia and poor access to the airway by the anesthesiologist.

The lateral decubitus position, originally described by O'Driscoll and Morrey,[32] has advantages similar to those of the prone position, including improved arm stability and posterior joint access. However, in the lateral decubitus position, the anesthesiologist's access to the airway is not compromised. The main disadvantage is that access to the anterior compartment may require repositioning by placing the patient in a lateral position with the shoulder flexed forward at 90 degrees over a padded bolster.

The supine-suspended position, originally described by Andrews and Carson,[25] positions the shoulder in 90 degrees of abduction, with the elbow flexed 90 degrees and the forearm, wrist, and hand suspended by a mechanical traction device. We prefer a modification of this position with the shoulder flexed

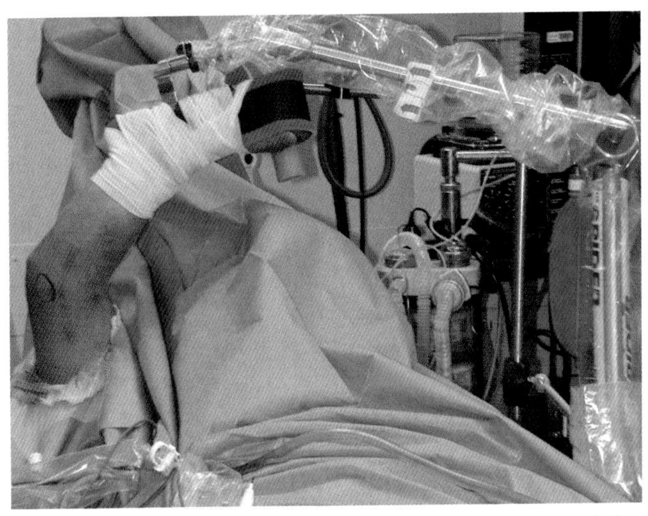

FIGURE 13-6 The modified supine position, with the arm suspended over the chest, is used for elbow arthroscopy. This position facilitates patient positioning and allows easy conversion to an open procedure when necessary.

90 degrees such that the forearm and humerus are suspended over the patient's chest for arthroscopic evaluation of the elbow. This position requires a mechanical arm holder, and it securely positions the arm in space and eliminates the need for an additional assistant. Several options are available, including the McConnell arm holder (McConnell Orthopaedic Manufacturing, Greenville, TX) and the Spider hydraulic arm holder (Spider Limb Positioner, Tenet Medical Engineering, Calgary, Alberta, Canada). We prefer the Spider hydraulic arm holder because it more rigidly suspends the arm in space and can be easily adjusted to allow for any desired changes in position (Fig. 13-6). This allows easy access to the anterior and posterior compartments, which facilitates arthroscopic work. With the forearm and humerus flexed over the chest, the anterior neurovascular structures effectively drop away from the anterior capsule, allowing for easier and safer work to be done on the anterior compartment.

The supine position also provides clear access to the posterior compartment when performing osteophyte débridement or microfracture to address posteromedial impingement in the throwing athlete. The supine position affords the anesthesiologist excellent access to the airway. Conversion to an open procedure can be easily performed by removing the arm from the holder and placing it across the arm board, where the seated surgeon can proceed with an open surgical procedure.

We have found this technique to be very successful and have not experienced the disadvantages reported in the literature, such as arm instability, difficult orientation, and poor access to the posterior compartment.[33] A tourniquet should be placed around the proximal aspect of the arm, but it should be inflated only when blood loss impairs arthroscopic visualization.

Portal Placement

The most common portals used for elbow arthroscopy include the anterolateral, midlateral, anteromedial, proximal medial, proximal lateral, and straight posterior.[29,34] We most commonly use the midlateral, proximal lateral, posterolateral, and trans-triceps portals (Figs. 13-7 to 13-9)

The midlateral portal, also known as the soft spot portal or direct lateral portal, is located in the center of the triangle formed by the lateral epicondyle, the tip of the olecranon, and the radial head. The anconeus is penetrated in this portal, and the nearest neurovascular structure is the posterior antebrachial cutaneous nerve.[35] This portal is often used to inject fluid to distend the capsule, but it can also be used to remove loose bodies stuck in the lateral gutter.[34]

The proximal lateral portal, originally described by Field and colleagues[36] and by Stothers and coworkers,[37] is located 2 cm proximal to the epicondyle and lies directly on the anterior surface of the humerus. The capsular attachments are such that, in flexion, the radial nerve is carried away from the nerve when the joint is distended. This enables clear visualization of the medial and lateral sides of the joint, the anterior and lateral aspects of the radial head and capitellum, and the lateral gutter.[38]

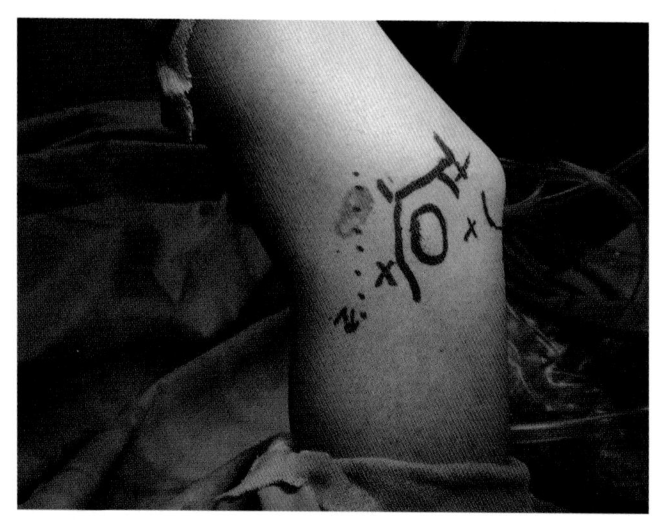

FIGURE 13-7 Lateral view of the elbow demonstrates the portals we typically use; each is marked with an X. The midlateral (soft spot) portal is upper right, the posterolateral portal is lower right, and the proximal lateral portal is lower left. The radial nerve *(dotted line)* is carried away from the proximal lateral portal in flexion when the joint is distended.

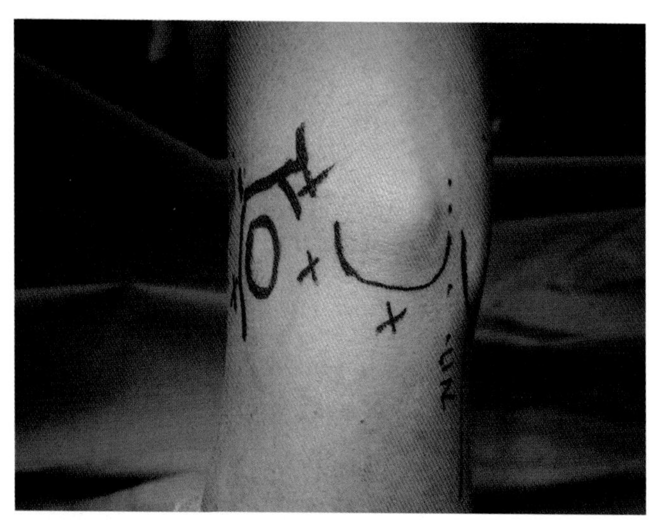

FIGURE 13-8 Posterior view of the elbow demonstrates the posterolateral portal *(left)* and the trans-triceps portal *(center)*.

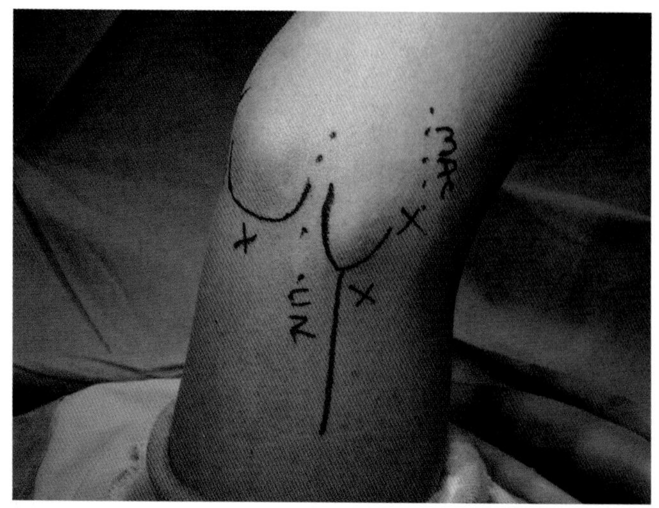

FIGURE 13-9 Medial view of the elbow shows the proximal medial portal *(proximal)* and the anteromedial portal *(distal)*. These portals are made after the scope is in the elbow joint under direct spinal needle localization. When making the proximal medial portal, it is important to stay above the intermuscular septum *(straight line)* to avoid injury to the ulnar nerve *(dotted line)*. The anteromedial portal is close to the medial antebrachial cutaneous (MAC) nerve, which should also be avoided.

The posterolateral portal is located 3 cm proximal to the tip of the olecranon and immediately lateral to the triceps tendon. The nearest neurovascular structures are the posterior brachial cutaneous and posterior antebrachial cutaneous nerves.[29] This portal provides unobstructed visualization of the entire posterior compartment.[34]

The trans-triceps portal is a straight posterior portal located in the midline and 3 cm proximal to the tip of the olecranon. It is mostly used to débride the posteromedial olecranon of osteophytes and the olecranon fossa of chondral lesions and for the removal of loose bodies.[34]

Operative Technique

After anesthesia administration and proper patient positioning, the elbow joint is insufflated with 20 to 30 mL of saline, which is injected through the soft spot in the midlateral portal. Distending the joint in this manner shifts the neurovascular structures away from the penetrating instruments and ensures safe entry of the instruments. Avoiding overdistention of the capsule is important because it can lead to capsular rupture and an inability to effectively maintain adequate fluid pressure for the ensuing arthroscopy.

Anterior Arthroscopy. The arthroscope is introduced through the proximal lateral portal into the anterior compartment (Fig. 13-10). Diagnostic arthroscopy is then performed anteriorly to evaluate the articular cartilage and synovium and to look for loose bodies. The coronoid process is examined for the presence of bone spurs, and the anterior trochlea and coronoid fossa are examined for cartilage lesions. The anterior radiocapitellar joint is evaluated for osteochondral lesions of the capitellum and any matching pathology of the radial head. The radial nerve lies on

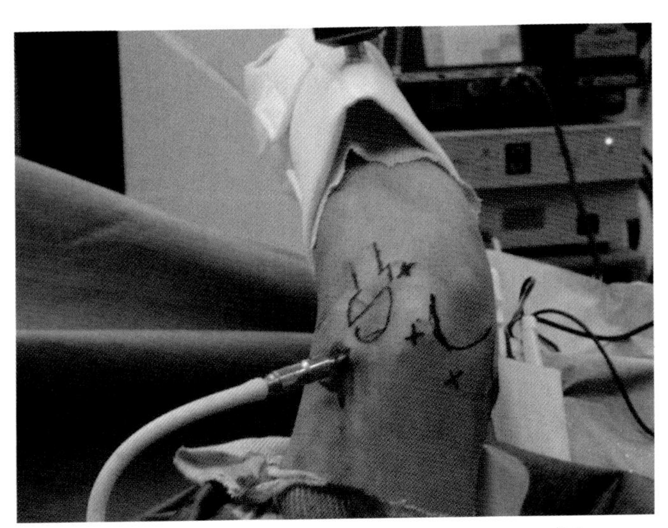

FIGURE 13-10 After the joint as been distended by means of the midlateral portal, the arthroscope is introduced into the anterior compartment through the proximal lateral portal.

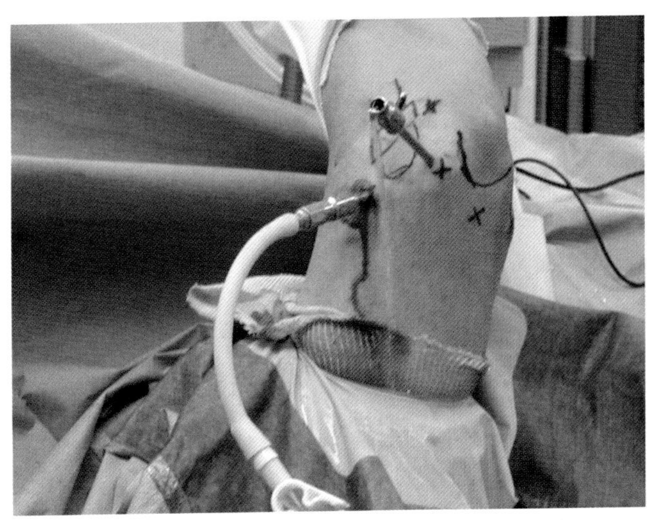

FIGURE 13-12 After completion of the anterior arthroscopy, the posterolateral portal is established. The camera is switched from the anterior cannula to this portal, but the anterior cannula is maintained to facilitate reentry into the anterior compartment if necessary.

or within a few millimeters of the anterolateral joint capsule. Débridement in this area therefore requires considerable caution. The anterior capsule is then evaluated for thickening or contracture in the context of a loss of passive extension.

To confirm the diagnosis of MCL insufficiency, the arthroscopic valgus stress test is performed during assessment of the anterior compartment. With the arthroscope in the proximal lateral portal visualizing the medial compartment, valgus stress is applied manually to the elbow. A gap between the ulna and humerus of more than 3 mm is consistent with ulnar collateral ligament insufficiency (Fig. 13-11). A probe of known dimensions can be inserted through the proximal medial portal to aid in the measurement of the ulnohumeral opening. If the portal is not necessary, a valgus opening can be visualized and appropriately estimated. If work needs to be performed in the anterior compartment, such as débridement, synovectomy, capsular release, or removal of loose bodies, a proximal medial portal is established under direct visualization.

Posterior Arthroscopy. After completion of the anterior arthroscopy, the cannula and its camera are retained, with fluid inflow attached to maintain distention of the joint (Fig. 13-12). A posterolateral portal is then established, and the camera is removed from the anterior cannula and inserted through this portal. We typically maintain the anterior cannula to facilitate reentry into the anterior compartment if necessary and to ultimately drain the elbow of fluid at the conclusion of the procedure.

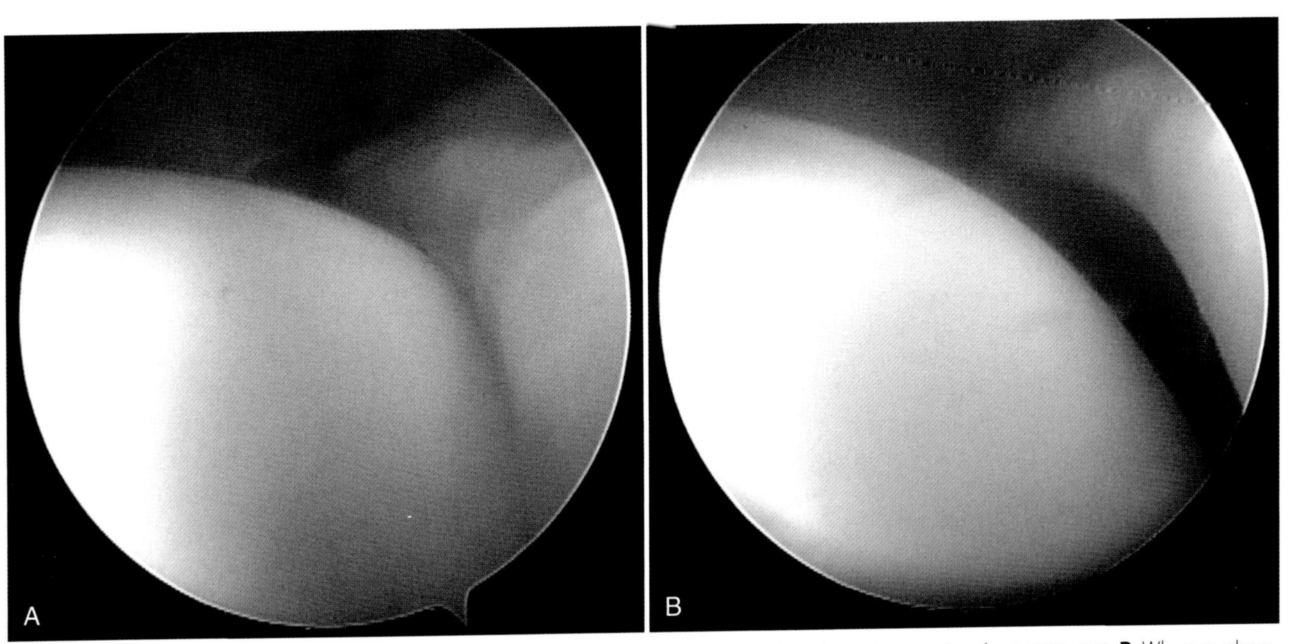

Figure 13-11 A, In cases of suspected medial collateral ligament insufficiency, we perform the arthroscopic valgus stress test. **B,** When a valgus stress is applied in this setting, the gap between the ulna and the humerus is more than 3 mm.

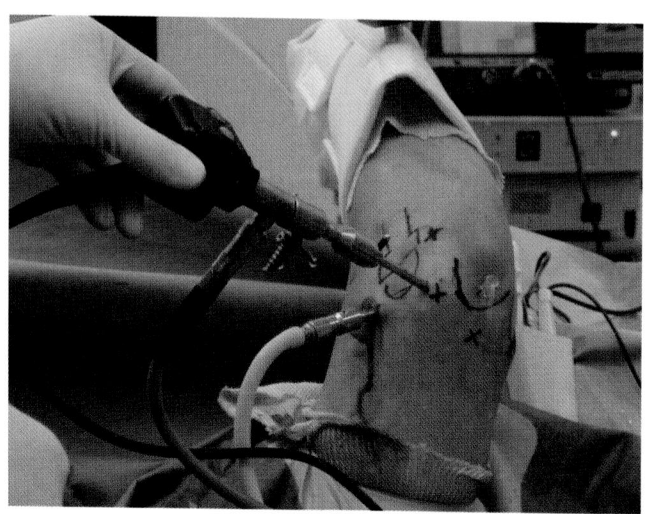

FIGURE 13-13 After the posterolateral has been established, the trans-triceps portal is established by spinal needle localization. The trans-triceps portal is the working portal in the posterior compartment.

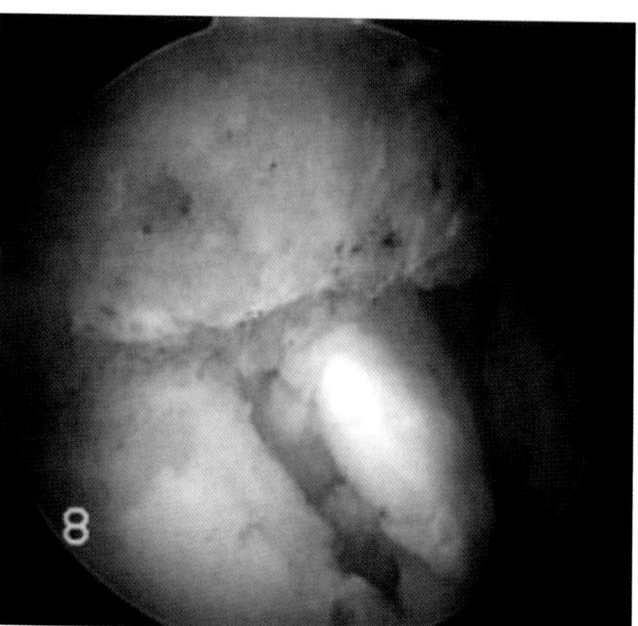

FIGURE 13-14 In throwing athletes, it is not uncommon to encounter posteromedial osteophytes *(top)* with a concomitant kissing lesion, which indicates chondral abrasion *(bottom)* opposite the osteophyte.

If work needs to be performed posteriorly, a trans-triceps portal is established (Fig. 13-13). The medial, lateral, and central aspects of the olecranon are then evaluated for the presence of osteophytes. The corresponding olecranon fossa and posteromedial aspect of the humeral condyle are evaluated for matching chondral defects. The posterior radiocapitellar joint is evaluated by advancing the arthroscope down the lateral gutter. One of the most common errors made in elbow arthroscopy is to miss a loose body that is caught in the posterior radiocapitellar joint.[39] An accessory midlateral portal through the soft spot often is necessary for removal of the loose body.[38]

In the throwing athlete, the most common problem encountered is a fragmented spur on the posteromedial olecranon as a result of posterior shear stresses seen in valgus extension overload (Fig. 13-14).[38] These spurs should be anticipated because they can be seen on the preoperative radiographs and MRI scans. With the camera in the posterolateral portal and the shaver in the trans-triceps portal, the extent and dimensions of the osteophyte can be evaluated. Excess soft tissues, including synovial reflections, are removed from the olecranon tip by carefully using a radiofrequency device.[38] The osteophyte is removed from the posteromedial olecranon using a gentle medial-to-lateral movement (Fig. 13-15).

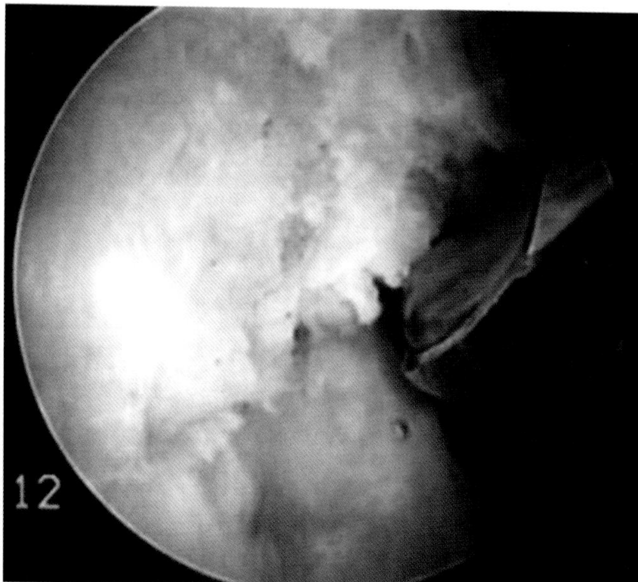

FIGURE 13-15 A shaver is introduced into the posterior compartment through the trans-triceps portal and is used to resect the osteophyte. As much native bone as possible should be preserved, but the offending pathology must be removed.

The optimal amount of olecranon to be débrided has been a matter of debate. Common surgical practice involves débridement of the osteophyte along with some amount of native olecranon bone. Biomechanical studies have demonstrated that excessive olecranon resection can lead to elbow instability and MCL strain in the throwing athlete.[40,41] Resections should be limited to approximately 3 mm, because resections greater than this may jeopardize the native or the reconstructed MCL. Practically speaking, our goal of arthroscopic débridement is to remove the osteophyte only and preserve as much native bone as possible.

After the osteophyte is removed, the humeral chondral surface can be visualized more completely and the kissing lesion of chondral abrasion opposite the osteophyte will be in direct view. Loose chondral flaps are débrided, and if necessary, microfracture is performed (Fig. 13-16). On completion of the posterior arthroscopy, the portals are briefly irrigated and closed with interrupted nylon sutures.

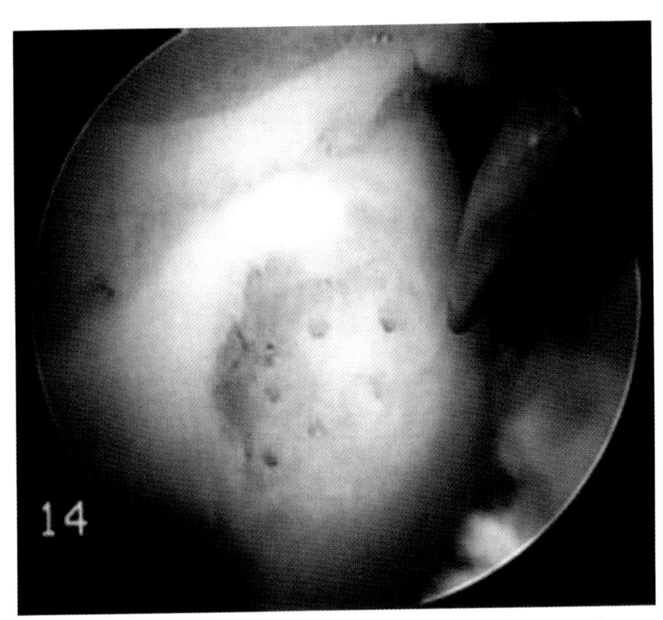

FIGURE 13-16 After the osteophyte has been adequately excised, any loose chondral flaps can be débrided and microfractured when necessary.

Open Medial Ulnar Collateral Ligament Reconstruction. If MCL reconstruction is needed, the forearm is easily removed from the arm holder and is placed onto the table extension. When the palmaris longus tendon is absent, the gracilis tendon is harvested at this time. Otherwise, the ipsilateral palmaris longus tendon is harvested through a 1-cm incision in the volar wrist flexion crease over the tendon. The visible portion of the tendon is then tagged with locking Krakow sutures, and the remaining tendon is then harvested using a tendon stripper. The incision is irrigated and closed using interrupted nylon sutures.

After the arm is exsanguinated to the level of the tourniquet, an 8- to 10-cm incision is made starting 2-cm proximal to the medial epicondyle in line with the intermuscular septum. The incision is carried distally, approximately 2 cm beyond the sublime tubercle. When exposing the flexor-pronator mass, the median antebrachial cutaneous nerve is often observed and should be identified and protected. A muscle-splitting approach is used through the posterior one third of the common flexor-pronator mass within the most anterior fibers of the flexor carpi ulnaris muscle. This is located at the raphe between the flexor carpi ulnaris muscle and the anterior portion of the flexor bundle. The advantage of this particular approach is that it uses a true internervous plane.[42] The anterior bundle of the MCL is excised to expose the joint.

The ulna tunnel sites are exposed first. The anterior and posterior portions of the sublime tubercle are exposed subperiosteally while carefully protecting the ulnar nerve. A 3-mm burr is then used to create tunnels anterior and posterior to the sublime tubercle. A curette is used to connect two tunnels while preserving the body bridge.

To expose the humeral tunnel position, the incision within the native MCL is extended proximally to the level of the epicondyle. A longitudinal tunnel is created along the axis of the medial epicondyle using a 4-mm burr. Care is taken not to violate the posterior cortex of the proximal epicondyle. Using a 1.5-mm burr, two small exit punctures are created on the anterior surface of the epicondyle anterior to the intermuscular septum. This allows the sutures on each end of the graft to be passed from the humeral tunnel.

With the forearm supinated and a mild varus stress applied to the elbow, the graft is passed through the ulnar tunnel from anterior to posterior. The posterior limb of the graft with sutures is then docked into the humeral tunnel, with the sutures exiting through one of two exit holes in the anterior portion of the epicondyle. With the elbow reduced, the graft is tensioned in flexion and extension to determine the optimal length by placing the graft adjacent to the humeral tunnel. Final length is determined by referencing the graft to the exit hole in the humeral tunnel. This point is marked on the graft, and another Krakow stitch is placed. Excess graft is excised above this point, and the end of the graft is securely docked in the anterior humeral tunnel, with the second set of graft sutures exiting the second puncture hole in the anterior portion of the epicondyle. Because a graft that is too long cannot be properly tensioned, it is essential that the final length be short of where the graft suture will exit the epicondyle.

Final tensioning is performed by taking the elbow through a complete range of motion while a varus stress is applied. After the surgeon is satisfied, the two suture ends are tied over the medial epicondyle with the elbow in approximately 20 degrees of flexion and full supination (Fig. 13-17). This position is chosen because it reduces excessive tension or laxity in either of the two limbs. After the tourniquet is deflated and hemostasis achieved, an ulnar nerve transposition is performed if indicated. Otherwise, the fascia over the flexor-pronator mass is reapproximated, and the remaining wound is closed in layers. The elbow is placed in a plaster splint at 45 degrees of flexion to reduce excessive laxity or tension on either limb and forearm supination to keep the joint reduced.

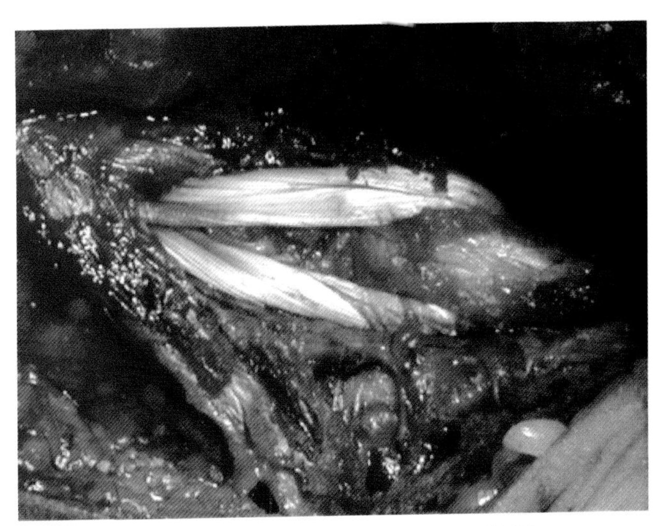

FIGURE 13-17 In cases of medial collateral ligament (MCL) insufficiency, an MCL reconstruction is performed after the arthroscopic component of the procedure has been completed. We have had excellent results using the docking technique for MCL reconstruction.

PEARLS & PITFALLS

PEARLS

- We prefer the supine, suspended position with the arm flexed over the chest (see Figs. 13-5 and 13-6), because the anterior neurovascular structures effectively drop away from the anterior capsule.
- The anterior and posterior compartments can be easily accessed.
- This position also facilitates conversion to an open surgical procedure when necessary (e.g., MCL reconstruction).

PITFALLS

- A common error is to miss a loose body that is caught in the posterior radiocapitellar joint. Use an accessory midlateral portal through the soft spot to aid in removal.
- Identify and mark bony landmarks before the capsule is distended, which can make palpation of landmarks more difficult.
- The joint should be distended with 20 to 40 mL of fluid through the midlateral portal before establishing the initial viewing portal. This significantly increases the distance between the joint surfaces and neurovascular structures.
- When creating portals, avoid penetrating the subcutaneous tissues. A hemostat or clamp should be used to spread the tissue down to the capsule.
- Avoid using any local anesthetic, which can prevent appropriate postoperative assessment of the neurologic status.
- Avoid multiple penetrations of the capsule to prevent excessive fluid extravasation, which can lead to excessive swelling and can injure neurovascular structures.
- When removing osteophyte from the olecranon, limit the resection to the osteophyte only; excessive posteromedial resection of the olecranon can lead to valgus instability, particularly in the throwing athlete.

Postoperative Rehabilitation

The specific physical therapy regimen chosen depends on the procedure performed, especially if arthroscopy is followed by reconstruction the MCL. The following description is a general guideline for rehabilitation after only elbow arthroscopy.

Postoperatively, we prefer a compressive dressing for 48 hours, cryotherapy, and routine wound care. Sling immobilization is minimal and used for comfort only. We then proceed in a triphasic rehabilitation program that focuses on the restoration of joint range of motion and flexibility within the healing parameters of the structures involved in the surgery (Box 13-1). Rehabilitation progresses through each phase only after the major goals of the previous phase have been successfully achieved. We recommend the athlete achieve the following criteria to safely return to play: painless and full range of motion, no elbow pain or tenderness, satisfactory isokinetic muscular strength testing, and a satisfactory clinical examination. Rehabilitation after elbow arthroscopy can be somewhat aggressive because the procedure causes minimal postoperative morbidity. For a more comprehensive review of nonoperative and postoperative rehabilitation of the athlete's elbow, we recommend the chapter by Wilk and Levinson in *The Athlete's Elbow*.[43] The authors outline the three-phase approach to rehabilitation in detail and explain how such a program allows the surgeon and therapist to tailor the program to the individual patient's needs.

Table 13-1 presents an interval throwing program. Age-related pitch counts according to days rest are listed in Table 13-2.

Box 13-1 Postoperative Rehabilitation Program

PHASE I: 0 TO 6 WEEKS

Sling immobilization (physician directed)*
- Codman's or pendulum exercises
- Wrist or elbow range-of-motion exercises
- Gripping exercises
- FF-AAROM, supine (limit to 90 degrees)
- Passive ER to neutral
- Passive elbow abduction to 30 degrees
- Scapula tightening
- Other modalities as needed

Discontinue sling (physician directed)
- Continue FF-AAROM (wand or pulleys)
- ER-AAROM to 30 degrees
- Manual scapular stabilization exercise, sidelying
- Begin pain-free IR and ER isometrics in modified neutral
- Other modalities as needed

PHASE II: 6 TO 10 WEEKS

Begin biceps and triceps strengthening
Progress scapular strengthening in protective arcs (emphasis on closed-chain activities)
Begin isotonic IR and ER strengthening in modified neutral
Begin latissimus strengthening below 90 degrees of elevation
Begin FF in plane of scapula and add weights as tolerated (emphasis on scapulohumeral rhythm)
Continue to increase AAROM for ER and FF
Begin upper body ergometer below 90 degrees of elevation
Begin humeral head stabilization exercises (must have adequate strength and range of motion)
Continue aggressive scapula strengthening
Advance strengthening for deltoid, biceps, triceps, and latissimus as tolerated
Begin PNF stretching patterns
Continue humeral head stabilization exercises
Advance IR and ER to elevated position in overhead athletes (must be pain free and have good proximal strength)
Continue upper body exercise for endurance training
Begin general flexibility exercises

PHASE III: 10 TO 24 WEEKS

Continue full upper extremity strengthening
Restore normal shoulder flexibility
Begin activity-specific polymeric program
Continue endurance training
Continue flexibility exercises
Continue full strengthening program
Begin return to interval throwing (physician directed)

*Patient begins this as directed by a physician starting on the first postoperative day.
AAROM, active assisted range of motion; ER, external rotation; FF, forward flexion; IR, internal rotation; PNF, proprioceptive neuromuscular facilitation.

TABLE 13-1 Interval Throwing Program

- Use interval throwing to 120-ft phase as a warm-up
- Throwing is performed every other day
- Do not rush through each stage—quicker is not better
- To move to the next step, you need to have no pain and good control. If pain does occur you will probably need to rest a few days and back up to the previous step
- Before and after throwing exercises must be performed. This includes stretching your shoulder once warm
- All throwing off the mound should be done in the presence of your pitching coach to stress proper throwing mechanics
- Use speed gun to aid in effort control

Interval Throwing Program: Phase I

	45-ft Phase
Step 1	Warm-up throwing 45 ft (25 throws) Rest 15 min Warm-up throwing 45 ft (25 throws)
Step 2	Warm-up throwing 45 ft (25 throws) Rest 10 min Warm-up throwing 45 ft (25 throws) Rest 10 min Warm-up throwing 45 ft (25 throws)
	80-ft Phase
Step 3	Warm-up throwing 60 ft (25 throws) Rest 15 min Warm-up throwing 60 ft (25 throws)
Step 4	Warm-up throwing 60 ft (25 throws) Rest 10 min Warm-up throwing 60 ft (25 throws) Rest 10 min Warm-up throwing 60 ft (25 throws)
	90-ft Phase
Step 5	Warm-up throwing 90 ft (25 throws) Rest 15 min Warm-up throwing 90 ft (25 throws)
Step 6	Warm-up throwing 90 ft (25 throws) Rest 10 min Warm-up throwing 90 ft (25 throws) Rest 10 min Warm-up throwing 90 ft (25 throws)
	120-ft Phase
Step 7	Warm-up throwing 120 ft (25 throws) Rest 15 min Warm-up throwing 120 ft (25 throws)
Step 8	Warm-up throwing 120 ft (25 throws) Rest 10 min Warm-up throwing 120 ft (25 throws) Rest 10 min Warm-up throwing 120 ft (25 throws)
	150-ft Phase
Step 9	Warm-up throwing 150 ft (25 throws) Rest 15 min Warm-up throwing 150 ft (25 throws)
Step 10	Warm-up throwing 150 ft (25 throws) Rest 10 min Warm-up throwing 150 ft (25 throws) Rest 10 min Warm-up throwing 150 ft (25 throws)
	180-ft Phase
Step 11	Warm-up throwing 180 ft (25 throws) Rest 15 min Warm-up throwing 180 ft (25 throws)
Step 12	Warm-up throwing 180 ft (25 throws) Rest 10 min Warm-up throwing 180 ft (25 throws) Rest 10 min Warm-up throwing 180 ft (25 throws)
Step 13	Warm-up throwing 180 ft (25 throws) Rest 10 min Warm-up throwing 180 ft (25 throws) Rest 10 min Warm-up throwing 180 ft (25 throws)
Step 14	Begin throwing off the mound or return to respective position

Continued

TABLE 13-1 Interval Throwing Program—cont'd

Interval Throwing Program Starting Off the Mound: Phase II			
Stage One	***Fastball Only***	***Stage Two***	***Fastball Only***
Step 1	Interval throwing 15 throws off mound at 50%	Step 9	45 throws off mound at 75% 15 throws in batting practice
Step 2	Interval throwing 30 throws off mound at 50%	Step 10	45 throws off mound at 75% 30 throws in batting practice
Step 3	Interval throwing 45 throws off mound at 50%	Step 11	45 throws off mound at 75% 45 throws in batting practice
Step 4	Interval throwing 60 throws off mound at 50%	***Stage Three***	
Step 5	Interval throwing 30 throws off mound at 75%	Step 12	30 throws off mound 75% warm-up 15 throws in batting practice
Step 6	30 throws off mound at 75% 45 throws off mound at 50%	Step 13	30 throws off mound 75% warm-up 30 breaking balls 75% 30 throws in batting practice
Step 7	45 throws off mound at 75% 15 throws off mound at 50%	Step 14	30 throws off mound 75% 60-90 throws in batting practice, with 25% breaking balls
Step 8	60 throws off mound at 75%	Step 15	Simulated game, progressing by 15 throws per workout

TABLE 13-2 Suggested Recovery Days

Age-Related Pitch Counts According to Days of Rest				
Age	***One Day***	***Two Days***	***Three Days***	***Four Days***
8-10 yr	21 pitches	34	43	51
11-12 yr	27	35	55	58
13-14 yr	30	36	56	70
15-16 yr	25	38	62	77
17-18 yr	27	45	62	89

CONCLUSIONS

Elbow arthroscopy is a powerful tool in the diagnosis and treatment of the various pathologies seen in the throwing athlete's elbow. Preoperative evaluation should consist of a complete history and physical examination and the use of appropriate imaging modalities to make a prompt diagnosis and facilitate a rapid return to play for the athlete. The arthroscopic recognition and treatment of related pathology correlates with appropriate surgical technique, particularly proper portal placement and adequate surgical instrumentation. The clinician who wishes to use arthroscopy as a tool for treating the thrower's elbow must be proficient in basic arthroscopic techniques, coupled with a thorough understanding of elbow anatomy and biomechanics.

REFERENCES

1. O'Holleran JD, Altchek DW. Elbow arthroscopy: treatment of the thrower's elbow. *Instr Course Lect.*. 2006;55:95-107.
2. Chen A, Youm T, Ong B, et al. Imaging of the elbow in the overhead throwing athlete. *Am J Sports Med.* 2003;31:466-473.
3. Cain E, Dugas J, Wolf R, Andrews J. Elbow injuries in throwing athletes: a current concepts review. *Am J Sports Med.* 2003;31:621-635.
4. Schickendantz M. Diagnosis and treatment of elbow disorders in the overhead athlete. *Hand Clin.* 2002;18:65-75.
5. Ball C, Galatz L, Yamaguchi K. Elbow instability: treatment strategies and emerging concepts. *Instr Course Lect.* 2002;51:53-61.
6. Rizio L, Uribe J. Overuse injuries of the upper extremity in baseball. *Clin Sports Med.* 2001;20:453-468.
7. Miller C, Savoie F III. Valgus extension injuries of the elbow in the throwing athlete. *J Am Acad Orthop Surg.* 1994;2:261-269.
8. Chen F, Rokito A, Jobe F. Medial elbow problems in the overhead throwing athlete. *J Am Acad Orthop Surg.* 2001;9:99-113.
9. Morrey BF, An KN. Articular and ligamentous contributions to the stability of the elbow joint. *Am J Sports Med.* 1983;11:315-319.
10. Callaway GH, Field LD, Deng XH, et al. Biomechanical evaluation of the medial collateral ligament of the elbow. *J Bone Joint Surg Am.* 1997; 79:1223-1231.
11. Hotchkiss RN, Weiland AJ. Valgus stability of the elbow. *J Orthop Res.* 1987;5:372-377.
12. Hechtman KS, Tjin-A-Tsoi EW, Zvijac JE, et al. Biomechanics of a less invasive procedure for reconstruction of the ulnar collateral ligament of the elbow. *Am J Sports Med.* 1998;26:620-624.
13. Regan WD, Korinek SL, Morrey BF, et al. Biomechanical study of ligaments around the elbow joint. *Clin Orthop.* 1991;271:170-179.
14. Fleisig GS, Andrews JR, Dillman CJ, et al. Kinetics of baseball pitching with implications about injury of mechanisms. *Am J Sports Med.* 1995; 23:233-239.

15. Pappas A, Zawacki R, Sullivan T. Biomechanics of baseball pitching: a preliminary report. *Am J Sports Med*. 1985;13:216-222.
16. Wilson FD, Andrews JR, Blackburn TA, et al. Valgus extension overload in the pitching elbow. *Am J Sports Med*. 1983;11:83-88.
17. King JW, Brelsford HJ, Tullos HS. Analysis of the pitching arm of the professional baseball pitcher. *Clin Orthop*. 1969;67:116-123.
18. Schickendantz MS, Ho CP, Koh J. Stress injury of the proximal ulna in professional baseball players. *Am J Sports Med*. 2002;30:737-741.
19. Antuna SA, O'Driscol SW. Snapping plicae associated with radiocapitellar chondromalacia. *Arthroscopy*. 2001;17:491-495.
20. O'Driscoll SW, Lawton RL, Smith AM. The "moving valgus stress test" for medial collateral ligament tears of the elbow. *Am J Sports Med*. 2005; 33:231-239.
21. Potter HG. Imaging of posttraumatic and soft tissue dysfunction of the elbow. *Clin Orthop*. 2000;370:9-18.
22. Gaary EA, Potter HG, Altchek DW. Medial elbow pain in the throwing athlete: MR imaging evaluation. *AJR Am J Roentgenol*. 1997;168:795-800.
23. Potter HG, Ho ST, Altchek DW. Magnetic resonance imaging of the elbow. *Semin Musculoskelet Radiol*. 2004;8:5-16.
24. Potter HG, Linklater JM, Allen AA, et al. Magnetic resonance imaging of articular cartilage in the knee. An evaluation with use of fast-spin-echo imaging. *J Bone Joint Surg Am*. 1998;80:1276-1284.
25. Andrews JR, Carson WG. Arthroscopy of the elbow. *Arthroscopy*. 1985; 1:97-107.
26. Baker CL. The elbow. In: Whipple TL, ed. *Arthroscopic Surgery: The Shoulder and Elbow*. Philadelphia, PA: JB Lippincott; 1993:239-300.
27. Yadao MA, Field LD, Savoie FH III. Osteochondritis dissecans of the elbow. *Instr Course Lect*. 2004;53:599-606.
28. Takahara M, Shundo M, Kondo M, et al. Early detection of osteochondritis dissecans of the capitellum in young baseball players: report of three cases. *J Bone Joint Surg Am*. 1998;80:892-897.
29. Walcott GD, Savoie FH, Field LD. Arthroscopy of the elbow: setup, portals and diagnostic technique. In: Altchek DW, Andrews JR, eds. *The Athlete's Elbow*. Philadelphia, PA: Lippincott Williams & Wilkins; 2001: 209-217, 249-273.
30. Andrews JR, St Pierre RK, Carson WG Jr. Arthroscopy of the elbow. *Clin Sports Med*. 1986;5:653-662.
31. Poehling GG, Whipple TL, Sisco L, Goldman B. Elbow arthroscopy: a new technique. *Arthroscopy*. 1989;5:222-224.
32. O'Driscoll SW, Morrey, BF. Arthroscopy of the elbow: diagnostic and therapeutic benefits and hazards. *J Bone Joint Surg Am*. 1992;74:84-94.
33. Abboud JA, Ricchetti ET, Tjoumakaris F, Ramsey ML. Elbow arthroscopy: basic setup and portal placement. *J Am Acad Orthop Surg*. 2006; 14:312-318.
34. Dodson CC, Nho SJ, Williams RJ III, Altchek DW. Elbow arthroscopy. *J Am Acad Orthop Surg*. 2008;16:574-585.
35. Adolfsson L. Arthroscopy of the elbow joint: a cadaveric study of portal placement. *J Shoulder Elbow Surg*. 1994;3:53-61.
36. Field LD, Altchek DW, Warren RF. Arthroscopic anatomy of the lateral elbow: a comparison of three portals. *Arthroscopy*. 1994;10:602-607.
37. Stothers K, Day BD, Regan WR. Arthroscopy of the elbow: anatomy, portal sites and a description of the proximal lateral portal. *Arthroscopy*. 1995;11:449-457.
38. O'Holleran JD, Altchek DW. Throwers elbow: arthroscopic treatment of valgus extension overload syndrome. *HSS J*. 2006;2:83-93.
39. Altchek DW, Hyman J, Williams R, et al. Management of MCL injuries of the elbow in throwers. *Tech Shoulder Elbow Surg*. 2000;1:73-81.
40. Kamineni S, Hirahara H, Pomianowski S, et al. Partial posteromedial olecranon resection: a kinematic study. *J Bone Joint Surg Am*. 2005;85A: 1005-1011.
41. Kamineni S, ElAttrache NS, O'Driscoll SW, et al. Medial collateral ligament strain with partial posteromedial olecranon resection: a biomechanical study. *J Bone Joint Surg Am*. 2004;86A:2424-2430.
42. Smith GR, Altchek DW, Pagnani MJ, et al. A muscle-splitting approach to the ulnar collateral ligament of the elbow: neuroanatomy and operative technique. *Am J Sports Med*. 1996;24:575-580.
43. Wilk KE, Levinson M. Rehabilitation of the athlete's elbow. In: Altchek DW, Andrews JR, eds. *The Athlete's Elbow*. Philadelphia, PA, Lippincott Williams & Wilkins; 2001:249-273.

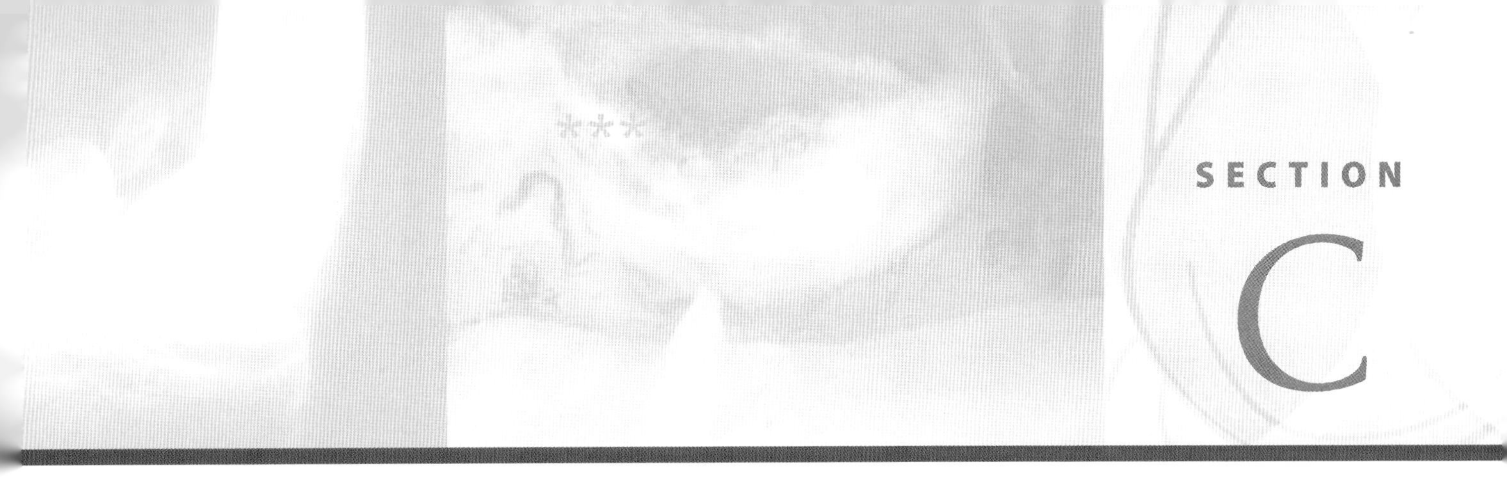

SECTION C

The Future of Elbow Arthroscopy

CHAPTER

14

Endoscopic Distal Biceps Repair

Gregory I. Bain • Luke Johnson • Adam C. Watts

Tears of the distal biceps tendon represent a diagnostic and imaging challenge for the orthopedic surgeon and sports physician.[1-8] Complete tears of the distal tendon account for approximately 3% of all tears involving the muscle, and partial tears are less common, although their exact incidence is unknown.[1-5] The symptoms may be subtle (e.g., antecubital pain) and signs difficult to illicit (e.g., weakness of elbow flexion and supination). Physicians who remain alert to the possibility are most likely to suspect the diagnosis. Use of correct imaging and of surgical endoscopy can lead to the correct diagnosis and management of the condition.

ANATOMY

Biceps brachii is the most superficial of the muscles in the anterior compartment of the arm, and it has two heads of origin. It acts across three articulations: the shoulder, the elbow, and the proximal radioulnar joint.[9] The short head takes a tendinous origin from the tip of the coracoid process of the scapula, immediately lateral to the origin of the coracobrachialis muscle. The long head arises from the supraglenoid tubercle and adjacent glenoid labrum. The two tendons expand into fleshy fusiform bellies, held together by loose epimysial tissue.[9,10] As they traverse parallel through the upper arm, the belly of the short head always remains to the ulnar side and the long head to the radial side.[9] It was once held that the two bellies fused below their main convexity, just above the elbow joint,[4,9,10] but anatomic cadaver studies have revealed a variable amount of interdigitation.[10] Eames and Bain[10] also described the distal tendon as having two distinct components held together by loose adventitia, one arising from each belly. Eames and Bain[10] further divide the distal biceps tendon into three zones.

In zone 1, the *pre-aponeurosis*, a variable amount of muscular interdigitation of the two bellies occurs, with many cadavers showing none at all (7 of 17 specimens). Where it was present, the raphe was easily overcome by blunt finger dissection (Fig. 14-1).

Zone 2, the *aponeurosis or lacertus fibrosus*, consists of three layers. The superficial layer arises from the anterior, radial aspect of the long head at the level of the distal musculotendinous junction. It spreads distally and ulnarward, coursing anterior to

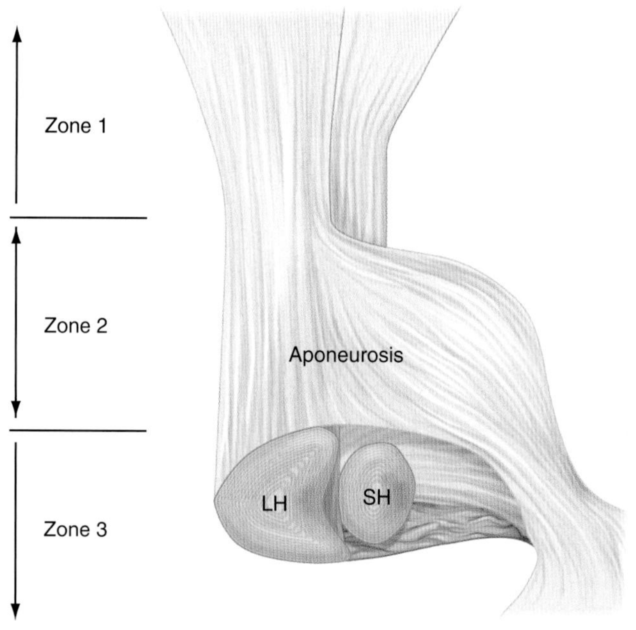

FIGURE 14-1 Anatomic zones of tendon injury are shown in the cross-sectional drawing of the two components of the distal biceps tendon, including the short head (SH) and long head (LH). The three layers of the aponeurosis stabilize the tendon of the short head. The three zones of the distal biceps tendon are also shown: zone 1 (pre-aponeurosis), zone 2 (biceps aponeurosis and lacertus fibrosus), and zone 3 (post-aponeurosis). *(Modified from Eames MH, Bain GI, Fogg QA, van Riet RP. Distal biceps tendon anatomy: a cadaveric study.* J Bone Joint Surg. *2007;89:1044-1049.)*

the musculotendinous junction of the short head. The middle layer acts as a mesentery to the short head tendon, embracing it before it passes distally and ulnarward and merges with the superficial layer. The deep layer arises from the deep radial aspect of the long head and sweeps distally and ulnarward, deep to the short head tendon. The three layers subsequently merge and continue distally as a single aponeurosis. The lacertus fibrosus has wide and deep involvement in the flexor compartment of the forearm—it completely encircles the flexors and has fascial attachments, particularly to the ulnar flexors, and it incorporates the median nerve and brachial artery.[10]

In zone 3, the *post-aponeurosis*, the two tendons continue distally past the lacertus fibrosus and insert onto the radial tuberosity. The distal biceps tendon footprint on the radial tuberosity is 2 × 14 mm.[11] In all specimens, the long head tendon passed deep to the short and inserted more proximally.[10] This point is also farthest away from the point of rotation of the radius. The tendon of the short head curves anterior to the long and inserts in a fanlike fashion on the distal portion of the radial tuberosity and extends distal to it (Fig. 14-2). With these different insertions, the long head provides greater supination power, and the short head may provide more flexion power, which can help in clinical evaluation of partial tears to localize the tear by power testing.

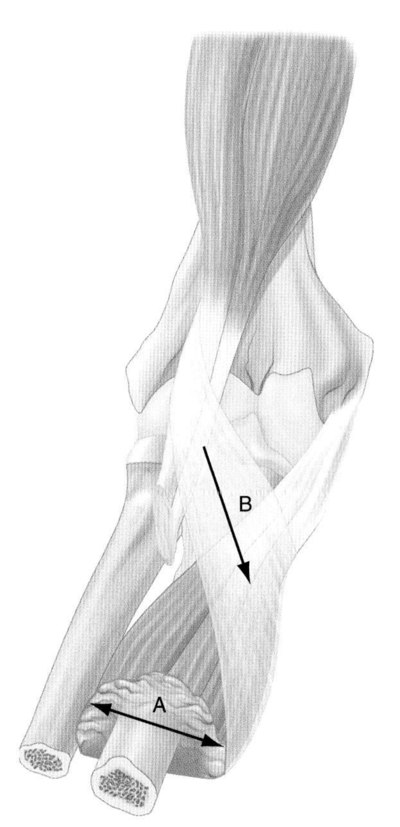

FIGURE 14-2 Prosection of the distal biceps tendon demonstrates separate insertions of the short and long heads and the pattern of insertion of the distal biceps lacertus fibrosis. As the forearm muscles contract, the flexor muscle mass migrates proximally, increasing the cross-sectional area (a). This tenses the aponeurosis, pulling the biceps tendons medially (b). This increases the force on the biceps tendon to provide a supramaximal force. This may be an important factor in the cause of tendon ruptures. *(Modified from Eames MH, Bain GI, Fogg QA, van Riet RP. Distal biceps tendon anatomy: a cadaveric study.* J Bone Joint Surg. *2007;89:1044-1049.)*

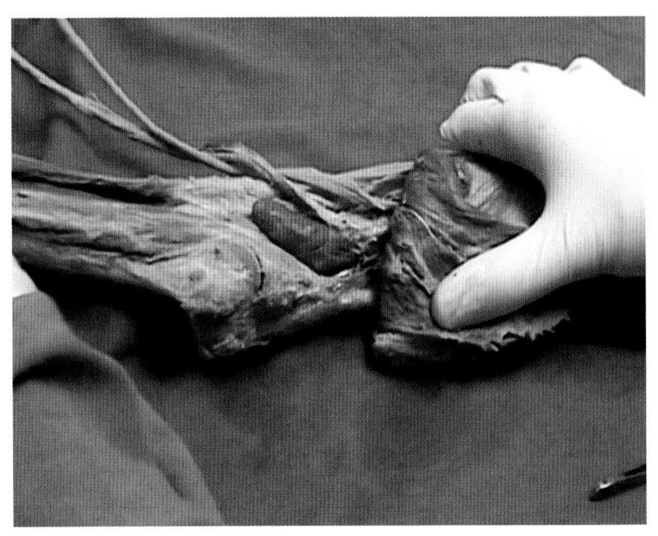

FIGURE 14-3 The biceps bursa is demonstrated by latex injection. A red latex mold was formed for the bicipitoradial bursa in a cadaveric specimen of the elbow.

Surrounding the tendon insertions is the bicipitoradial bursa.[7,8,10,12] This structure is of great clinical importance in endoscopic evaluation of the distal tendon after injury. Eames and Bain[10] found that the bursa encircled the tendons in all cases of their anatomic study. They observed that the bursa was easily distended by approximately 7 mL of normal saline from its deep radial side. The bursa drapes over the tendons, is teardrop shaped, and lies between the groove in the brachialis muscle and the distal tendons with the elbow extended and between the proximal radius and biceps tendon during pronation (Fig. 14-3).[8,10]

PATIENT EVALUATION

History and Physical Examination

Complete tears of the distal biceps tendon are uncommon, accounting for 3% of all tears involving the biceps.[1-3] Partial tears are less common, but descriptions of this type of tear in the literature is increasing, probably as recognition of the pathology improves. Maintaining clinical suspicion of tears of the distal tendon (particularly partial tears) is likely key, particularly in the presence of sometimes very subtle clinical signs.

The age of presentation of patients with partial tears is slightly higher than that of those with complete tears—mid-50s and mid-40s, respectively.[10,13] Almost all complete tears reported in the literature have occurred in male patients, whereas partial tears have been reported for both sexes.[1-3]

In complete and partial tears, the dominant limb is most often affected.[4] In the case of complete tears, the injury occurs through sudden, forced, eccentric contraction of the biceps muscle, such as a sudden and unexpected extension load on a flexed elbow.[4,6,10,13] Partial tears are associated with mixed etiologic factors.

Partial tears are caused by acute traumatic and chronic degenerative mechanisms.[1,2,4,13] The mechanism of injury of acute partial tears is the same as for complete tears, but the force causing the

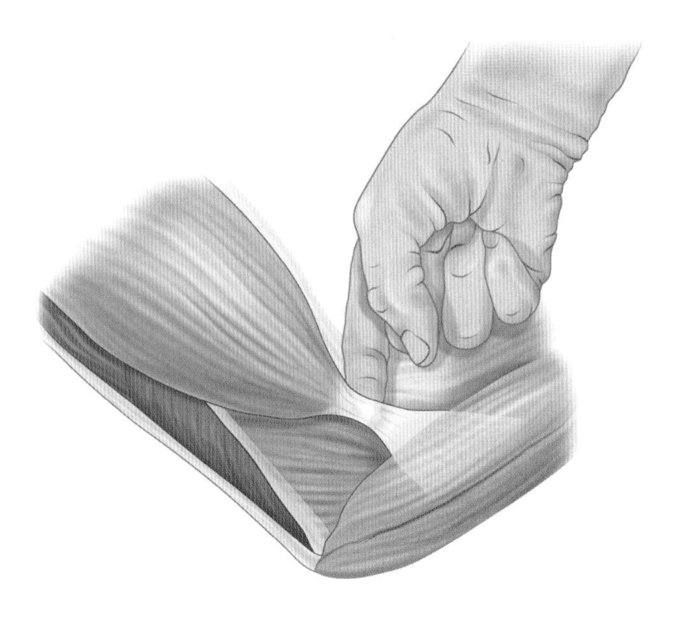

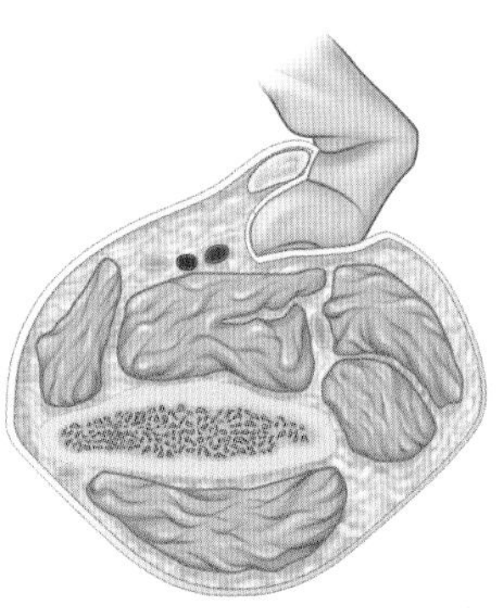

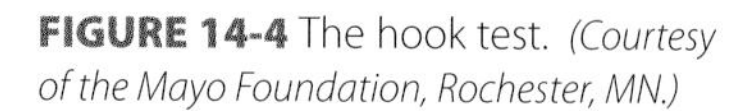

FIGURE 14-4 The hook test. *(Courtesy of the Mayo Foundation, Rochester, MN.)*

injury is interrupted before complete avulsion occurs. Various mechanisms for degeneration have been proposed, including abnormal friction forces, impingement, repetitive strain with supination and pronation, and vascular changes in the tendons.[4,10] It is our experience that degenerate tears of the biceps tendon can occur in the older patient and occurs more often in female patients.

The patient often reports pain in the antecubital fossa, weakness of flexion or supination and possible limitation of elbow range of motion, particularly flexion.[1-6,8,10,13] Inspection may reveal swelling and bruising at the antecubital fossa. This can be an inconsistent finding, particularly in partial tears.[4] Tenderness is elicited on palpation of the antecubital fossa. Pain with resisted supination is a common finding. With complete ruptures, the distal biceps tendon is not palpable in the antecubital fossa, and the physician must be careful that the biceps tendon is being examined, not mistakenly an intact lacertus fibrosus.

The hook test for distal biceps was described by O'Driscoll and colleagues.[14] While the patient actively supinates with the elbow flexed 90 degrees, a positive hook test result permits the examiner to hook his or her index finger under the intact biceps tendon from the lateral side. With an abnormal hook test result, indicating distal avulsion, there is no cordlike structure under which the examiner may hook a finger (Fig. 14-4).[14] The hook test is highly sensitive and specific for complete tears of the distal biceps tendon (as good as or better than magnetic resonance imaging), and it is easy to perform.

A large area of bursitis can compress the median nerve[3] and may produce neurologic signs distally. Imaging can differentiate other diagnoses in the absence of trauma (e.g., antecubital lipoma, other tender lesions) from distal biceps tendinitis or bursitis.

Diagnostic Imaging

For complete tears confirmed by clinical examination, imaging is not required. For partial tears, assessment is difficult, and further investigation can be of assistance. This includes radiologic imaging with magnetic resonance imaging (MRI) or ultrasound and sometimes includes surgical endoscopic examination.

Plain radiography usually is not helpful in the diagnosis of distal biceps tendon tears. Some calcification of degenerate tendons may be seen at the radial tuberosity, but this is not a reliable diagnostic finding and has been reported only for complete tears.[15]

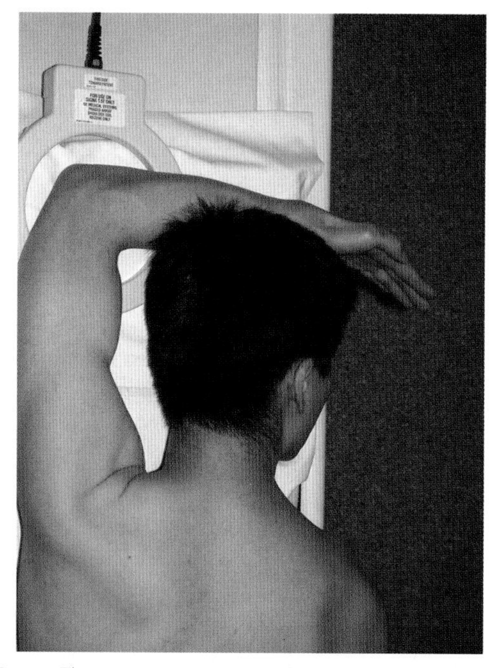

FIGURE 14-5 The patient is positioned for the flexed abducted supinated (FABS) MRI view. This viewing position is used for imaging the distal biceps throughout its length. The patient is prone, with the elbow flexed (F) to 90 degrees, the shoulder is abducted (AB) 180 degrees, and the forearm supinated (S). *(From Giuffre BM, Moss MJ. Optimal positioning for MRI of the distal biceps brachii tendon: flexed abducted supinated view.* AJR Am J Roentgenol. *2004;182:944-946.)*

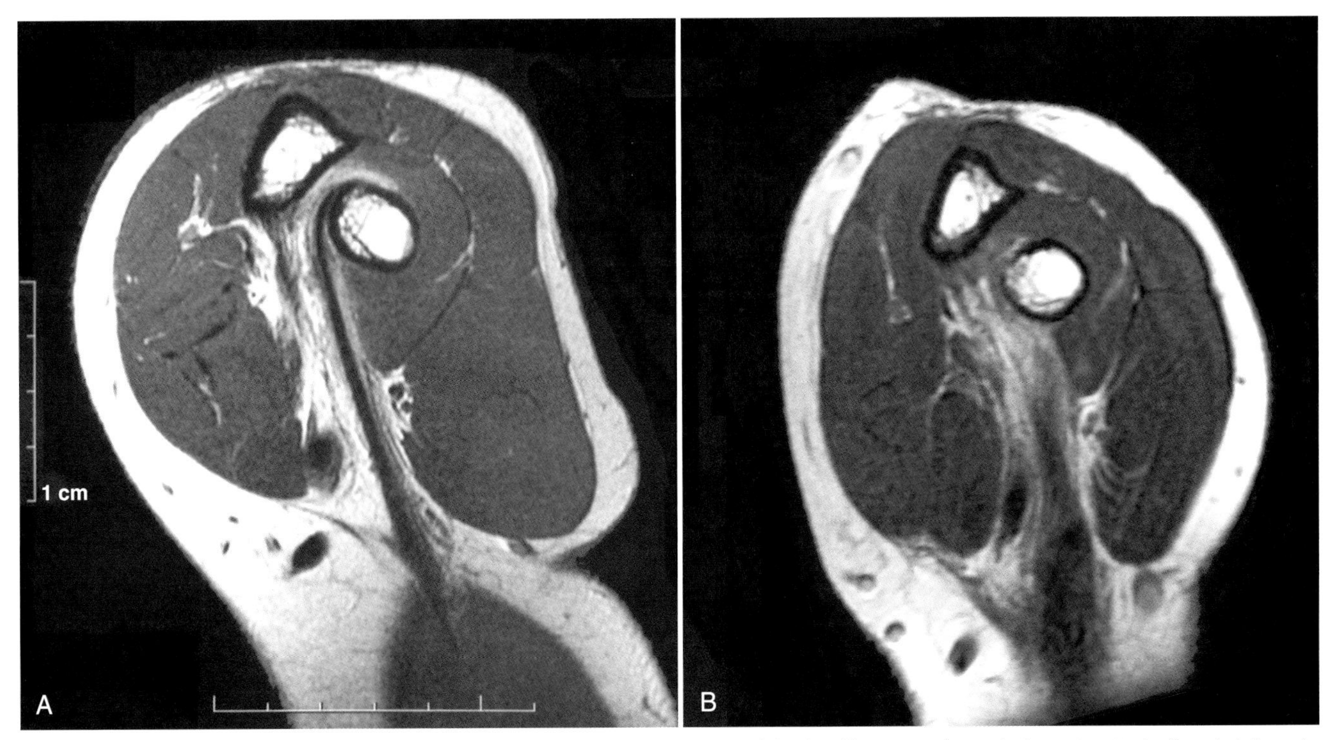

FIGURE 14-6 A, The proton-density magnetic resonance image shows a partial tear of the distal biceps tendon with the patient in the flexed abducted supinated (FABS) position. The image shows a linear, abnormal signal adjacent to the intact tendon, extending from the insertion to the middle part of the tendon, and blurring of fat adjacent to the tendon. **B,** The proton-density magnetic resonance image shows a complete tear of the distal biceps tendon with the patient in the FABS position. The image shows discontinuity of the tendon and an abnormally thickened proximal part of the tendon. *(From Giuffre BM, Moss MJ. Optimal positioning for MRI of the distal biceps brachii tendon: flexed abducted supinated view.* AJR Am J Roentgenol. *2004;182:944-946.)*

Traditional positioning techniques for MRI of the distal biceps tendon yielded images that were difficult to interpret,[5,6] because axial images are obtained from an extended arm for a tendon with an oblique course in the antecubital fossa. Giuffre and Moss[5] described a method for optimal patient positioning that allows full-length views of the biceps brachii tendon from the musculotendinous junction (i.e., Eames and Bain's zone 1) to its insertion on the radial tuberosity (Eames and Bain's zone 3) in one or at most two sections.[5,6,8] This position has become known as the *flexed abducted supinated* (FABS) view, and it is used in addition to conventional views of the biceps brachii (Fig. 14-5).[5,6]

The patient is positioned prone with the shoulder abducted 180 degrees and the arm positioned adjacent to the head. The elbow is then flexed to 90 degrees, with the forearm supinated and the patient's thumb pointing upward. A shoulder phased-array coil is placed at the elbow, making it the center-of-magnet position; this makes fat-suppressed imaging optimal, allowing improved visualization of small amounts of fluid (Fig. 14-6).[6]

Partial tears can be difficult to assess with MRI. The use of T3 MRI with the FABS technique may demonstrate a bicipital effusion and synovitis with adjacent edema.

Ultrasonography has several advantages over other modalities. It is far cheaper than MRI and can be performed in most clinical circumstances. It can be used to confirm continuity of the distal tendon or measure changes in the caliber of the tendinous structures. Dynamic ultrasound evaluation of the distal tendon can differentiate partial from complete ruptures.[6] Peritendinous fluid, such as blood or edema, can be visualized.[6] However, it is operator dependent and therefore less reproducible. Imaging is often performed from the antecubital fossa and volar surface of the elbow, where the anatomic structures are easily palpable. Positioning the forearm in supination brings the distal tendon and its insertion on the radial tuberosity into view on the medial aspect of the radius.[6] Dynamic assessment can then be performed by moving through slight flexion-extension and supination-pronation ranges of motion. The pronator window can be used from the medial side of the proximal forearm through the pronator teres muscle bed (Fig. 14-7).

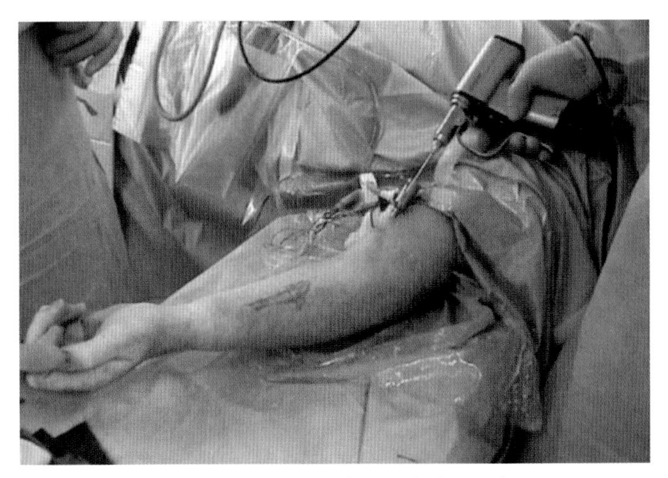

FIGURE 14-7 Patient positioning and setup for biceps bursoscopy. *(From Sharma S, MacKay G. Endoscopic repair of distal biceps tendon using an EndoButton.* Arthroscopy. *2005;21:897.e891-897.e894.)*

TREATMENT

Indications and Contraindications

A complete tear of the distal biceps tendon can be diagnosed clinically with more ease than partial tears, and imaging can aid in clarifying the diagnosis in both instances. Endoscopic investigation of the bicipitoradial bursa allows dynamic assessment of the distal biceps tendon, giving a clear magnified view of the pathology by a comparatively minimally invasive procedure.[8,12]

Patients who have been diagnosed with a complete tear of the distal biceps tendon are usually managed with an open procedure to repair the torn tendon and therefore do not require endoscopic evaluation. For patients who have been diagnosed with a partial tear or tenosynovitis of the distal biceps tendon, we perform an endoscopic assessment. This approach for patients with abnormal anatomy, such as from previous injury or surgery at the elbow and antecubital fossa, is relatively contraindicated.[12] The functional demands and comorbidities of the patient must also be taken into account.

Treatment Alternatives

Although complete tears of the distal biceps tendon require immediate surgical repair to maximize functional outcome, the same may not be true of partial tears.[3,4,8,10,12] Quantifying the percentage of tendon involved in the injury is important. The literature states that tears involving less than 50% of the total insertional footprint do not require surgical reattachment because no functional deficit results.[3,12] Tears involving more than 50% of the insertional footprint require formal surgical division and reattachment using standard techniques.[1-3,8,12,13,16] What is not known is the functional outcomes of tears of long head versus short head tears with regard to operative or nonoperative management.[8] Distal biceps endoscopy allows further assessment of the pathology and treatment of partial tears. Classification of the injury can aid management decisions (Table 14-1).

Conservative Management

Tears of less than 50% of the insertional footprint may not require initial surgical management.[3,8,12] Bourne and Morre[1] treated clinically diagnosed partial tears with 3 weeks of immobilization, 3 weeks of flexion, and then assisted brace with modified duties for 3 months. Durr and colleagues[3] reported treatment with a plaster splint in neutral for 2 weeks in conjunction with systemic anti-inflammatory drugs, followed by physiotherapy. This study found that conservative management of these injuries was successful for patients not requiring forearm strength for professional activities.[3] Local anesthetic injected into the distal tendon insertion site has had satisfactory effects.[3] Each of these series reports decreased pain and functional improvement over the course of several months after the initial injury.

TABLE 14-1 Classification of Insertional (Zone 3) Distal Biceps Tendon Injury

Grade	Injury	Signs	Examples	Treatment
0	Distal biceps tendinosis	Pain on resisted supination and flexion		Nonoperative
1	Distal biceps tendon partial tear	Pain and weakness on resisted supination and flexion		Biceps endoscopy
2	Combined short and long head avulsion, lacertus intact, minimal muscle retraction	Marked weakness of resisted supination and flexion; positive hook test result		Biceps tendon repair
3	Complete tendon rupture with torn lacertus fibrosus and muscle retraction	Marked weakness of resisted supination and flexion positive hook test; "empty" cubital fossa		Biceps tendon repair ± lacertus repair
4	Delayed presentation	Persistent weakness of resisted supination and flexion; positive hook test; proximal retraction of muscle belly		Autograft or allograft reconstruction procedure

Arthroscopic Technique

The benefits of immediate surgical repair for complete ruptures are well established.[4] Through the course of its evolution, surgical treatment of partial tears has involved double- and single-incision open techniques, which were used to complete the partial tear, débride the insertion and torn tendon, and proceed with primary anatomic repair of tendon to bone. Débridement alone of the tendon with a tear greater than 50% of its fibers is not successful.[1,4,15] The various techniques described over the years are directed at reducing the complications encountered by repair (see Table 14-1).[16]

Endoscopy and Partial Tears

Endoscopic investigation of the bicipitoradial bursa enables dynamic assessment of the distal biceps tendon (which cannot be achieved with open techniques), giving a clear, magnified view of the pathology by means of a comparatively minimally invasive procedure.[8,12]

Our preferred technique[8,12] consists of endoscopy of the bicipitoradial bursa performed with the patient under general anesthesia. The arm is exsanguinated, and a proximal tourniquet is inflated to 250 mm Hg. The arm is positioned in extension and supination. A small (2.5-cm), longitudinal incision is made over the palpable biceps tendon 2 cm distal to the elbow crease (Fig. 14-8). The lateral cutaneous nerve of the forearm needs to be identified and protected. Using this mini-open approach, the distal biceps tendon and its bursa are identified with finger dissection. The bursa is insufflated with 7 to 10 mL of normal saline, and a small entry point is made on its radial side at the apex for the arthroscope. Constant insufflation of the bursa is achieved by gravity feed only to avoid excessive extravasation into the forearm. Keeping radial to the entry point enables the surgeon to avoid damaging the median nerve and brachial artery that lie on the ulna aspect of the tendon.

The tendons are identifiable in the field of view and can be followed distally to their insertion into the radial tuberosity, with the long head tendon inserting proximally and the short head distally.[8-10,12] Because the bursa encircles the tendons at their insertion, evaluation can be obtained for tendon patency and for any synovitis and bursitis. The tendons can be viewed dynamically through forearm rotation or with traction applied to a nylon tape placed around the tendon. A hook probe may be introduced through the same portal to examine the distal insertion. A practice point is to appreciate that the bursa may be adherent to tendon on the ulnar side, and it may not inflate on this side in some individuals. Carefully reviewing the tendon, the extent (percentage) of rupture can be determined (Fig. 14-9).

After the extent of injury has been determined, further treatment decisions can be made. Synovitis and tears involving less than 50% of the insertion may be débrided by employing an oscillating chondrotome through the same portal. To avoid damaging neurovascular structures, a full-radius resector without teeth and without suction is used, minimizing the chance of these structures being suctioned into the resector's aperture.[12] By moving the forearm through supination and pronation during the procedure, the surgeon can inspect the entire area of injury and débride it under endoscopic vision. Tears found to be larger than 50% of the tendon insertion can be formally repaired with an open technique by extending the existing endoscopy incision.

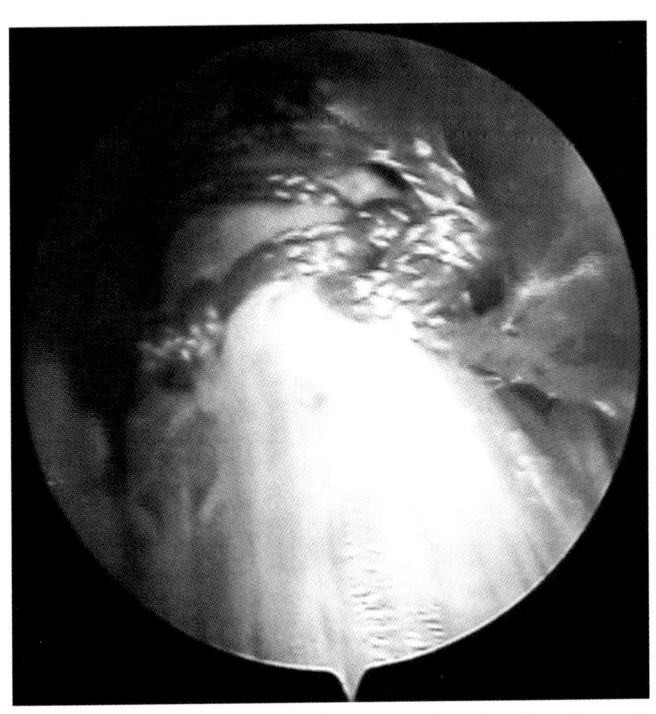

FIGURE 14-8 Arthroscopic view of the repaired tendon. *(From Sharma S, MacKay G. Endoscopic repair of distal biceps tendon using an EndoButton.* Arthroscopy. *2005;21:897.e891-897.e894.)*

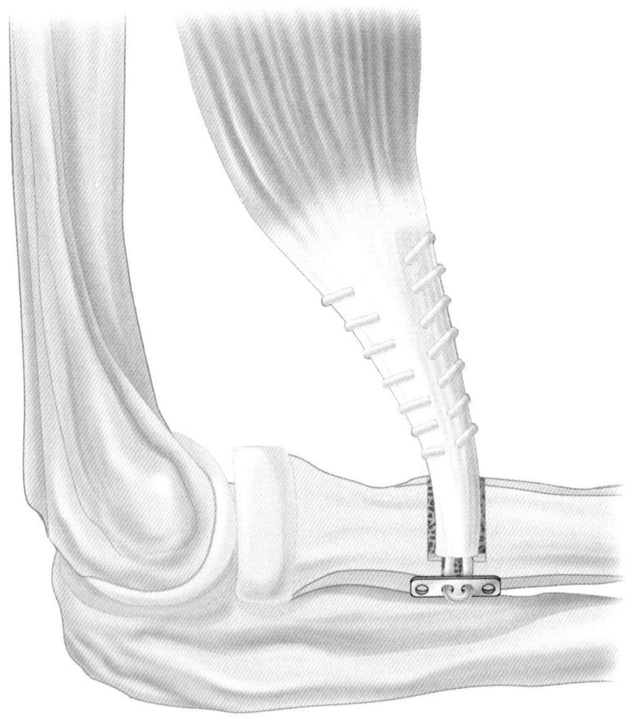

FIGURE 14-9 EndoButton technique for repair of a distal biceps tendon tear. *(Modified from Bain GI, Prem H, Heptinstall RJ, Verhellen R, Paix D. Repair of distal biceps tendon rupture: a new technique using the Endobutton.* J Shoulder Elbow Surg. *2000;9:120-126.)*

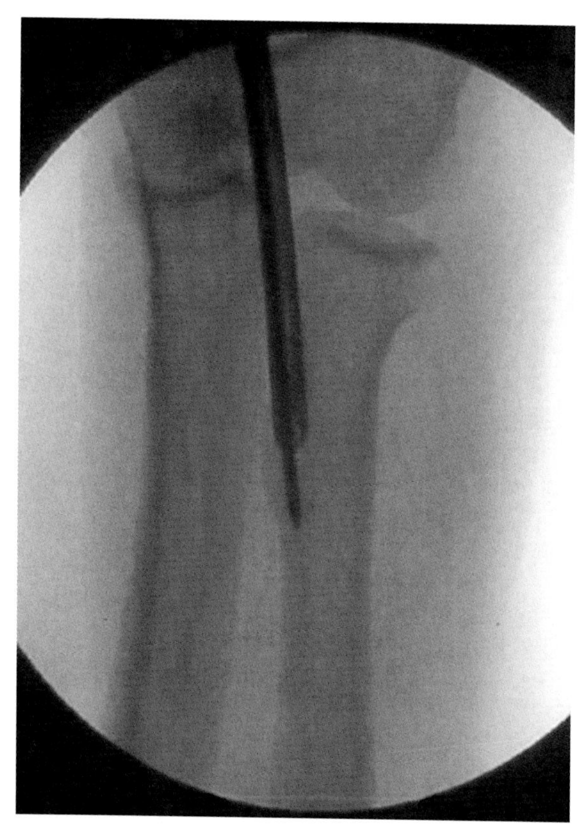

FIGURE 14-10 Intra-operative fluoroscopic confirmation of guidewire placement through an arthroscope cannula into the radial tuberosity. *(From Sharma S, MacKay G. Endoscopic repair of distal biceps tendon using an EndoButton.* Arthroscopy. *2005;21: 897.e891-897.e894.)*

A systematic review of repair techniques concluded that EndoButton repairs consistently performed biomechanically better than other repair methods.[17] The same review found that a significantly larger proportion of unsatisfactory results were obtained for the two-incision approach group for repairs to the distal biceps tendon. It appears that single-incision repairs using an EndoButton give the best results in terms of biomechanical stability and strength and produce fewer unsatisfactory results.

Bain and colleagues[17] described a technique for repair using the EndoButton (Accufex Microsurgical, Mansfield, MA). It is a relatively simple technique that minimizes many of the complications associated with repair, such as stiffness, radioulnar synostosis, and weakness of supination (Fig. 14-10).[16] The superior mechanical strength of this technique compared with other methods of repair allows early active mobilization.

After endoscopic evaluation of the distal biceps tendon, the anterior portal incision can be lengthened, and open repair can be performed if more than 50% of the insertional footprint has been involved by the injury. If there is an incomplete tear that requires release and repair, a hooked monopolar cautery device can be used to perform the release from the radial tuberosity.

Endoscopy and Complete Tears

Sharma and MacKay[18] described an endoscopic technique for repair of complete tears using the EndoButton technique. The technique is performed with the patient under general anesthesia and with the patient's arm on an arm board. A 1.5-cm, longitudinal incision is made in the midline of the anterior aspect of the arm at a point 5 cm proximal to the transverse anterior elbow crease. The ruptured distal end of the biceps tendon is then delivered out of the wound. The ruptured end of the tendon is freshened and sutured to a fixed-loop 20-mm EndoButton using a continuous loop of no. 5 Ethibond (Ethicon, Somerville, NJ), which is interlocked and secured 3 cm proximal to the end of the ruptured tendon.[18] Leading and trailing sutures are applied to the EndoButton as previously described.

The endoscope is then inserted into the sheath of the biceps and the tract of the tendon can be visualized. The tract is followed to its base, where the radial tuberosity can be clearly seen. The camera is removed, leaving the endoscope sheath in situ and positioned against the radial tuberosity. The sheath acts as a tissue protector for the surrounding neurovascular structures while the guidewire and reamers for the EndoButton are employed. A 2.4-mm drill-tipped guidewire that is 15 inches long (Acufex, Smith & Nephew, London, UK) is inserted and its position confirmed using an image intensifier. The guidewire is then drilled through to exit from the extensor aspect of the forearm. A 4.5-mm endoscopic cannulated drill bit (Smith & Nephew) is placed over the guidewire. This is followed by a 6-mm cannulated drill bit for the near cortex of the radial tuberosity to create a socket to accept the distal biceps tendon. The socket should be at least 5 mm deep to achieve tendon-bone interface. The leading and trailing sutures are passed through the eye of the guidewire, and the guidewire is extracted from the extensor surface of the forearm.

The EndoButton is toggled as previously described, and the endoscope is again introduced into the portal to confirm reattachment. The native footprint of the biceps tendon is ulnar in the fully supinated forearm. With the cannulated technique described by Sharma and McKay,[18] it is not possible to place the tunnel at the ulnar side, in addition to risking the radial nerve on the posterolateral forearm. As a consequence, we continue to use the open repair technique for distal biceps repair as originally described.

PEARLS & PITFALLS

PEARLS

- Arm exsanguination facilitates visualization at endoscopy.
- Enter the bursa on the radial side under direct vision to avoid damage to median nerve and brachial artery lying immediately ulnar to the distal biceps tendon.
- Gravity feed fluid only to minimize soft tissue extravasation.
- Do not use suction if using a chondrotome to avoid damaging neurovascular structures.
- Avoid the posterior interosseous nerve by aiming the Beath needle ulnarward when passing through the drill hole in the radius.

PITFALLS

- The bursa encircles the tendons at their insertion but may not inflate on the ulnar side in all individuals.
- Failure to identify and protect the lateral cutaneous nerve of the fore arm leads to neuropraxia.

Postoperative Rehabilitation

Partial tears of the distal biceps tendon that undergo endoscopic débridement only may be mobilized as comfort allows immediately postoperatively.[12] Heavy lifting and resistance activities should be avoided for 6 weeks, and a short course of nonsteroidal anti-inflammatory drugs may be considered for patients with considerable synovitis or those who have a history of heterotopic ossification.[12] Strengthening activities may commence after 6 weeks.

Partial or complete tears that have undergone repair using the EndoButton technique are routinely provided with a sling for comfort.[8,16] After the first postoperative appointment at 1 week, the patient is encouraged to perform range-of-motion exercises as tolerated. The patient is advised not to perform heavy lifting or heavy-resistance work for 3 months, but light duties can commence at 3 weeks.[8,16] Nonsteroidal anti-inflammatory drugs are not routinely used because they may compromise tendon healing, but they should be considered for patients with considerable synovitis or those who have a history of heterotopic ossification.[12]

CONCLUSIONS

We suggest that distal biceps tendon endoscopy be undertaken only by surgeons who are thoroughly familiar with elbow anatomy and who have a high proficiency with endoscopic equipment.[8] The proximity of major neurovascular structures to working portals must be appreciated.

The 50% Rule provides a guide. Tears involving less than 50% of the total insertional footprint do not require surgical reattachment, and tears involving more than 50% of the insertional footprint require surgical division and reattachment using standard techniques.

It is unknown whether short or long head distal biceps tendon tears are important subgroups with regard to nonoperative management. The surgeon must to take into account patient factors (e.g., age, occupation) and tendon tear factors (e.g., percentage, dominant arm, chronic or acute injury) before a final decision is made about treatment.[8]

REFERENCES

1. Bourne MH, Morrey BF. Partial rupture of the distal biceps tendon. *Clin Orthop Relat Res*. 1991;(271):143-148.
2. Rokito AS, McLaughlin JA, Gallagher MA, Zuckerman JD. Partial rupture of the distal biceps tendon. *J Shoulder Elbow Surg*. 1996;5:73-75.
3. Durr HR, Stabler A, Pfahler M, et al. Partial rupture of the distal biceps tendon. *Clin Orthop Relat Res*. 2000;374:195-200.
4. Bernstein AD, Breslow MJ, Jazrawi LM. Distal biceps tendon ruptures: a historical perspective and current concepts. *Am J Orthop*. 2001;30:193-200.
5. Giuffre BM, Moss MJ. Optimal positioning for MRI of the distal biceps brachii tendon: flexed abducted supinated view. *AJR Am J Roentgenol*. 2004;182:944-946.
6. Chew ML, Giuffre BM. Disorders of the distal biceps brachii tendon. *Radiographics*. 2005;25:1227-1237.
7. Sassmannshausen G, Mair SD, Blazar PE. Rupture of a bifurcated distal biceps tendon. A case report. *J Bone Joint Surg Am*. 2004;86A:2737-2740.
8. Bain GI, Johnson LJ, Turner PC. Treatment of partial distal biceps tendon tears. *Sports Med Arthrosc*. 2008;16:154-161.
9. McMinn RMH. Last's Anatomy, Regional and Applied. 9th ed. New York, NY: Churchill Livingstone; 2003.
10. Eames MH, Bain GI, Fogg QA, van Riet RP. Distal biceps tendon anatomy: a cadaveric study. *J Bone Joint Surg Am*. 2007;89:1044-1049.
11. Mazzocca AD, Burton KJ, Romeo AA, et al. Biomechanical evaluation of 4 techniques of distal biceps brachii tendon repair. *Am J Sports Med*. 2007;35:252-258.
12. Eames MHA, Bain GI. Distal biceps tendon endoscopy and anterior elbow arthroscopy portal. *Tech Shoulder Elbow Surg*. 2006;7:139-142.
13. Vardakas DG, Musgrave DS, Varitimidis SE, et al. Partial rupture of the distal biceps tendon. *J Shoulder Elbow Surg*. 2001;10:377-379.
14. O'Driscoll SW, Goncalves LB, Dietz P. The hook test for distal biceps tendon avulsion. *Am J Sports Med*. 2007;35:1865-1869.
15. Ramsey ML. Distal biceps tendon injuries: diagnosis and management. *J Am Acad Orthop Surg*. 1999;7:199-207.
16. Bain GI, Prem H, Heptinstall RJ, et al. Repair of distal biceps tendon rupture: a new technique using the EndoButton. *J Shoulder Elbow Surg*. 2000;9:120-126.
17. Chavan PR, Duquin TR, Bisson LJ. Repair of the ruptured distal biceps tendon: a systematic review. *Am J Sports Med*. 2008;36:1618-1624.
18. Sharma S, MacKay G. Endoscopic repair of distal biceps tendon using an EndoButton. *Arthroscopy*. 2005;21:897.e891-897.e894.

CHAPTER

15

New Techniques in Elbow Arthroscopy

Adam C. Watts • Gregory I. Bain

Elbow arthroscopy was pioneered during the early 1980s, but it came to increased prominence after Andrews and Carson's 1985 paper,[1] which described the anatomy of the elbow joint as seen through the arthroscope and demonstrated the feasibility of arthroscopic diagnosis and treatment of disorders of the elbow. Further works by Morrey,[2] Lynch and colleagues,[3] Poehling and coworkers,[4] and O'Driscoll and Morrey[5] secured the procedure as an accepted orthopedic practice. Initial concerns about the potential for neurologic injury remain the primary concern of elbow arthroscopists today, and thorough knowledge of the neurovascular anatomy of the elbow is essential for performing elbow arthroscopy safely.

Improvements and innovations in instrumentation, patient positioning, and arthroscopic techniques have led to a greatly expanded role of the arthroscope in the management of disorders of the elbow. A broad spectrum of indications for elbow surgery can be considered as indications for elbow arthroscopy or arthroscopically assisted management. This list is limited by the experience of the operating surgeon and includes the classic indications of diagnostic arthroscopy, treatment of osteochondritis dissecans, removal of loose bodies, and irrigation or débridement of septic joints. Widely accepted additional indications include capsular release, débridement, and osteophyte removal for osteoarthritis; synovectomy for rheumatoid arthritis or other inflammatory arthropathies; extensor carpi radialis brevis (ECRB) débridement for lateral epicondylitis; excision of symptomatic synovial plicae; and arthroscope-assisted repair of radial head fractures.

Further indications include a repair of other intra-articular fractures; assessment and arthroscope assisted repair of biceps tendon tears; management of posterolateral rotatory instability and the sequelae of thrower's elbow; débridement of olecranon bursa in olecranon bursitis; and cubital tunnel release in cubital tunnel syndrome. Evidence for these procedures is limited to early reports from centers with an interest in elbow arthroscopy, and indications remain largely at the discretion of the expert arthroscopist based on individual experience and a limited number of case series.

In this chapter, we discuss newer surgical techniques that we employ for elbow arthroscopy and published procedures not covered in other chapters.

THE STIFF ELBOW

Familiarity with the classic open techniques of capsular release is essential before arthroscopic surgery can be considered. These procedures and approaches are necessary fallbacks and are still considered to set the standards by which arthroscopic surgical outcomes are measured. The procedures of arthroscopic capsular release remain the domain of experienced arthroscopic surgeons, who are thoroughly familiar with the regional anatomy and elbow arthroscopy. Before surgical intervention, the cause of the elbow stiffness must be determined. It may be classified according to the anatomic location of the tissue causing contracture:

- Intra-articular pathology, such as intra-articular fibrosis, causing elbow stiffness may be amenable to arthroscopic treatment, but the prognosis may be limited.
- Capsular contracture is the pathology most easily treated with arthroscopy, and it therefore carries the best prognosis.
- Extra-articular causes of elbow stiffness, such as heterotopic ossification, are not amenable to arthroscopic management. The prognosis is mixed.

We prefer to position the patient in a lateral position with the arm flexed at the elbow 90 degrees over a fixed bolster (Fig. 15-1). A 30-degree, 4.0-mm arthroscope without side-venting cannulas is most often used, but a 2.7-mm arthroscope can make visualization of the lateral gutter easier, and a 70-degree scope may add perspective in tight joints.

Capsule distention is performed easily and safely through the lateral soft spot. The normal joint can accommodate about 30 mL

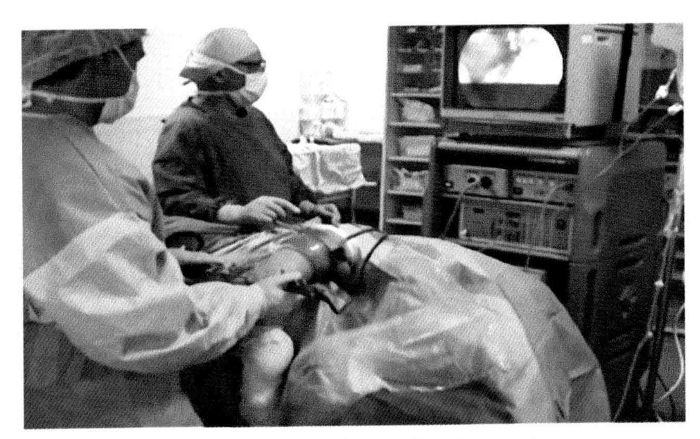

FIGURE 15-1 Our preferred setup for elbow arthroscopy.

of fluid at 70 degrees of flexion, but in patients with joint contracture, this amount is significantly decreased and averages only 6 mL at 85 degrees. The capsule is also about 15% less compliant in these cases, and it is often thickened.[6] Although capsule distention can increase the safety of portal placement by increasing the distance from the articulation to related neurovascular structures, the distance from the capsule to these structures remains unchanged and does not protect the neurovasculature during capsulectomy or capsular release.

We think the safest method of making portals is to incise sharply through the epidermis and dermis and bluntly dissect through the depths of the subcutaneous fat layers. This minimizes damage to cutaneous nerves that are found in the very depth of the subcutaneous fat (Fig. 15-2).[7]

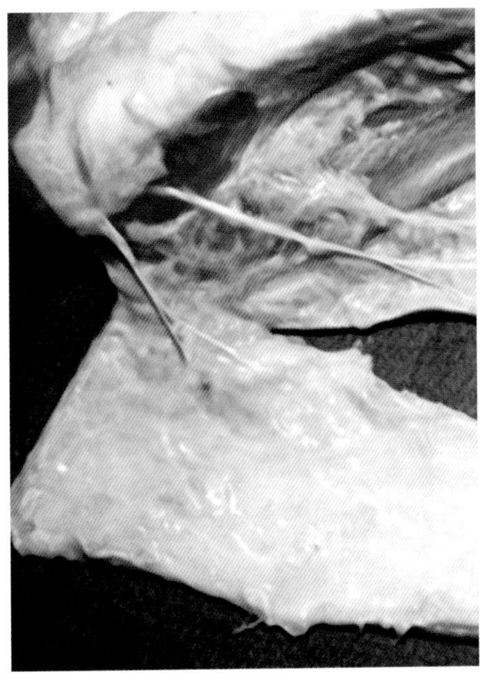

FIGURE 15-2 Cadaveric dissection shows the superficial cutaneous nerves in the deep subcutaneous fat layers about the elbow.

Advanced therapeutic arthroscopy requires the ability to view the anatomy from multiple portals. Switching the arthroscope and other instruments between portals is necessary so the joint can be perceived in three dimensions. The joint is like a three-dimensional box. The use of retractors to increase arthroscopic exposure is a major advance in therapeutic arthroscopy of the elbow, but cutting instruments should only be used with direct visualization of the instruments and adjacent structures. Suction should be avoided near nervous tissue, and shaver blades should always point away from nerves. Patients with contracture greater than 90 degrees of flexion require open ulnar nerve release before any capsular release to prevent neurologic deficit.

Three types of anterior capsular releases have been reported:

- A *capsulotomy* is performed superiorly from medial to lateral. It is performed proximally to minimize the chance of radial nerve injury, and it is usually performed with cautery or a hook knife.
- In a *linear capsulectomy*, a strip of the proximal capsule is excised with a basket forceps or a resector.[8]
- In a *radical capsulectomy*, the entire anterior capsule is excised. To perform this safely, the radial nerve requires exploration.[9]

We strongly recommend that these procedures be considered only by an experienced arthroscopist. Surgeons should first perform the procedure on a cadaveric model.

We prefer to perform a capsulectomy rather than a simple release to reduce the risk of recurrence. If the surgeon wishes to identify the radial nerve before excising the adjacent capsule, we recommend the use of two medial portals and a lateral retractor to protect nervous tissue (Fig. 15-3). Our preferred technique is to excise the medial one half of the capsule first. A mini-Hohmann retractor is then introduced through the medial portal. An arthroscope is placed in the medial superior portal with the

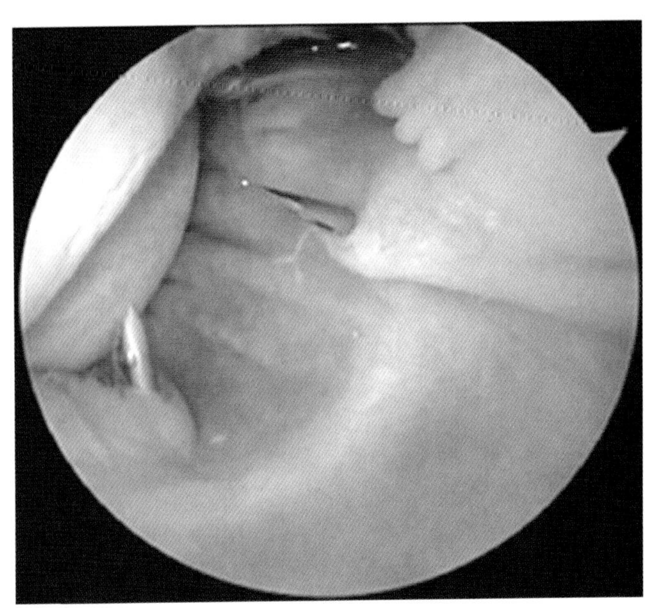

FIGURE 15-3 In this cadaveric specimen, the radial nerve has been exposed by an open technique. The course of the nerve where it is in direct contact with the elbow joint capsule has been identified by the two needles that are seen in the arthroscopic view.

retractor in the medial inferior portal. The capsule can then be teased off the brachialis muscle using blunt dissection. The blunt-ended retractor can be rotated to identify this natural interval. The radial nerve can be safely retracted anteriorly by advancing the retractor toward the lateral side. After this interval is developed, a second retractor is passed through the anterolateral portal and passed between the capsule and the first retractor, which can be removed. At this point, the capsulectomy can be safely completed. The capsulectomy should not proceed unless the nerve can be clearly visualized and protected with the Hohmann retractor.

A common cause of limited elbow flexion in an elbow with degenerative change is a coronoid osteophyte. Adequate excision of this osteophyte with a chondrotome can be challenging, and it may be associated with chondral damage to the trochlea. We prefer to introduce a narrow osteotome from an anteromedial working portal, with the arthroscope in the anterolateral portal. The osteotome can be placed at the chosen level of resection, and under arthroscopic vision, it is advanced into the bone with a mallet. This is most easily performed with the elbow flexed to 120 degrees. The osteotome can be rotated to complete the osteotomy of the coronoid (a wrench applied to the handle of the osteotome may be necessary to perform this maneuver). The resected bone is removed from the joint using an arthroscopic clamp or pituitary rongeur. We do not use a motorized resector because the shape of the blade prevents adequate excision.

PEARLS & PITFALLS

- Commence the capsulectomy from the medial side with a second medial viewing portal, and use a mini-Hohmann retractor interposed between the capsule and brachialis muscle.
- Use an osteotome to resect the tip of the coronoid.
- The radial nerve lies on the anterior capsule laterally and may be injured if not visualized when performing the capsulectomy.

Postoperative Management and Rehabilitation

The range of motion achieved intraoperatively should be accurately recorded. The aim is to achieve this range as early as possible postoperatively. Good postoperative analgesia is essential, and the use of nerve blocks can be useful. Range-of-motion exercises should be active whenever possible. Continuous passive motion (CPM) or night splinting is advocated by some surgeons, but it is not used in our practice. Although CPM has been shown to mildly improve active flexion in open capsulectomy, mean active extension is unaffected, and it is often poorly tolerated.[10] We implement a 14-day course of nonsteroidal anti-inflammatory medication to minimize the risk of heterotopic bone formation and to reduce pain and swelling. We have used turnbuckle splints in more severe cases and for patients for whom rehabilitation has been slow.

ASSESSMENT OF ELBOW INSTABILITY

In our practice, elbow arthroscopy has an important role in the assessment of elbow instability. At the outset of any reconstructive procedure, the elbow is examined clinically through a range of movement, varus-valgus loading, and a pivot shift test. Fluoroscopic examination is performed to look for widening of the ulnohumeral joint on valgus loading. With the forearm held in supination, a lateral view is obtained to look for the tilt sign, which suggests lateral ligament instability.

Elbow arthroscopy is performed in all patients. The elbow is assessed with the arthroscope in the anteromedial portal. A rent may be seen of the lateral ligament complex from the humerus, which often tears off as a sleave.[11] This rent is the best sign of posterolateral rotatory instability (PLRI) when viewing from the anterior compartment. The capsule sits on the capitellum and therefore does not heal back to the lateral epicondyle. Scuffing of the radial head or capitellum humeri may be seen.

The arthroscope is then moved to the anterolateral portal to visualize the coronoid-trochlea articulation. Abnormal widening of this joint may be seen with varus or valgus loading in the unstable elbow. Widening of the joint of more than 1 mm is abnormal on the medial and lateral sides. This varus-valgus instability is best assessed anteriorly. PLRI is difficult to assess in the anterior compartment because the radial head is seen to slide of the capitellum. It can be impossible to determine whether this is normal or pathologic, because the radiocapitellar joint appears to close.

Another portal is created posteriorly to inspect the ulnohumeral articulation. With lateral instability, the joint may be seen to open laterally with forearm supination, and with medial instability, forearm pronation may cause the joint to open medially. The rotatory instability is best assessed from the posterior compartment. In the normal elbow, the olecranon-trochlea articulation may open and admit the probe medially and laterally. In patients with PLRI, the arthroscope can be introduced between the trochlea and trochlea notch. The bare area of the olecranon can often be seen, as can the radial head and a rent in the lateral capsule.

We use arthroscopy to classify patients with PLRI in three groups. Those with isolated PLRI are managed with a lateral reconstruction. Those with associated medial joint space opening are managed with a circumferential graft to reconstruct the medial and lateral collateral ligaments.[12] The third group of patients has degenerative changes, and their management is governed by the degree of instability and osteoarthrosis.

PEARLS & PITFALLS

- Rotational instability is most reliably assessed form the posterior compartment of the elbow.

SOFT TISSUE LESIONS OF THE ELBOW

Ulnar Neuritis

Ulnar neuritis is the second most common entrapment neuropathy of the upper limb. Various techniques have been described for performing endoscopic ulnar nerve decompression at the elbow. We prefer to use the Agee Micro-Aire device (LMT, Taringa, Queensland, Australia). A cadaveric study demonstrated the safety and efficacy of this technique.[13]

With the patient under general anesthesia and placed in the lateral position with the elbow flexed over a padded bar and an upper arm tourniquet inflated, a 3-cm incision is made between the olecranon and medial epicondyle. Blunt dissection is performed to the cubital retinaculum. A small fenestration is performed to allow insertion of the Agee device adjacent to the nerve under direct vision. The device is used proximally and distally to divide the cubital retinaculum. The device is gently manipulated until the retinaculum is clearly visible and inspection shows that the nerve and its branches are not threatened. Activating the trigger mechanism advances the blade, and the entire device is carefully withdrawn to incise the retinaculum. The blade can be rapidly retracted by release of the trigger if any important structures come into view. The endoscope is then reintroduced to assess the adequacy of the decompression.

We performed a prospective study that compared the outcomes of this technique with open, in situ decompression and found no differences in the patient-reported outcomes at 12 months after surgery. The rate of complications was lower in the endoscopic group than in the open group. Complications included elbow pain, numbness, and scar tenderness. No patients had injury to the ulnar nerve, and there were no infections.

Biceps Tendon Bursoscopy

Distal biceps tendon bursoscopy may be indicated for patients presenting with symptoms of biceps bursitis or those with a suspected partial-thickness tear of the distal biceps tendon. The bicipitoradial bursa surrounds the distal biceps tendon. It is adherent to the radial aspect of the biceps tendon and drapes around the tendon before attaching circumferentially to the radius at the tendon-bone interface.[14]

The procedure is performed under general anesthesia with an inflated upper arm tourniquet. The arm is positioned in extension and supination. A 2.5-cm longitudinal incision commencing 2 cm distal to the anterior elbow crease is performed over the palpable biceps tendon. Care is taken to protect the lateral cutaneous nerve of the forearm. The bursa is identified surrounding the distal biceps tendon. The bursa can be inflated with 7 to 10 mL of saline. The trocar and cannula of the arthroscope are inserted into the apex of the bursa on its radial side, and the arthroscope is inserted. Inflation is maintained with saline by gravity feed.[15]

The bursa can be visualized to confirm the diagnosis of bursitis (Fig. 15-4). The biceps tendon insertion is examined for partial tears. Bursectomy or débridement of partial-thickness tears can be performed using a toothless, full-radius oscillating chondrotome. This should be performed without suction to avoid injury to neurovascular structures.

With this approach, care must be taken to avoid the median nerve and brachial artery. These structures lie on the ulnar side of the tendon and can be avoided by entering the bursa on its radial side. The chondrotome should not be used unless a clear field is visible, and suction should not be used. The lateral cutaneous nerve is at risk because it lies radial to the tendon. Neurapraxia has been witnessed with retraction, and care is required to protect it.

Olecranon Bursoscopy

Olecranon bursoscopy is discussed in detail in Chapter 5. We have modified our technique to protect the overlying skin when resecting the inflamed or infected bursa.

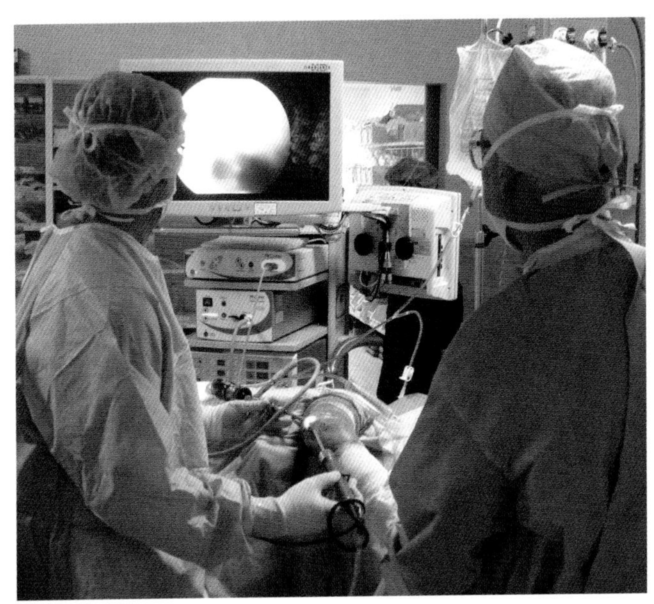

FIGURE 15-4 Olecranon bursectomy. *(Photograph courtesy of Adam C. Watts, MD, Adelaide, Australia.)*

With the patient placed in the lateral position under general anesthesia and an upper arm tourniquet inflated, two 1.5-cm longitudinal incisions are made in the midline 3 cm proximal and distal to the margins of the bursa (Fig. 15-5). Blunt dissection is performed in the subcutaneous plane using Metzenbaum scissors to connect the two incisions, separating the cutaneous tissue from the bursa. Bursectomy can be safely performed using a toothed, oscillating chondrotome, which should be used with the jaws facing the bursa, away from the skin. The bursectomy is performed from the subcutaneous plane and directed toward the olecranon. The procedure is complete when the fibers of the triceps tendon are visible. Care must be taken not to weaken this insertion. Distention of the subcutaneous field can be facilitated by passing a tape or suture through from one portal to the other and applying traction or with the use of disposable arthroscopy portals placed in the dependent (distal) incision.

Ganglia

Synovial cysts (i.e., ganglia) of the elbow joint can rarely be found in patients with osteoarthrosis or rheumatoid arthritis (Fig. 15-6). Most can be managed nonoperatively. For patients with persistent symptoms, surgery may be advised. Other indications include compression of neurologic structures of the elbow by the mass affect of the ganglion.[16] Feldman reported the first case of a ganglion cyst of the elbow treated with arthroscopic excision.[17]

The procedure is performed through standard arthroscopy portals. Excision can be facilitated by the addition of another portal anterior and distal to the anterolateral portal, through which a transfixing Wissinger rod can be inserted to distract the anterior neurovascular bundle away from the operating field.[16,18] The transfixing rod can protect neurologic structures, improve the arthroscopic view, and facilitate excision. We emphasize the importance of complete excision of the cyst lining to prevent recurrence (Fig. 15-7).

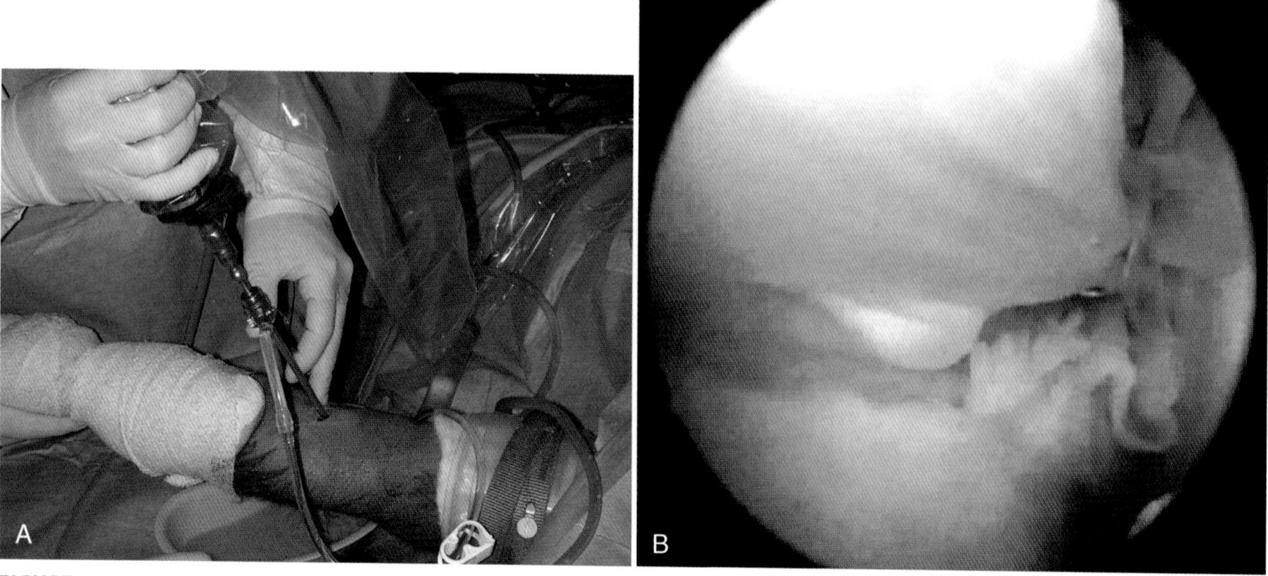

FIGURE 15-5 A, Biceps bursoscopy intraoperative setup. **B,** Endoscopic view of the bursa. *(From Eames MH, Bain GI. Distal biceps tendon endoscopy and anterior elbow arthroscopy portal.* Tech Shoulder Elbow Surg. *2006;7:139-142.)*

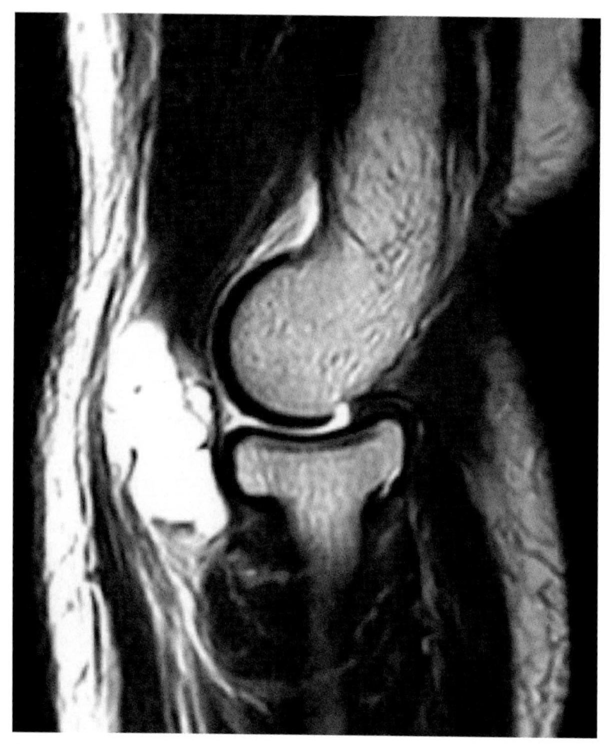

FIGURE 15-6 Sagittal, T2-weighted magnetic resonance image shows a multilocular ganglion cyst arising from the elbow joint. *(From Kirpalani PA, Lee HK, Han CW. Transarticular arthroscopic excision of an elbow cyst.* Acta Orthop Belg. *2005;71:477-480.)*

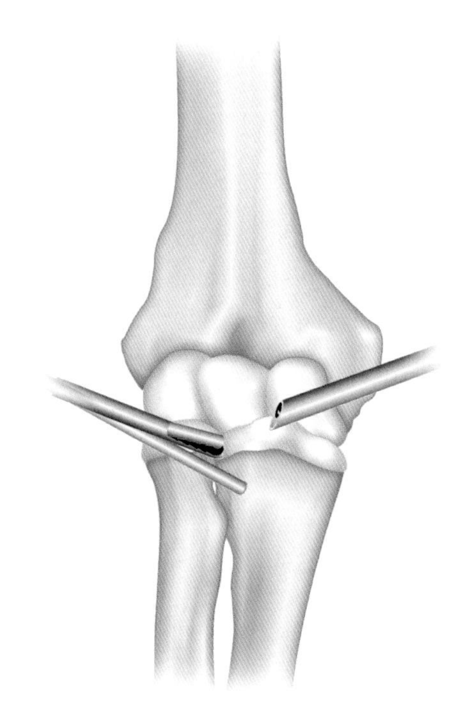

FIGURE 15-7 Diagrammatic view of the Wissinger rod inserted anterior and distal to the anterolateral portal. *(Modified from Kirpalani PA, Lee HK, Han CW. Transarticular arthroscopic excision of an elbow cyst.* Acta Orthop Belg. *2005;71:477-480.)*

PEARLS & PITFALLS

PEARLS

- For soft tissue lesions of the elbow, enter the bursa on its radial side after inflation with up to 10 mL of saline.
- Subcutaneous dissection between the skin and bursa can protect the dermis during olecranon bursectomy.
- A Wissinger rod can be inserted anterior and distal to the anterolateral portal to protect neurovascular structures when addressing a ganglion.

PITFALLS

- In treating soft tissue lesions, neurapraxia of the lateral cutaneous nerve of the forearm can occur with overzealous retraction.
- Care must be taken not to weaken the triceps insertion during olecranon bursectomy.
- Avoid skin perforation by working toward the olecranon.
- Incomplete excision of the lining of the ganglion cyst may lead to recurrence.

BENIGN INTRA-ARTICULAR LESIONS

Osteoid Osteoma

Arthroscopic techniques can be used for the treatment of intra-articular osteoid osteoma of the elbow. Although this diagnosis is rare, the location of the lesions can render them entirely suitable for arthroscopic excision (Fig. 15-8).

Osteoid osteoma is a benign neoplasm that typically affects the diaphysis of long bones. Patients typically present with nocturnal symptoms of elbow pain that may be relieved by nonsteroidal anti-inflammatory analgesia. The elbow may be stiff because of pain or synovitis. Computed tomography showing a lesion less than 1 cm in diameter with a dense central nidus is diagnostic. The lesion may be visible on plain radiographs. Medical treatment of osteoid osteoma with nonsteroidal anti-inflammatory analgesia is possible, but it may take several years for the symptoms to resolve, and the location of the lesion may be associated with elbow stiffness that may not be tolerated.

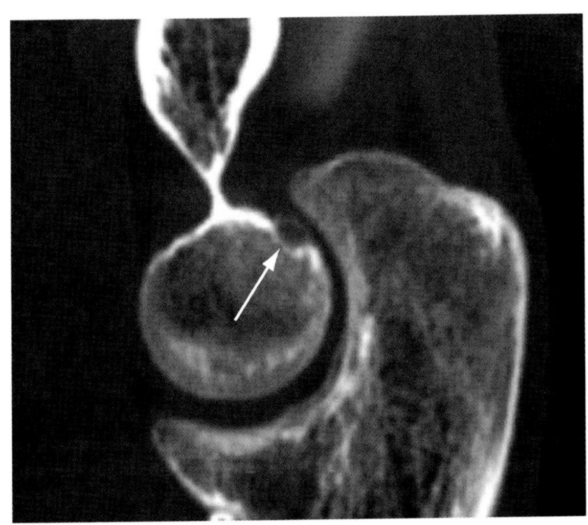

FIGURE 15-8 Computed tomography of the elbow shows an osteoid osteoma of the posterior aspect of the capitellum in a 20-year-old man. *(From Nourissat G, Kakuda C, Dumontier C. Arthroscopic excision of osteoid osteoma of the elbow.* Arthroscopy. *2007;23:799e1-799e4.)*

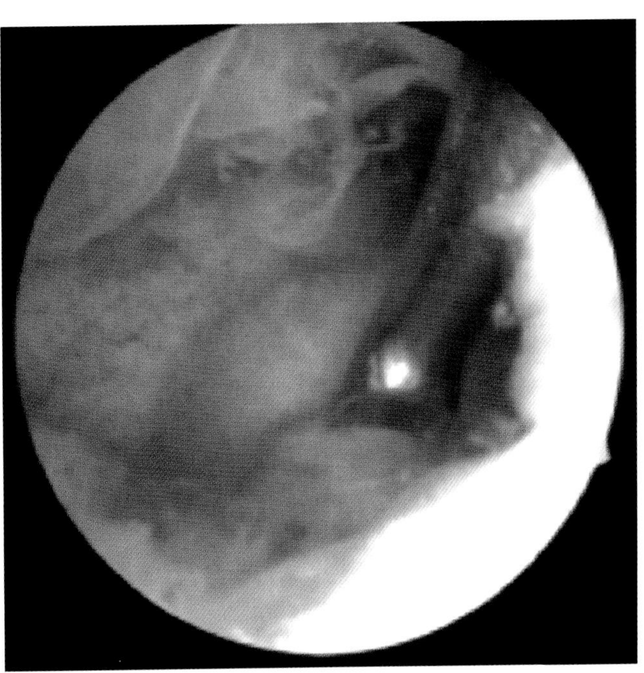

FIGURE 15-9 The arthroscopic view demonstrates the use of a curette for en bloc excision. *(From Nourissat G, Kakuda C, Dumontier C. Arthroscopic excision of osteoid osteoma of the elbow.* Arthroscopy. *2007;23: 799e1-799e4.)*

Nourissat and colleagues[19] reported two cases of osteoid osteoma, one on the capitellum and the other on the trochlea in patients 20 and 27 years old, respectively. The procedure was performed with the patient under general anesthesia and in the lateral decubitus position. The lesion was removed with a curette (Fig. 15-9), producing complete resolution of symptoms by 2 weeks. One patient had an early, symptomatic recurrence of the lesion. This was attributed to the surgical technique. The surgeons thought that use of the chondrotome shaver for excision led to incomplete excision.

Patients with osteoid osteoma in the elbow joint can be offered arthroscopic excision, but the surgeon must ensure that incomplete excision does not occur. Complete excision may be aided with the use of fluoroscopy. A shaver should not be used for excision but may be used to expose the lesion. Excision biopsy should be performed with a curette, and the specimen should be sent for histologic evaluation. The surrounding hyperemic bone should be removed with a burr. The appropriate arthroscopic portals for safe excision should be tailored to the site of the lesion and can be planned from preoperative radiologic imaging.

The surgeon also should consider image-guided percutaneous radiofrequency ablation. It is an established technique for the treatment of osteoid osteoma when accessible.[20]

Synovial Chondromatosis

Synovial chondromatosis is a rare condition that can be a primary condition or result from an underlying pathology, such as osteoarthrosis or osteochondritis dissecans. It is caused by metaplasia of synoviocytes. Histologically, the condition is characterized by synovitis with foci of newly formed cartilage. The patient presents with pain and swelling of the elbow. Epi-

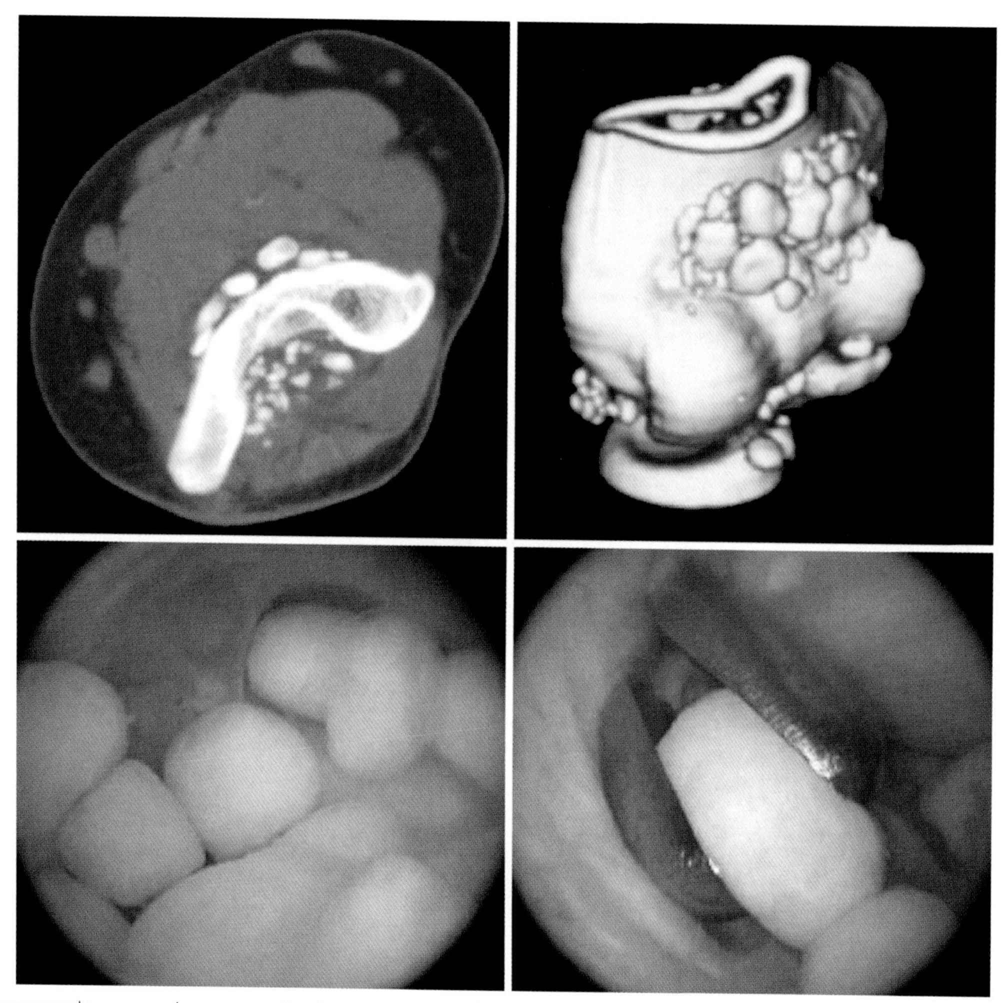

FIGURE 15-10 Computed tomography scans and arthroscopic views of primary chondromatosis. *(From Flury MP, Goldhahn J, Drerup S, Simmen BR. Arthroscopic and open options for surgical treatment of chondromatosis of the elbow.* Arthroscopy. *2008;24:520-525e1.)*

sodes of locking occur because of cartilage bodies that develop within the joint.

Standard care involves removal of chondral bodies (often described as loose, although most remain bound to the synovium) and partial synovectomy, which may be performed as an open or an arthroscopic procedure. Arthroscopy is advocated because synovectomy can be performed with less trauma to the surrounding tissues,[21] but it does require advanced arthroscopic skills to perform safely and adequately.

The procedure is performed through standard arthroscopy portals. Removal of sizeable chondral lesions that cause mechanical symptoms is mandatory (Fig. 15-10). The synovectomy should be as extensive as is safe to perform, but affected tissue often remains in the medial and lateral gutters.[21,22]

Flury and colleagues[23] reported the largest series of arthroscopic treatment of synovial chondromatosis. Fourteen adult patients with a mixture of primary and secondary chondromatosis of the elbow were reviewed retrospectively at an average of 39 months (range, 11 to 70 months) after arthroscopic synovectomy. This group was compared with five patients treated at the same center using open techniques. No differences in outcome were reported using validated outcome measures, although the investigators acknowledged the power limitations of the study. None of the patients had recurrence of chondral lesions on radiographic review. Two patients had some recurrence of symptoms that were attributed to underlying osteoarthrosis. The study authors suggest that the rehabilitation time was shorter for the arthroscopic group.

PEARLS & PITFALLS

PEARLS

- Intra-articular osteoid osteoma of the elbow can be treated with surgical excision using a curette and a burr to remove surrounding hyperemic bone.
- Synovial chondromatosis of the elbow is best treated with arthroscopic synovectomy.

PITFALLS

- Excision with a shaver may be associated with incomplete excision and recurrence. The shaver may be used to expose the osteoid osteoma.
- Incomplete synovial resection may be associated with recurrence.

REFERENCES

1. Andrews JR, Carson WG. Arthroscopy of the elbow. *Arthroscopy*. 1985; 1:97-107.
2. Morrey BF. Arthroscopy of the elbow. *Instr Course Lect*. 1986;35:102-107.
3. Lynch GJ, Meyers JF, Whipple TL, Caspari RB. Neurovascular anatomy and elbow arthroscopy: inherent risks. *Arthroscopy*. 1986;2:190-197.
4. Poehling GG, Whipple TL, Sisco L, Goldman B. Elbow arthroscopy: a new technique. *Arthroscopy*. 1989;5:222-224.
5. O'Driscoll SW, Morrey BF. Arthroscopy of the elbow. Diagnostic and therapeutic benefits and hazards. *J Bone Joint Surg Am*. 1992;74:84-94.
6. O'Driscoll SW, Morrey BF, An KN. Intraarticular pressure and capacity of the elbow. *Arthroscopy*. 1990;6:100-103.
7. Dowdy PA, Bain GI, King GJ, Patterson SD. The midline posterior elbow incision. An anatomical appraisal. *J Bone Joint Surg Br*. 1995;77: 696-699.
8. Ball CM, Meunier M, Galatz LM, et al. Arthroscopic treatment of post-traumatic elbow contracture. *J Shoulder Elbow Surg*. 2002;11:624-629.
9. O'Driscoll SW. Operative treatment of elbow arthritis. *Curr Opin Rheumatol*. 1995;7:103-106.
10. Gates HS 3rd, Sullivan FL, Urbaniak JR. Anterior capsulotomy and continuous passive motion in the treatment of post-traumatic flexion contracture of the elbow. A prospective study. *J Bone Joint Surg Am*. 1992; 74:1229-1234.
11. Mehta JA, Bain GI. Posterolateral rotatory instability of the elbow. *J Am Acad Orthop Surg*. 2004;12:405-415.
12. van Riet RP, Bain GI, Baird R, Lim YW. Simultaneous reconstruction of medial and lateral elbow ligaments for instability using a circumferential graft. *Tech Hand Up Extrem Surg*. 2006;10:239-244.
13. Bain GI, Bajhau A. Endoscopic release of the ulnar nerve at the elbow using the Agee device: a cadaveric study. *Arthroscopy*. 2005;21:691-695.
14. Eames MH, Bain GI, Fogg QA, van Riet RP. Distal biceps tendon anatomy: a cadaveric study. *J Bone Joint Surg Am*. 2007;89:1044-1049.
15. Eames MH, Bain GI. Distal biceps tendon endoscopy and anterior elbow arthroscopy portal. *Tech Shoulder Elbow Surg*. 2006;7:139-142.
16. Mileti J, Largacha M, O'Driscoll SW. Radial tunnel syndrome caused by ganglion cyst: treatment by arthroscopic cyst decompression. *Arthroscopy*. 2004;20:e39-44.
17. Feldman MD. Arthroscopic excision of a ganglion cyst from the elbow. *Arthroscopy*. 2000;16:661-664.
18. Kirpalani PA, Lee HK, Lee YS, Han CW. Transarticular arthroscopic excision of an elbow cyst. *Acta Orthop Belg*. 2005;71:477-480.
19. Nourissat G, Kakuda C, Dumontier C. Arthroscopic excision of osteoid osteoma of the elbow. *Arthroscopy*. 2007;23:799e1-799e4.
20. Venbrux AC, Montague BJ, Murphy KP, et al. Image-guided percutaneous radiofrequency ablation for osteoid osteomas. *J Vasc Interv Radiol*. 2003;14:375-380.
21. Bynum CK, Tasto J. Arthroscopic treatment of synovial disorders in the shoulder, elbow, and ankle. *J Knee Surg*. 2002;15:57-59.
22. Byrd JW. Arthroscopy of the elbow for synovial chondromatosis. *J South Orthop Assoc*. 2000;9:119-124.
23. Flury MP, Goldhahn J, Drerup S, Simmen BR. Arthroscopic and open options for surgical treatment of chondromatosis of the elbow. *Arthroscopy*. 2008;24:520-525e1.

CHAPTER

16

Arthroscopic Triceps Repair

Felix H. Savoie III • Larry D. Field • Michael O'Brien

Injuries to the triceps tendon were once thought to occur only in patients performing extremely heavy lifting exercises or those using supplementation to artificially enhance their ability to perform these types of exercises. However, as our population has aged and attempted to maintain an extremely active lifestyle, many such injuries have become more commonplace in the average population. The increased number of older, more active individuals has increased the incidence of injury to the triceps.

ANATOMY

The triceps tendon takes its name from the three sites of its origin from the humerus and inferior glenoid. The triceps muscle courses distally along the posterior aspect of the humerus to insert in a fanlike fashion on the proximal and posterior aspects of the olecranon process of the ulna. The insertion lies beneath the olecranon bursa and blends with the forearm muscle origins arising from the ulna. The main function of the triceps is to extend the elbow. Injuries to the triceps muscle-tendon unit may take many forms, including partial or complete avulsion from the bone, intrasubstance tears, and muscle-tendon junction tears.

PATIENT EVALUATION

History and Physical Examination

Most patients have experienced pain or a "pop" when performing a press-type activity or after a fall on an outstretched and slightly flexed elbow. In heavy-weight lifters, this usually occurs during a bench press activity, with resultant loss of control of the bar. In less active individuals, it can occur while pushing up from a seated position. Partial tears may begin with a subtle pain noticed in the beginning of extension from a fully flexed position. Dips and overhead triceps extension exercises, as often performed in body pump or weight-lifting classes, may represent the first time a patient begins to notice pain in the back of the elbow. This is especially true in cases of degenerative, dysvascular tear patterns.

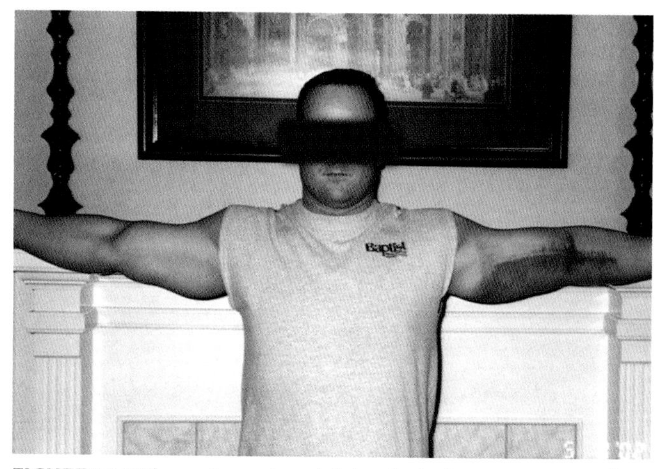

FIGURE 16-1 The ecchymosis and deformity in the upper arm resulted from a triceps injury sustained during heavy bench press activity.

The physical examination begins with observation for swelling or ecchymosis (Fig. 16-1). Patients with complete tears may have a complete loss of the ability to extend the elbow, whereas those with partial or degenerative tears may retain active extension but in a weakened state. In those with the more subtle tears, trying to extend the elbow from a fully flexed position reproduces pain directly over the site of the injury (i.e., triceps stress test), which can then be palpated for a defect.

Diagnostic Imaging

Radiographs may show a small fragment of bone pulled off the tip of the olecranon or a fracture of a preexisting traction spur with superior migration up the arm. Magnetic resonance imaging may be more helpful in cases of incomplete or partial tears.

TREATMENT

Conservative Management

In partial and degenerative tears, the elbow may be splinted in extension for a brief period, followed by bracing to prevent hyperflexion. Massage with anti-inflammatory cream may decrease swelling and stimulate blood flow in the tendon. As pain and inflammation subside, a rehabilitation program can be initiated to regain strength. The patient should refrain from excessive stress on the tendon for at least 3 months.

Arthroscopic Technique

The patient is placed in the prone or lateral decubitus position. The entire course of the ulnar nerve is carefully marked out. If there is too much swelling or the anatomy is distorted, a small incision is made, and the nerve is located and protected before beginning the arthroscopy.

The initial portal is a proximal anterior medial or lateral portal for a diagnostic arthroscopy of the anterior compartment. Because many of these patients use the arm for heavy lifting, there may be pathology anteriorly involving loose bodies or coronoid spurring that requires treatment before the repair procedure begins.

The initial portal into the posterior aspect of the elbow is the posterior central portal, located approximately 3 cm above the tip of the olecranon. In most triceps avulsions, this portal goes through the tear. A posterior lateral portal is then established, and the injury to the tendon is visualized (Fig. 16-2). The arthroscope is moved to the posterior lateral portal, and the shaver is introduced through the posterior central portal. The ulnar insertion is identified and lightly débrided, as are the edges of the torn tendon. A central olecranon bursa portal is then established, and a dual-sutured anchor is inserted at the proximal olecranon tip, angling toward the coronoid base to prevent inadvertent penetration through the articular surface (Fig. 16-3).

A retrograde retriever is then placed percutaneously through the medial and lateral aspects of the muscle-tendon junction of the triceps and is used to retrieve a suture through this area of the tendon (Fig. 16-4). Two mattress stitches are usually required to complete the proximal part of the repair (Fig. 16-5). The first set of sutures is retrieved percutaneously, and a sliding knot is tied to lock down the proximal attachment of the triceps and seal the joint. The second set of sutures is retrieved through the tendon and tied. The arthroscope is then placed into the olecranon bursa, and a second anchor is placed more distally in the ulna. These sutures are retrieved through the end of the tendon in a simple fashion to complete the repair (Fig. 16-6).

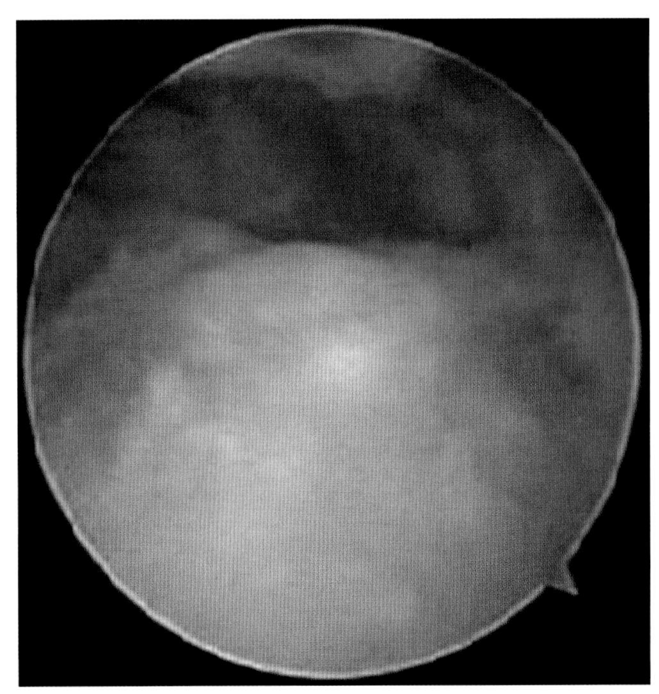

FIGURE 16-2 The triceps tear is visualized through a posterior lateral portal. Notice the exposure of the entire proximal olecranon.

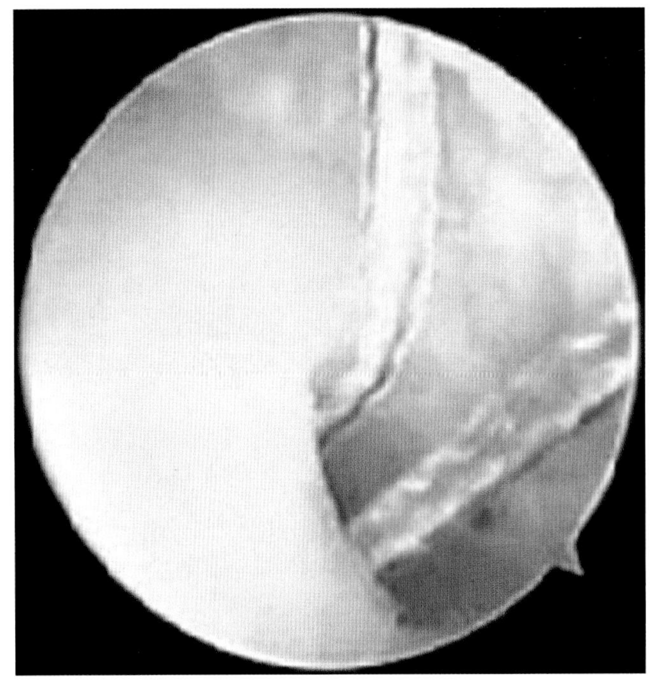

FIGURE 16-3 The first anchor is placed into the proximal part of the olecranon in preparation for repair.

In an alternative technique, both anchors are placed before any suture shuttle or retrieval is undertaken. The proximal and distal sutures are then retrieved and tied. The sutures may be crossed to create a suture bridge that holds the tendon down to the bone.

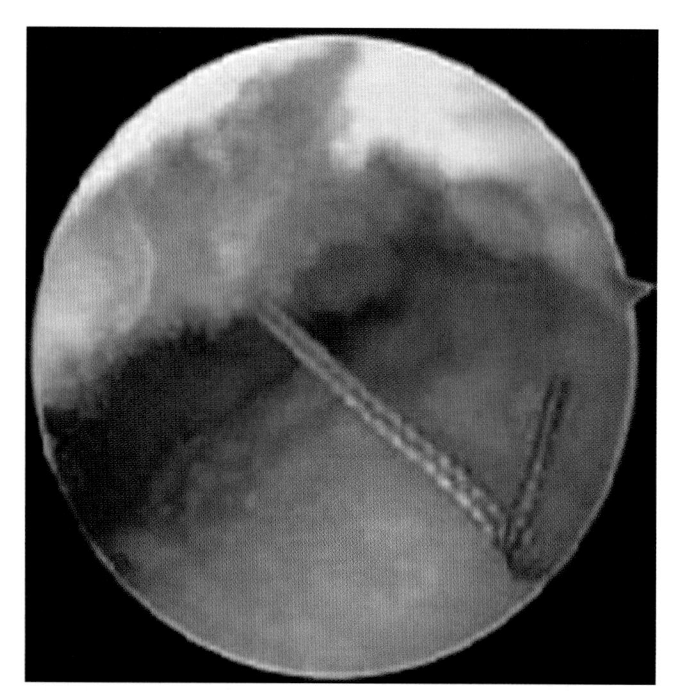

FIGURE 16-4 The sutures from the anchor are moved superiorly into the olecranon fossa and then retrieved through the proximal aspect of the triceps tendon.

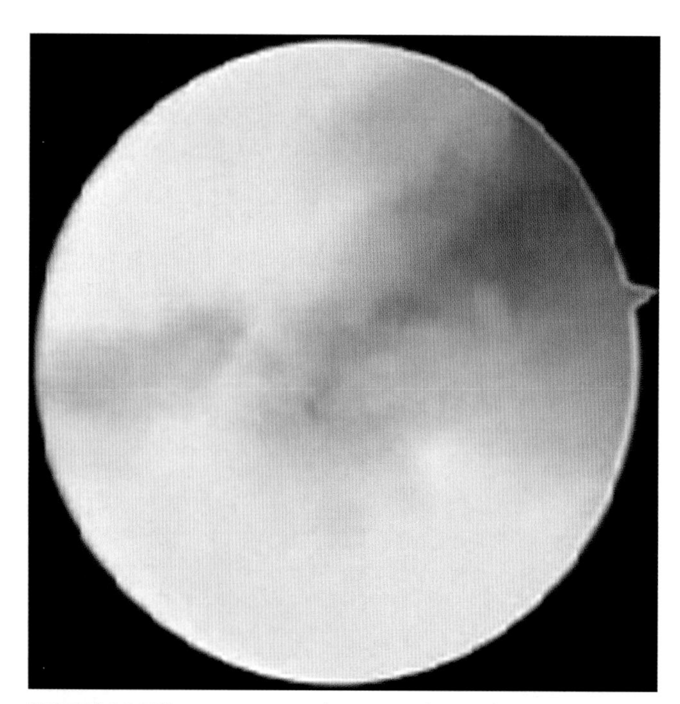

FIGURE 16-5 The sutures are tied, repairing the tendon to the bone of the olecranon.

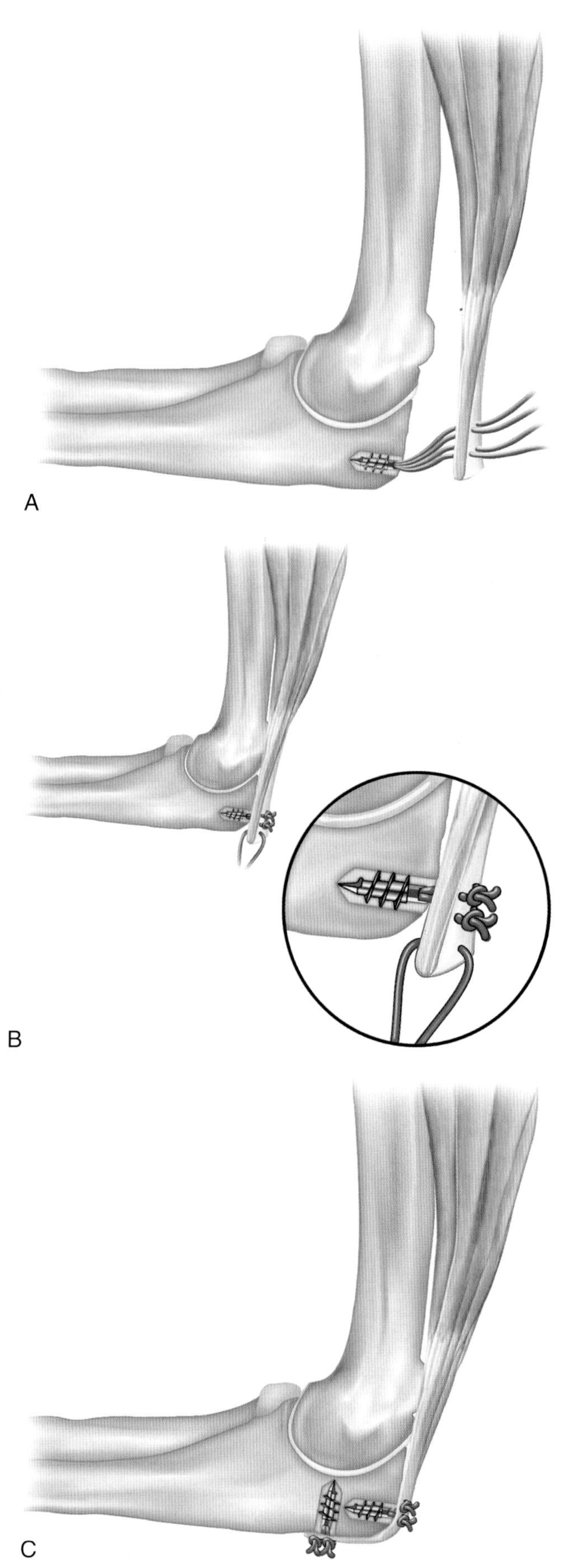

FIGURE 16-6 A-C, Repair technique for triceps avulsion injuries.

PEARLS & PITFALLS

PEARLS

- Map out the ulnar nerve.
- Free the muscle and tendon from the underlying humerus.
- Separate the mattress stitches to get adequate repair and avoid suture pull-out.
- Oversize the pilot hole, and tap deeply into the bone, or use an expansion anchor, because the bone can be extremely hard in this area.
- If only the central slip is involved, placing a traction stitch and pulling it into a pilot hole in the olecranon may allow interference screw fixation.

PITFALLS

- Failure to stop and convert to an open procedure if swelling becomes too great
- Losing orientation of the ulnar nerve
- Breaking off the anchors during insertion into hard bone and damaging the potential repair site

Postoperative Management

The patient is placed in anterior and posterior splints with the elbow in almost full extension. On the first postoperative visit, a motion-limiting brace is applied, and an arc of 0 to 30 degrees is allowed. Each week, an additional 10 degrees is allowed until 6 to 8 weeks postoperatively, when the brace is discontinued.

REFERENCES

1. Morrey B. Rupture of the triceps tendon. In: Morrey B, ed. *The Elbow and its Disorders: Expert Consult*. 4th ed. Philadelphia, PA: WB Saunders; 2009:536-546.
2. Armando F, Vidal AF, Drakos MC, Allen AA. Biceps tendon and triceps tendon injuries. *Clin Sports Med*. 2004;23:707-722.
3. Daglar B, Delialioglu OM, Ceyhan E, et al. Combined surgical treatment for missed rupture of triceps tendon associated with avulsion of the ulnar collateral ligament and flexor-pronator muscle mass. *Strat Traum Limb Recon*. 2009;4:35-39.
4. Rineer CA, Ruch DS. Elbow tendinopathy and tendon ruptures: epicondylitis, biceps and triceps ruptures. *J Hand Surg Am*. 2009;34:566-576.
5. Belentani C, Pastore D, Wangwinyuvirat M, et al. Triceps brachii tendon: anatomic-MR imaging study in cadavers with histologic correlation. *Skeletal Radiol*. 2009;38:171-175.
6. Morrey B. Rupture of the triceps tendon. In: Morrey B, ed. *The Elbow and its Disorders*. 3rd ed. Philadelphia, PA: WB Saunders; 2000;479-484.

CHAPTER

17

Arthroscopic Treatment of Elbow Fractures

John P. Peden • Felix H. Savoie III • Larry D. Field

Arthroscopic techniques are having a dramatic impact in the arenas of trauma and fracture management. Proponents are advocating arthroscopically assisted treatment of intra-articular and other periarticular injuries throughout the appendicular skeleton, including management of triangular fibrocartilage complex injuries, distal radius fractures, and carpal fractures. During the past decade, the indications for elbow arthroscopy have expanded to encompass the management of various elbow fractures. Little has been published on the subject, because the field is in its infancy. This chapter offers an overview of this innovative frontier of elbow arthroscopy to the advanced arthroscopist and encourages an appreciation of the creativity that is leading to future developments in the field.

ANATOMY

Careful attention to the regional anatomy is essential to prevent direct or indirect injury to the neurovascular structures of the elbow, the most feared complication of elbow arthroscopy. The surgeon should be thoroughly familiar and agile with portal placement and the use of retractors. The various fracture classifications and their relevance are discussed in more detail in the sections on surgical management that follow.

PATIENT EVALUATION

History and Physical Examination

Clinical assessment is often limited or impaired by pain, soft tissue swelling, and hemarthrosis. In these circumstances, aspiration of the hemarthrosis, followed by an intra-articular infusion of bupivacaine, may provide sufficient analgesia to facilitate the assessment of motion and stability. The technique may also provide a means to differentiate patient guarding from a true mechanical block to elbow motion.

Diagnostic Imaging

At presentation, patients often have imaging studies offering suboptimal radiographic detail because of limited emergency room evaluation. Imaging may also be limited by the inability of patients to tolerate positioning of the injured joint for adequate assessment. As with the physical examination, aspiration and infiltration of the joint with an anesthetic may facilitate positioning for optimal radiography. A surgeon should have a low threshold for the application of computed tomography or magnetic resonance imaging for preoperative planning when interpreting fracture lines and the three-dimensional relationships of fracture fragments or loose bodies. Magnetic resonance imaging provides further detail regarding ligament integrity in the setting of coronoid fractures and elbow dislocations.

TREATMENT

Indications and Contraindications

Arthroscopic management of elbow fractures is a rapidly evolving indication for the use of elbow arthroscopy in the identification and treatment of intra-articular pathology. The technique provides for a minimally invasive surgical exposure, minimizing further soft tissue trauma in a region notorious for wound complications. Arthroscopic débridement of fibrinous and osseous debris facilitates postoperative elbow range of motion. Visualization of fracture fragments and chondral injuries is often superior to that achieved with open approaches, and it minimizes the requirements for intraoperative fluoroscopy. Identification of intra-articular pathology not evident on preoperative imaging enables appropriate treatment measures and a more accurate prognosis. Elbow arthroscopy can be used in combination with indirect reduction techniques to maximize articular congruity, or it can be used for direct arthroscopic reduction with fixation devices passed into the joint.

Absolute contraindications to arthroscopic treatment of acute elbow fractures include infection or gross contamination, neurovascular injuries, concomitant chest wall injuries in which positioning would interfere with ventilation, and severely osteoporotic bone for which fixation will be inadequate. Relative contraindications include severe soft tissue swelling and severely displaced intra-articular fractures in which altered anatomic landmarks and orientation compromise safe arthroscopic access. Open nerve exploration may be necessary in patients with previous ulnar nerve transposition. Arthroscopic treatment of open fractures is controversial but may facilitate irrigation and débridement and minimize further soft tissue injury in selected cases.

Open exploration of the posterior interosseous nerve is recommended for radial head fractures in which fracture fragments penetrate the capsule and the brachialis muscle anteriorly. Injury to the nerve is possible with arthroscopic extraction of fracture fragments from this location because of the proximity to or entanglement with the nerve. Open removal of these fragments is essential to eliminate nerve entrapment in scar tissue that may result in shearing and traction injuries during the rehabilitation process.

Conservative Management

Most intra-articular fractures of the distal humerus can be effectively treated with open reduction and internal fixation (ORIF), and superior results are achieved with this approach compared with skeletal traction or cast immobilization. Khalfayan and colleagues[1] concluded that patients with displaced Mason type II radial head fractures who were treated conservatively had more pain, decreased strength, and decreased elbow motion compared with patients treated with open osteosynthesis. Radial head fracture treatment depends on the fracture pattern and displacement and includes early mobilization, ORIF, and resection or prosthetic replacement. Open treatment options for displaced olecranon fractures include tension band wiring, lag screw placement, neutralization plating, and excision with extensor mechanism reconstruction. Capitellar fractures can likewise be excised or stabilized with standard open techniques. Cadaveric research has drawn attention to the important stabilizing role of the coronoid and has provided compelling evidence for surgical management of these fractures in various circumstances.[2,3]

Arthroscopic Technique

The patient is placed prone or in the lateral decubitus position. The lateral decubitus position typically requires a supportive device to provide arm suspension. With the patient in the prone position, the arm is elevated on a 4-inch padded block with the elbow flexed to 90 degrees over an arm board located at the patient's side parallel to the table (Fig. 17-1). This method avoids compression of neurovascular structures in the axilla and facilitates medial or lateral access (in case an open procedure becomes necessary) by internal or external rotation of the forearm onto the arm board. The forearm and hand should be wrapped with compressive wrapping material to restrict swelling and fluid extravasation. Intravenous prophylactic antibiotics are routinely administered preoperatively.

Most procedures can be accomplished with the 4.0-mm, 30-degree arthroscopic camera. A 70-degree camera can provide visualization of the capitellum or radial head from a posterior portal when instrumentation is required from the soft spot portal. Graspers with teeth and smooth outer surfaces are preferred to prevent hang-up on soft tissue. A 3.5-mm, full-radius arthroscopic shaver is useful for removal of organized fracture hematoma and debris (Fig. 17-2). Various implants can be used for fixation, contingent on the fracture configuration (discussed later).

After fracture stabilization has been achieved, the surgeon should thoroughly evaluate elbow stability. This can be accomplished with the assistance of fluoroscopy, but it can also be read-

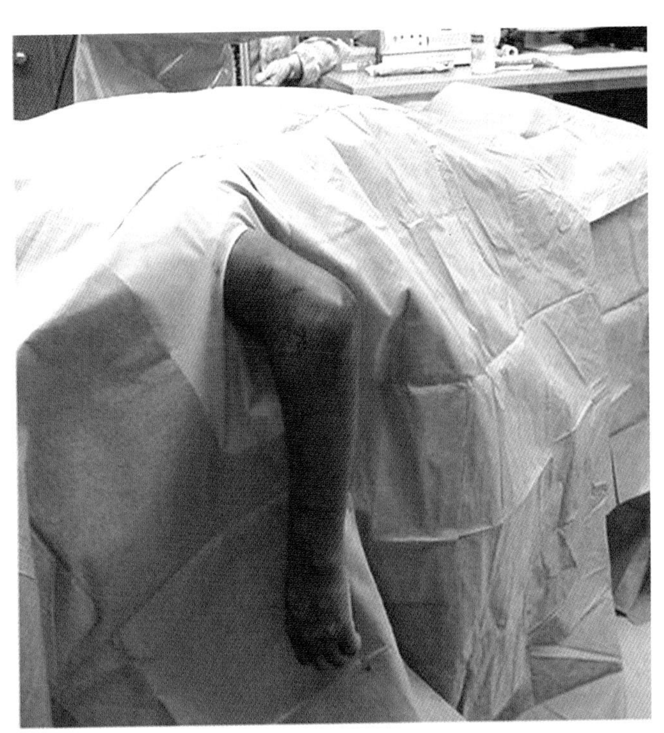

FIGURE 17-1 The prone position with a bump under the arm is demonstrated.

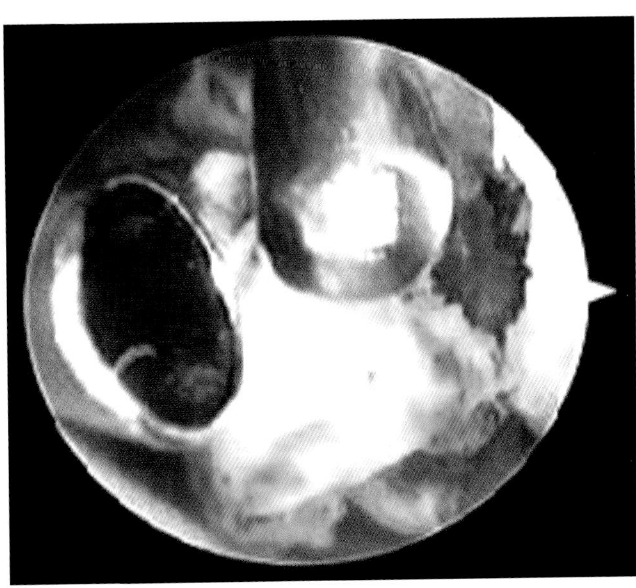

FIGURE 17-2 Débridement and removal of fracture debris are possible arthroscopically, as shown by the use of a shaver in this intercondylar humerus fracture.

ily assessed arthroscopically. Diagnosis and management of associated ligamentous injuries of the elbow are discussed in Chapters 13 and 14.

A small drain can be placed through one of the elbow joint portals at the conclusion of the procedure. Portals can be closed with a locked horizontal mattress stitch to minimize prolonged drainage, which is a frequent minor complication. Concomitant elbow incisions or lacerations should be managed in the manner deemed appropriate by the surgeon and should be considered carefully, given the propensity of the traumatized soft tissue envelope of the elbow to develop wound problems.

Radial Head Fractures

Radial head fractures are the most common type of elbow fracture in adults, and they offer an excellent opportunity for arthroscopic evaluation and management (Fig. 17-3A). In patients with persistent locking and pain despite radiographic evidence of minimally displaced radial head fractures, diagnostic arthroscopy enables accurate assessment of articular cartilage, identification of any osteochondral flaps or loose bodies, and débridement with minimal morbidity. Displaced two-part radial head fractures can be visualized through a proximal anteromedial or posterolateral portal to assess the degree of articular incongruity, fracture fragment stability,

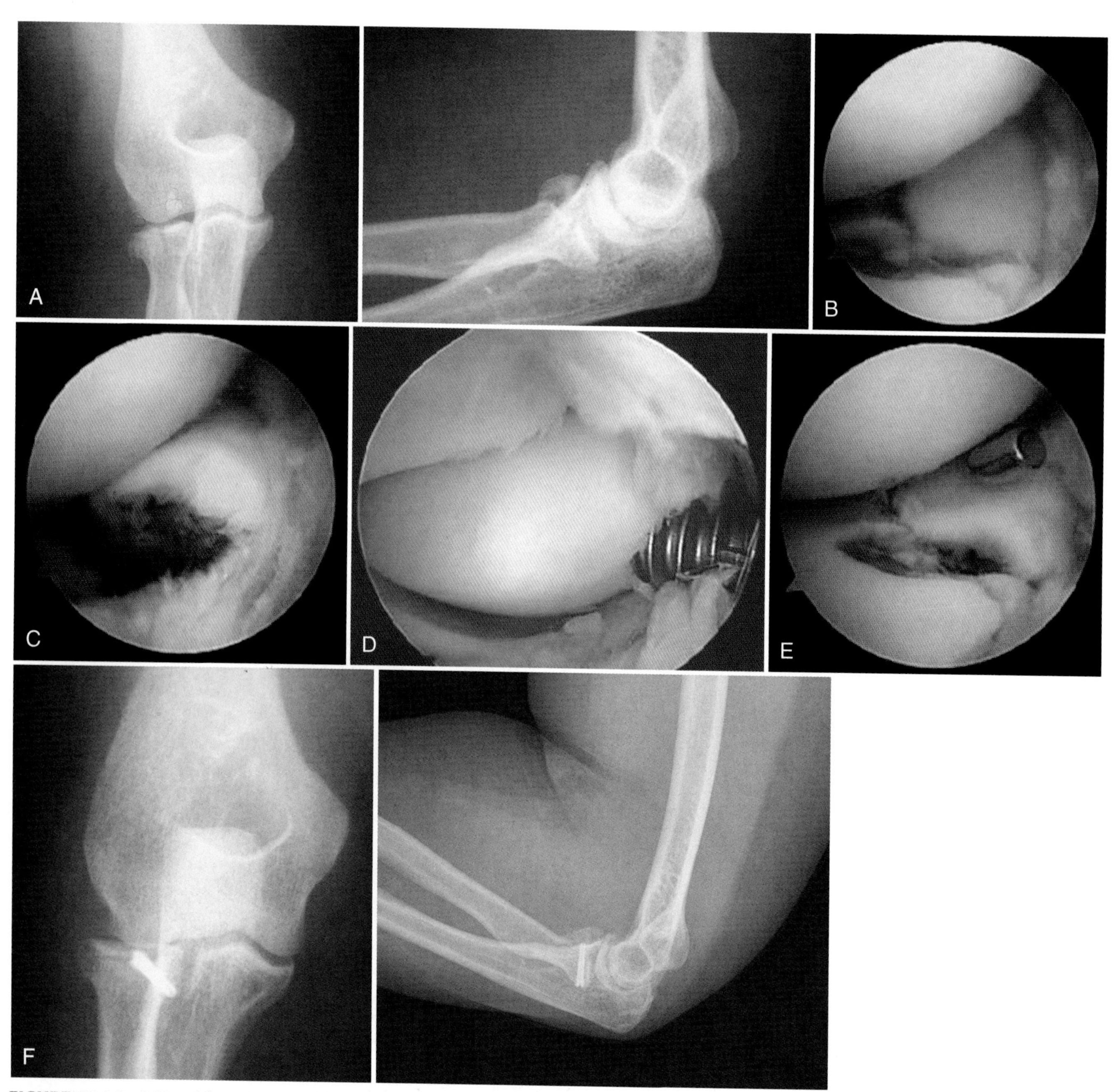

FIGURE 17-3 Radial head fractures are easily visualized arthroscopically and can be accessed for internal fixation through several portals. **A,** Posteroanterior *(left)* and lateral *(right)* radiographs show a radial head fracture. **B,** The initial view shows the fracture after the hematoma has been removed. **C,** The depressed fragments are mobilized using a Kirschner wire joystick technique. **D,** The screw fixation device is inserted. **E,** The final fixation was obtained by means of arthroscopically assisted techniques. **F,** Final radiographs show the fracture with internal fixation in place.

and any impingement to forearm rotation. A direct lateral portal can also provide visualization of the posterior aspect of the radial head during confirmation of fracture reduction. If arthroscopic reduction with internal fixation is desired, visualization is best achieved with a 70-degree camera from a posterolateral portal, with instruments and implants introduced through a soft spot portal.

After débridement and lavage, Kirschner wires can be positioned through the anterolateral or soft spot portals in conjunction with arthroscopic probes, graspers, and occasionally, a reduction tenaculum to allow for manipulation, reduction, and provisional fixation of larger fracture fragments. Visualization can often be facilitated by rotating the forearm into maximal supination. Definitive fixation can then be performed using absorbable pins or cannulated screws (see Fig. 17-3D). Herbert-Whipple screws (Zimmer, Inc., Warsaw, IN) and headless variable-pitch screws (Acutrak screws, Acumed, LLC, Hillsboro, OR) are advantageous in providing secure fixation with compression to allow early motion, while being buried beneath the articular surface to avoid impingement. Reduction and stability of the fixation can be directly assessed during full rotation of the elbow (see Fig. 17-3E).

Rolla and colleagues[4] reported preliminary results for six patients who underwent arthroscopic reduction and internal fixation for radial head fractures classified as Mason[5] type II (3), type III (2), or type IV (1). All patients returned to their preinjury level of function within 6 months. The Mayo Elbow Performance (MEP) scores were excellent for three and good for the other three patients at mean follow-up of 12 months.

Michels and associates[6] presented longer-term results of an arthroscopic technique for treatment of Mason type II radial head fractures in 14 patients. The MEP scores were excellent for 11 and good for the other 3 patients at a mean follow-up of 5 years 6 months. The procedure was refined to the use of only a midlateral viewing portal and an anterolateral working portal. A potential advantage of this arthroscopic technique was the observation that a single screw was usually sufficient to obtain stability. The investigators concluded that the capsular dissection required by an open technique might increase fracture fragment instability, resulting in the requirement for additional fixation.

Dawson and Inostroza[7] have published a case report in which they described a technique of arthroscopic reduction and percutaneous pinning to treat an angulated radial neck fracture, an entity encountered in the developing elbow and occurring most commonly in patients between 9 and 13 years old. The fracture is reduced through an anterolateral portal with a hemostatic forceps while a Kirschner wire is percutaneously inserted to obtain fixation of the radial head to the diaphysis. A cast is applied for 3 weeks, and the Kirschner wire is then removed.

Arthroscopic excision of acute radial head fractures should not be performed in high-demand patients or when the fracture is associated with instability. Radial head resection in the setting of post-traumatic arthritis of radial head fractures remains controversial. If conservative or primary surgical treatment results in an unsatisfactory clinical outcome, delayed radial head excision is an effective option. Broberg and Morrey[8] documented significant relief of pain and recovery of motion with late resection of the radial head after nonoperative treatment of Mason type II and III fractures in a review of 21 patients.

Menth-Chiari and colleagues[9,10] demonstrated similar positive benefits for delayed radial head resection by an arthroscopic technique in a mixed series that included 10 patients with post-traumatic arthritis after type II and III fractures. The procedure begins with a partial resection of the anterior three fourths of the radial head and 2 to 3 mm of radial neck using a hooded abrader in the anterolateral portal and the arthroscope in the proximal medial portal. The abrader is then transferred to the mediolateral portal to complete the resection. No subjective or objective evidence of instability was documented in this series. The surgeons advocated that preservation of the annular ligament complex should be an important consideration in maintaining the stability at the proximal radioulnar joint.

Coronoid Fractures

Operative intervention for coronoid process fractures is recommended for Regan and Morrey[11] type III fractures and any type of fracture that interferes with joint motion. When comminution precludes fixation, loose debris can be removed arthroscopically. However, larger coronoid fractures can be effectively treated with the use of arthroscopic reduction techniques. The fracture can be manipulated into reduction by a tibial anterior cruciate ligament guide inserted through the anteromedial portal while viewing through a lateral portal (Fig. 17-4).[12] A guide pin can then be drilled through the ulnar shaft to engage the fragment, followed by definitive fixation with a small, cannulated screw placed in antegrade fashion. Fragments that are too small for screw fixation

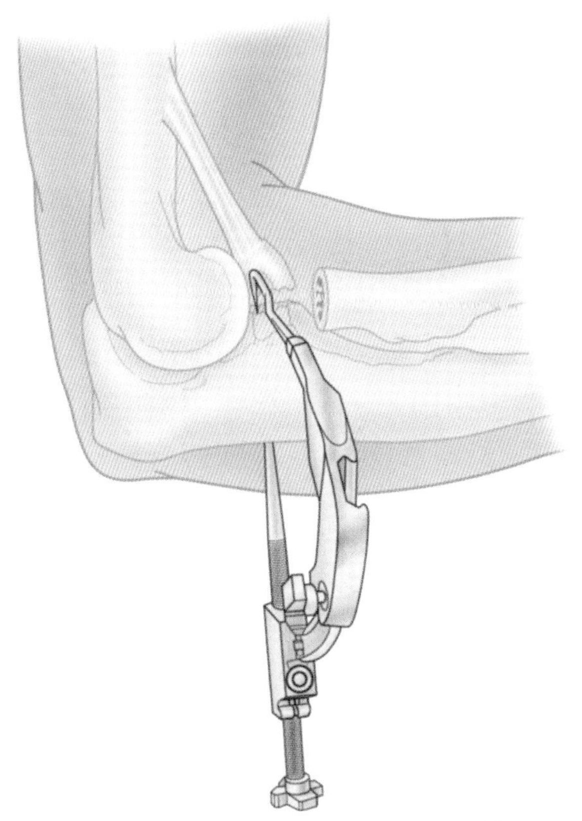

FIGURE 17-4 An anterior cruciate ligament guide is used for coronoid fractures. *(Modified from Adams JE, Merten SM, Steinmann SP. Arthroscopic-assisted treatment of coronoid fractures.* Arthroscopy. *2007;23:1060-1065.)*

can be stabilized with the application of suture anchors placed within the base of the fracture. A hinged brace or external fixator may be necessary to maintain joint stability and offload the repair until adequate healing has occurred.

Lui and coworkers[13] described successful arthroscopic outcomes in two athletes with type I coronoid fractures after initial conservative management had failed. Treatment consisted of excision of loose bodies in one patient and excision of a fibrous nonunion in the other. Adams and colleagues[12] reported their experience with arthroscopically assisted reduction and fixation of four type II and three type III coronoid fractures. Cannulated screw fixation was achieved antegrade over pins placed with the use of an anterior cruciate ligament guide. The surgeons observed that all five of the patients available for follow-up at an average 2 years and 8 months had MEP scores of 100%.

Capitellar and Coronal Shear Fractures

Capitellar fractures account for less than 1% of all elbow fractures. They are divided into type I (i.e., Hahn-Steinthal fragment), type II (i.e., Kocher-Lorenz fragment), and type III (i.e., markedly comminuted) fractures (Fig. 17-5A).[14] However, a high incidence of osteochondral capitellar defects has been associated with radial head fractures. Types I and II capitellar and coronal shear fractures can be treated with an antegrade arthroscopically assisted technique similar to that used for coronoid fractures (see Fig. 17-5B). Alternatively, provisional reduction can be carried out in a retrograde fashion with Kirschner wires, followed by cannulated screw fixation (see Fig. 17-5C). The anterolateral portal can provide access for bioabsorbable pin fixation of Kocher-Lorenz fragments and reparable osteochondral flaps considered too fragile for screw fixation. Osteochondral defects that are not reparable should be arthroscopically débrided.[15]

A 70-degree camera introduced through a posterior portal may provide the optimum view of the capitellum when instrumenting from the soft spot portal. Alternatively, Hardy and colleagues[16] found that the proximal lateral portal provided effective visualization in a case report in which a type I fracture was reduced by manipulating the fragment through an anterolateral working portal. Reduction required traction through the axis of the forearm with the elbow flexed at 30 degrees. The surgeon may consider partial release of the lateral collateral ligament to facilitate visualization and reduction of shear-type fractures. Repair can be later achieved arthroscopically with a suture anchor.

Lateral Condylar Fractures

Fractures of the lateral humeral condyle represent approximately 15% of elbow fractures in the pediatric population.[17] To ensure articular congruity, these fractures historically have been treated with a closed reduction with arthrography or an open lateral Kocher approach for displaced fractures. Milch type I and II

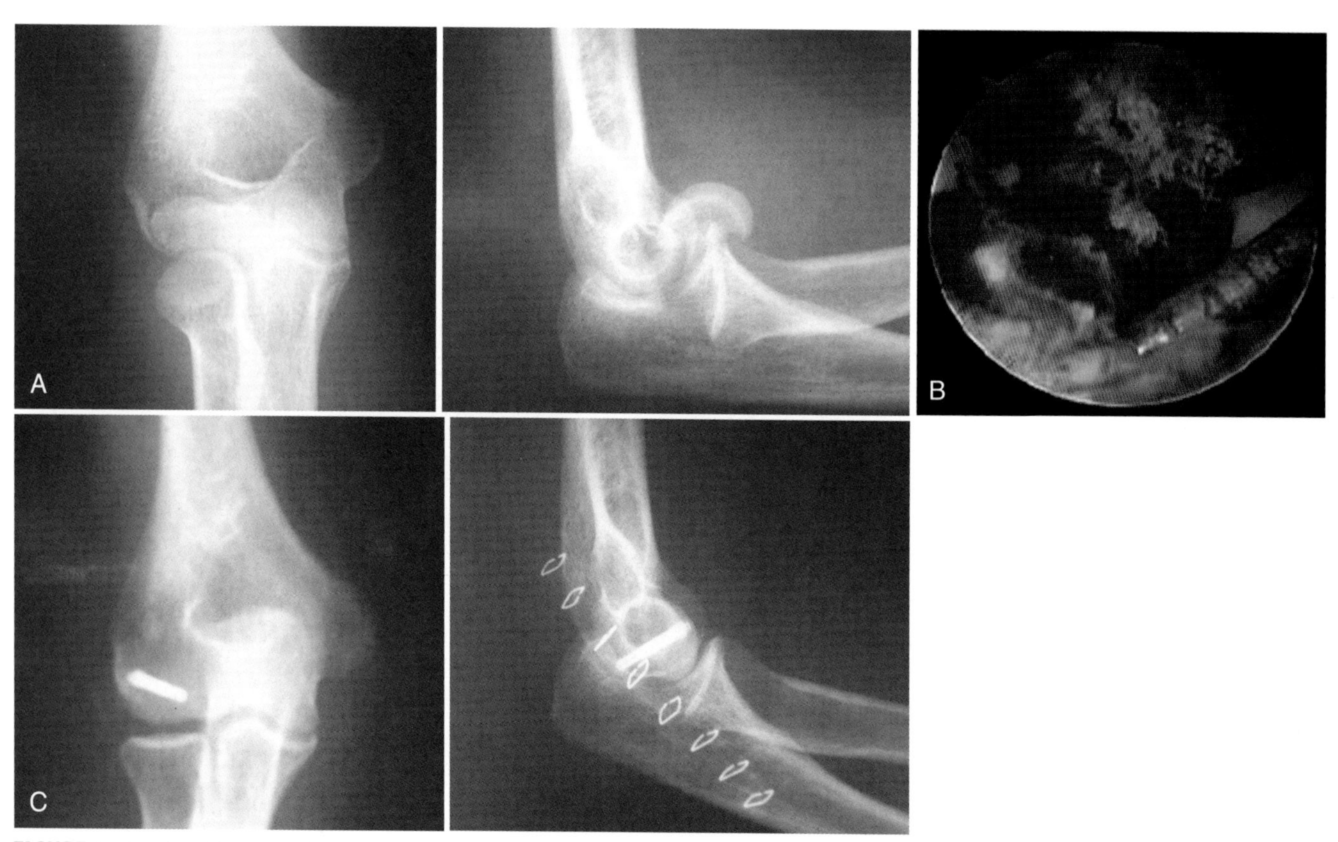

FIGURE 17-5 Isolated fractures of the capitellum are an excellent indication for arthroscopic techniques, eliminating the need for an extensive open procedure. **A,** A displaced, shear-type capitellar fracture was documented on elbow radiographs and confirmed on magnetic resonance imaging. **B,** Arthroscopic evaluation and reduction was achieved with various instruments, including the nerve hook to pull the fragment back to its original bed in this elbow. **C,** Ultimate fixation was attained with the use of a Herbert screw, as shown in these postoperative radiographs.

fractures are often amenable to arthroscopic evaluation and arthroscopically assisted percutaneous screw or pin fixation. Arthroscopic reduction has the advantage of avoiding the elevation of the capsulosynovial and periosteal attachments that may occur during a Kocher approach, potentially reducing the risk of compromise to the vasculature of the distal fragment that may lead to avascular necrosis and cubitus valgus deformity.

Hausman and associates[18] retrospectively reviewed their results from arthroscopically assisted treatment of six pediatric lateral condyle fractures. Standard anteromedial and anterolateral portals were used. The fracture fragment was reduced under direct visualization with the assistance of percutaneous 0.062-inch Kirschner wire joysticks, including a Kirschner wire placed transversely through the axis of the capitellum to facilitate rotational control of the reduction. The Kirschner wire fixation was maintained for 4 weeks postoperatively in a long arm cast. Although the mean follow-up was only 32 weeks, all patients achieved full active range of motion with no radiographic evidence of nonunion or malunion. Perez Carro and coworkers[19] described similar results in their series of four patients.

Intercondylar and Supracondylar Fractures

Intercondylar and supracondylar fractures usually require open reduction with plate fixation. Of the three AO North America group C classification subtypes, only the C1 type is amenable to arthroscopically assisted reduction with percutaneous fixation as previously described (Fig. 17-6A and B). Kirschner wires are drilled from a medial to lateral direction to reduce and provisionally secure each condyle. Wires are then drilled proximally into each column to secure this construct to the distal humerus.

Arthroscopic evaluation must confirm anatomic reduction anteriorly and posteriorly before definitive screw fixation is performed (see Fig. 17-6C through E). Single-column screw fixation limits this technique to individuals with bone quality sufficient to allow for early, protected motion. Visualization can be augmented with an arthroscopic triceps reflection, if necessary. A retractor strategically placed through a superior portal can be used to lift the triceps and facilitate the exposure.

Epicondylar Fractures

Medial apophyseal avulsion fractures can occur in young throwing athletes and lead to instability. Arthroscopic evaluation demonstrates valgus laxity. After arthroscopically assisted percutaneous fixation, the elbow should be reassessed for valgus laxity to confirm ligament integrity. Only 3 mm of ulnohumeral widening is consistent with instability. Careful attention must be paid to the ulnar nerve, which should be palpated well posterior to any incisions.

Olecranon Fractures

Olecranon process fractures typically develop a hemorrhagic elbow effusion because of their intra-articular involvement. Arthroscopic débridement allows visualization of the trochlear notch in arthroscopically assisted percutaneous reduction techniques and treatment of osteochondral flaps or loose bodies that may obstruct motion. Access to this area through posterior, posterolateral, and direct lateral portals minimizes the risk to the collateral ligaments, which may be greater with open approaches.

Principles of Arthroscopic Fracture Management of the Elbow

Elbow arthroscopy has a higher complication rate than that for any other joint, with an overall rate of major and minor complications of approximately 10% reported in the literature. Moreover, the wound complication rate is substantial in the acutely traumatized elbow. Adherence to the few important principles can minimize the risk of these potential complications.

Principle 1: Keep it simple. An effective technique for managing elbow trauma involves starting on the less traumatized side and working from what is normal and identifiable to what is abnormal and displaced. Smaller and double-port cannulas are valuable for initial viewing and irrigation, and additional portals are established based on the anticipated procedure.

Principle 2: Know the portals. Ten primary access portals are dictated by the local neurovascular and musculotendinous anatomy, a discussion of which is beyond the scope of this chapter. A thorough understanding of anatomic landmarks is critical for achieving successful results and avoiding neurologic injury, especially because soft tissue swelling can distort these landmarks in the acute setting. The surgeon must ensure adequate intracapsular pressure before portal placement, injecting the joint with 10 to 15 mL of saline through the soft spot or posterocentral portal if distention provided by hemarthrosis is inadequate. Needle localization of portal placement is always recommended. Skin is sharply incised, but subcutaneous tissue should be penetrated by means of cannula and obturator.

Principle 3: Maintain visualization at all times. If necessary, use additional portals to introduce a Freer elevator or similar specialized instrument to retract capsule and muscle. A proximal posterocentral portal can be used to retract over the ulnar nerve in the posteromedial gutter, and a proximal anterolateral portal can be used to retract the brachialis muscle and underlying posterior interosseous nerve when working near the anterior radial head. Retraction is especially important when the capsule is disrupted and nerves are exposed. The suction should be turned off when a shaver is used in proximity to an exposed nerve. Use of arthroscopic punches and baskets for débridement is encouraged in these circumstances. Arthroscopic identification and, if necessary, exploration of nerves can be undertaken to ensure safe arthroscopic fracture manipulation and reduction.

Principle 4: Monitor flow. Injury can be avoided by limiting fluid extravasation, and this is particularly relevant in the acute traumatic setting, in which capsular disruption may have occurred. Gravity inflow is preferred to a pump. Cannulas should be exchanged over Wissinger rods, and correct inflow position should be visually confirmed before the flow is restarted. The camera may be used dry if concern warrants. Indwelling catheters should not be used postoperatively.

Principal 5: Know the limits. A surgeon must make a realistic appraisal of the technical demands imposed by each case and be especially cognizant of time constraints with regard to fluid extravasation and tourniquet use. A good strategy is to enforce time limits set at the beginning of a case. The use of limited incisions should be considered in preoperative planning, and conversion to conventional open techniques should take precedence over arthroscopic measures whenever the principles of fracture management require.

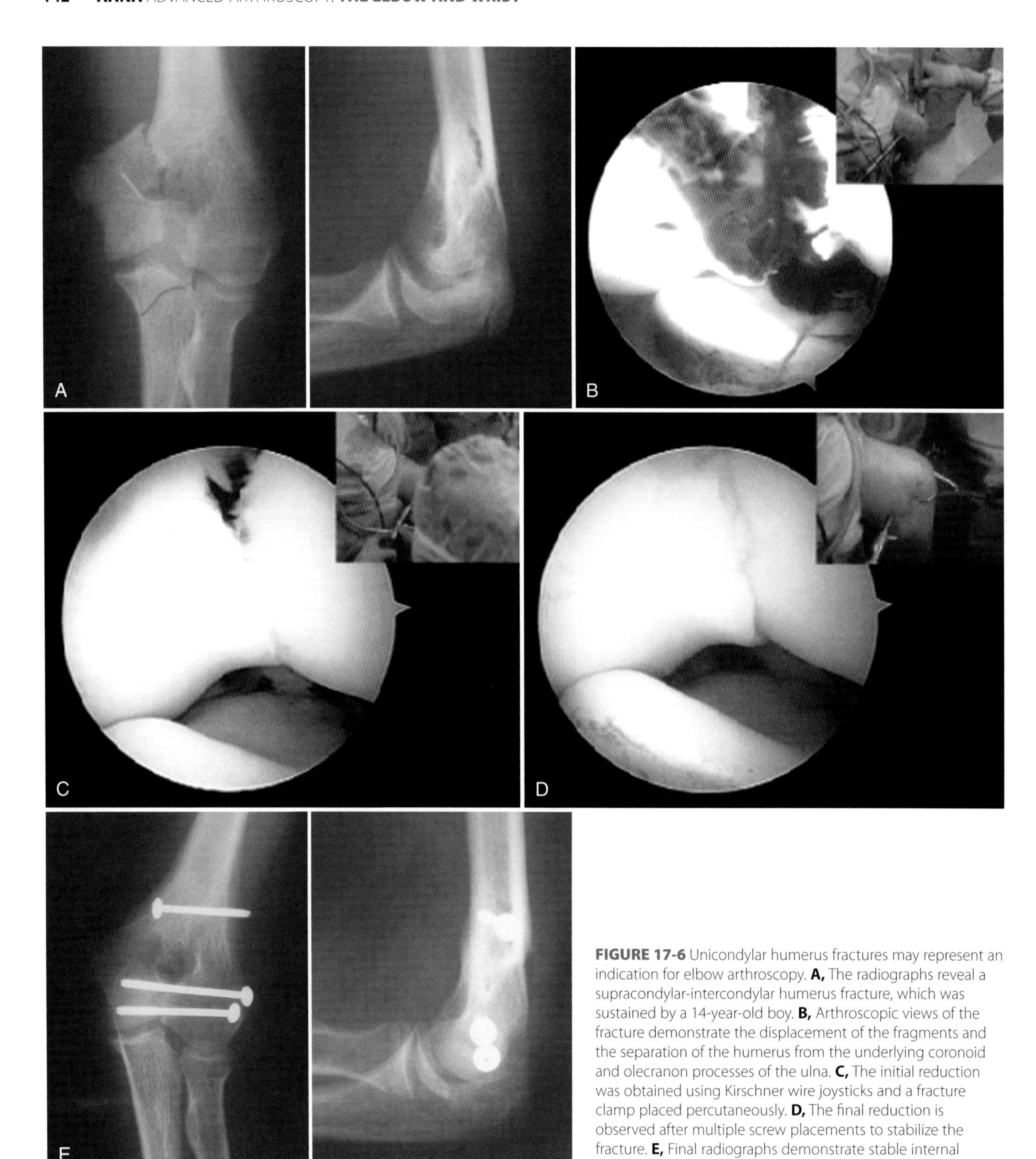

FIGURE 17-6 Unicondylar humerus fractures may represent an indication for elbow arthroscopy. **A,** The radiographs reveal a supracondylar-intercondylar humerus fracture, which was sustained by a 14-year-old boy. **B,** Arthroscopic views of the fracture demonstrate the displacement of the fragments and the separation of the humerus from the underlying coronoid and olecranon processes of the ulna. **C,** The initial reduction was obtained using Kirschner wire joysticks and a fracture clamp placed percutaneously. **D,** The final reduction is observed after multiple screw placements to stabilize the fracture. **E,** Final radiographs demonstrate stable internal fixation.

PEARLS & PITFALLS

PEARLS

- Keep it simple. Work from what is normal and identifiable to what is abnormal and displaced.
- Smaller cannulas are valuable for initial viewing and irrigation, and additional portals are established based on the anticipated procedure.
- Know the portals. Ten primary access portals are dictated by the local neurovascular and musculotendinous anatomy, and a thorough understanding of anatomic landmarks is critical to achieving successful results and avoiding neurologic injury.
- Draw the ulnar nerve in every case.
- Needle localization of portal placement and access sites for fracture fixation helps with proper placement and orientation.
- Maintain visualization at all times. If necessary, use additional portals to introduce specialized instruments.
- Monitor flow. Injury can be avoided by limiting fluid extravasation, and this is particularly relevant in the acute traumatic setting, in which capsular disruption may have occurred. Gravity inflow is recommended in preference to a pump. Cannulas should be exchanged over Wissinger rods, and correct inflow position should be visually confirmed before flow is restarted. The camera may be used dry if concern warrants.
- Respect the limits of skill and time. Make a realistic appraisal of the technical demands imposed by each case, and be especially cognizant of time constraints with regard to fluid extravasation and tourniquet use. A good strategy is to enforce time limits set at the beginning of a case.
- Be prepared. Conversion to conventional open techniques should take precedence over arthroscopic measures whenever the principles of fracture management require.
- Start the initial placement of Kirschner wires into the fragments to be manipulated before there is edema distortion of the anatomy.

PITFALLS

- Fracture displacement and soft tissue swelling can distort anatomic landmarks in acute cases. If there is any doubt, make a small incision and find the nerves before proceeding with the case.
- Capsular tearing from the trauma can result in low intracapsular pressure and a lack of distention, with concomitant loss of the safety zone protecting the nerves. Ensure adequate intracapsular pressure before portal placement, injecting the joint with 10 to 15 mL of saline through the soft spot or posterocentral portals if distention provided by hemarthrosis is inadequate.
- Whereas skin is sharply incised, subcutaneous tissue should be penetrated by means of blunt dissection with a hemostat and by using only blunt trocars in the cannula.
- Pay attention to the nerves. Retraction is especially important if the capsule is disrupted and nerves are exposed. Turn off the suction when using a shaver in proximity to an exposed nerve. Use of arthroscopic punches and baskets for débridement is encouraged in these circumstances. If there is any question, make an incision, and put a protective retractor around the nerve.

Postoperative Rehabilitation

A light compressive dressing in applied, and gentle, protected range of motion is encouraged on the first postoperative day. The rehabilitation process is coordinated by the surgeon and depends on the fracture pattern. Passive activities are encouraged, and resisted exercises are avoided for a minimum of 6 weeks. A passive motion machine may be of some benefit if the patient is unable to comply with the rehabilitation protocols. A hinged brace may be used within designated motion guidelines when concern for stability and protection of the soft tissues is warranted. Union is assessed radiographically at 6 to 8 weeks or sooner, depending on concern regarding stability of the fixation.

REFERENCES

1. Khalfayan EE, Culp RW, Alexander AH. Mason type II radial head fractures: operative versus nonoperative treatment. *J Orthop Trauma*. 1992;6:283-289.
2. Closkey RF, Goode JR, Kirschenbaum D, Cody RP. The role of the coronoid process in elbow stability: a biomechanical analysis of axial loading. *J Bone Joint Surg Am*. 2000;82:1749-1753.
3. Schneeberger AG, Sadowski MM, Jacob HA. Coronoid process and radial head as posterolateral rotatory stabilizers of the elbow. *J Bone Joint Surg Am*. 2004;86:975-982.
4. Rolla PR, Surace MF, Bini A, Pilato G. Arthroscopic treatment of fractures of the radial head. *Arthroscopy*. 2006;22:233 e1-233 e6.
5. Mason ML. Some observations on fractures of the head of the radius with a review of one hundred cases. *Br J Surg*. 1954;42:123-132.
6. Michels F, Pouliart N, Handelberg F. Arthroscopic management of Mason type 2 radial head fractures. *Knee Surg Sports Traumatol Arthrosc*. 2007; 15:1244-1250.
7. Dawson FA, Inostroza F. Arthroscopic reduction and percutaneous fixation of a radial neck fracture in a child. *Arthroscopy*. 2004;20(suppl 2): 90-93.
8. Broberg MA, Morrey BF. Results of delayed excision of the radial head after fracture. *J Bone Joint Surg Am.*, 1986;68:669-674.
9. Menth-Chiari WA, Poehling GG, Ruch DS. Arthroscopic resection of the radial head. *Arthroscopy*. 1999;15:226-230.
10. Menth-Chiari WA, Ruch DS, Poehling GG. Arthroscopic excision of the radial head: clinical outcome in 12 patients with post-traumatic arthritis after fracture of the radial head or rheumatoid arthritis. *Arthroscopy*. 2001;17:918-923.
11. Regan W, Morrey B. Fractures of the coronoid process of the ulna. *J Bone Joint Surg Am*. 1989;71:1348-1354.
12. Adams JE, Merten SM, Steinmann SP. Arthroscopic-assisted treatment of coronoid fractures. *Arthroscopy*. 2007;23:1060-1065.
13. Liu SH, Henry M, Bowen R. Complications of type I coronoid fractures in competitive athletes: report of two cases and review of the literature. *J Shoulder Elbow Surg*. 1996;5:223-227.
14. Bryan RS, Morrey BF. Fractures of the distal humerus. In: Morrey, BF, ed. *The Elbow and Its Disorders* Philadelphia, PA: WB Saunders; 1985:302-309.
15. Feldman MD. Arthroscopic excision of type II capitellar fractures. *Arthroscopy*. 1997,13:743-748
16. Hardy P, Menguy F, Guillot S. Arthroscopic treatment of capitellum fracture of the humerus. *Arthroscopy*. 2002;18:422-426.
17. Milch H. Fractures and fracture dislocations of the humeral condyles. *J Trauma*. 1964;4:592-607.
18. Hausman MR, Qureshi S, Goldstein R, et al. Arthroscopically assisted treatment of pediatric lateral humeral condyle fractures. *J Pediatr Orthop*. 2007;27:739-742.
19. Perez Carro L, Golano P, Vega J. Arthroscopic-assisted reduction and percutaneous external fixation of lateral condyle fractures of the humerus. *Arthroscopy*. 2007;23:1131 e1-1131 e4.

SELECTED READINGS

Brown TD, Peden JP, Savoie FH, Field LD. Arthroscopic reduction internal fixation of elbow fractures. In: Levine WN, Blaine TA, Ahmad CS, eds. *Minimally Invasive Shoulder and Elbow Surgery*. New York, NY: Informa Healthcare USA; 2007:375-383.

Holt MS, Savoie FH 3rd, Field LD, Ramsey JR. Arthroscopic management of elbow trauma. *Hand Clin*. 2004;20:485-495.

Moskal MJ, Savoie FH 3rd, Field LD. Elbow arthroscopy in trauma and reconstruction. *Orthop Clin North Am*. 1999;30:163-177.

Savoie FH, Peden JP, Field LD. Arthroscopic reduction and internal fixation of elbow fractures. In: Yamaguchi K, King GJW, McKee MD, O'Driscoll SW, eds. *Advanced Reconstruction: Elbow*. Evanston, IL: American Academy of Orthopaedic Surgeons; 2007:85-92.

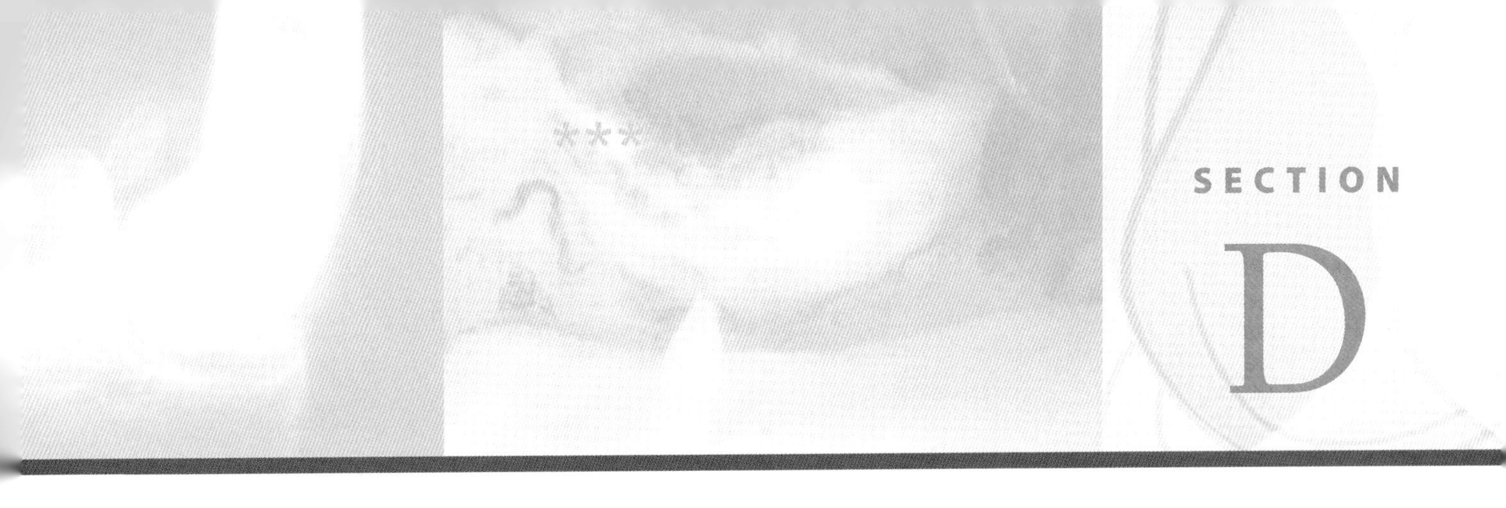

SECTION D

Complications

CHAPTER

18

Complications of Elbow Arthroscopy

Richard J. Thomas • Felix H. Savoie III • Larry D. Field

Arthroscopic surgery is increasingly used in the treatment of elbow pathology, including loose bodies, synovitis, degenerative joint disease, osteochondritis dissecans, arthrofibrosis, lateral epicondylitis, olecranon bursitis, fractures, and plica.[1,2] Advantages of elbow arthroscopy over open surgery include decreased scarring, decreased risk of infection, less postoperative pain, and better visualization of the joint.[2] Elbow arthroscopy is considered one of the most challenging types of arthroscopic surgery, most likely because of the high congruence of the joint and the proximity of neurovascular structures.[2]

Little research has been done in regard to complications in elbow arthroscopy. Most studies in the literature are case reports or case series that do not specifically look at the incidence of complications of arthroscopic surgery of the elbow. Few large series studies have looked at complications in elbow arthroscopy. In a review of the literature, Savoie[3] found 16 reported complications in 465 elbow arthroscopic surgeries, or a 3% incidence. Micheli and colleagues[4] described elbow arthroscopy performed on an athletically active pediatric population and found no complications for 47 patients. The members of the Arthroscopy Association of North America were surveyed about the complications of arthroscopic surgery. For the 1569 elbow arthroscopies in the survey, only three complications were reported.[5]

Kelly and coworkers[2] looked at 473 elbow arthroscopies over an 18-year period done by 12 different surgeons and reported an 11% minor complication rate and a 0.8% major complication rate. Savoie and associates[6] found an overall complication rate of 7% in a series of 269 consecutive elbow arthroscopies over a 3-year period. In this chapter, we discuss the complications associated with elbow arthroscopy, their possible causes, and tips on how to prevent them.

COMPLICATIONS

The anatomy of the elbow makes arthroscopy a technically difficult procedure that is predisposed to complications.[7] The reported complications of elbow arthroscopy include infection, heterotopic ossification, complex regional pain syndrome, nerve injury, fistula, and olecranon bursitis.[2,6-10]

Infection

One of the most common complications of elbow arthroscopy is infection. The anatomy of the elbow makes it more vulnerable than other joints to infection. The soft tissue envelope around the elbow is extremely thin, and the capsule is separated from the skin by a thin layer of subcutaneous tissue, predisposing the site to prolonged drainage,[7] which may precede cellulitis, abscesses, intraarticular infections, or portal fistulas.

Superficial infections and persistent drainage after elbow arthroscopy are much more common than deep infections.[2,10,11] Superficial infections of the elbow after arthroscopy typically manifest as prolonged serous drainage or erythema around a portal site. Patients may have low-grade fevers and tenderness around portal sites. The erythema and drainage usually resolve with 2 weeks of oral antibiotics. Immobilization may be beneficial in the setting of prolonged drainage.

Kelly and colleagues[2] reported a 5% incidence of prolonged drainage from portal sites and a 2% incidence of superficial infection in their series of 473 procedures. These minor infections resolved with a short course of oral antibiotics. Reddy and associates[12] reported a 1% incidence of persistent drainage from arthroscopic portals. Drainage was treated successfully with 7 days of oral antibiotics. Thomas and coworkers[6] found a 2.2% incidence of superficial infections, which resolved within

7 to 14 days with oral antibiotics. Several reports[2,6,7] indicate that the lateral portals, including the soft spot portal and the anterolateral portal, are more susceptible to infection and prolonged drainage than the medial portals. This finding is probably reflects the fact that the skin is thinner on the lateral side of the elbow.[2,7] Suture closure of the portal sites has been recommended to decrease the incidence of prolonged drainage and infection.[2,13]

Extreme pain with minimal elbow motion, high fevers, and purulent drainage after elbow arthroscopy should alert the clinician to the possibility of a septic joint. Because of the catastrophic results of a missed septic joint, the clinician should be ready to aspirate the elbow to rule out an intra-articular infection.. A septic joint should be treated with emergent irrigation and débridement of the joint, drain placement, and a course of intravenous antibiotics.

Deep infections are rare after elbow arthroscopy. Micheli and colleagues,[4] Reddy and associates,[12] and Lynch and coworkers[14] reported no deep infections in their series of 47, 187, and 21 respective elbow arthroscopies. Thomas and colleagues[6] reported one deep infection in their series of 269 patients (0.4% incidence) that resolved with arthroscopic irrigation and débridement, drain placement, and 6 weeks of intravenous antibiotics. Kelly and associates[2] reported a 0.8% incidence of intra-articular infections after elbow arthroscopy. They theorized that immediate postoperative steroid injections might increase the risk of joint infections.

Portal fistula formation, although rare, has been reported in the literature. Thomas and colleagues[5] reported one soft spot portal fistula formation in a paraplegic patient with a prior instance of methicillin-resistant *Staphylococcus aureus* infection. The patient was treated successfully with open irrigation, débridement, fistula excision, and closure. The patient also received a course of oral antibiotics.

Nerve Injury

Of all the complications resulting from elbow arthroscopy, nerve injuries are the most feared and the most reported. Most reported nerve injuries associated with elbow arthroscopy are transient, although permanent nerve injuries have been reported.[11]

Knowledge of the anatomy of the elbow is crucial to the avoidance of neurologic injury in elbow arthroscopy. All three nerves that cross the elbow joint are close to the capsule, and capsular distention does not protect the nerves from capsular procedures, such as a release or synovectomy.[7] Lynch and coworkers[14] performed cadaveric dissections and found that the radial nerve lay within an average of 5 mm of the joint and that distention of the joint increased this distance to 10 mm. The median nerve was also found to be within 5 mm of the anterior joint. Lindenfeld[20] reported that the radial nerve was an average of 7.8 mm from the anterolateral portal when the portal was made 3 cm distal and 1 cm anterior to the lateral epicondyle (Fig. 18-1). The radial nerve and the posterior interosseous nerve are therefore at risk when making an anterolateral portal. The ulnar nerve is at risk when creating the anteromedial portal. The median nerve is at risk when débriding or performing a capsulectomy of the anterior capsule.[7] O'Driscoll

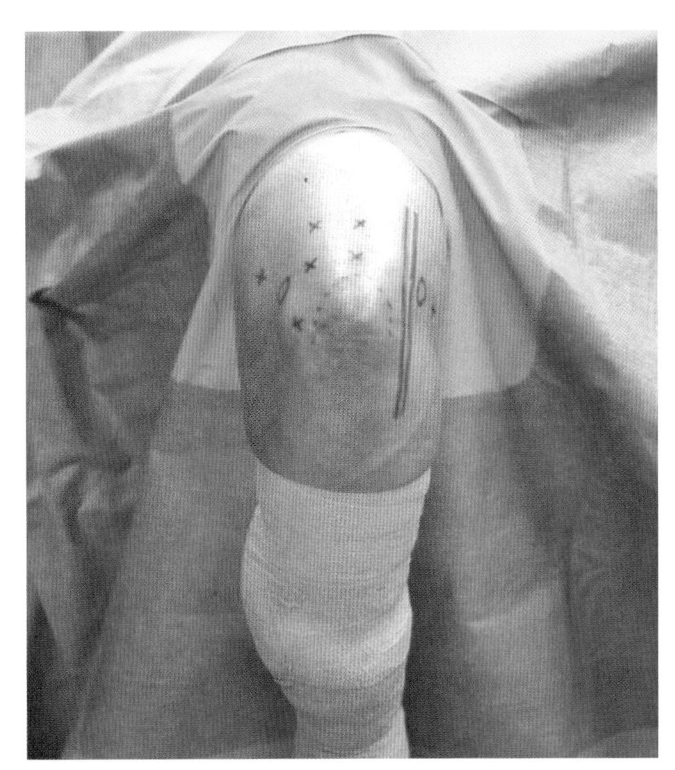

FIGURE 18-1 The radial nerve is an average of 7.8 mm from the anterolateral portal when the portal is made 3 cm distal and 1 cm anterior to the lateral epicondyle.

and Morrey[10] reported three patients with transient radial nerve palsies lasting several hours in their series of 71 elbow arthroscopies. They attributed these palsies to local anesthetic extravasation. Lynch and associates[14] reported a 14% incidence of nerve injuries in their series of 21 arthroscopies, including a transient radial nerve palsy, a transient median nerve palsy, and a neuroma of the medial antebrachial cutaneous nerve.

Kelly and colleagues[2] had a 2% incidence of transient nerve palsies in their series of 473 consecutive elbow arthroscopies. These palsies included four superficial radial, five ulnar, one posterior interosseous, one anterior interosseous, and one medial antebrachial cutaneous nerve palsies. All palsies resolved within 6 weeks after arthroscopy, except for one case, which resolved within 6 months. They reported that rheumatoid arthritis and capsular release were risk factors for nerve injury. Thomas and coworkers[6] reported a 1.9% incidence of transient nerve palsies in a series of 269 arthroscopies and identified an increased risk of nerve injury with capsular release. The nerve palsies in this series required an average of 6.1 months to completely resolve.

Permanent nerve injuries after elbow arthroscopy are a rare complication. Neither series by Kelly and colleagues[2] or Thomas and associates[6] reported a permanent nerve injury. Reddy and coworkers[12] reported a complete transection of the ulnar nerve after an arthroscopic synovectomy and loose body removal. The injury was not noticed during the initial procedure, but after reexploration of the ulnar nerve 3 days postoperatively, a 1.5-cm defect in the ulnar nerve was found and repaired. The patient regained some light touch and pinprick sensation but did not regain strength in the intrinsic musculature. Casscells[16] reported an irreparable injury to the ulnar nerve when using a motorized shaver posteromedially. Jones and Savoie,[17] Papilion and colleagues,[18] and Thomas and associates[19] reported permanent posterior interosseous nerve injuries that occurred during arthroscopic procedures. Jones and Savoie[17] described the injury in a patient who had a displaced radial head fracture that healed to the anterior capsule. During arthroscopic débridement and manipulation, the capsule separated in this area rather than near the humerus, where it had been excised, and it severed the nerve. Jones and Savoie[17] recommended avoiding arthroscopic capsular release in patients with excessive scarring in the vicinity of the posterior interosseous nerve without first dissecting out the nerve.

To avoid nerve injuries in elbow arthroscopy, several principles should be followed. Joint distention should be used before portal placement to move the nerves farther away from the joint. Even so, the nerves remain close to the capsule, and distention does not protect the nerves during capsular procedures. Proximal portals are safer than more distal portals, and the radial nerve is most at risk when making the anterolateral portal. The ulnar nerve should be palpated before anteromedial portal placement. Posteromedial and direct anterior portals should never be used. The elbow should be flexed to 90 degrees during portal placement. Retractors may increase the safety of elbow arthroscopic procedures, especially in capsulectomies and synovectomies. Particular caution should be used when working posteromedially because of the proximity of the ulnar nerve. Suction should be avoided around nerves, and instrument tips should be visualized at all times. Knowledge of elbow anatomy and proficiency in arthroscopy are keys to avoiding neurologic injury in elbow arthroscopy.[7,15,20]

Other Complications

Although nerve injuries and infection are the most common complications associated with elbow arthroscopy, several others have been reported. Olecranon bursitis, heterotopic ossification, contracture, and complex regional pain syndrome have been associated with elbow arthroscopy.

A 1.1% incidence of olecranon bursitis was reported by Thomas and colleagues[6] in their series. Most cases were benign and responded to conservative therapy (Fig. 18-2). No other incidents of olecranon bursitis associated with elbow arthroscopy have been reported in the literature.

Kelly and associates[2] reported seven cases of minor postoperative contracture in their series of 473 elbow arthroscopies. The patients lost less than 20 degrees, and the contractures only affected the flexion-extension plane. No heterotopic ossification occurred. Thomas and colleagues[6] reported one case of anterior heterotopic ossification after an arthroscopic ulnohumeral arthroplasty and capsular release. Less than 20 degrees of motion was lost due to the heterotopic ossification.

Complex regional pain syndrome is another rare complication that has been reported after elbow arthroscopy.[6] These cases have responded to physical therapy, pain management, and sympathetic blocks.

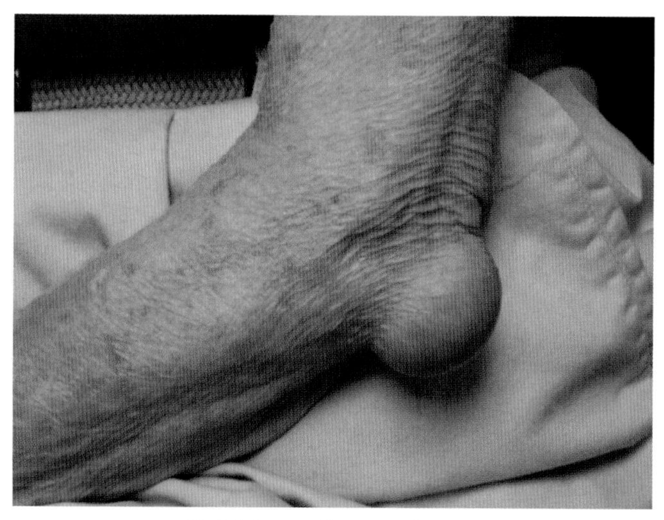

FIGURE 18-2 Olecranon bursitis.

PEARLS & PITFALLS

- Suturing portals may decrease incidence of prolonged drainage or infection.
- Proximal portals are safer than more distal ones.
- Nerves remain close to the capsule in the distended joint, and they are at risk during capsular procedures.
- Posteromedial and direct anterior portals should never be used.
- Extreme care should be used in the posteromedial elbow because of the proximity of the ulnar nerve.
- Suction should not be used near nerves, and the tips of instruments should always be visualized.
- The ulnar nerve should be palpated before creation of the anteromedial portal.
- Portals should be created with the elbow flexed to 90 degrees.
- Knowledge of anatomy and proficiency in arthroscopy is crucial for preventing complications.

CONCLUSIONS

Elbow arthroscopy is a safe procedure when performed by experienced surgeons. Major complications, including permanent nerve injuries, are rare, and the incidence of minor complications is comparable to that for other forms of arthroscopy.

REFERENCES

1. Baker CL, Jones GL. Arthroscopy of the elbow. *Am J Sports Med*. 1999; 27:251-264.
2. Kelly EW, Morrey BF, O'Driscoll SW. Complications of elbow arthroscopy. *J Bone Joint Surg Am*. 2001;83:25-34.
3. Savoie FH. Complications. In: Savoie FH, Field LD, eds. *Arthroscopy of the Elbow*. New York, NY: Churchill Livingstone; 1996:151-156.
4. Micheli LJ, Luke AC, Mintzer CM, Waters PM. Elbow arthroscopy in the pediatric and adolescent population. *Arthroscopy*. 2001;17:694-699.
5. Small NC. Complications in arthroscopy: the knee and other joints. *Arthroscopy*. 1986;2:253-258.
6. Thomas RJ, Savoie FH, Field LD. Complications in elbow arthroscopy. 2010. *Am J Sports Med*. In Press.
7. Morrey BF. Complications of elbow arthroscopy. *Instr Course Lect*. 2000; 49:255-258.

8. Angelo RL. Advances in elbow arthroscopy. *Orthopedics*. 1993;16:1037-1046.
9. Redden JF, Stanley D. Arthroscopic fenestration of the olecranon fossa in the treatment of osteoarthritis of the elbow. *Arthroscopy*.1993;9:14-16.
10. O'Driscoll SW, Morrey BF. Arthroscopy of the elbow: diagnostic and therapeutic benefits and hazards. *J Bone Joint Surg Am*. 1992;74:84-94.
11. Phillips BB. Arthroscopy of the upper extremity. In: Canale ST, Beaty JH, eds. *Campbell's Operative Orthopaedics*. Philadelphia, PA: Mosby Elsevier; 2008:2923-3014.
12. Reddy AS, Kvitne RS, Yocum LA, et al. Arthroscopy of the elbow: a long term clinical review. *Arthroscopy*. 2000;16:588-594.
13. Morrey BF, Askew LJ, An KN, et al. A biomechanical study of normal functional elbow motion. *J Bone Joint Surg Am*. 1981;63:872-877.
14. Lynch GJ, Meyers JF, Whipple TL, et al. Neurovascular anatomy and elbow arthroscopy: inherent risks. *Arthroscopy*. 1986;2:190-197.
15. Lindenfeld TN. Medial approach in elbow arthroscopy. *Am J Sports Med*. 1990;18:413-417.
16. Casscells SW. Neurovascular anatomy and elbow arthroscopy: inherent risks [editor's comment]. *Arthroscopy*. 1987;2:190.
17. Jones GS, Savoie FH III. Arthroscopic capsular release of flexion contractures (arthrofibrosis) of the elbow. *Arthroscopy*. 1993;9:277-283.
18. Papilion JD, Neff RS, Shall LM. Compression neuropathy of the radial nerve as a complication of elbow arthroscopy: a case report and review of the literature. *Arthroscopy*. 1988;4:284-286.
19. Thomas MA, Fast A, Shapiro DL. Radial nerve damage as a complication of elbow arthroscopy. *Clin Orthop*. 1987;215:130-131.
20. Wiesler ER, Poehling GG. Elbow arthroscopy: introduction, indications, complications, and results. In: McGinty JB, ed. *Operative Arthroscopy*. Philadelphia, PA: Lippincott Williams & Wilkins; 2003:661-664.

PART

II

The Wrist

SECTION

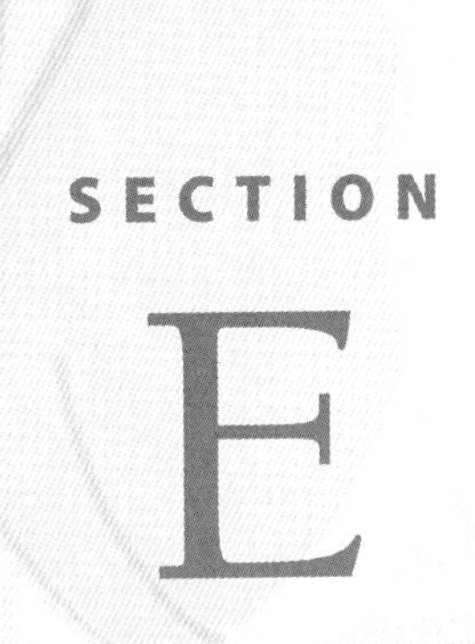

Basics

CHAPTER

19

Wrist Arthroscopy: Setup, Anatomy, and Portals

Mark Morishige • Larry D. Field • Felix H. Savoie III

Wrist arthroscopy has been used since it was first described by Chen in 1979.[1] In the early stages of development, it provided only partial evaluation of the articular surfaces, and it was not used therapeutically. Few investigators routinely used arthroscopic techniques.[2] It was not until 1986, when Whipple advocated distraction techniques and precise portal placement, that the exposure necessary to perform an extensive evaluation of the wrist joint became an option.[3] Even then, diagnosis was the primary function, and therapeutic indications were minimal. Since that time, innovations in wrist arthroscopy have expanded treatment indications and promoted widespread acceptance.

Diagnostic and operative forms of arthroscopy have advanced our understanding of wrist anatomy and function, and arthroscopic techniques have facilitated the repair of previously unrecognized pathology. Continued advances in instrumentation and technology will improve the ability to perform challenging and innovative procedures as the principles of open surgical procedures become adapted to arthroscopy.[4]

Wrist arthroscopy allows close visual examination of the carpal articular surfaces and wrist ligaments, which is often inadequate with open procedures and which can be performed in a less invasive manner than traditional arthrotomy.[5] The extremely close evaluation of details provides many benefits and increases appreciation of the subtle differences between normal and pathologic anatomy.[6] This fact alone underscores the importance of a thorough understanding of arthroscopic anatomy.

ANATOMY

The wrist is made up of the eight carpal bones, each with multiple articular surfaces and the intrinsic and extrinsic ligaments, and a triangular fibrocartilage complex (TFCC) that is surrounded by tendons and neurovascular structures (Fig. 19-1).[7,8] A thorough understanding of the relationship between the surface anatomy of the wrist and these underlying structures is essential to perform accurate arthroscopic portal placement and adequate arthroscopy. Understanding these relationships helps to prevent injury to the cutaneous nerves, tendons, and vascular structures and can minimize the risk to the articular surfaces in the wrist. It also facilitates the use of instruments during procedures, enabling the completion of increasingly complicated arthroscopic wrist procedures.

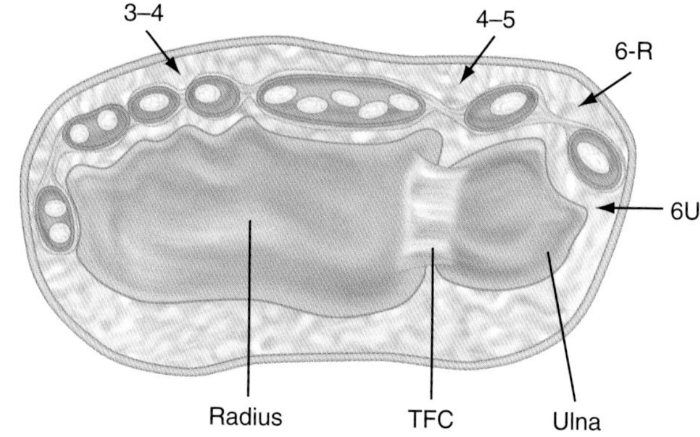

FIGURE 19-1 Cross-sectional anatomy of the dorsal compartments. *(Modified from Geissler WB, Freeland AE, Weiss AP, Chow JC. Techniques of wrist arthroscopy.* Instr Course Lect. *2000:49:225-237.)*

To accurately place portals, the surface anatomy should be mapped and labeled before making the first incision. Bony landmarks that should be familiar to the surgeon include Lister's tubercle, the radius and ulna with their styloids, the radiocarpal joint level, the radial border of the third ray, and the central portion of the fourth ray. The capitate sulcus (i.e., soft spot) also should be palpated.

The extensor retinaculum is an obliquely oriented structure that spans the dorsal distal radius and ulna. It overlies the 12 extensor tendons, which are partitioned into six compartments to prevent bowstringing of the extensor tendons.[4] The extensor pollicis longus (EPL) is the only tendon in the third compart-

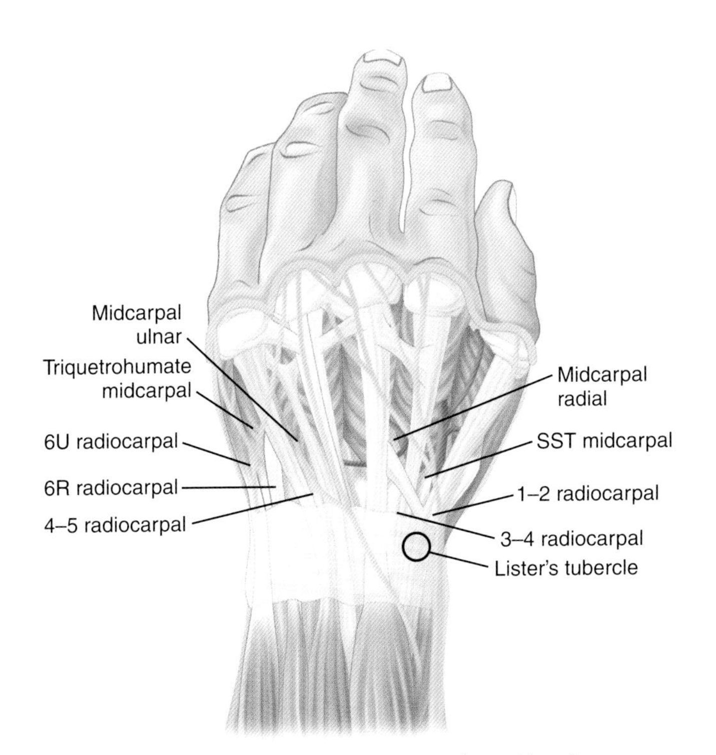

FIGURE 19-2 Dorsal wrist anatomy and portal locations.

ment, and it is easily palpated, especially after application of traction. This structure passes just ulnar to Lister's tubercle and should be appropriately marked. The area bordered by the EPL and extensor pollicis brevis together and the extensor carpi radialis longus (ECRL) define the margins of the anatomic snuffbox. The extensor digitorum communis (EDC) is just ulnar to the EPL. The extensor carpi ulnaris (ECU) and the ECRL and ECRB tendons are easily palpated and should be marked. The intersection of these tendons and the bony structures allows accurate identification and precise placement arthroscopy portals (Fig. 19-2).

PATIENT EVALUATION

History and Physical Examination

A thorough history and physical examination are essential before proceeding with arthroscopic evaluation of the wrist. It has been said that if no diagnosis can be made after a thorough clinical assessment, little additional information can be obtained from arthoscopy.[9] A meticulous history helps focus the examiner on the cause and directs the physical examination to the suspected pathology. The examiner must determine the activities that exacerbate or lessen the problem, the functional loss, and the ability of the patient to perform daily activities, including work and leisure activities. The mechanism of injury should be ascertained.

Physical examination is the most accurate method for diagnosing pathology.[2] A systematic approach to the wrist examination is essential. All joints must be carefully inspected, palpated, and appropriately stressed with the use of provocative tests. Areas of swelling, tenderness, or pain can focus attention on the specific pathology. Examination includes palpation of the tendons and evaluation of the patient's neurologic and vascular status.

Diagnostic Imaging

The initial evaluation should include routine radiographs, including standard posteroanterior, lateral, and oblique views. The radiographs should be examined for fractures, misalignments, and joint space problems. Advanced radiographs, which may be needed if specific pathologies are suspected, include pronation, supination, clenched fist, and carpal tunnel views, and stress radiographs should be obtained.

Occasionally, the diagnosis remains unclear after an adequate history, physical examination, and routine radiographic studies have been completed. Further diagnostic studies may be indicated. Computed tomography (CT) is useful for evaluating osseous and articular morphology. Magnetic resonance imaging (MRI) provides important information about the soft tissues of the wrist and the vascularity of bones. The most definitive study is magnetic resonance arthrography, which begins with a radiocarpal injection followed by a distal radioulnar joint injection.[10]

TREATMENT

Indications and Contraindications

Wrist arthroscopy provides an accurate complement to the probable diagnosis obtained from the physical examination. Arthroscopy is useful for evaluation of patients with wrist pain and motion loss when noninvasive studies have failed to provide a diagnosis, and it is more sensitive than arthrography for evaluating pathology.[8] Diagnosis of interosseous ligaments tears and the degree of carpal instability can be accurately determined using arthroscopy. It is also useful in patients with well-defined pathology, such as nonunions, Kienbock's disease, and scapholunate or lunotriquetral dissociations, for which evaluation of the articular surfaces is of prognostic and therapeutic importance.

Although once used almost exclusively for diagnostic purposes, the therapeutic indications for wrist arthroscopy continue to expand. Arthroscopic treatment is indicated for loose body removal, synovectomy, intra-articular adhesion release, lavage of a septic wrist, debridement of chondral lesions, hypertrophic or torn ligaments, and tears of the TFCC. It has also been used for dorsal ganglion excision and provides a useful adjunct in the reduction of distal radius and scaphoid fractures. Bone excision procedures, such as radial styloidectomy and partial resection of the distal ulna (i.e., wafer procedures), have been performed arthroscopically. Arthroscopy has been described for advanced procedures, such as proximal row carpectomy, excision of the proximal pole of the scaphoid, lunate excision in Kienbock's disease, and capitolunate arthrodesis.[7,8]

Contraindications to wrist arthroscopy are limited mainly to conditions of trauma or swelling that distorts the normal anatomy or significantly damages capsular integrity, leading to fluid extravasation.

Conservative Management

Before arthroscopy, nonoperative measures should usually be exhausted. Temporary immobilization and anti-inflammatory medication may be helpful. Diagnostic and therapeutic injections frequently provide some benefit. A physical therapy regimen for wrist range of motion and strengthening may prove definitive for some wrist pathology.

Arthroscopic Technique

Setup

A significant improvement in wrist arthroscopy came with the innovation of wrist distraction. This key element enhanced the surgeon's ability to perform arthroscopic procedures in the confined wrist joint. Distraction is essential to improve visualization and provide adequate space for maneuverability during wrist arthroscopy, because distention of the joint alone does not provide adequate room for instrumentation.[2] Several options exist to provide the necessary distraction. A dedicated sterile or nonsterile traction tower is a popular choice. Alternatives include the use of horizontal traction with a pulley and weight system and a nonsterile traction boom device (Figs. 19-3 to 19-5).

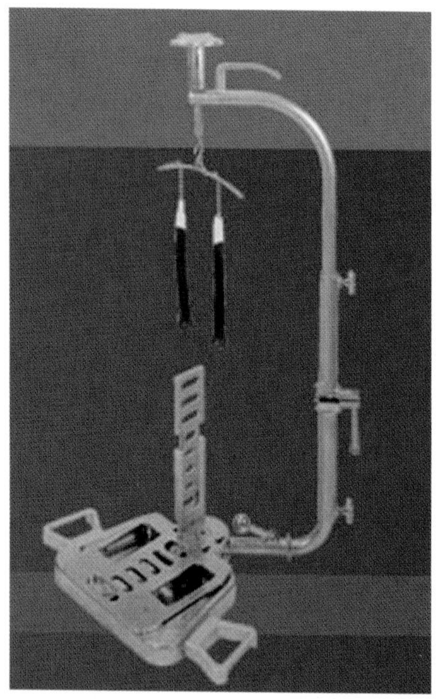

FIGURE 19-3 Traction tower.

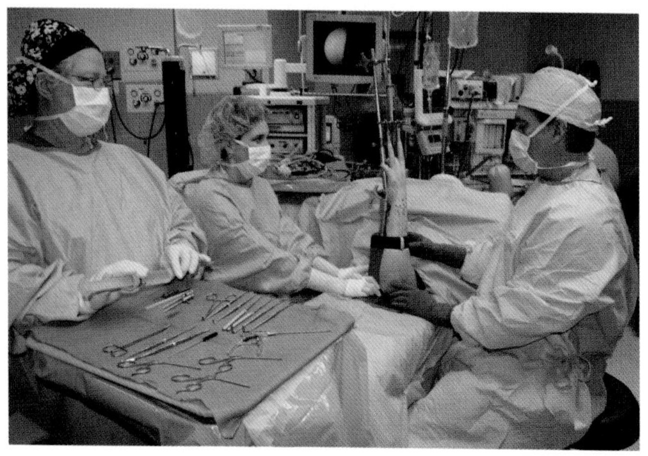

FIGURE 19-4 Operating room setup, showing the positions of the assistant and surgical assistant.

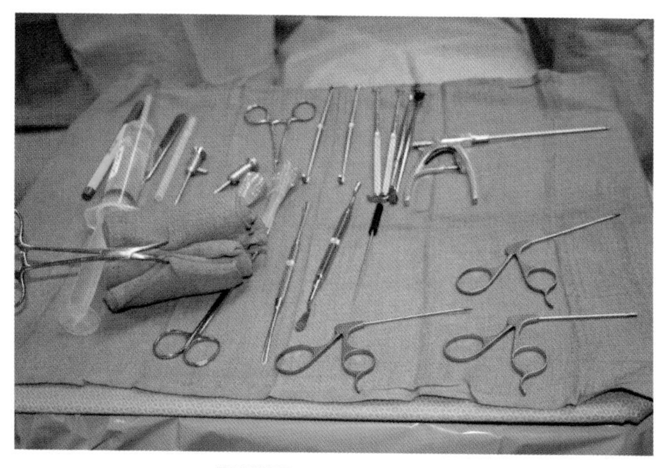

FIGURE 19-5 Mayo setup.

We prefer a sterile traction tower with nylon finger traps. It provides convenient application of wrist distraction in flexion, extension, and radial and ulnar deviation. This system allows adjustability to the distraction force and the position of the wrist, and it permits easy conversion to open procedures if necessary. The traction tower system maintains the wrist in a stable position for portal preservation during the exchange of instruments.[2]

The arm is placed in an abducted position, and the upper arm is secured to the traction tower. A nonsterile tourniquet is applied, and the arm and hand are prepared and draped with the forearm in a vertical position (Fig. 19-6). We use sterile soft nylon finger traps to secure the index and long finger to the tower for most procedures. Soft traps increase the surface area and distribute the

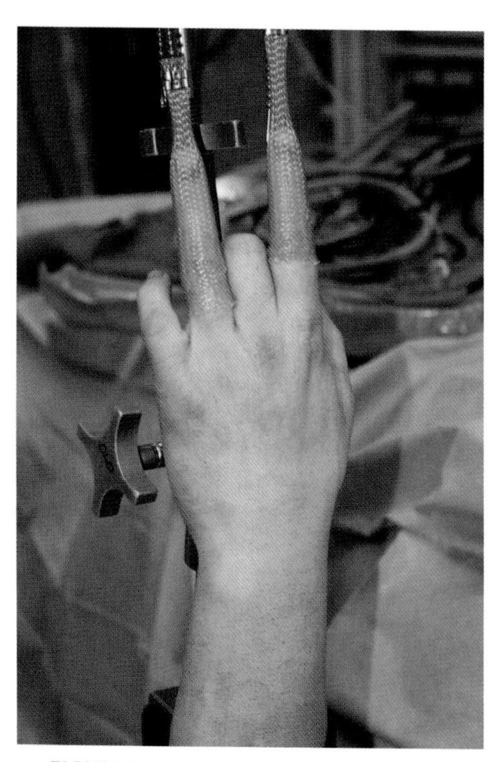

FIGURE 19-6 Draping and tower placement.

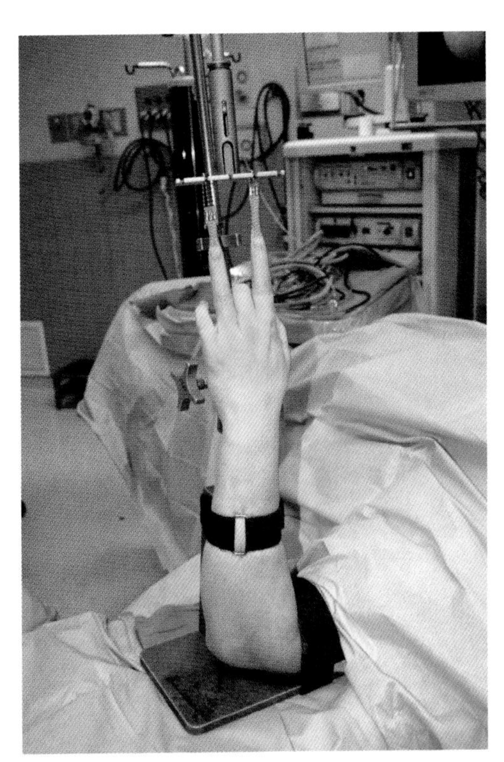

FIGURE 19-7 Soft finger trap placement for ulnar-sided procedure.

force better than wire devices. For patients with poor or fragile skin, additional fingers in the traps can decrease the force to the skin.[2] To improve visualization for ulnar-sided pathology, we frequently use the index and ring fingers (Fig. 19-7). Most procedures require 5 to 10 pounds of traction.

Equipment

Proper equipment is essential to perform a quality wrist arthroscopy. A video arthroscope and monitor with printer and video recorder are used to document the intra-articular findings. In addition to adequate visualization, a major improvement came with the innovation of instruments specifically designed for use in small joints. Larger instrumentation used for knee and shoulder arthroscopy is not adequate for procedures in the wrist. A 2.0- to 3.0-mm-diameter arthroscope is essential to allow adequate mobilization without the risk of injury to surrounding structures and articular surfaces. In addition to the standard 30-degree arthroscope, a 70-degree arthroscope is occasionally useful.

Other small joint arthroscopy equipment is available and necessary for mastery of wrist arthroscopy. Equipment includes a small joint shaver (2.7 or 2.9 mm) with multiple tips, a wrist probe (1.7 or 2.0 mm), and many of the smaller versions of large joint arthroscopic instruments.[5,7] As arthroscopy has advanced, more specialized equipment has become available, including TFCC repair kits, retrograde retrievers, ablation shrinkage devices, and fracture fixation devices. Spinal needles and passing sutures are helpful tools that have been adapted from other arthroscopic repair techniques.

Clear physiologic crystalloid solution, such as lactated Ringer's solution, is preferable because it can be rapidly absorbed into the tissues and can prevent overdistention. Irrigant can be introduced through the sheath of the arthroscope or by separate inflow and outflow portals. Gravity inflow has proved adequate in our practice. Pinch chambers can introduce small boluses of irrigant to clear the visual field.[2] Fluid pumps that can precisely control the pressure in the joint are available. However, pressurized injection increases the risk of fluid extravasation into subcutaneous tissue and is usually unnecessary.

Portals

Wrist arthroscopy portals include radiocarpal, midcarpal, distal radioulnar, and volar portals. Traditionally, arthroscopic viewing portals are described by their relation to the six extensor compartments of the wrist. Eleven historical access portals typically are used. They include five radiocarpal, four midcarpal, and two distal radioulnar portals. Two additional volar portals have become increasingly popular.

Precise portal placement is essential for performing a complete wrist arthroscopy and for minimizing iatrogenic injury to the wrist joint and surrounding structures. Placing the portals in an incorrect manner can result in damage to neurovascular structures and the articular cartilage. All portals and surface landmarks should be marked on the skin. Marking portals after the application of traction helps to prevent distortion and improperly placed portal sites (Fig. 19-8).

Radiocarpal Portals. Radiocarpal portals include the 3-4, 4-5, 6-R, 6-U, and 1-2 portals. Radiocarpal portals show smooth carpal articulations, whereas the midcarpal portals show more irregular articulations.[5] Portals are named according to the interspace between extensor compartments. The 3-4 portal divides the third and fourth extensor compartments. The 6-R and 6-U

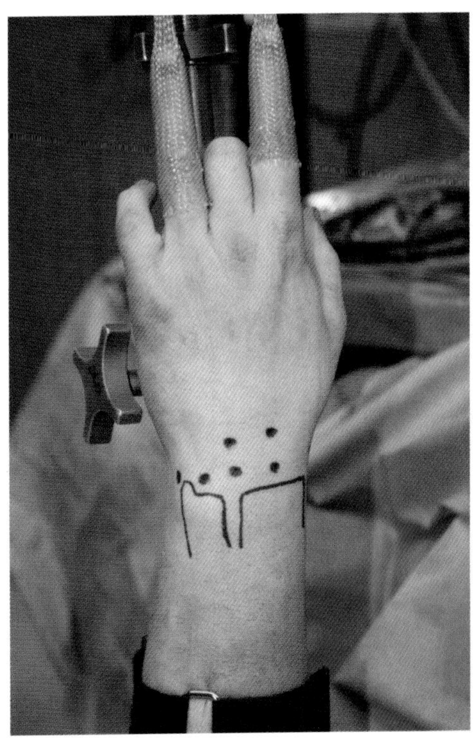

FIGURE 19-8 Marking portals and landmarks on the skin.

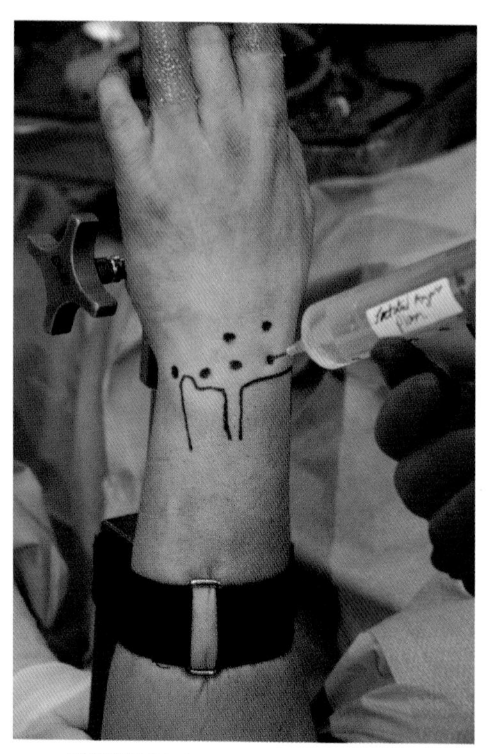

FIGURE 19-9 Injection of the 3-4 portal.

portals are named by their relationship to the ECU, with the 6-R on the radial aspect and the 6-U on the ulnar aspect.[7] Palpation between these compartments demonstrates soft spots of the wrist, which provide the least traumatic entry points into the joint.

The 3-4 Portal. The 3-4 portal is usually the first portal established, and it is the primary viewing portal. It is bordered on the radial side by the EPL and ECRB, on the ulnar side by the EDC, on the proximal side by the distal radius, and on the distal side by the scapholunate ligament. The 3-4 portal is established 1 cm distal to Lister's tubercle, and it is located by palpating the distal edge of the radius between the ulnar border of the ECRB and the radial margin of the EDC in line with the radial border of the long finger. This is the soft spot between the third and fourth compartments.[7] A spinal needle is then inserted parallel to the radial articular surface at about 10 degrees, matching the palmar tilt (Fig. 19-9).

This portal is the workhorse of standard wrist arthroscopy and provides a broad view of most of the radiocarpal joint on the volar side. The portal is relatively safe, with the sensory branch of the radial nerve (SBRN) a mean distance of 16 mm and a mean distance from the radial artery of 26.3 mm.[11]

The 4-5 Portal. The 4-5 portal is bordered on the radial side by EDC, on the ulnar side by the extensor digiti quinti (EDQ), proximally by the attachment of the radius and the TFCC, and distally by the lunate. It is established 1 cm ulnar and slightly more proximal to the 3-4 portal because of the inclination of the radius.[7] It can be found by palpating the soft spot directly ulnar to the EDC. A spinal needle should then be placed just proximal to the lunate. Entry through this portal places instruments directly adjacent to the midportion of the TFCC.[12] The 4-5 portal is typically the main working portal for instrumentation on the ulnar side of the wrist. It may also be used as a viewing portal for ulnar sided structures. This portal has minimal neurovascular risk unless there is an aberrant branch of the SBRN.[11]

The 6-R Portal. Frequently used as an alternative to the 4-5 portal, the 6-R portal is bordered radially by the EDQ, ulnarly by the ECU, proximally by the TFCC, and distally by the lunotriquetral joint. It enters the wrist joint just distal to the ulnar attachment of the TFCC. This portal is found by using the proximal border of the triquetrum rather than distal ulna as a surface landmark to avoid damaging the TFCC. It is establish under arthroscopic guidance by introducing a needle just radial to the ECU. The 6-R portal is typically used for instrumentation or for outflow. It also provides visualization of the TFCC and the ulnolunate, ulnotriquetral, and interosseous lunotriquetral ligaments. The 6-R has a mean distance of 8.2 mm from the dorsal sensory branch of the ulnar nerve (DBUN).[11]

The 6-U Portal. The 6-U portal is established volar to the ECU tendon, but because of its proximity to the DBUN, it is not routinely used. The skin incision may be placed as far volar as the dorsal border of the ECU tendon. The portal enters the wrist joint through the prestyloid recess between the ECU tendon and the ulnar styloid. The portal is distal to the TFCC and dorsal ulnar to the ulnotriquetral ligament. The 6-U portal is typically used for the inflow or outflow cannula. It may be used as an accessory portal for viewing ulnar-sided structures or for instrumentation during TFCC repairs. The mean distance of the portal to the DBUN is 4.5 mm, but the nerve can have multiple branches in some patients.[11]

The 1-2 Portal. The 1-2 portal is not used frequently. It is established between the first and second extensor compartments 1 to 2 mm distal to the radial styloid. This portal is placed by finding the soft spot between the first extensor compartment containing the abductor pollicis longus and extensor pollicis brevis and the second compartment with the ECRL and ECRB tendons along the far ulnar part of the anatomic snuffbox. It is located just proximal to the waist of the scaphoid. The radial artery is located at the volar and radial aspect of the anatomic snuffbox. This necessitates placement of this portal as far dorsal as possible to avoid injury to the artery.[12]

The 1-2 portal provides access to the radial styloid, scaphoid, and articular surface of the distal radius, but it allows only a limited view of the lunate.[4] There is significant risk with the placement of this portal. Two branches of the SBRN are a mean distance of 3 mm radial and 5 mm ulnar to the portal, and the radial artery is a mean distance of 3 mm radial to the portal.[11]

Midcarpal Portals. Midcarpal evaluation should be done as a routine part of wrist arthroscopy. The four midcarpal portals include the midcarpal radial, midcarpal ulnar, triquetrohamate, and triscaphe portals. The most commonly used are the radial and ulnar midcarpal portals. The less common ones are the triscaphe and the triquetrohamate portals. The very limited room in the midcarpal space requires extra care when entering the joint. Once established, these portals should be maintained to minimize the difficulty in re-establishing them due to fluid extravisation.[7] Normally, there is no communication between the radiocarpal and midcarpal spaces.

Evaluation of wrist instability with midcarpal arthroscopy is better than with radiocarpal arthroscopy alone. Studies show that instability of the scapholunate or lunotriquetral ligament diagnosed with radiocarpal arthroscopy was always seen on midcarpal arthroscopy, but instability seen by midcarpal arthroscopy was not always noticed when performing radiocarpal arthroscopy alone. Grading of the instability was equal to or greater than that done by midcarpal examination.[13]

Visualization of the scaphoid-trapezoid-trapezium (STT) joint, the midcarpal extrinsic ligaments, the capitohamate joint, and the articular surfaces of the midcarpal bones is improved with midcarpal arthroscopy. Midcarpal arthroscopy can be mastered quickly and adds little time to wrist arthroscopy. It has a low morbidity rate and should be used routinely for a thorough evaluation of the wrist.[13]

Midcarpal Radial Portal. The radial midcarpal portal is the most commonly used midcarpal portal. It is bordered radially by the ECRB, ulnarly by the EDC, proximally by the scapholunate ligament, and distally by the capitate. It should be established in line with the radial border of the third metacarpal, 1 cm distal to the 3-4 portal. A soft spot may be palpated on the radial side of the proximal capitate between the base of the third metacarpal and the dorsal margin of the distal radius. The arthroscope enters between the capitate and scaphoid. This allows evaluation of the midcarpal space and the scapholunate, lunotriquetral, and STT articulations. This portal is relatively safe, with branches of the SBRN found radially at a mean distance of 15.8 mm.[11]

Midcarpal Ulnar Portal. The midcarpal ulnar portal is bordered radially by the EDC, ulnarly by the EDQ, proximally by the lunotriquetral joint, and distally by the capitate hamate joint. It is in line with the center of the fourth metacarpal. As with the radial midcarpal portal, it is placed approximately 1 cm distal to the 4-5 portal and at about the same level as the radial midcarpal portal. This portal enters through capitate-hamate-triquetral-lunate interval. It is used primarily for instrumentation within the midcarpal joint. There is minimal risk when making this portal because the SBRN branches are usually remote to this portal.[11]

Triquetrohumate Portal. The triquetrohumate portal is established on the ulnar side of the wrist, distal to the triquetrum and ulnar to the midcarpal ulnar portal. The EDQ borders it on the radial side and the end of the ECU on its ulnar side. It enters the triquetrohumate joint just ulnar to the ECU tendon. It provides excellent access for an inflow or outflow canula and can be used for instrumentation in the triquetrohumate joint.

Triscaphe Portal. The triscaphe portal (STT) is on the radial side of the midcarpal space. It is established ulnar to the EPL or radial to the abductor pollicis longus in line with the radial margin of the second metacarpal at the level of the distal pole of the scaphoid. The STT-R portal provides an additional view and access to the STT joint.[14] Staying ulnar to EPL helps to avoid the radial artery. The ulnar aspect of the ECRL tendon can be used to check the location of this portal, because the EPL is quite mobile at the level of the STT joint. Care must be taken to prevent displacing the tendon radially while establishing the STT portal to protect the radial artery. The STT joint can be entered directly through this portal, and it is used primarily for instrumentation in this joint.[12] Care should be taken to avoid the small terminal branches of the SBRN.

Volar Portals. Volar portals have become increasingly popular to complete the view of diagnostic wrist arthroscopy and to provide access for procedures that are not feasible from the dorsal entry sites. Bain and colleagues suggested a box approach to wrist arthroscopy (Fig. 19-10).[4] By using portals around the circumference of the wrist, visualization and access to all surfaces within the wrist are improved.[15] The viewing and working portals can then be adjusted for the specific diagnostic or therapeutic procedure.[4] The volar portals allow improved treatment for dorsal pathology, such as dorsal rim fractures of the distal radius, dorsal rheumatoid synovial proliferation, and volar segment tears of the scapholunate and lunotriquetral interosseous ligaments.[15]

Volar Radial Portal. To place the volar radial (VR) portal, a mini-open technique is used over the flexor carpi radialis on the radial side of the volar proximal wrist crease. An anatomic study found that there was a safe zone that included the width of the flexor carpi radialis and at least 3 mm in all directions at this level from the palmar cutaneous branch of median nerve (ulnarly) and the radial artery (radially).[16] Because of this safe zone, a 2-cm transverse incision can be made over the flexor carpi radialis tendon. The transverse incision provides superior cosmesis while maintaining minimal risk for the volar structures. The tendon sheath is divided, the radial artery is retracted radially, and the flexor carpi radialis and median nerve are retracted ulnarly. The radiocarpal joint is identified with a spinal needle, and the portal is opened with a blunt instrument. This portal is used to assess the dorsal aspect of the scapholunate interosseous ligament and the dorsal radiocarpal ligament.[16]

Volar Ulnar Portal. Placement of the volar ulnar portal uses a mini-open technique. A 2-cm longitudinal incision is centered over the proximal wrist crease along the ulnar edge of the common flexors. The interval between the flexor carpi ulnaris and common flexor tendons is then used. The common flexors are retracted radially, and the flexor carpi ulnaris and the ulnar nerve are retracted ulnarly. The joint space is identified with a spinal needle, and the capsule is again opened bluntly. Because there is no true safe zone for the volar ulnar portal, it requires a careful dissection and spread technique (Fig. 19-11).[17] This portal provides access for reduction of a distal radius fracture and a view of the dorsal articular surfaces and dorsal ligaments.

Distal Radioulnar Portals. The distal radioulnar joint (DRUJ) is difficult to examine, and arthroscopy is not frequently used in

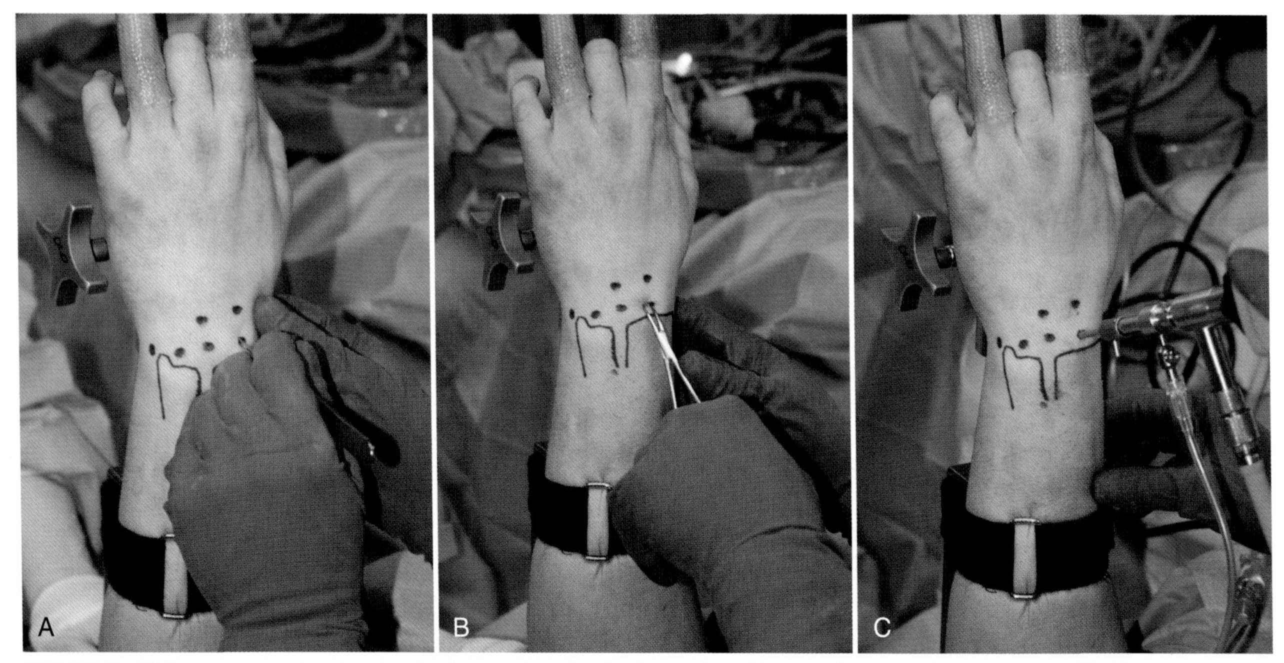

FIGURE 19-10 Box concept using dorsal and volar portals as the viewing and working portals to encircle the wrist. *(Modified from Bain GI, Munt J, Turner PC. New advances in wrist arthroscopy.* Arthroscopy. *2008:24:355-367.)*

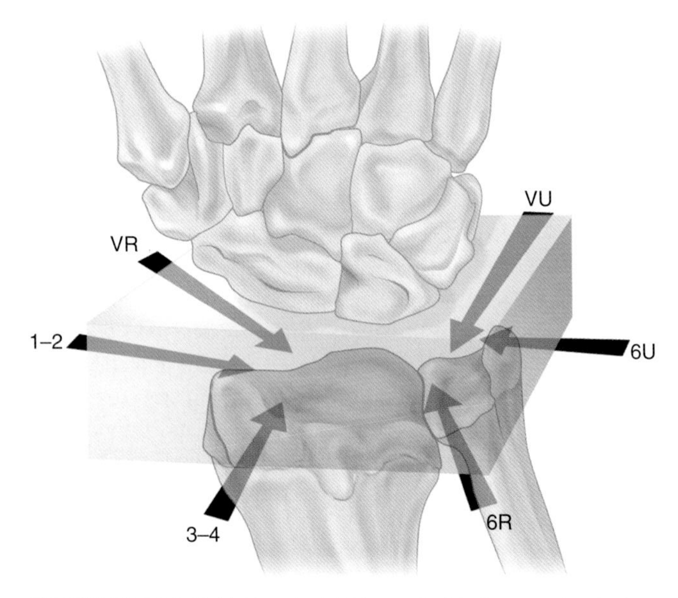

FIGURE 19-11 A-C, Making the initial portal with the spread technique and placement of the arthroscope.

these cases. The proximal and distal DRUJ portals are named according to their location proximal or distal to the ulnar head. The DRUJ portals are bordered radially by the EDC and ulnarly by the ECU. The joint is entered from at the base of the DRUJ, bordered by the radius and ulna. The proximal portal is placed in this line just proximal to the DRUJ. The forearm is supinated to relax the dorsal capsule, and the arthroscope is then introduced between the radius and ulna underneath the TFCC and proximal to the articular surface. The radioulnar articular surfaces can then be seen. Pronation and supination increase the available surface area during examination.

The distal portal is not always accessible. Use of this portal allows the surgeon to examine the distal articular surface of the ulna and the undersurface of the TFCC. The DRUJ portal uses a mini-open approach. It is located just proximal to the TFCC, and care must be taken to stay below the TFCC to prevent injury to this structure. There is some risk to the posterior interosseous nerve.[8] There is minimal risk to sensory nerves, with the closest 17.5 mm distally.[11]

Neurovascular Structure Risk

Because of the absence of major neurovascular structures, most wrist arthroscopy uses the dorsum of the wrist. Only the deep branch of the radial artery and the superficial dorsal sensory branches of the radial, ulnar, and lateral antebrachial cutaneous nerves are located on the dorsal side of the wrist.[8] Injury to these structures can cause numbness and, at worst, a painful neuroma and complex regional pain syndrome. Certain portals have an increased risk of iatrogenic neurovascular injury. The greatest risk to the radial artery and dorsal radial and ulnar sensory nerve branches occur with the 1-2, 6R, and 6-U portals. The midcarpal, 3-4, 4-5, and distal radioulnar joint portals are relatively safe.

Risk does exists even in safe portals because aberrant sensory nerve branches can be dangerously close.[11] This usually necessitates incisions that are longitudinal and are made by pulling only the skin over a blade and bluntly spreading through the subcutaneous tissue. When piercing the capsule, only a blunt trocar should be used. This technique helps protect structures between the dermis and capsule from injury.[11]

Diagnostic Arthroscopy

The details of the diagnostic arthroscopy are covered in a later chapter, but we include some thoughts about evaluating the wrist. To perform an adequate diagnostic arthroscopy requires familiarity with the normal-appearing structures. This includes the ability to differentiate normal from pathologic structures. The appearance of the normal, white, smooth articular cartilage must be differentiated from the more yellow fibrocartilage.

The surgeon should be able to identify cracked and fibrillated tissue and eburnated bone. Ligaments should have a white or yellow appearance and should be taut when probed, especially under traction. Pathologic ligaments may become attenuated with fraying due to injury or degeneration. Inflammation may cause the synovium to become hypertrophic and reddish. A discolored or brown tinge to synovial fluid likely represents a pathologic problem. Joints should be congruous without step-offs, and ligaments should be tight without the ability to pass a probe from the radiocarpal joint.[12]

Dry Wrist Arthroscopy

A newer technique that uses wrist arthroscopy without irrigation has been tried. Proponents claim that there are benefits to arthroscopy without water, including limiting loss of vision and compartment syndrome. Another possible advantage is the ability to do open procedures without soft tissue infiltration. The investigators also suggest the possibility of less pain and swelling after surgery.[18] No prospective studies have evaluated these reported benefits, and this technique is still in its early stages.

Postoperative Management

For débridement and resection procedures, a compressive wrap is used in the postoperative phase. Range of motion is started immediately, and exercises are initiated 1 week postoperatively. If necessary, formal physical therapy is started 3 to 4 weeks postoperatively. Normal use is allowed as pain and strength dictate.

In repair procedures, we favor the use of a Muenster cast for approximately 6 weeks. The wrist is placed in slight dorsiflexion and neutral pronation or supination. This cast prevents pronation or supination of the forearm. Approximately 4 weeks postoperatively, a removable Muenster splint is used, and gentle range of motion is initiated. The splint is discontinued, and exercises begin 6 to 8 weeks postoperatively. Full recovery takes 3 to 9 months.

COMPLICATIONS

Complications during and after wrist arthroscopy are rare. Most physicians report rates of less than 2%.[4,5] A study of 210 patients reported only two (0.9%) major complications and nine (4.3%) minor complications, all of which resolved with observation. The most common complication was dorsal ulnar sensory neuropraxia, and it was associated with open procedures.[19] Complications can be the result of traction and arm positioning or related to establishment of portals. They can be procedure-specific complications or general arthroscopic complications. Major complications include compartment syndrome, permanent nerve injury, postsurgical joint infection, vascular injury, complex regional pain syndrome, permanent stiffness, and tendon rupture.[19]

Most complications can be prevented if the risks are understood and simple precautions are used when performing the surgery. Large instrumentation within a small joint space predisposes to iatrogenic injuries to nerves, the radial artery, and extensor tendons. The EPL and EDQ are the tendons most at risk during wrist arthroscopy. Flexible nylon finger traps help prevent skin damage for patients with friable skin.[4] Using a spinal needle ensures an adequate pathway, and blunt trocars help to minimize risk to the articular surfaces.

Excessive extravasation of fluid may occur in recently injured patients with torn capsules or if the inflow cannula is placed extra-articularly. If extravasation occurs, the causative factor should be addressed, or the arthroscopic portion of the procedure should be stopped. Pressure diminishes quickly when the inflow is halted, and elevating the extremity is usually all that is necessary for correction. Physiologic solutions allow better fluid absorption in the soft tissues and further decrease the risk of extravasation.[7] Whipple reports the risk of compartment syndromes is minimal to none because, even in the case of intra-articular fractures, extravasated fluid is rapidly absorbed by clysis and does not increase compartment pressures long enough to compromise circulation. Caution is advised if pressure pumps are used.[20]

Postoperative infection is uncommon. If there is any evidence of superficial infection, oral antibiotics are usually sufficient. If a deep intra-articular infection develops, irrigation, arthroscopic débridement, and intravenous antibiotic therapy are usually required.[21]

PEARLS & PITFALLS

- Use only soft finger traps. If skin quality is poor, minimize traction, and limit the duration of the procedure.
- To protect neurovascular structures, incise only the dermis by pulling the skin against a scalpel; bluntly spread tissues before cannula placement; use care with all portals, but use extreme caution with high-risk portals; and pace the 1-2 portal in the most dorsal portion of the snuff box to protect the radial artery.
- To protect the articular surfaces, know the precise portal location and anatomy, localize the joint space with a spinal needle before establishing a portal, insert with the angle of radial inclination and volar tilt, and use only blunt instruments and cannulas.
- Visualize the work area. Use volar and dorsal portals to see the area required, maintain a clear visual field, and prevent or remove bubbles.
- Probe articular surfaces, ligaments, and the TFCC for tears and pathology.
- Evaluate the midcarpal joint space.
- Prevent fluid extravasation. Use adequate outflow, and use gravity inflow if possible.

CONCLUSIONS

Wrist arthroscopy provides an accurate supplement to a complete wrist examination. Although once used as a tool for diagnosis only, this is no longer the case. As technology advances, arthroscopy can be used in more complicated cases, and our ability to master new and advanced procedures will continue to improve. Although simple to learn and relatively easy to master, arthroscopy requires a thorough understanding of surgical principles and anatomy to perform procedures successfully. With adherence to standard precautions, wrist arthroscopy will continue to prove beneficial in the management of disorders of the wrist.

REFERENCES

1. Chen YC. Arthroscopy of the wrist and finger joints. *Orthop Clin North Am*. 1979;10:723-733.
2. Whipple TL, Cooney WP 3rd, Osterman AL, Viegas SF. Wrist arthroscopy. *Instr Course Lect*. 1995;44:139-145.
3. Whipple TL, Marotta JJ, Powell JH 3rd. Techniques of wrist arthroscopy. *Arthroscopy*. 1986;2:244-252.
4. Bain GI, Munt J, Turner PC. New advances in wrist arthroscopy. *Arthroscopy*. 2008;24:355-367.
5. Haisman JM, Matthew B, Scott W. Wrist arthroscopy: standard portals and arthroscopic anatomy. *J Am Soc Surg Hand*. 2005;5:175-181.
6. Berger RA. Arthroscopic anatomy of the wrist and distal radioulnar joint. *Hand Clin*. 1999;15:393-413, vii.
7. Geissler WB, Freeland AE, Weiss AP, Chow JC. Techniques of wrist arthroscopy. *Instr Course Lect*. 2000;49:225-237.
8. Gupta R, Bozentka DJ, Osterman AL. Wrist arthroscopy: principles and clinical applications. *J Am Acad Orthop Surg*. 2001;9:200-209.
9. Jones WA, Lovell ME. The role of arthroscopy in the investigation of wrist disorders. *J Hand Surg Br*. 1996;21:442-445.
10. Maizlin ZV, Brown JA, Clement JJ, et al. MR arthrography of the wrist: controversies and concepts. *Hand (N Y)*. 2009;4:66-73.
11. Abrams RA, Petersen M, Botte MJ. Arthroscopic portals of the wrist: an anatomic study. *J Hand Surg Am*. 1994;19:940-944.
12. Bettinger PC, Cooney WP 3rd, Berger RA. Arthroscopic anatomy of the wrist. *Orthop Clin North Am*. 1995;26:707-719.
13. Hofmeister EP, Dao KD, Glowacki KA, Shin AY. The role of midcarpal arthroscopy in the diagnosis of disorders of the wrist. *J Hand Surg Am*. 2001;26:407-414.
14. Carro LP, Golano P, Farinas O, et al. The radial portal for scaphotrapeziotrapezoid arthroscopy. *Arthroscopy*. 2003;19:547-553.
15. Abe Y, Doi K, Hattori Y, et al. A benefit of the volar approach for wrist arthroscopy. *Arthroscopy*. 2003;19:440-445.
16. Slutsky DJ. Wrist arthroscopy through a volar radial portal. *Arthroscopy*. 2002;18:624-630.
17. Slutsky DJ, Nagle DJ. Wrist arthroscopy: current concepts. *J Hand Surg Am*. 2008;33:1228-1244.
18. del Pinal F, Garcia-Bernal FJ, Pisani D, et al. Dry arthroscopy of the wrist: surgical technique. *J Hand Surg Am*. 2007;32:119-123.
19. Beredjiklian PK, Bozentka DJ, Leung YL, Monaghan BA. Complications of wrist arthroscopy. *J Hand Surg Am*. 2004;29:406-411.
20. Whipple TL. Precautions for arthroscopy of the wrist. *Arthroscopy*. 1990;6:3-4.
21. Botte MJ, Cooney WP, Linscheid RL. Arthroscopy of the wrist: anatomy and technique. *J Hand Surg Am*. 1989;14:313-316.

CHAPTER

20

Diagnostic Wrist Arthroscopy

Robert Dews • Larry D. Field

During the past 20 years, wrist arthroscopy has evolved into one of the most reliable and productive means of diagnosing, qualifying, and treating wrist pathology. As the arthroscopic surgeon's instrumentation and technical ability improves, wrist arthroscopy is increasingly being presented as a necessary, routine, and safe procedure.[1] Although it is a relatively new modality, it is an easily learned skill with ever-increasing indications.

An arthroscopic view allows excellent access to the articular surfaces of the carpal bones and ligaments that is not possible with arthrotomy.[2] However, a thorough knowledge of wrist anatomy is essential for the safe arthroscopic identification and treatment of wrist pathology. This chapter emphasizes the standard elements of a diagnostic arthroscopic evaluation of the wrist.

ANATOMY

The standard portals for wrist arthroscopy are located on the dorsum of the wrist, primarily because of the lack of neurovascular structures at risk in this area. The dorsal portals are named by their location in relation to the six dorsal compartments of the wrist. The 1-2 portal lies between the first extensor compartment, which includes the extensor pollicis brevis (EPB) and the abductor pollicis longus (APL), and the second dorsal compartment, which contains the extensor carpi radialis brevis (ECRB) and longus (ECRL). The 3-4 portal, which is the primary viewing portal, is located between the third dorsal compartment, which contains the extensor pollicis longus (EPL) tendon, and the fourth dorsal compartment, which contains the extensor digitorum communis (EDC) tendon. The bony landmark for this portal is Lister's tubercle, which is approximately 1 cm proximal to the wrist joint. The 4-5 portal is located between the EDC and the extensor digiti minimi (EDM). The 6-R portal lies on the radial side of the extensor carpi ulnaris (ECU) tendon, and the 6-U portal is located on the ulnar side of the ECU.

Two primary portals and two accessory portals have been described for use in the midcarpal space. The portal most commonly used for viewing is the radial midcarpal (RMC), which is located approximately 1 cm distal to the 3-4 radiocarpal portal and in line with the third metacarpal. The ulnar midcarpal portal is located on the midaxial line of the fourth metacarpal, approximately 1 to 1.5 cm distal to the 4-5 portal, enters the joint at the four-corner intersection between the lunate, triquetrum, hamate, and capitate. One of the two accessory portals is on the radial side of the midcarpal space and enters the scaphotrapeziotrapezoid (STT) joint. It is located just ulnar to the EPL tendon, at the level of the articular surface on the distal pole of the scaphoid. Staying on the ulnar side of this tendon usually maintains a safe margin between the portal and the radial artery at this level. Another accessory portal can be used, entering the triquetrohamate joint just ulnar to the ECU tendon, for a probe or instrument to access the joint or proximal pole of the hamate.[3]

PATIENT EVALUATION

History and Physical Examination

A thorough history is essential. This should include the patient's medical and surgical history; medications; allergies; family history; trauma history, including duration of symptoms, location, intensity, and any aggravating or relieving factors; and the effects of various treatment modalities already used. Contact sports and noncontact sports with repetitive activity should be identified. The mechanism of injury should be fully detailed, and specifics such as position of the hand, direction of force, and resultant area of pain should be kept in mind during the diagnostic evaluation.

The patient's age and sex should be considered when evaluating a painful wrist. The young patient (<40 years) is more prone to post-traumatic carpal injuries, whereas the older patient is more susceptible to the late effects of systemic and degenerative processes. The patient's medical history and the family medical history are helpful for diagnosing patients with many of the systemic and hereditary disorders that can manifest in the wrist. Laboratory values combined with this history is often helpful in this situation. Knowledge of the effect of the wrist pain on the patient's daily activities, including work and leisure activities, is also essential for treatment planning.[4]

The physical examination begins with a careful inspection for specific areas of swelling, erythema, warmth, nodules, skin lesions, and obvious deformities or prior surgical incisions. If possible, tenderness is localized to a specific anatomic structure. Wrist range of motion should be examined, paying careful attention to any snapping or clicking. Clicks, which may indicate carpal instability, can sometimes be felt throughout the wrist range of motion but are usually not significant unless they reproduce the patient's clinical symptoms.

A systematic approach is essential for palpation of the wrist. All joints must be palpated and appropriately stressed with the use of some of the many provocative tests that have been described. Radially, carpometacarpal thumb arthritis can be assessed with the grind test. Just proximal to this, the STT joint should be palpated to assess for arthritis. Anatomic snuff box tenderness may indicate scaphoid or scapholunate ligament pathology. This ligament can be further assessed by Watson's scaphoid shift test.[5] The distal pole of the scaphoid is stabilized to restrict palmer flexion while the wrist is moved from ulnar to radial deviation. Dorsal wrist pain indicates subluxation of the scaphoid and scapholunate ligament instability. Ulnarly, lunotriquetral instability can be assessed by manipulating the two bones relative to each other (i.e., shear or ballottement test). Ulnocarpal abutment and triangular fibrocartilage complex (TFCC) tears are tested by axial loading and ulnar wrist deviation. Pain just distal to the ulnar styloid and reproduction of symptoms with this maneuver indicate these conditions.

Instability of the midcarpal joint is suggested by the catch-up clunk, which is produced when the wrist is moved from radial to ulnar deviation during axial loading. The clunk is produced by sudden change in position of the proximal carpal row from a flexed position to an extended position as the triquetrum engages the hamate without the synchronizing effect of the attenuated ulnar ligaments. A painful response or crepitation on compressing the distal radioulnar joint (DRUJ) suggests instability or arthritic changes of the joint. Volarly, tenderness with palpation of the pisiform or hook of the hamate may represent pisotriquetral arthritis or hamate fracture, respectively.[6]

To complete the wrist examination, the tendons are palpated and stressed to rule out tenosynovitis on the dorsal and volar aspects. The nerves are evaluated to rule out compressive neuropathies, and the vascular status is assessed by evaluating capillary refill along with Allen's test to rule out insufficiency or thrombosis.

Diagnostic Imaging

Unless otherwise indicated by clinical evaluation, the initial radiographic evaluation should consist of standard posteroanterior, oblique, and lateral views of the wrist. They should be examined for bony disruptions such as fractures, alignment and congruence of joint spaces, and evidence of arthritic changes and mineralization. The lateral view is important for assessment of the carpal alignment. A scapholunate angle of greater than 60 degrees suggests possible scapholunate instability, and an angle of less than 30 degrees suggests ulnar-sided wrist instability. Additional radiographs may be needed depending on the clinical scenario. The clenched fist view is valuable for better visualization of possible scapholunate dissociation, and a carpal tunnel view can better elucidate the bony tubercles of the carpal tunnel.

Musculoskeletal ultrasound may be useful for the evaluation of soft tissue abnormalities, such as tendinopathy, ganglia, and synovial cysts. However, it is highly operator dependent.

Arthrography is useful to evaluate the integrity of capsular structures and interosseous ligaments, especially the scapholunate, lunotriquetral, and triangular fibrocartilage (TFC).[2] It may show localized synovitis or abnormal leaks between normally compartmentalized spaces.

Computed tomography (CT) is useful to evaluate osseous and articular morphology. It is most effective in the evaluation of bone healing in the carpus after fracture or surgery, and CT can provide images in any plane needed (e.g., oblique axis of the scaphoid). Likewise, because fractures of the hook of the hamate are difficult to visualize with plain radiographs, CT provides clear detail to assist with decision making and treatment.[6]

Magnetic resonance imaging (MRI) provides important information about the soft tissues of the wrist and the vascularity of the bones. Avascular necrosis of the carpal bones, such as the lunate and scaphoid, and occult ganglions, soft tissue tumors, tendonitis, and joint effusions are well visualized using MRI. It is also the most accurate modality for evaluating bone bruises and microfractures. MRI has a sensitivity of 90% in evaluating the integrity of the TFCC. The accuracy of MRI for identifying tears of the scapholunate ligament has also approached 90%, but it drops significantly to 50% for lunotriquetral tears.[6]

To evaluate the bony architecture and overall wrist alignment, we prefer the use of standard radiographs, usually with additional radiographic views based on clinical presentation. This is commonly followed by standard MRI to further evaluate the wrist for occult fractures, avascular necrosis, and soft tissue pathology.

TREATMENT

Indications and Contraindications

Wrist arthroscopy is a useful tool for diagnosis in patients who present with wrist pain, motion loss, and weakness, for which noninvasive diagnostic and treatment protocols have failed. It is also useful in patients with well-defined pathology such as nonunions, Kienbock's disease, and scapholunate or lunotriquetral dissociations, for which evaluation of the articular surfaces is of prognostic and therapeutic importance.

Many forms of wrist pathology, such as cartilage flaps or tears of the (TFC), can be treated during arthroscopy.[1] Wrist arthroscopy is a useful adjunct in the reduction of intra-articular fractures of the distal radius and percutaneous pinning of scaphoid fractures. Innovative surgeons have described partial carpal resections for posttraumatic arthritis and arthroscopically guided capitolunate fusions. Using the midcarpal, DRUJ, and volar portals has further expanded the arthroscope's use as a tool for evaluation and treatment of midcarpal chondral lesions of the hamate, articular damage to the ulnar head or surrounding synovitis, and improved visualization of volar articular surfaces and dorsal capsular structures.[7]

Contraindications to wrist arthroscopy are limited mainly to conditions of trauma or swelling that distorts the normal anatomy or significantly damages capsular integrity, leading to fluid extravasation.

Conservative Management

Before operative management, nonoperative measures should be exhausted. Depending on the pathology, temporarily immobilizing the wrist in a splint or brace and administering anti-inflammatory medication may be the only treatment necessary. Diagnostic and therapeutic injections can be helpful. A small amount of local anesthetic may confirm the source of pain and provide relief for the patient. A structured therapy regimen for wrist range of motion and strengthening may help in treating certain types of wrist pathology.

Arthroscopic Technique

Regional or general anesthesia may be used. The patient is positioned supine, with the operative extremity on an arm table. A tourniquet is placed proximally on the upper arm. A 2.5- or 3-mm, 30-degree arthroscope; small joint arthroscopic instruments; and gravity flow are used for the procedure. The operating table is angled so that the surgeon is positioned above the arm table and near the patient's head, and the assistant is positioned directly across the arm table within the patient's axilla.

After preparing and draping, the arm is exsanguinated before inflation of the tourniquet and placed in position in the traction tower. We prefer a sterile traction tower with nylon finger traps to provide convenient application of wrist distraction in flexion, extension, and radial and ulnar deviation. We use soft nylon finger traps to secure the index and long finger to the tower in a sterile fashion for most procedures. However, for ulnar-sided pathology, we frequently use the index and ring fingers. Five to ten pounds of traction is adequate for most procedures.

Radiocarpal Evaluation

Diagnostic wrist arthroscopy begins with the 3-4 portal and is the primary viewing portal. Palpation and spinal needle localization of this portal are essential before the skin incision is made. Through the 3-4 portal, a needle is inserted, and the joint is distended with 5 to 7 mL of saline. The skin is incised with a no. 15 or 11 blade, and a small hemostat is used spread the soft tissues. Next, the blunt trocar should be inserted at approximately a 20-degree proximal angle to match the distal radius articular slope. This angle can avoid damaging the dorsal articular surface.[2,8,9] Only blunt trocars are used in establishing portals. The inflow and outflow are interchangeable and can be maintained through the arthroscopic cannula or a separate 6-U portal established under direct arthroscopic visualization. We prefer the inflow through the arthroscope to push debris away instead of pulling it toward the camera. After a 3-4 portal is established, a diagnostic radiocarpal arthroscopy is performed.

The radial styloid and radial capsule are examined first. The scaphoid superiorly and the radial styloid inferiorly can be evaluated for signs of arthritic change or articular injury (Fig. 20-1). The proximal border of the radial facet is examined, as are the volar extrinsic ligaments, the radioscaphocapitate ligament, and long radiolunate ligament (Fig. 20-2). The long radiolunate ligament is a wide structure usually two to three times the width of the radioscaphocapitate ligament.[9,10]

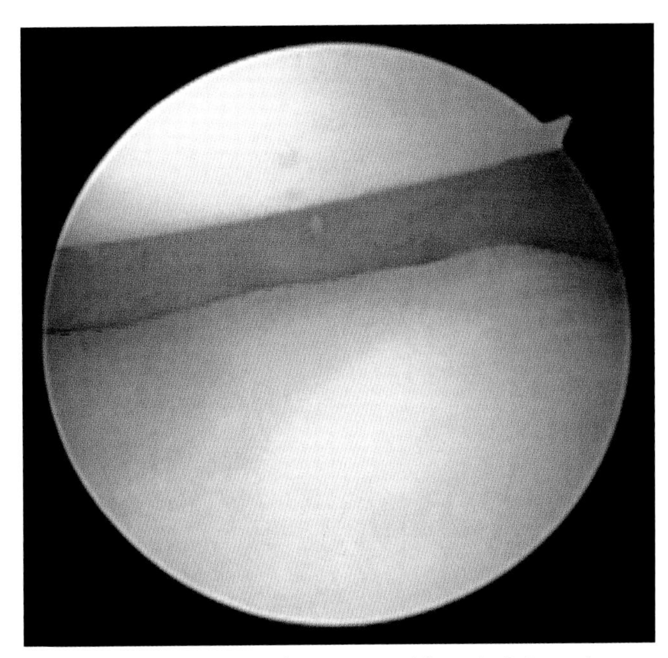

FIGURE 20-1 The radiocarpal joint is viewed from the 3-4 portal, showing the scaphoid superiorly and distal radius inferiorly.

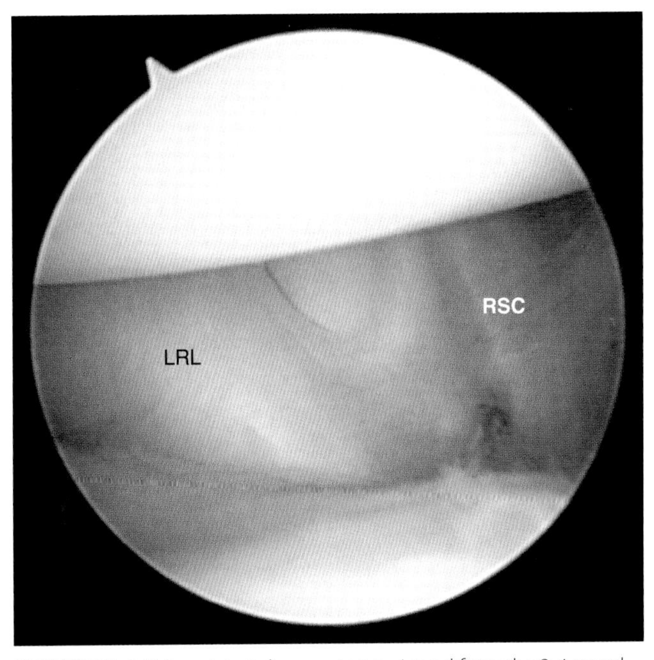

FIGURE 20-2 Volar extrinsic ligaments are viewed from the 3-4 portal, showing the radioscaphocapitate ligament (RSC) and the long radiolunate ligament (LRL).

The ligaments should be taut on probing because of the traction applied to the wrist. Ulnar to these is the radioscapholunate ligament, also called the ligament of Testut, which is a vascularized tuft of tissue without any significant structural integrity. This tuft marks the scapholunate interval and sagittal ridge.[10-12] Blood vessels are frequently seen along this ligament, and there is a natural redundancy to this ligament that should not be mistaken for a tear.

Following the scaphoid ulnarly, the slightly concave scapholunate interosseous ligament can be examined for tears or scapho-

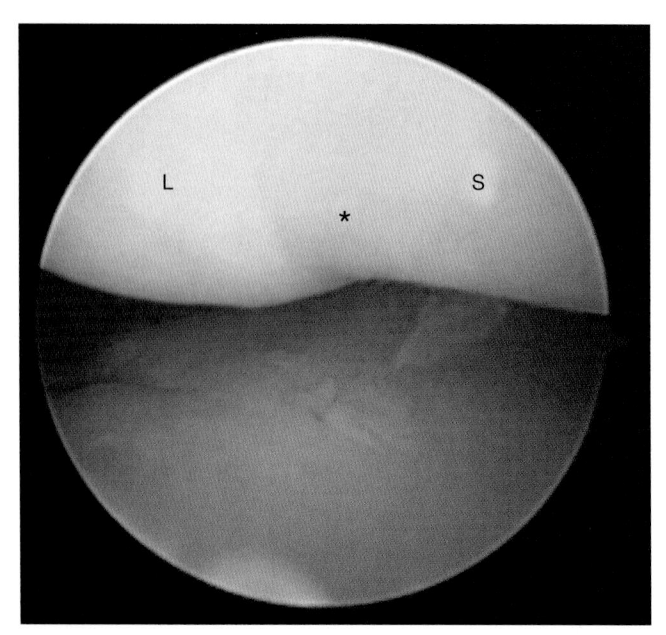

FIGURE 20-3 The convexity of the scapholunate interosseous ligament (asterisk), scaphoid (S), and lunate (L) can be seen.

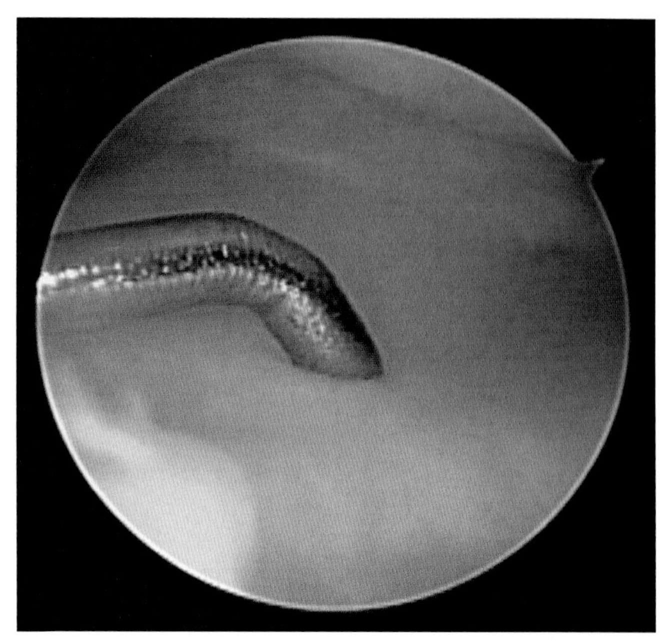

FIGURE 20-4 For the trampoline test, a probe is used to test the tension of the triangular fibrocartilage.

lunate diastasis (Fig. 20-3). An intact ligament may not be immediately obvious because it mimics the appearance of cartilage. Complete injury to this ligament, however, allows the arthroscope to pass between the scaphoid and the lunate (i.e., drive-through sign).[2]

The proximal surface of the lunate and the distal surface of the radius can be evaluated next. The two fossae of the distal radius, the scaphoid and the lunate fossae, are separated by a sagittal ridge. Fraying or fissuring of this area, suggestive of chondromalacia, should be documented. Normally, in the neutral wrist position, one half of the lunate articulates with the lunate facet, and one half articulates with the TFC.[10]

The radial attachment of the TFC is evaluated, as are the volar and dorsal radioulnar ligaments. The lunotriquetral interosseous ligament is evaluated by identifying a sulcus or concavity in the otherwise convex articular surfaces of the lunate and triquetrum.[13] A probe can be inserted through the 4-5 or 6-R portal to evaluate the integrity of the lunotriquetral ligament. Next, the peripheral attachment of the TFC and the ulnar prestyloid recess should be examined. The TFC is wedge shaped in the coronal plane, with a thickened periphery and a thin radial attachment.[12] A probe can be used to evaluate the tension of the TFCC by ballottement (i.e., trampoline test) (Fig. 20-4).[11,13] The TFC, also known as the articular disk, should be taut, and lack of tension raises suspicion of a central or peripheral TFCC tear. The peripheral 15% to 20% of the TFCC is vascularized and therefore has healing potential if torn.[2] The prestyloid ulnar recess is a normal anatomic finding that is approximately 3 to 4 mm wide, and it should not be mistaken for a peripheral tear.[10] The ulnolunate and ulnotriquetral ligaments may be more easily evaluated by placing the arthroscope in the 4-5 or 6-R portal. These ligaments are identified as capsular thickenings in the volar aspect of the ulnar capsule.

Midcarpal Evaluation

After a complete examination of the radiocarpal joint has been performed, the arthroscope can be used to evaluate the midcarpal space. The radial midcarpal portal, located approximately 1 cm distal to the 3-4 radiocarpal portal, is typically used to establish a diagnostic arthroscopy portal. The midcarpal joint can be distended with 3 to 5 mL of fluid through any of the portals. This allows easier access into the joint with a blunt trocar and minimizes the risk of damaging the articular cartilage.[10] Normally, there is no communication between the radiocarpal and midcarpal spaces.[3]

Care must be taken when entering the radial midcarpal space, because it is less than one half of the depth of the radiocarpal space.[2] The ulnar midcarpal portal is created for instrumentation and visualization of the ulnar portion of the midcarpal joint. The arthroscopic evaluation in this area begins with visualization of the convexity of the capitate (superiorly) and the scapholunate joint (inferiorly). The scapholunate joint should be perfectly congruous (Fig. 20-5). The scapholunate ligament is not present on the distal edge of the scapholunate joint, and the joint is best viewed from this perspective. Intraoperatively, the stability of the joint may be assessed by performing Watson's scaphoid shift test.[3,14]

The distal surfaces of the lunate and the triquetrum are then evaluated, as is the concave proximal surface of the hamate (Fig. 20-6). The lunotriquetral joint is also well visualized from this view, and a ballottement test can be performed to assess stability. Within the distal row, the capitate and capitohamate articulation can be examined from this portal. Farther ulnarly, the triquetrohamate joint may be used to establish an accessory portal. The triquetrohamate joint is a saddle-shaped joint that is normally quite tight and difficult to view across unless pathologic laxity exists.[3]

The STT joint can be seen by passing the arthroscope radially, and early osteoarthritic changes, common in this area, should be identified.[15] In the STT joint, the trapezoid is in the foreground,

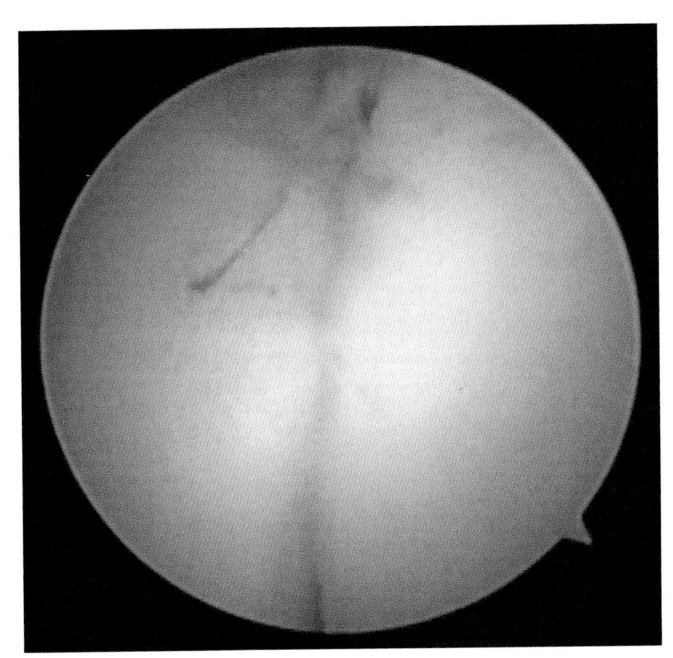

FIGURE 20-5 The congruent scapholunate joint is viewed from the radial midcarpal portal.

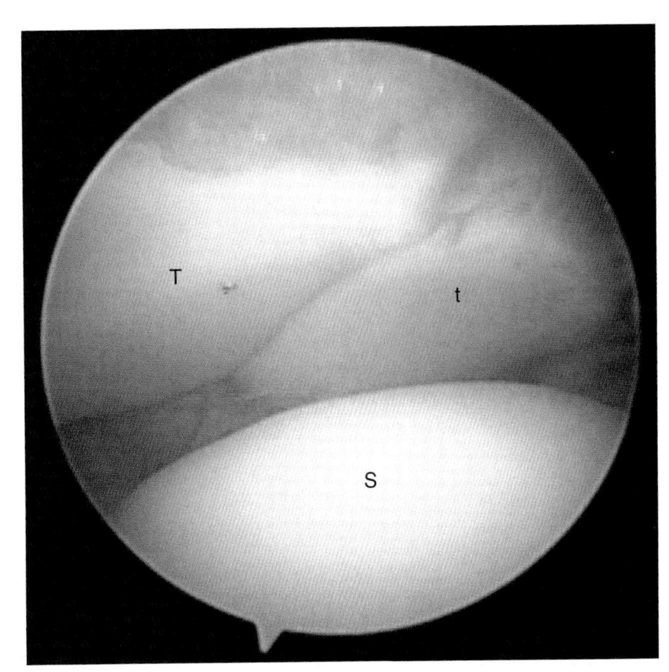

FIGURE 20-7 The scaphotrapeziotrapezoid joint, including the scaphoid (S), trapezoid (T), and trapezium (t), is viewed from the radial midcarpal portal.

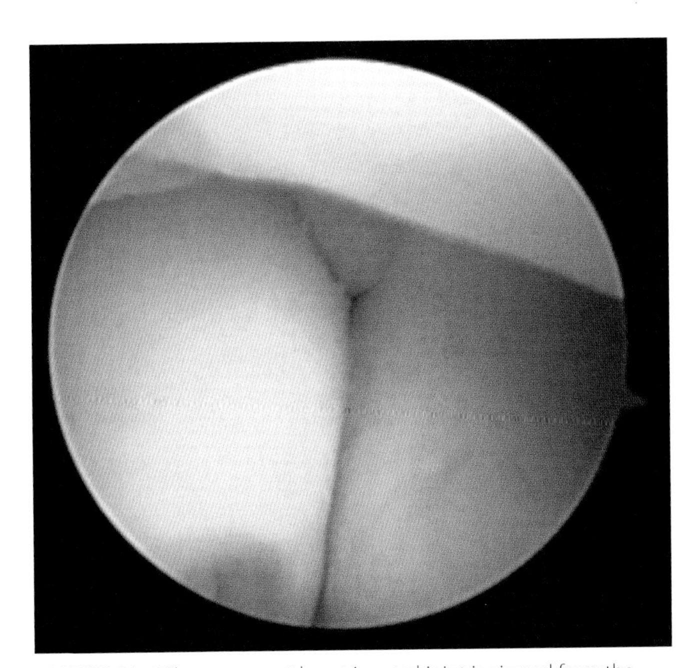

FIGURE 20-6 The congruent lunotriquetral joint is viewed from the radial midcarpal portal.

and the trapezium is in the background (Fig. 20-7). Bubbles frequently collect here and may impair visualization of the joint. These bubbles may be evacuated with a 21-guage needle, and débridement can be performed with a small, motorized shaver through an accessory STT portal.[3]

Distal Radioulnar Joint Evaluation

On completion of the diagnostic midcarpal arthroscopy, a proximal distal radial ulnar joint portal can be established, and the ulnar surface of the radius, the radial surface of the ulna, the distal surface of the ulnar head, and the proximal surface of the TFCC can be evaluated. DRUJ arthroscopy is performed with the forearm in supination and suspended in the wrist traction device but without any traction applied. A blunt trocar is angled slightly distal and placed in the joint. If required, outflow can be created by placing an 18-gauge needle into the distal portion of the joint. Through pronation and supination of the wrist, the articular margin of the ulna can be passed in front of the arthroscope lens. This approach is useful for lysis of adhesions, débridement, exostectomy, or capsulotomy of the DRUJ.[2,16]

PEARLS & PITFALLS

PEARLS

- After the initial skin incision, use a small, blunt hemostat to enter the joint capsule and spread the tissues.
- Angle the trocar to coincide with the radial tilt to avoid damage to the articular surface.
- Have an assistant maintain fluid flow through the joint with a finger pressure pump.
- Place the inflow on the camera to push debris away from the scope.

PITFALLS

- Draw portals and landmarks after applying traction to the wrist because anatomic structures may change.
- Avoid positioning the camera within the joint because the depth of the wrist is relatively small.
- Incise only the skin for portal placement, and use a hemostat to dissect through the soft tissue or risk iatrogenic injury to the superficial nerves and extensor tendons.

CONCLUSIONS

Arthroscopy of the wrist has become a commonly employed technique for the evaluation and treatment of intra-articular wrist disorders. It enables evaluation of the intercarpal structures under bright, magnified conditions with minimal morbidity compared with arthrotomy.[9] A systematic approach combined with a thorough knowledge of wrist anatomy allows the surgeon to optimize the probability of a successful outcome while minimizing the potential for complications of wrist arthroscopy.

REFERENCES

1. Sennwald G. Diagnostic arthroscopy: indications and interpretations of findings. *J Hand Surg Br*. 2001;26:241-246.
2. Geissler WB. *Wrist Arthroscopy*. New York, NY: Springer; 2005:1-13.
3. Viegas SF. Midcarpal arthroscopy; anatomy and portals. *Hand Clin*. 1994;10:577-587.
4. Brown DE, Lichtman DN. The evaluation of chronic wrist pain. *Orthop Clin North Am*. 1984;15:184.
5. Watson HK, Ashmead D IV, Makhlouf MV. Examination of the scaphoid. *J Hand Surg Am*. 1988;13:657-660.
6. Nagle DJ. Evaluation of chronic wrist pain. *J Am Acad Orthop Surg*. 2000;8:45-55.
7. Slutsky DJ. Wrist arthroscopy portals, volar and dorsal. In: Trumble TE, Budoff JE, eds. *Master Skills: Wrist and Elbow Arthroscopy Reconstruction*. Rosemont, IL: American Society of Surgery of the Hand; 2006:31-46.
8. Roth JH. Radiocarpal arthroscopy. *Orthopedics*. 1988;11:1309-1312.
9. Geissler WB, Freeland AE, Weiss AP, et al. Techniques in wrist arthroscopy. *J Bone Joint Surg Am*. 1999;81:1184-1197.
10. Bettinger PC, Cooney WP 3rd, Berger RA. Arthroscopic anatomy of the wrist. *Orthop Clin North Am*. 1995;26:707-719.
11. North ER, Thomas S. An anatomic guide for arthroscopic visualization of the wrist capsular ligaments. *J Hand Surg Am*. 1988;13:815-822.
12. Roth JH, Poehling GG, Whipple TL. Arthroscopic surgery of the wrist. *Instr Course Lect*. 1988;37:183-194.
13. Berger RA. Arthroscopic anatomy of the wrist and distal radioulnar joint. *Hand Clin*. 1999;15:393-413, vii.
14. Hofmeister EP, Dao KD, Glowacki KA. The role of midcarpal arthroscopy in the diagnosis of disorders of the wrist. *J Hand Surg Am*. 2001; 26:407-414.
15. Viegas SF. Advances in skeletal anatomy of the wrist [review]. *Hand Clin*. 2001;17:1-11, v.
16. Whipple TL, Cooney WP 3rd, Osterman AL, et al. Wrist arthroscopy. *Instr Course Lect*. 1995;44:139-145.

SECTION

F

Basic Procedures

CHAPTER

21

Injuries to the Triangular Fibrocartilage Complex

Kane Anderson • Thomas Trumble

In 1981, Palmer and Werner used the term *triangular fibrocartilage complex* (TFCC) to describe the set of related structures at the distal ulnar aspect of the wrist.[1] The TFCC physically separates the distal radioulnar joint (DRUJ) from the radiocarpal joint. The TFCC must be simultaneously robust and flexible. It must have the strength to transmit 20% of the load of the carpus to the ulna and to stabilize the DRUJ and ulnar carpus in conjunction with the bony architecture of the sigmoid notch. It is must also be supple enough to accommodate the significant, complex motion that occurs during forearm rotation. The motion of the DRUJ is a combination of approximately 150 degrees of rotation and sliding. This occurs because the radius of curvature is 50% larger on the radial side of the DRUJ (15 versus 10 mm) (Fig. 21-1A). The axis of rotation passes through the fovea of the ulnar head, which is a major attachment site for the TFCC.

The five structures that comprise the TFCC are the articular disk, the distal radioulnar ligaments (palmar and dorsal), the meniscal homologue, and the extensor carpi ulnaris (ECU) sub-

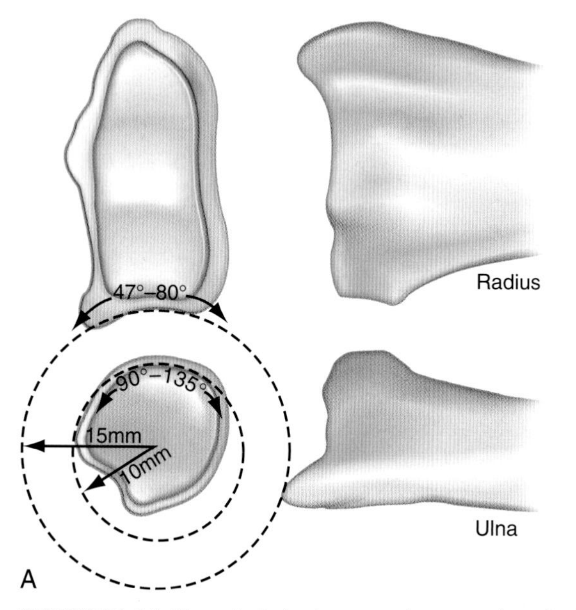

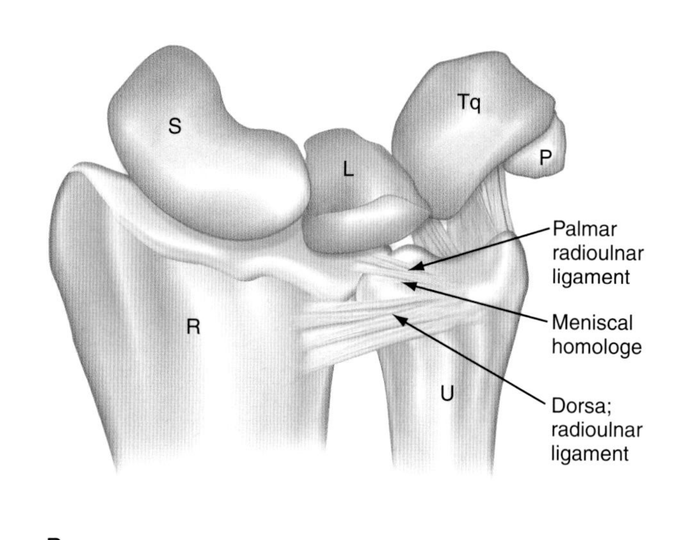

FIGURE 21-1 A, The articulation between the sigmoid notch of the radius and the ulnar head is viewed end-on *(left)* and dorsally *(right)*. The arc covered with articular cartilage is greater for the ulnar head than for the sigmoid notch, whereas the radius of curvature is greater for the sigmoid notch. This results in rotational and sliding motions during supination and pronation. **B,** The triangular fibrocartilage complex (TFCC) consists of the triangular fibrocartilage, meniscal homologue, extensor carpi ulnaris tendon sheath, and dorsal and palmar radioulnar ligaments. L, lunate; P, pisiform; R, radius; S, scaphoid; Tq, triquetrum; U, ulna; UL, ulnolunate ligament; UT, ulnotriquetral ligament. (**A,** *Modified from Chidgey LK. The distal radioulnar joint: problems and solutions.* J Am Acad Orthop Surg. *1995;3:95-109;* **B,** *Modified from Trumble TE. Distal radioulnar joint and triangular fibrocartilage complex. In: Trumble TE, ed.* Principles of Hand Surgery and Therapy. *Pennsylvania, PA: WB Saunders; 1999:128.)*

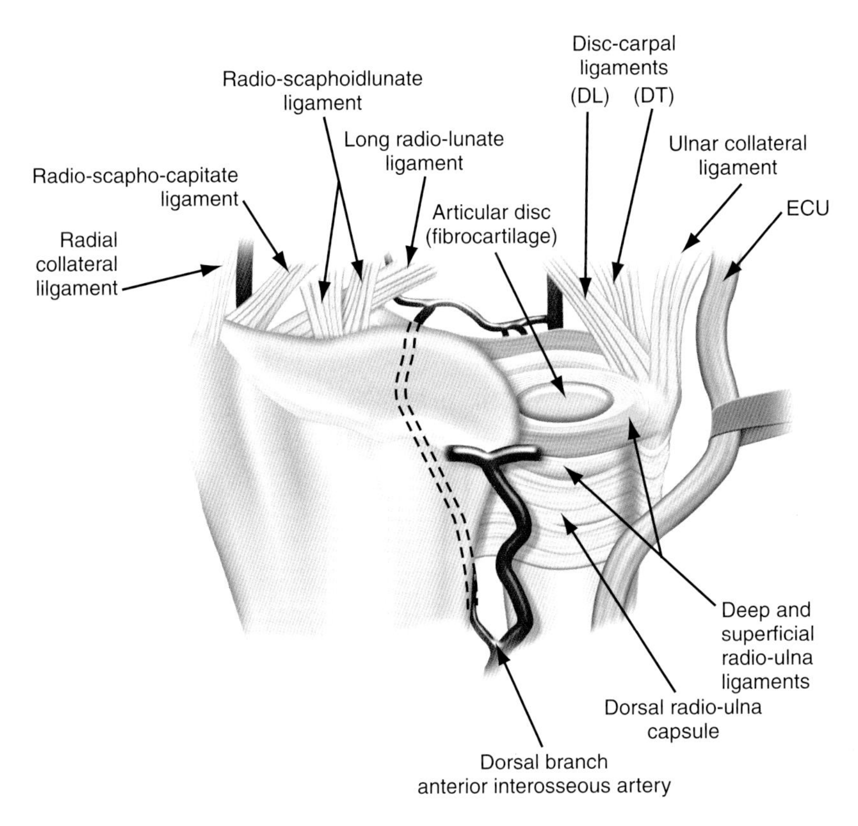

FIGURE 21-2 The prime intrinsic stabilizer of the distal radioulnar joint is the triangular fibrocartilage (TFC). The TFC complex consists of superficial *(green)* and deep *(blue)* radioulnar fibers, the two disk-carpal ligaments (disk-lunate and disk-triquetral), and the central articular disk *(white)*. The articular disk is responsible for transferring load from the medial carpus to the pole of the distal ulna. The vascularized, peripheral radioulnar ligaments *(green and blue)* are nourished by dorsal and palmar branches of the posterior interosseous artery and are responsible for guiding the radiocarpal unit around the seat of the ulna. *(Modified from Kleinman WB: Stability of the distal radioulna joint: biomechanics, pathophysiology, physical diagnosis, and restoration of function: what we have learned in 25 years.* J Hand Surg. *2007;32:1086-1106.)*

sheath, which is confluent with the (ulnocarpal collateral ligament (see Fig. 21-1B).[2] The central portion of the complex consists of an articular disk called the triangular fibrocartilage (TFC). The disk is composed predominately of type II collagen, which is consistent with its role in distributing compressive forces. It lies in the axial plane and structurally represents an extension of the articular surface of the distal radius. Dorsally and palmarly, the TFC is surrounded by the radioulnar ligaments, which are transverse bands that derive their broad origin from the sigmoid notch of the distal radius and insert on the base of the ulnar styloid. The ulnotriquetral and ulnolunate ligaments form the palmar border of the TFCC, and, although Palmer and Werner did not include them in their original description of the TFCC, they serve an important role in the stability of the ulnar side of the wrist.

The ulnar and dorsal edges of the complex consist of the ECU tendon subsheath and dorsal radial triquetral ligament, respectively. When viewed in the axial plane, these borders form a stout pyramid that attaches the TFCC to the ulnar side of the carpus. Stability of the TFCC is a prerequisite for smooth pronosupination and pain-free load bearing through the articular disk. The vestigial meniscal homologue derives from synovium. Its function is unclear, and it is often absent.

The blood supply of TFCC enters from the periphery (Fig. 21-2). Thiru and colleagues evaluated cadaveric specimens and identified three main branches of the TFCC.[3] The ulnar periphery of the TFCC has the richest blood supply and, consequently, the greatest potential for healing. It is fed predominantly via the dorsal and palmar radiocarpal branches of the ulnar artery. Dorsal and palmar branches of the anterior interosseous artery supply the more radial part of the complex.

CLASSIFICATION OF TRIANGULAR FIBROCARTILAGE COMPLEX INJURIES

Palmer's original classification divides injuries of the TFCC into degenerative and acute tears (Box 21-1).[4] The classification is anatomically subdivided into radial, central, and ulnar tears. This classification bears consideration, because the vascular anatomy dictates the healing potential and therefore the treatment and prognosis for TFCC tears, similarly to tears of the knee's meniscus.

Palmer class 1 injuries are acute, traumatic injuries. They are subdivided into four types, based on the site of injury (Fig. 21-3):

Type 1A lesions involve the central avascular portion; the rim is still attached to the radius. This lesion usually is not amenable to direct repair. Arthroscopic treatment is limited to débridement of the central tear to remove any flaps that may impede movement (Fig. 21-4).

Type 1B (ulnar-avulsion) lesions are peripheral tears that occur when the ulnar side of the TFCC complex is avulsed from its capsule; they can be associated with ulnar styloid fractures.

Type 1C (ulnar-distal) injuries involve ruptures along the volar attachment of the TFCC or distal ulnocarpal ligaments; they are variably amenable to repair.

Type 1D (radial-avulsion) injuries are rare injuries with tears from the radial attachment. These represent traumatic avulsions of the TFCC from the attachment at the sigmoid notch, with or without a fracture of the sigmoid notch (Fig. 21-5).

Degenerative TFCC lesions (Palmer class 2) all involve the central portion and are staged from A to E, depending on the

Box 21-1 Classification of Triangular Fibrocartilage Complex Injury

CLASS 1: TRAUMATIC	CLASS 2: DEGENERATIVE (ULNOCARPAL ABUTMENT SYNDROME)
A. Central perforation	**Stage**
B. Ulnar avulsion	A. TFCC wear
With distal ulnar fracture	B. TFCC wear
Without distal ulnar fracture	+ Lunate and/or ulnar chondromalacia
C. Distal avulsion	C. TFCC perforation
D. Radial avulsion	+ Lunate and/or ulnar chondromalacia
With sigmoid notch fracture	D. TFCC perforation
Without sigmoid notch fracture	+ Lunate and/or ulnar chondromalacia
	+ LT ligament perforation
	E. TFCC perforation
	+ Lunate and/or ulnar chondromalacia
	+ LT ligament perforation
	+ Ulnocarpal arthritis

LT, lunotriquetral; TFCC, triangular fibrocartilage complex.

From Palmer AK. Triangular fibrocartilage complex lesions: a classification. *J Hand Surg Am.* 1989;14:594.

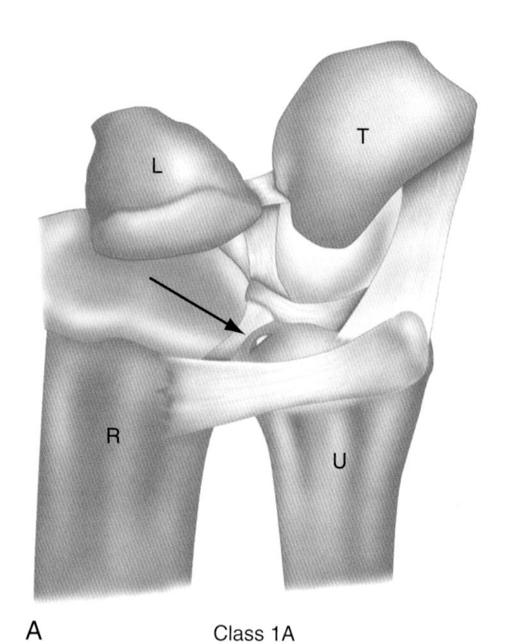

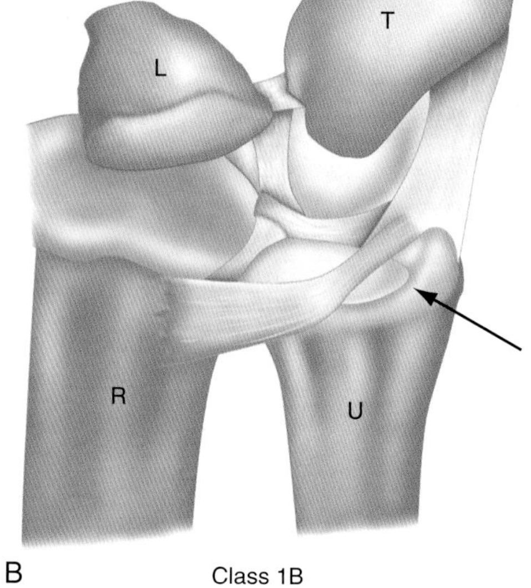

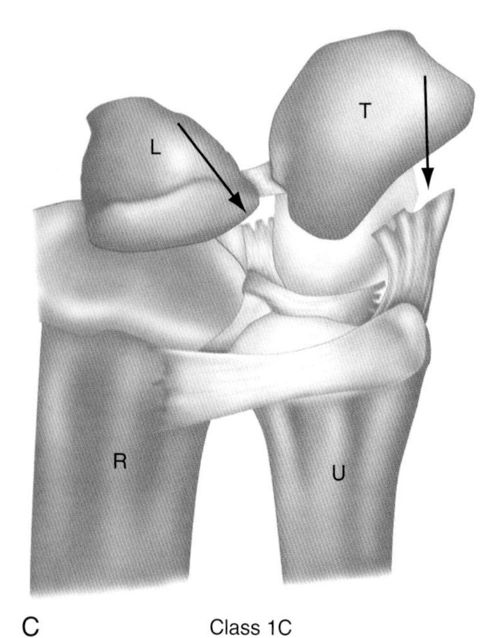

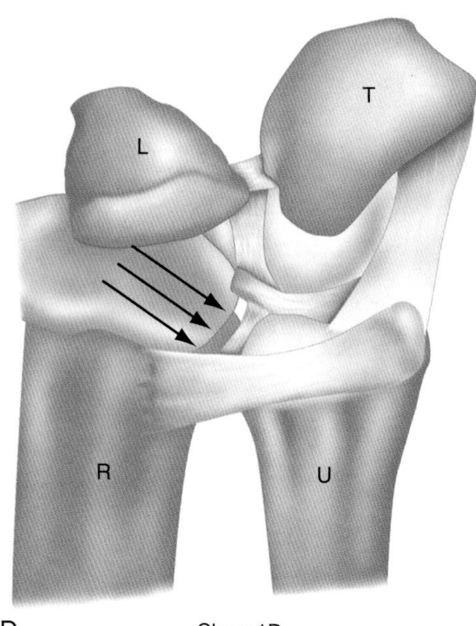

FIGURE 21-3 Four types of class 1 lesions of the triangular fibrocartilage complex. L, lunate; R, radius; T, triquetrum; U, ulna. *(Modified from Palmer AK. Triangular fibrocartilage complex lesions: a classification.* J Hand Surg Am. *1989;14:594-606.)*

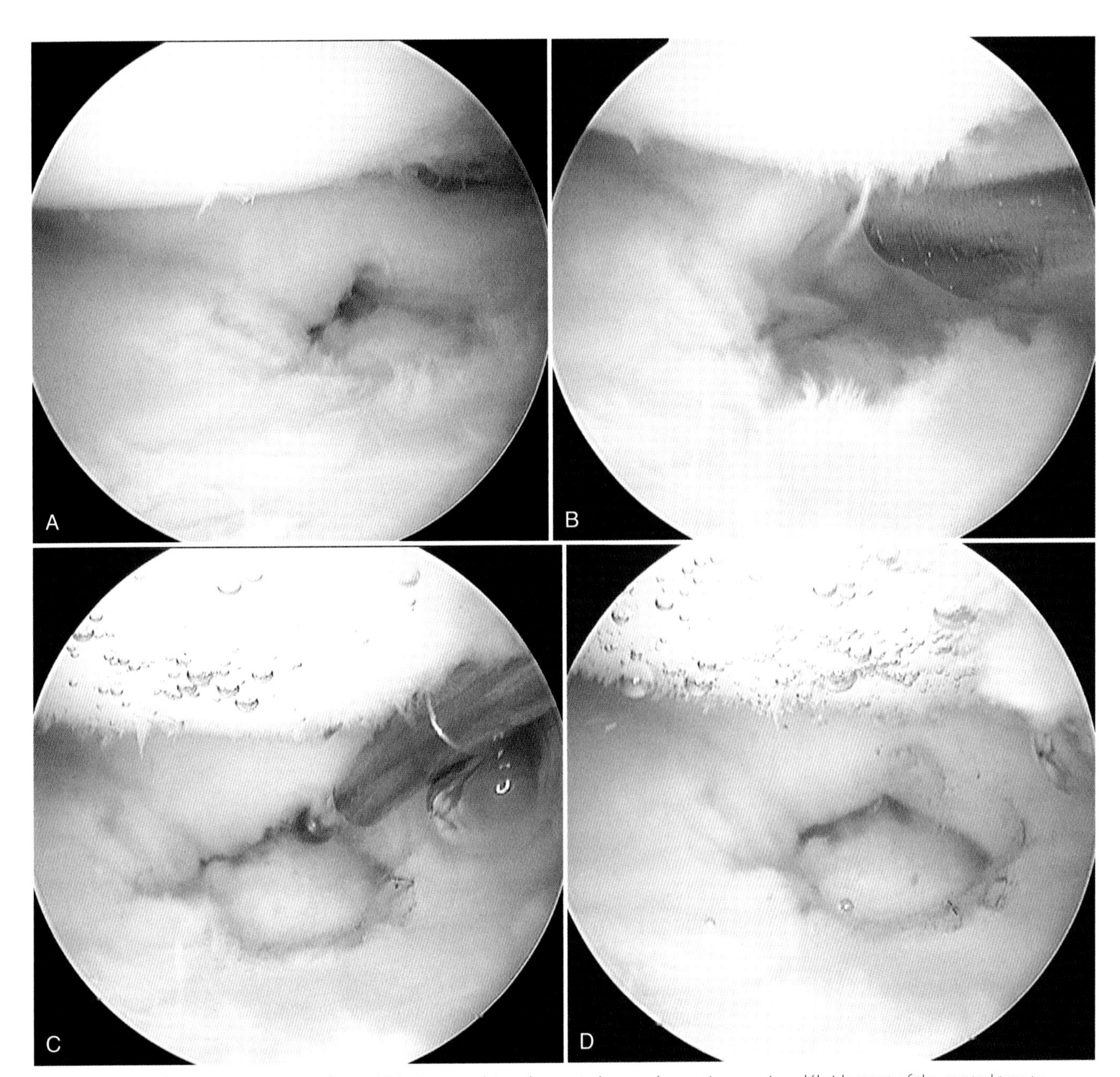

FIGURE 21-4 Arthroscopic treatment of type 1A lesions involving the central avascular portion requires débridement of the central tear to remove any flaps that may impede movement. **A,** Lesion in the central portion of the triangular fibrocartilage complex (TFCC). **B,** Central tear of the TFCC is débrided using a 2.5-mm arthroscopic shaver. **C,** Ablation at the edge of the lesion using a small joint radiofrequency probe. **D,** Smooth surface of the lesion after débridement.

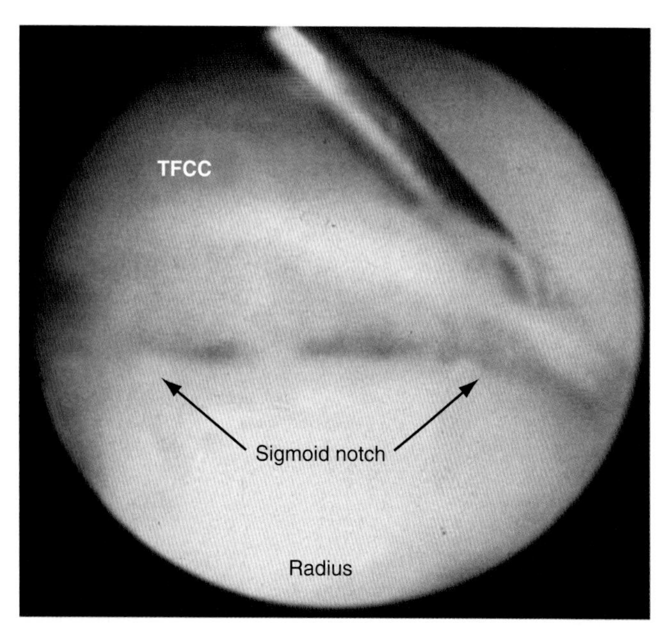

FIGURE 21-5 Arthroscopic image demonstrates an avulsion of the triangular fibrocartilage complex (TFCC) from the sigmoid notch of the distal radius (i.e., type 1D TFCC tear).

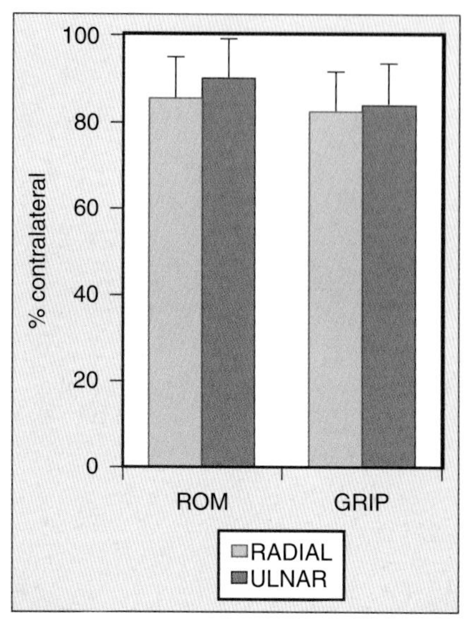

FIGURE 21-6 Arthroscopic repairs of acute triangular fibrocartilage complex tears have resulted in the return of 80% of the grip strength and range of motion of the contralateral uninjured wrist. *(Modified from Trumble TE, Gilbert M, Vedder N. Isolated tears of the triangular fibrocartilage: management by early arthroscopic repair.* J Hand Surg Am. *1997; 22:57-65.)*

presence or absence of a TFCC perforation, lunate and ulnar chondromalacia, a lunotriquetral ligament perforation, or degenerative radiocarpal arthritis. These degenerative lesions usually arise from ulnar abutment. Class 2 lesions usually are not amenable to surgical repair and are treated with débridement.

TFCC tears can be further subdivided by their acuteness. The chronicity has prognostic implications, and addressing tears in the acute phase usually provides better results.[5-7]

Acute tears (0 to 3 months): Arthroscopic repair of these injuries results in the recovery of 80% of grip strength and range of motion (ROM) compared with the contralateral side (Fig. 21-6). Trumble and associates showed that there was a significant relief of pain postoperatively. Postoperative ROM averaged 89% ± 9% SD of the contralateral side, and grip strength averaged 85% ± 20% SD of the contralateral side.[6]

Subacute tears (3 to 12 months): These tears are amenable to direct repair of the TFCC, but these patients usually regain less strength and ROM than those with acute injuries.

Chronic tears (>1 year): These tears are *reparable,* but, presumably because of contraction of the ligaments and degeneration of the torn fibrocartilage margins, outcomes lag behind those for acute or subacute tears. The treatment of chronic injuries frequently requires an ulnar shortening osteotomy, with or without TFCC débridement, to decrease load distribution to the distal ulna.[7,8]

The incidence of asymptomatic TFCC tears increases with age. Wright and coworkers, in a study of 62 wrists from cadavers of individuals whose average age at death was 78 years and found a tear of the TFCC in 33 wrists (11 lesions were central, and 21 were vertical radial).[9-11] Mikic observed an age-related correlation with disk perforation in his cadaveric study of 180 wrists from fetuses to the elderly. He found the prevalence of perforations to be zero among patients younger than 20 years; 7.6% among those in the third decade; 18.1% in the fourth decade; 40.0% in the fifth decade; 42.8% in the sixth decade, and 53.1% (26 wrists) among patients older than 60 years.[9] These degenerative changes correlated with magnetic resonance imaging (MRI) findings from healthy volunteers.[12] This illustrates the necessity of correlating imaging with history and examination findings in these patients.

PATIENT EVALUATION

History, Signs, and Symptoms

Ulnar-sided wrist pain has been referred to as the low back pain of the hand surgeon. The multitude of structures and diagnoses that can contribute to a patient's symptoms are often subtle and require precise physical examination and correlation with history and imaging. Causes of ulnar-sided wrist pain are listed in Box 21-2.

The typical history for an acute TFCC tear involves a fall on an outstretched hand. The literature is controversial regarding which ligaments are tightest in varying positions of forearm supination or pronation, but acute or delayed complaint of ulnar-sided wrist pain, often radiating dorsally and exacerbated by firm grasp and push-off (wrist extended, getting up from a table) is a characteristic features of the patient's history. Aching with repetitive supination and pronation tasks is also common. The pain is often characterized as diffuse, deep, and sometimes burning.

Chronic attritional injuries and degenerative changes of the ulnocarpal joint, including the TFCC, result from repetitive overloading. Ulnar deviation of the wrist, along with forearm supination and power grasp, increase the damage from axial loads. Pa-

Box 21-2 Common Causes of Ulnar-Sided Wrist Pain

Fractures and nonunions
- Sigmoid notch
- Ulnar head
- Ulnar styloid
- Hook of hamate
- Triquetrum
- Pisiform

TFCC tears
- Traumatic tears
- Degenerative lesions (ulnar impaction syndrome)

Luotriquetral interosseous ligament or meniscus homologue tears

DRUJ instability
- Acute Galeazzi fracture dislocation
- Acute or chronic Essex-Lopressti injury
- Chronic TFCC tear
- Distal radius malunion

ECU tendinopathy or subluxation

Arthritis
- DRUJ
- Pisotriquetral joint

DRUJ, distal radioulnar joint; ECU, extensor carpi ulnaris; TFCC, triangular fibrocartilage complex.

tients with acquired ulnar positive variance, discussed in greater detail later, are at higher risk for degenerative changes and recurrent injury from minor trauma.

A clicking sensation may be present with wrist pronation and supination. Patients may also complain of generalized weakness with and without wrist loading. Patients often delay treatment or are misdiagnosed as having a "wrist sprain" that fails to improve.

TFCC tears have been associated with distal radius fractures on imaging and direct arthroscopy. The incidence ranges between 13% and 60%.[13-17] The literature does not clearly indicate, in the absence of frank DRUJ instability, which tears should be fixed and by which methods, in part because it is unclear how many of these tears become symptomatic. It is likely that many of these tears are effectively treated by treatment of the concomitant fracture.[14] Nevertheless, several authors have endorsed the use of arthroscopy in the setting of distal radius fracture fixation to identify and treat concomitant soft tissue injuries. Varitimidis and associates reported that 60% of their patients with distal radius fracture had TFCC tears, half of which were ulnar sided.[17] All TFCC tears underwent débridement; 20% (2 of 12) had arthroscopic repair, and 1 patient required open repair. The arthroscopic group demonstrated improved ROM and Mayo wrist scores, compared with those treated with traditional external fixation. In 2003, Ruch and colleagues demonstrated good or excellent results with acute repair of the TFCC at the time of distal radius operative treatment in 56 patients, with only 2 patients with transient ulnar dorsal sensory irritation, but they lacked a control group.[18]

Lindau and coworkers reported that 10 of 11 patients with a documented complete peripheral TFCC tear associated with a distal radius fracture exhibited DRUJ instability at a 1-year follow-up examination, compared with 22% of those with no peripheral tear or only a partial tear.[19] This instability was correlated with worse clinical outcome.

Physical Examination

Patients with acute TFCC injuries frequently present with ulnar-sided wrist swelling that may reverse the normal convex shape of the ulnar wrist border. The soft, ballotable region between the ulnar styloid and the triquetrum can frequently be point tender (Fig. 21-7). Clicking can often be elicited with passive and active circumduction of the wrist. Specialized tests to distinguish TFCC injuries from other ulnar wrist injuries include the TFCC compression test, the ulnar impaction test, and the piano key test. Significant pain from axial loading of the TFCC, in conjunction with ulnar deviation, is a positive compression test. Similarly, pain with the combination of wrist hyperextension and the previous maneuvers indicates a positive ulnar impaction test.[20] Comparison of any dorsal-volar plane instability of the DRUJ with the normal contralateral side is the piano key test (Fig. 21-8). This should be performed in neutral position, in supination, and in pronation. The DRUJ typically has the most anteroposterior translation in the neutral position. Volar subluxation of the distal ulna with wrist supination can be appreciated by dimpling of the skin of the dorsal ulnar border (Fig. 21-9). Lunotriquetral ballottement tests ligament stability (Fig. 21-10). Pisotriquetral manipulation should be performed to rule out arthrosis of this joint.

Diagnostic Imaging

Acute or chronic ulnar-sided wrist pain warrants posteroanterior, lateral, and oblique radiographs of the wrist. True neutral rotation, posteroanterior radiographs are taken with the shoulder in 90 degrees of abduction and the elbow in 90 degrees of flexion. The ulnar styloid should be visible at the far ulnar portion of the distal ulna in a true posteroanterior view, in contradistinction to its location in the midportion of the distal ulna on radiographs taken in a supinated or pronated position. Others advocate the use of the pisiform's relationship to the scaphoid as a landmark, citing the variability of the position of the ulnar styloid. In a true

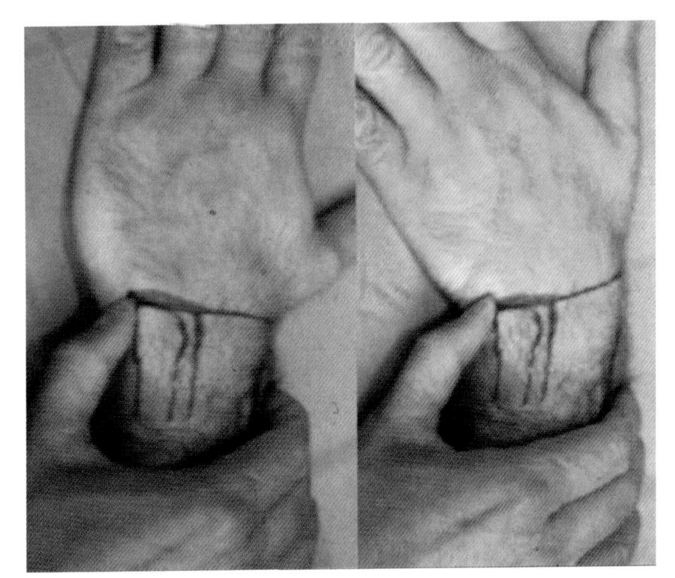

FIGURE 21-7 Tenderness elicited by direct pressure between the ulnar styloid and triquetrum is consistent with an injury to the triangular fibrocartilage complex.

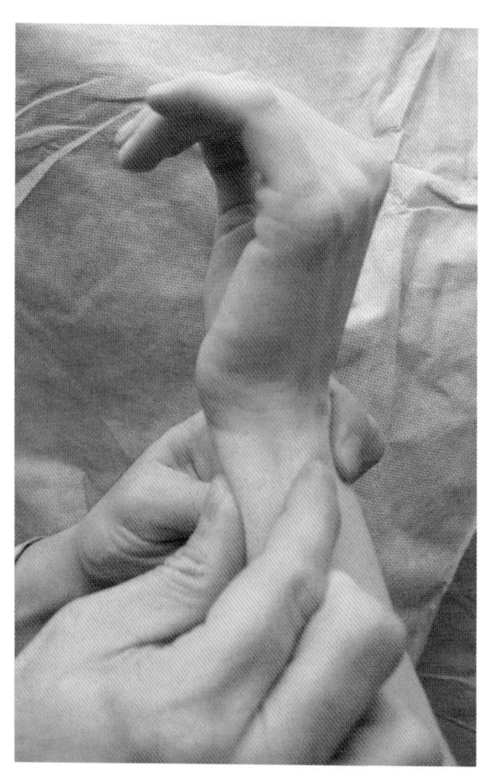

FIGURE 21-8 The piano key test evaluates distal radioulnar joint (DRUJ) stability. Anteroposterior translation of the ulna on the radius should be checked in neutral, pronation, and supination and then compared with the contralateral wrist. Excessive volar or dorsal motion indicates DRUJ instability.

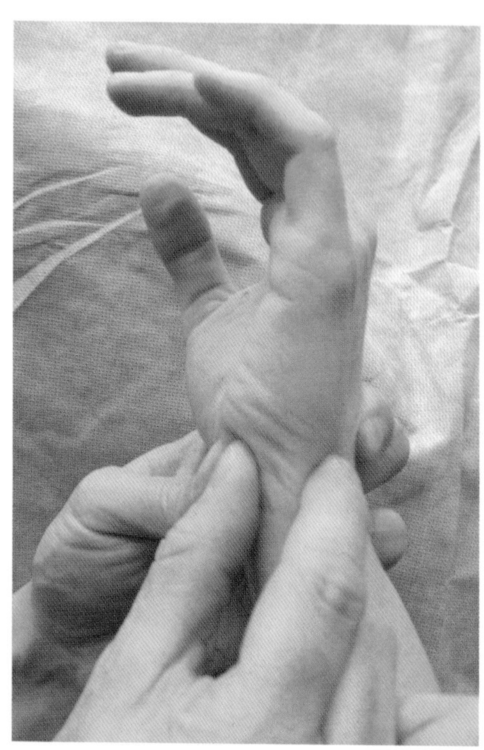

FIGURE 21-10 The ballottement test (i.e., shuck test) evaluates lunotriquetral motion with the lunate stabilized between the thumb and index finger of one hand and the triquetrum between the thumb and index finger of the other. Volar and dorsal forces are applied. Increased excursion (compared with the contralateral wrist) or pain with the maneuvers suggests injury to the lunotriquetral interosseous ligament.

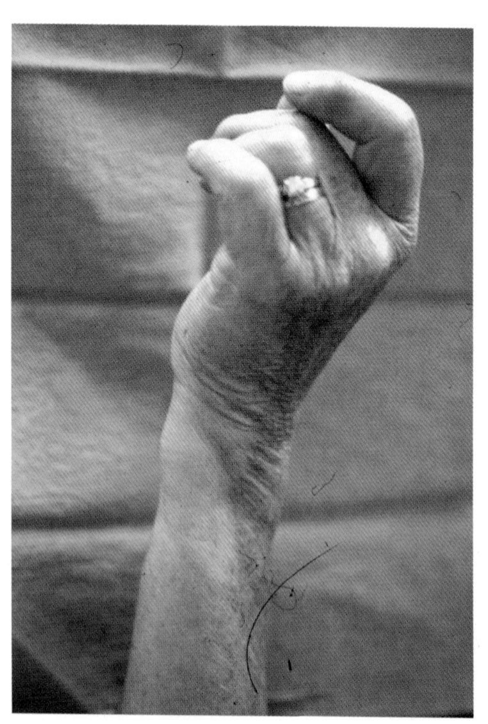

FIGURE 21-9 Dimpling along the dorsoulnar aspect of the wrist surface with supination indicates volar subluxation of the distal ulna and represents distal radioulnar joint instability.

lateral view, the pisiform should lie between the palmar surface of the scaphoid distal pole and the capitate.

Ulnar variance is the difference between the length of the ulna and the length of the radius at the wrist. Specifically, this distance is measured between lines drawn perpendicular to the shaft of the radius and the ulnar corner of the radius and a line drawn along the distal articular surface of the ulna. Ulnar-positive or -negative variance is defined as a distal ulna that is longer or shorter, respectively, than the radius (Fig. 21-11). This is clinically important for several reasons. Anatomically, Palmer showed that ulnar variance is inversely correlated with the thickness of the central portion of the TFC.[21] Cystic changes in the lunate and the distal ulna, especially in conjunction with ulnar-neutral or -positive variance, can be the hallmark of excessive loading through the ulnar carpus, as is the case with ulnar impaction syndrome (see Fig. 21-19). These changes may suggest the need for off-loading procedures, such as an ulnar shortening osteotomy, in conjunction with TFCC treatment. In this setting, encouraging results have been achieved by combining these treatments. Trumble and associates demonstrated significant relief of pain.[7] Grip strength and ROM averaged approximately 80% of the uninjured side. Central TFCC tears treated in the setting of ulnar-positive variance with ulnar shortening osteotomy alone showed 50% healing on second-look arthroscopy, with a spectrum of greatest to least healing on the more vascular ulnar side, compared with the less vascular radial side.[22]

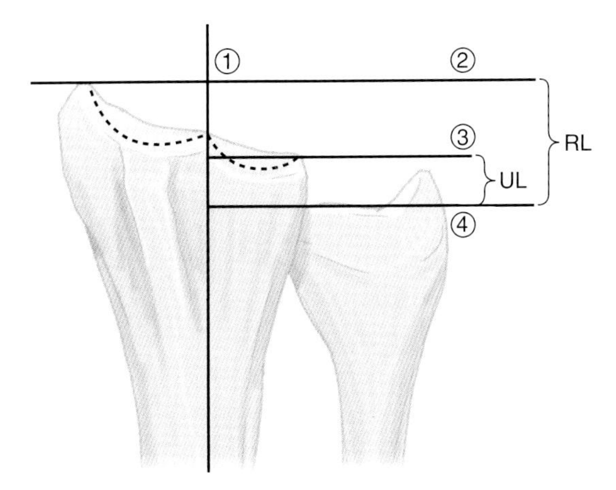

FIGURE 21-11 The relative length of the radius and ulna can be determined by measuring the distance between the tip of the radial styloid (line 2) drawn perpendicular to the longitudinal axis of the radius (line 1) and the distal end of the ulnar articular surface (line 4). The ulnar variance (UV) is measured as the distance between line 4 and line 3. *(Modified from Trumble TE. Distal radioulnar joint and triangular fibrocartilage complex. In: Trumble TE, ed.* Principles of Hand Surgery and Therapy. *Pennsylvania, PA: WB Saunders; 1999:130.)*

Radiography

Plain radiographs are undoubtedly important to rule out alternative causes of wrist pain, but the correlation between specific radiographic findings and injuries to the TFCC itself remains contentious. Although Geissler and colleagues concluded that TFCC tears had occurred in 26 of 60 patients in their series, representing the most common intracarpal soft tissue lesion found. They believed that radiographs were most helpful in the setting of scapholunate ligament injury and least helpful in TFCC tear. Nevertheless, radiographic findings of DRUJ dislocation and ulnar styloid fracture were the best surrogates to infer TFCC injury. Of the 25 patients with ulnar styloid fracture, 16 had TFCC tears, 14 of which were ulnar sided.[16] This finding was corroborated by Lindau and coworkers.[19] On the other hand, Richards and colleagues[22a] found no correlation between ulnar styloid fractures and TFCC injuries. Instead, tears were related to greater shortening and dorsal angulation of the distal radius on the preoperative radiographs in their study of 118 intra-articular and extra-articular wrist fractures. In 2008, Bombaci and associates compared MRI findings of TFCC tears with plain radiographs.[23] MRI revealed that 27 (45%) of the 60 patients had TFC lesions. No correlation was found between TFCC injury and the Melone classification system, the presence of an ulnar styloid fracture, comminution of the articular surface of the distal radius, more than 20 degrees of dorsal angulation of the distal radius, or subluxation or dislocation of the DRUJ on the plain radiographs. However, Frykman subtypes with distal radius fracture that extended to the DRUJ and/or the radiocarpal joint with an ulnar styloid fracture did have a statistically higher incidence of TFCC tears, compared with the remaining Frykman subtypes of injury after distal radial fractures.[23]

Arthrography

Wrist arthrography can be used to help diagnose tears of the scapholunate and lunotriquetral interosseous ligaments.[24-27] After midcarpal row injection, the contrast agent is injected into the radiocarpal joint. Contrast extravasation into the DRUJ indicates perforation of the TFCC (Fig. 21-12A). Injection directly into the DRUJ can demonstrate smaller tears and those with an overlying flap. Arthrograms more reliably diagnose TFCC radial detachment and lunotriquetral ligament tears than ulnocarpal ligament injuries and ulnar TFCC detachments.[24,25,28] Single-injection arthrograms have a high incidence of positive findings in asymptomatic patients.[24] It is important to correlate the presences of symptoms with the suspected findings on the study.

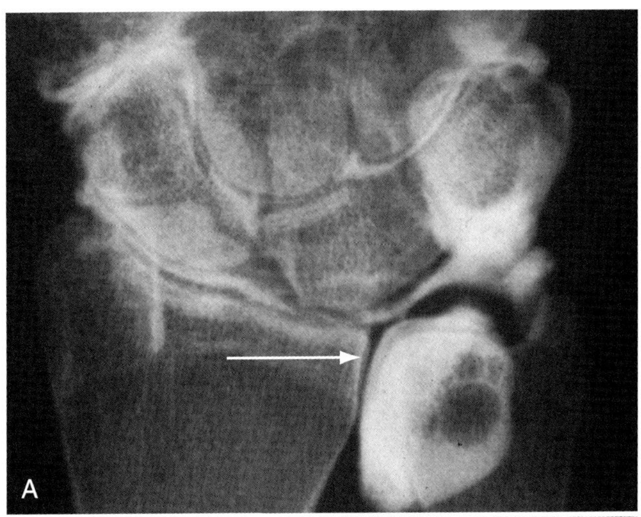

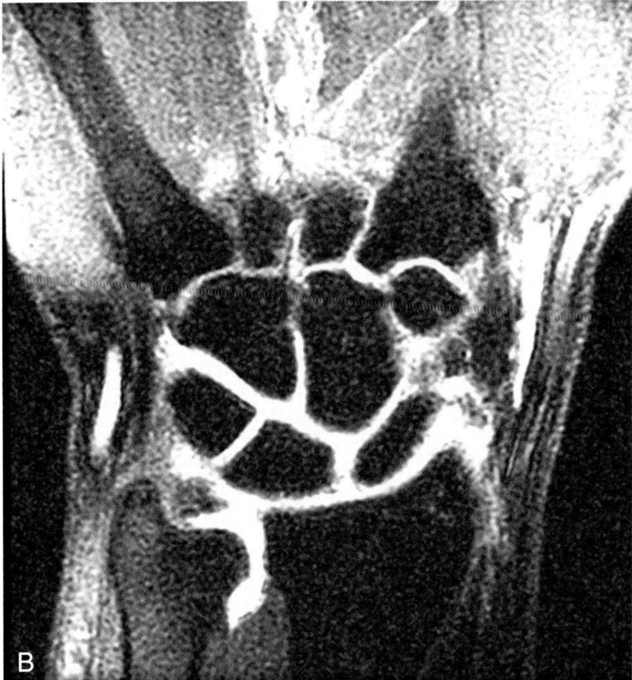

FIGURE 21-12 A, Wrist arthrogram demonstrates dye leakage from the radiocarpal joint into the distal radioulnar joint (DRUJ), indicating a perforation of the triangular fibrocartilage complex. **B,** MR arthrogram demonstrates leakage of dye from radiocarpal joint into the DRUJ, indicating a perforation of the triangular fibrocartilage complex. *(**A,** From Trumble TE. Distal radioulnar joint and triangular fibrocartilage complex. In: Trumble TE, ed.* Principles of Hand Surgery and Therapy. *Pennsylvania, PA: WB Saunders; 1999:130.)*

Magnetic Resonance Imaging

MRI for the diagnosis of TFCC injuries is a controversial issue. The specificity and sensitivity of MRI for detection of central and radial detachments vary but can be improved by dedicated musculoskeletal radiologists using specialized equipment such as wrist surface coils and higher Tesla magnets.[29] Golimbu and colleagues,[30] Joshy and associates,[31] Skahen and coworkers[32] detected TFCC injuries with an accuracy between 74% and 95%. In the study by Joshy and asociates,[31] in which patients underwent arthroscopy after MRI arthrography, the positive predictive value was 0.95, but the negative predictive value was only 0.50. This study used a 1.0-T magnet, whereas a Mayo clinic study using 3.0-T magnets showed improved accuracy.[33] Compared with arthroscopy for definitive diagnosis, MRI appears to understage some TFCC pathology, specifically the proximal and distal radioulnar ligaments, while overstaging others, such as radial-sided and disk tears.[29,34] In our experience, magnetic resonance arthrograms have been the most efficient and accurate nonoperative means of evaluating ulnar wrist pain (see Fig. 21-12B).

TREATMENT

Indications

The appropriate treatment for TFCC injuries depends on the type of injury and the stability of the DRUJ and the ulnar-sided carpus. If a patient's history and physical examination findings are consistent with a TFCC injury, but the patient has normal radiographs and clinical stability, immobilization in a long arm cast or brace for 3 to 4 weeks is usually successful. Other nonoperative measures include corticosteroid injections and administration of nonsteroidal anti-inflammatory drugs. We prefer to avoid steroid injection in young, active athletes. If the patient continues to have pain after 1 month of conservative treatment, further diagnostic studies, such as an arthrogram, MRI, or arthroscopy, are warranted. We recommend the magnetic resonance arthrogram as the most sensitive and accurate diagnostic study. If a patient presents with radiographic or clinical instability, arthroscopic evaluation and repair should be considered primarily.

Patients with TFCC tears that fail to respond to nonoperative therapy after 1 month and those with DRUJ instability warrant operative intervention. TFCC lesions can be divided into radial or ulnar detachments, with their specific approaches detailed later, and central attritional tears that are amenable to débridement.

Reparable tears of the TFCC: Peripheral tears, such as types 1B, 1C, and 1D, do exceptionally well, in part because of their excellent blood supply. Techniques of repairing type 1B tears along the ulnar border have been demonstrated by numerous authors. Arthroscopic repair techniques for type 1D tears are continuing to be honed.

Non-reparable tears of the TFCC: Central degenerative tears and central tears that that have a small rim attached to the radius (type 1A) usually cannot be repaired. In certain cases, the body of the TFCC can be advanced to the sigmoid notch and repaired, similar to a type 1D lesion. In these cases, the torn rim along the sigmoid notch can be excised, and the major body of TFCC can be advanced and sutured to the radius.

Preferred open treatment: TFCC injuries that are less amenable to arthroscopic intervention, for which an open approach should be considered, are those with combined ECU tendon instability, a large ulnar styloid avulsion fracture that requires open reduction and internal fixation to re-establish the primary ulnar attachment of the TFCC and lunotriquetral or other intercarpal instability.

Equipment and Implants

Required items include the following:

- Standard traction apparatus such as wrist distraction tower
- Arthroscope with pressure monitoring system
- Arthroscopic shaver, preferred 2.5-mm diameter with full-rnadius blade
- Small probe
- Small arthroscope grasping and basket forceps
- Wire suture grasper
- Small hypodermic needle
- 18-gauge needle
- Suction-tip cannula
- Small retractor
- 0.045-inch Kirschner wire
- 2-0 Maxon meniscal repair sutures
- 3-0 Dacron sutures
- Suture anchor
- Small-joint radiofrequency device for capsular shrinkage or ablation
- Mini-arthroscopic lasso
- Mini Push-lock

Optional items include the following:

- Touhy 20-gauge needle for arthroscopic cannula
- Wire suture passer for 18-gauge needle
- 2-0 biodegradable meniscal repair sutures

Although several authors contend that most TFCC tears, in the absence of DRUJ instability, can be treated nonoperatively, there is not strong support from the literature.[35] After a reasonable period of activity modification, steroid injections, and immobilization, if the patient's symptoms are unresolved, surgical intervention is warranted.

Arthroscopic Techniques and Results

Numerous authors have published case series regarding their experience with treatment of isolated TFCC tears and those that occur in conjunction with other wrist injuries. However, only a limited number of studies allow comparison of different methods of treatment or separate the results of Palmer's different types. The following paragraphs describe the techniques for addressing each subtype of tear and the results of treatment.

Type 1A

A wrist distraction tower is used to suspend the hand and wrist by means of finger traps with 10 to 15 pounds applied. Lidocaine with epinephrine is injected to distend the radiocarpal joint through the area of the planned 3-4 portal. The 3-4 portal is placed between the extensor pollicis longus (EPL) tendon and the extensor digitorum communis (EDC) tendon, 1 cm distal to Lister's

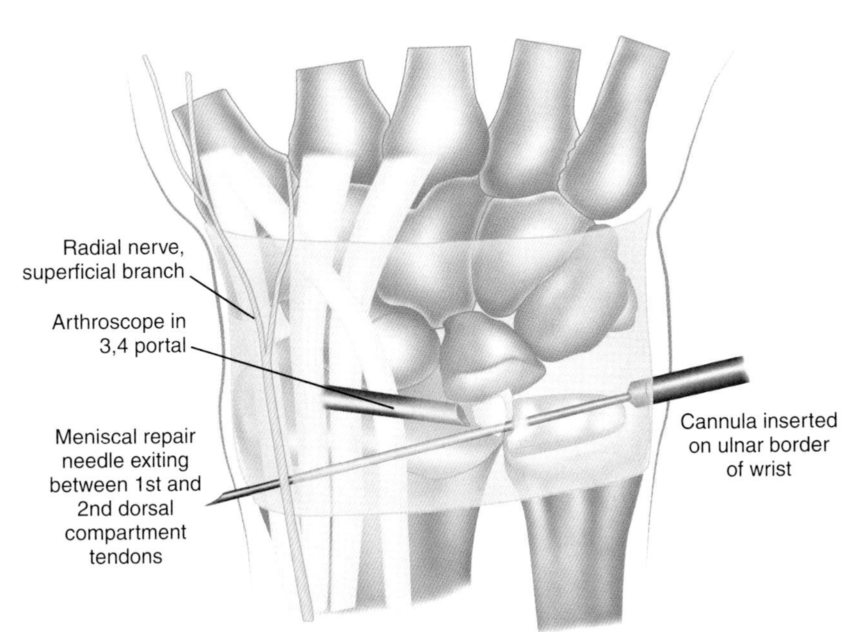

FIGURE 21-13 A radial-sided tear of the triangular fibrocartilage complex (type 1D) can be repaired using an arthroscope placed in the 3-4 portal and a suture-passing cannula in the 6-U portal. *(Modified from Trumble, TE, Gilbert M, Vedder N. Isolated tears of the triangular fibrocartilage: management by early arthroscopic repair.* J Hand Surg Am. *1997; 22:57-65.)*

tubercle between the scaphoid and the lunate. For the initial diagnostic examination, the arthroscope is placed into the 3-4 portal, and a small probe is placed into the 4-5 portal between the EDC and the extensor digiti minimi (EDM) (Fig. 21-13). A 2.7-mm Linvatec arthroscope is used with a 2.5-mm small-joint débrider (Stryker, Sunnyvale, CA) that has a full-radius blade for synovectomies and débridement of the central tear.

The goal in treating central tears is to débride the tear back to a stable rim. Various methods of doing so (e.g., shaver, thermal, laser) are available but have not been compared for efficacy. The results of treatment are good or excellent in 66% to 87% of patients with traditional débridement or with laser and radiofrequency probe ablation.[36] Results decline in patients with ulnar positivity, leading to failure rates as high as 60%, most likely because of sustained higher loads across the TFCC.[37] Hulsizer and colleagues demonstrated that even in the absence of ulnar positivity, good results can still be salvaged from patients who have poor results after TFCC débridement by performing a subsequent ulnar shortening osteotomy.[38]

Types 1B and 1C

Because type 1B and 1C injuries occur in the peripheral, well-vascularized portion of the TFCC, suture repair is likely to lead to healing. Repairs of this class of ulnar-sided avulsion injuries can be divided into inside-out and outside-in techniques.

The *inside-out technique* is occasionally used for small volar or peripheral tears. Diagnostic arthroscopy is performed in a similar fashion as for TFCC detachment from the radius. With the use of a small probe, the diagnosis of peripheral detachment is made by the trampoline test of the TFCC, as described by Hermansdorfer and Kleinman.[39] The normal TFCC should be taut when tested with the probe. If the TFCC is redundant and wavy when compressed by the arthroscopic probe (Fig. 21-14), a peripheral or ulnar-sided tear is indicated. In these cases, the arthroscope is placed in the 6-R portal. The arthroscopic shaver is placed into the 3-4 portal to débride any excess synovium that may be blocking the view needed for suture passage. The shaver should also be used to débride the frayed portions of the TFCC in the region of the tear. An arthroscopic cannula is then placed into the 3-4 portal to facilitate passage of the 2-0 Maxon meniscal repair sutures. A small longitudinal incision is made at the 6-U portal. The wrist capsule should be exposed but not incised, to avoid leakage of the intra-articular solution used to distend the joint. The ulnar nerve is identified and protected with the use of a retractor. The sutures are placed through the cannula and brought out through the ulnar incision. Two or three sets of sutures are used for repair of the peripheral detachment (Fig. 21-15). Tension is then placed on the sutures to re-establish the normal tension of the TFCC and obliterate any gapping between the meniscal homologue and portions of the peripheral capsule. The patient's hand is then taken out of the traction device, and the sutures are tied with the wrist in neutral rotation and slight ulnar deviation. In type IC lesions, the repair is almost directly under the flexor carpi ulnaris, and close to the ulnar nerve, so the use of a protective retractor is critical.

We prefer the *outside-in technique* for repair of ulnar sided or peripheral TFCC tears. It involves puncturing the ulnar wrist capsule through the edge of the torn TFCC and retrieving the suture from the ulnar side of the wrist (see Video 1: Ulnar-Sided TFCC Repair).

The repair suture is threaded into an 18-guage needle (Kendall, Argyle, NY) or a special passing needle and inserted into the wrist joint through the 6-U portal under arthroscopic control. The needle passes through the torn edge of the TFCC just radial to the edge (Fig. 21-16). The suture is threaded out through the needle and grasped with a small arthroscopic grasping forceps or wire suture grasper (Smith & Nephew, Inc., Andover, MA) (Fig. 21-17) placed through the 6-U portal. Two or three sutures are passed by this technique (Fig. 21-18). The incision for the portal is enlarged so that all the suture ends can be brought out through the 6-U portal incision and tied over the capsule under direct vision. This exposure helps to protect the small branches of the dorsal sensory branch of the ulnar nerve.

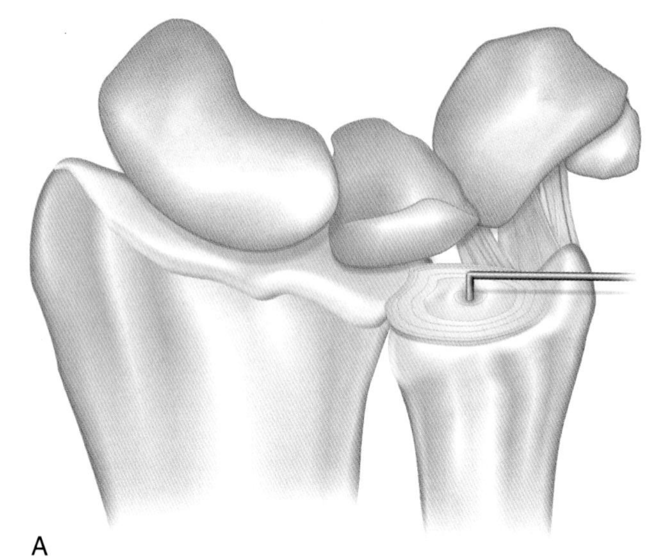

FIGURE 21-14 A, The trampoline test uses the arthroscopic probe to differentiate between the normal, taut triangular fibrocartilage complex (TFCC) *(left)* and the loose, redundant TFCC with a peripheral or ulnar-sided TFCC tear *(right)*. **B,** During the arthroscopic examination of the ulnar-sided TFCC tear, the loose, redundant TFCC can be detected by the trampoline test. (**A,** *Modified from Trumble TE. Distal radioulnar joint and triangular fibrocartilage complex. In: Trumble TE, ed.* Principles of Hand Surgery and Therapy. *Pennsylvania, PA: WB Saunders; 1999:136.)*

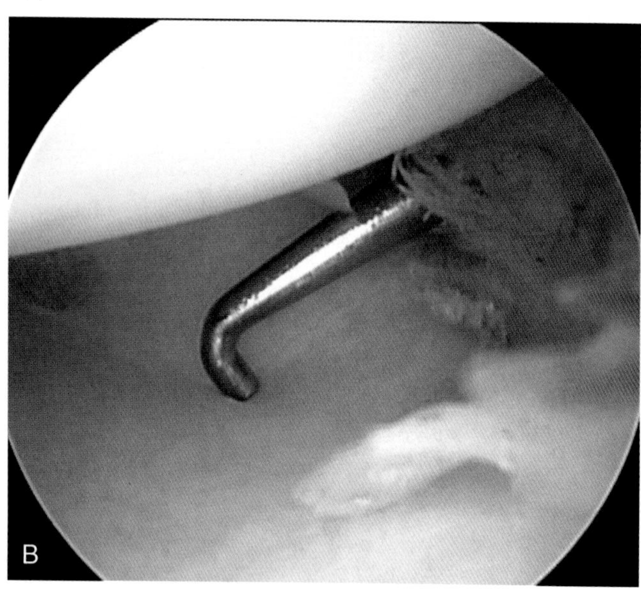

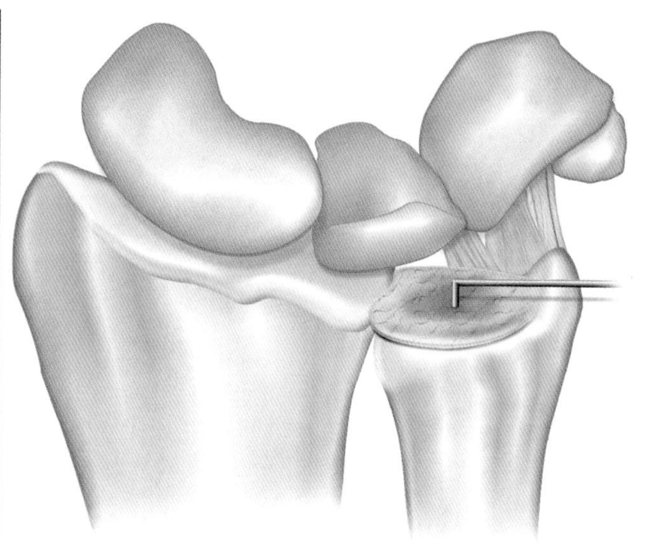

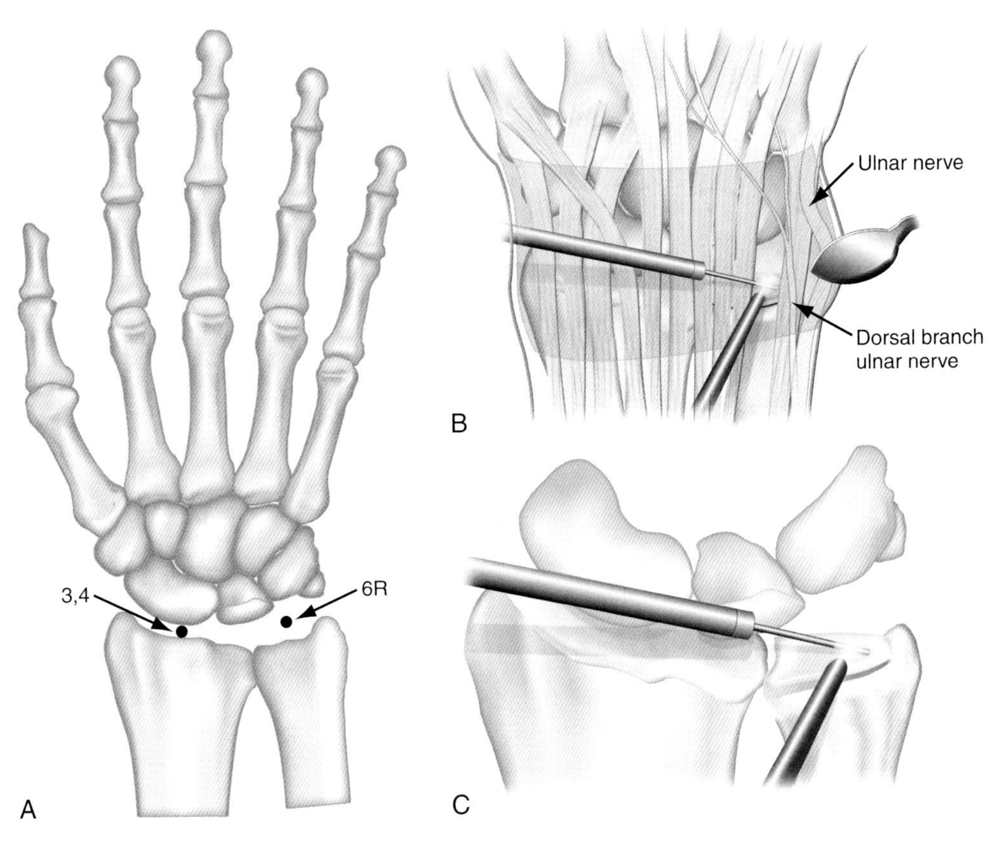

FIGURE 21-15 Peripheral tears of the triangular fibrocartilage complex can be repaired with an inside-out technique by passing sutures through a cannula in the 3-4 portal while the arthroscope is in the 4-5 portal. *(Modified from Trumble TE, Gilbert M, Vedder N. Isolated tears of the triangular fibrocartilage: Management by early arthroscopic repair.* J Hand Surg Am. *1997; 22:57-65.)*

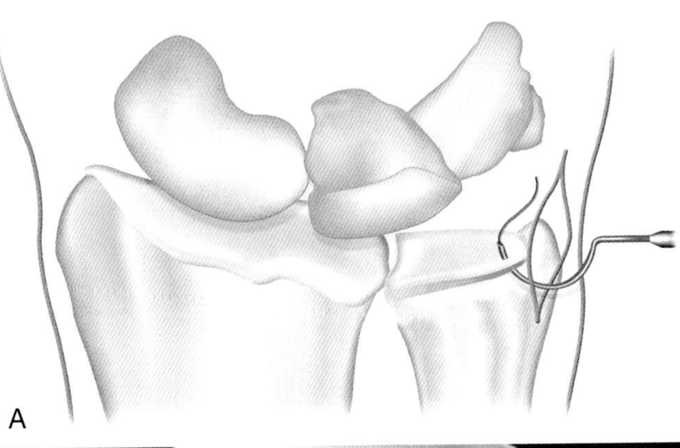

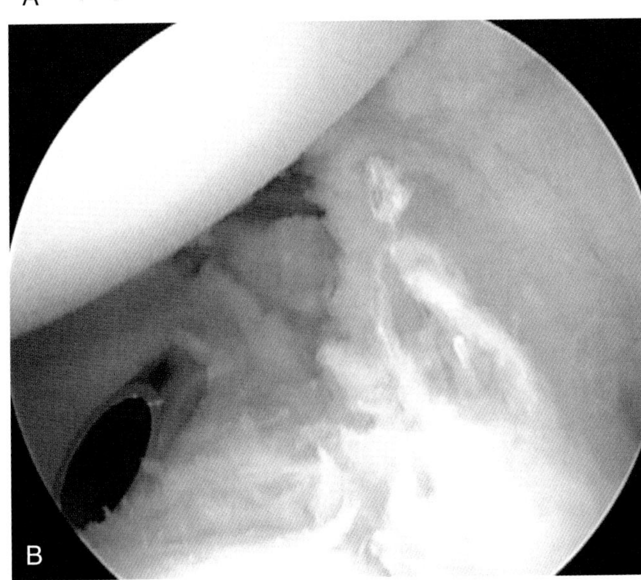

FIGURE 21-16 A, The outside-in technique for repairing peripheral tears of the TFCC is performed by placing an 18-gauge needle or curved suture cannula in the 6-U portal so that it pierces the detached edge of the triangular fibrocartilage complex (TFCC). **B,** During the arthroscopy, the hollow needle cannula is placed through the rim of the TFCC tear to pass the repair suture. (**A,** *Modified from Trumble TE. Distal radioulnar joint and triangular fibrocartilage complex. In: Trumble TE, ed.* Principles of Hand Surgery and Therapy. *Pennsylvania, PA: WB Saunders; 1999:137.)*

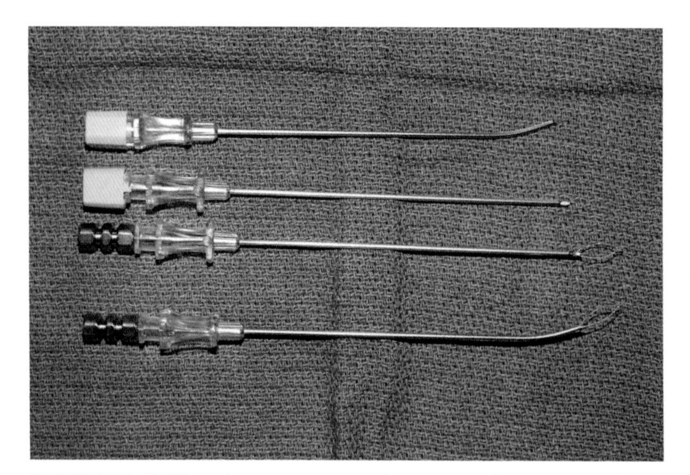

FIGURE 21-17 The wire suture grasper is an option for retrieving the suture during arthroscopic repair of the triangular fibrocartilage complex.

Ulnar-sided peripheral tears can be addressed with either open or arthroscopic techniques. Corso and associates reported that 42 (93%) of the 45 patients in their multicentered trial had a satisfactory outcome, with an average of 75% of the grip strength of the contralateral hand 3 years after repair.[40] However, 27 patients in that study had additional wrist injuries, including distal radius fractures and scapholunate ligament tears. Patients without these injuries would likely have improved outcomes. In 2002, Millants and colleagues published an outcome study of 35 patients who had arthroscopic surgical repair of ulnar-sided tears.[41] Patients were assessed using a visual analog scale the Disabilities of the Arm, Shoulder, and Hand (DASH) score. According to the DASH score, 29 patients had good results, 5 had fair results, and 1 had a poor result. Degreef and colleagues corroborated these results, showing 80% grip strength and minimal to no pain in 47 of 52 patients after ulnar-sided repair.[42]

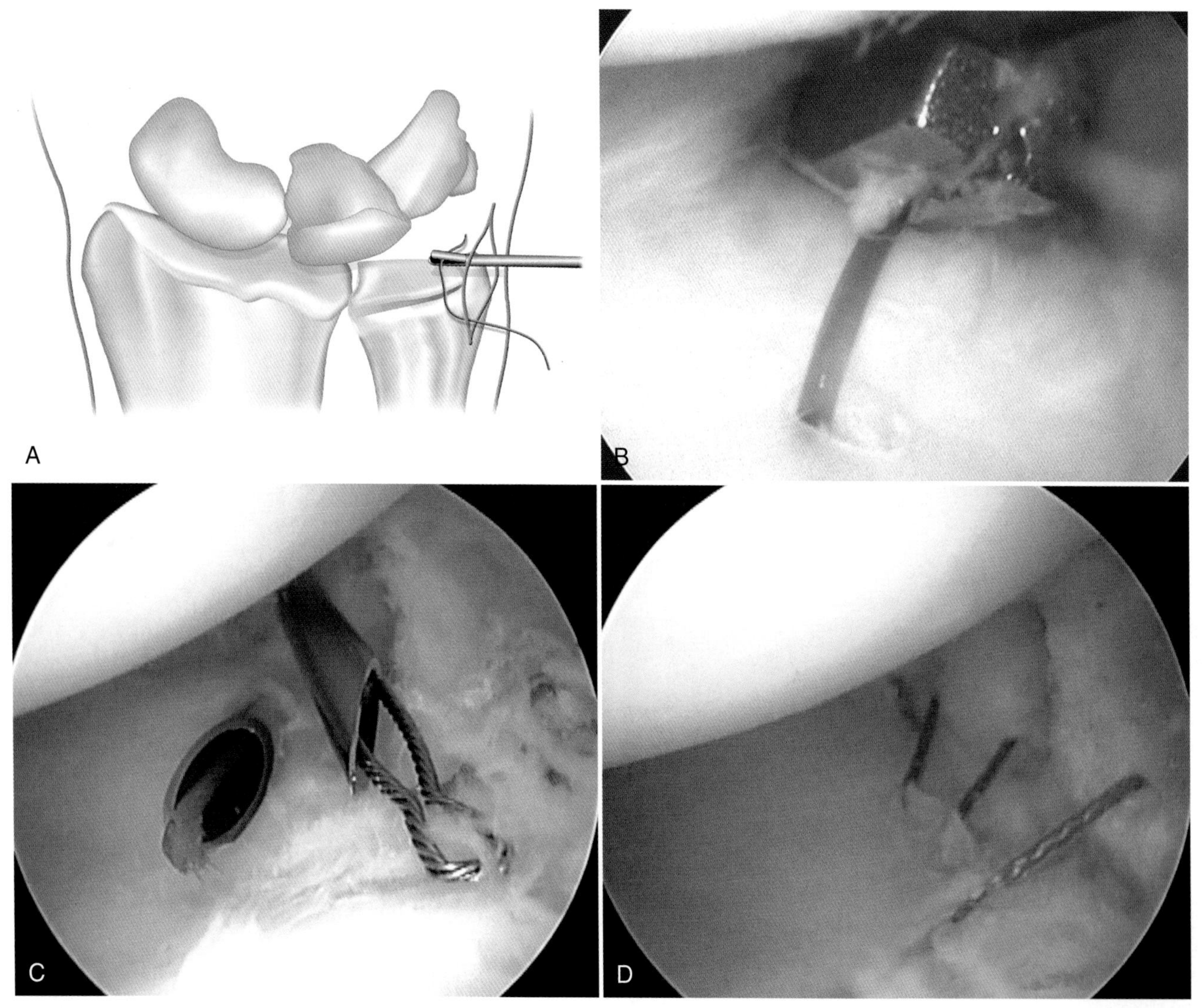

FIGURE 21-18 A and **B,** Using the arthroscopic grasping forceps, the suture is brought back out through the 6-U portal so that the suture can be tied over the portal site. Care should be taken to avoid injury to the dorsal sensory branch of the ulnar nerve. **C,** The wire suture grasper can be used to retrieve the repair suture during arthroscopy. **D,** The normal tension of the triangular fibrocartilage complex can be seen after two to three sutures are passed and tied. *(From Trumble TE. Distal radioulnar joint and triangular fibrocartilage complex. In: Trumble TE, ed.* Principles of Hand Surgery and Therapy. *Pennsylvania, PA: WB Saunders; 1999:137.)*

Results of type 1C injuries have not been specifically addressed in the literature. These lesions are uncommon and represent injuries to the extrinsic volar ulnar-sided ligaments caused by high-energy trauma. In 2007, Estrella and coworkers studied 35 patients with all subtypes, 5 of whom had type 1C; overall, 75% had good or excellent results and averaged 88% and 82% motion and grip strength, respectively.[43]

Type 1D

The technique for treatment of type 1D lesions was modified from the that described by Cooney for open repairs using sutures placed through the radius.[28] A wrist distraction tower and portals as previously described are used. The 2.5-mm, full-radius, small-joint débrider is used to prepare for the reattachment of the TFC.

After the tear is identified by the techniques described earlier, a small hypodermic needle is placed into the wrist joint through the 6-U portal. The needle tip determines the appropriate access point for introducing the repair sutures. The 6-U portal is located on the ulnar aspect of the ECU, just proximal to the triquetrum. The reattachment site of the TFCC on the distal radius is débrided down to bleeding bone with the use of an arthroscopic shaver inserted via the 4-5 portal. A small incision is then made in the region of the 6-U portal, and blunt dissection is carried down to bone to avoid injury to the dorsal sensory branch of the ulnar nerve. Meniscal repair sutures (2-0 Maxon , Davis & Geck, Manati, PA) are passed into the suction-tip cannula, placed into the central rim of the TFCC under arthroscopic guidance, and driven across the radius with the use of a power wire driver. Care is taken to avoid suture coiling when using this double-armed meniscal repair suture. When the first needle is passed, coiling is prevented by holding the suture and allowing the second needle to rotate. The second needle must be inserted into the wire driver with the attached suture folded alongside the suture needle. A curved retractor is placed around the loop of suture, between the tip of the wire driver and the patient. The suture coils along the needle as the needle is driven across the radius. After the suture has coiled along the length of the needle, the direction of the wire driver is reversed. This pattern is continued until the needle exits the skin along the radial side of the wrist. The suture needles should exit between the first and second dorsal compartments on the radial aspect of the wrist. The first suture is brought out through the skin, and then the second suture is passed through the radius. Two sets of repair sutures are used to secure the TFCC to the radius. The sutures are then placed under tension to ensure that the TFCC lines up with the surface of the distal radius. After correct positioning of the TFCC has been confirmed, the patient's hand is removed from the traction device, and an incision is made longitudinally between the two sets of exiting sutures. The extensor tendons in the first and second compartments are identified and retracted so that the suture can be placed under tension and tied onto the radius with the wrist in neutral rotation.

An alternative to the technique of drilling two holes, which can be difficult in a small wrist, is to use a cannulated 2.0-mm drill (Synthes Inc., Paoli, PA) to drill a single hole from the sigmoid notch to the base of the radial styloid (see Video 2: Cannulated Drill for Radial-Sided TFCC Tear). The guide pin is drilled first through the 6-U portal with the 2.0-mm guide inserted into the wrist joint. The radial-sided incision is made after the exit site of the guide pin has been determined. The double-armed sutures are passed through the cannula and through the TFCC. The sutures are secured by placing an absorbable anchor (Panalok Loop, Ethicon Inc., Norwood, MA) between the sutures for an interference fit. The sutures are then tied over the anchor.

In the 2007 study of Estrella and colleagues,[43] only 1 of 35 patients had a type 1D tear. Results were not given for that patient specifically.[43] In a 2002 study by Shih and colleagues, 8 of the 37 patients had type 1D tears and "showed the same results" as those with type 1B tears on Mayo wrist scores with 2-year follow-up.[44] Newer techniques are being developed that utilize a mini Push-lock anchor (Arthrex, Naples, FL) in a fully arthroscopic technique. Use of the mini-suture lasso and small arthroscopic cannulas to assist in passage of the anchor into the sigmoid notch can facilitate the technique.

Type 2 Tears

Most of Palmer's class 2 attritional lesions result from excessive loading of the distal ulna, triquetrum, and/or lunate (Fig. 21-19). After an TFCC tear has been identified by arthroscopic evaluation, non-reparable lesions can be débrided with the use of the 2.5-mm, full-radius shaver, with the device placed in the 6-R portal and the arthroscope in the 3-4 portal. In cases of positive ulnar variance, an ulnar shortening osteotomy in conjunction with TFCC débridement is recommended. The shortening osteotomy decompresses the ulnar side of the wrist by decreasing the impaction between the distal ulna and the carpus.

Although poor results have been associated with DRUJ arthritis, chronicity of symptoms, and worker's compensation claims, Bernstein and coworkers demonstrated that ulnar shortening osteotomy resulted in increased Mayo wrist scores, improved grip, better motion, and high patient satisfaction.[45,46]

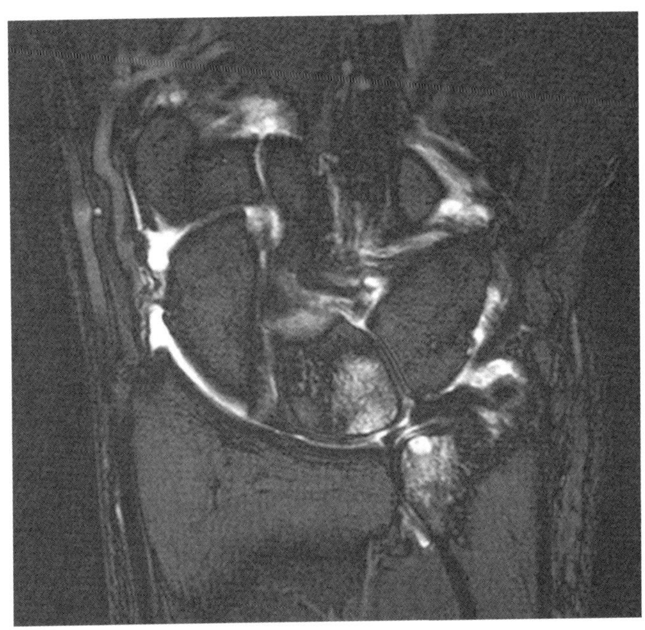

FIGURE 21-19 Coronal, T2-weighted MRI shows ulnar impaction syndrome with significant edema within the lunate and distal ulna.

PEARLS & PITFALLS

PEARLS

- Early diagnosis is helpful in patients with ulnar-sided wrist pain.
- Magnetic resonance arthrograms offer the best diagnosis but need to be correlated with symptoms.
- Central tears and class IA tears often benefit from débridement.
- Ulna shortening can help in delayed cases and with central tears that do not respond to débridement.

PITFALLS

- Avoid placing too many sutures through the TFCC, which can be fragile.
- Protect the dorsal sensory nerve on ulnar-sided repairs and the superficial sensory branch on radial-sided repairs.
- Place tension on untied sutures while tying the other sutures.
- Initiate ROM exercises earlier, rather than later, to avoid stiffness.

Postoperative Rehabilitation

After an TFCC repair is performed, forearm rotation and wrist motion should be restricted by an above-elbow splint applied with the wrist in a neutral position. Maintain the splint for 3 to 4 weeks, and begin finger ROM exercises during this period. After the long arm splint is removed, a removable wrist brace is used for an additional 2 weeks (postoperative weeks 4 through 6). Active wrist and forearm motion can be started at this time, but radial and ulnar deviation should be avoided to protect the repair. Flexion and extension usually are permitted at 4 weeks, and supination and pronation are permitted slightly later, at 6 weeks. Passive wrist ROM exercises are started (postoperative weeks 6 through 8), followed by strengthening (postoperative weeks 8 through 12). Overall, the period of immobilization is adjusted for severity of injury, strength of repair, and patient compliance.

CONCLUSIONS

TFCC tears are among the numerous causes of ulnar-sided wrist pain. Although tears often can be treated nonoperatively, early diagnosis is helpful for patients with ulnar-sided wrist pain that does not improve despite initial conservative efforts. Correlating the patient's history and symptoms with findings on the magnetic resonance arthrogram is critical to accurate diagnosis. After identification, peripheral tears on the radial or the ulnar side can be repaired, whereas central tears and class 1A tears benefit from débridement. If arthroscopic treatment fails to provided relief, ulna shortening can improve the symptoms.

REFERENCES

1. Palmer AK, Werner FW. The triangular fibrocartilage complex of the wrist: anatomy and function. *J Hand Surg Am*. 1981;6:153.
2. DiTano O, Trumble TE, Tencer AF. Biomechanical function of the distal radioulnar and ulnocarpal wrist ligaments. *J Hand Surg Am*. 2003; 28:622.
3. Thiru RG, Ferlic DC, Clayton ML, et al. Arterial anatomy of the triangular fibrocartilage of the wrist and its surgical significance. *J Hand Surg Am*. 1986;11:258.
4. Palmer AK. Triangular fibrocartilage complex lesions: a classification. *J Hand Surg Am*. 1989;14:594.
5. Trumble TE, Gilbert M, Vedder N. Arthroscopic repair of the triangular fibrocartilage complex. *Arthroscopy*. 1996;12:588.
6. Trumble TE, Gilbert M, Vedder N. Isolated tears of the triangular fibrocartilage: management by early arthroscopic repair. *J Hand Surg Am*. 1997;22:57.
7. Trumble TE, Gilbert M, Vedder N. Ulnar shortening combined with arthroscopic repairs in the delayed management of triangular fibrocartilage complex tears. *J Hand Surg Am*. 1997;22:807.
8. Labosky DA, Waggy CA. Oblique ulnar shortening osteotomy by a single saw cut. *J Hand Surg Am*. 1996;21:48.
9. Mikic ZD. Age changes in the triangular fibrocartilage of the wrist joint. *J Anat*. 1978;126:367.
10. Mikic ZD. Treatment of acute injuries of the triangular fibrocartilage complex associated with distal radioulnar joint instability. *J Hand Surg Am*. 1995;20:319.
11. Wright TW, Del Charco M, Wheeler D. Incidence of ligament lesions and associated degenerative changes in the elderly wrist. *J Hand Surg Am*. 1994;19:313.
12. Metz VM, Schratter M, Dock WI, et al. Age-associated changes of the triangular fibrocartilage of the wrist: evaluation of the diagnostic performance of MR imaging. *Radiology*. 1992;184:217.
13. Geissler WB. Arthroscopically assisted reduction of intra-articular fractures of the distal radius. *Hand Clin*. 1995;11:19.
14. Geissler WB. Intra-articular distal radius fractures: the role of arthroscopy? *Hand Clin*. 2005;21:407.
15. Geissler WB, Freeland AE. Arthroscopic management of intra-articular distal radius fractures. *Hand Clin*. 1999;15:455.
16. Geissler WB, Freeland AE, Savoie FH, et al. Intracarpal soft-tissue lesions associated with an intra-articular fracture of the distal end of the radius. *J Bone Joint Surg Am*. 1996;78:357.
17. Varitimidis SE, Basdekis GK, Dailiana ZH, et al. Treatment of intra-articular fractures of the distal radius: fluoroscopic or arthroscopic reduction? *J Bone Joint Surg Br*. 2008;90:778.
18. Ruch DS, Yang CC, Smith BP. Results of acute arthroscopically repaired triangular fibrocartilage complex injuries associated with intra-articular distal radius fractures. *Arthroscopy*. 2003;19:511.
19. Lindau T, Arner M, Hagberg L. Intraarticular lesions in distal fractures of the radius in young adults: a descriptive arthroscopic study in 50 patients. *J Bone Joint Surg Br*. 1997;22:638.
20. de Araujo W, Poehling GG, Kuzma GR. New Tuohy needle technique for triangular fibrocartilage complex repair: preliminary studies. *Arthroscopy*. 1996;12:699.
21. Palmer AK, Glisson RR, Werner FW. Relationship between ulnar variance and triangular fibrocartilage complex thickness. *J Hand Surg Am*. 1984;9:681.
22. Tatebe M, Horii E, Nakao E, et al. Repair of the triangular fibrocartilage complex after ulnar-shortening osteotomy: second-look arthroscopy. *J Hand Surg Am*. 2007;32:445.

22a. Richards RS, Bennett JD, Roth JH, Milne K Jr. Arthroscopic diagnosis of intra-articular soft tissue injuries associated with distal radial fractures. *J Hand Surg Am*. 1997;22(5):772.

23. Bombaci H, Polat A, Deniz G, et al. The value of plain x-rays in predicting TFCC injury after distal radial fractures. *J Hand Surg Eur*. 2008; 33:322.
24. Brown JA, Janzen DL, Adler BD, et al. Arthrography of the contralateral, asymptomatic wrist in patients with unilateral wrist pain. *Can Assoc Radiol J*. 1994;45:292.
25. Cerofolini E, Luchetti R, Pederzini L, et al. MR evaluation of triangular fibrocartilage complex tears in the wrist: comparison with arthrography and arthroscopy. *J Comput Assist Tomogr*. 1990;14:963.
26. Levinsohn EM, Palmer AK, Coren AB, et al. Wrist arthrography: the value of the three compartment injection technique. *Skeletal Radiol*. 1987;16:539.
27. Levinsohn EM, Rosen ID, Palmer AK. Wrist arthrography: value of the three-compartment injection method. *Radiology*. 1991;179:231.
28. Cooney WP, Linscheid RL, Dobyns JH. Triangular fibrocartilage tears. *J Hand Surg Am*. 1994;19:143.
29. Tanaka T, Amadio PC, Zhao C, et al. Effect of wrist and ulna head position on gliding resistance of the extensor digitorum minimi and extensor digitorum communis III tendons: a cadaver study. *J Orthop Res*. 2006;24:757.
30. Golimbu CN, Firooznia H, Melone CP Jr, et al. Tears of the triangular fibrocartilage of the wrist: MR imaging. *Radiology*. 1989;173:731.
31. Joshy S, Ghosh S, Lee K, et al. Accuracy of direct magnetic resonance arthrography in the diagnosis of triangular fibrocartilage complex tears of the wrist. *Int Orthop*. 2008;32:251.

32. Skahen JR 3rd, Palmer AK, Levinsohn EM, et al. Magnetic resonance imaging of the triangular fibrocartilage complex. *J Hand Surg Am*. 1990; 15:552.
33. Anderson ML, Skinner JA, Felmlee JP, et al. Diagnostic comparison of 1.5 Tesla and 3.0 Tesla preoperative MRI of the wrist in patients with ulnar-sided wrist pain. *J Hand Surg Am*. 2008;33:1153.
34. Fulcher SM, Poehling GG. The role of operative arthroscopy for the diagnosis and treatment of lesions about the distal ulna. *Hand Clin*. 1998;14:285.
35. Osterman A, Bednar M, Gambin K, et al. The natural history of untreated symptomatic tears in the triangular fibrocartilage. Paper presented at the 51st annual meeting of the American Society for Surgery of the Hand, October 1996, Nashville, TN.
36. Blackwell RE, Jemison DM, Foy BD. The holmium:yttrium-aluminum-garnet laser in wrist arthroscopy: a five-year experience in the treatment of central triangular fibrocartilage complex tears by partial excision. *J Hand Surg Am*. 2001;26:77.
37. Minami A, Ishikawa J, Suenaga N, et al. Clinical results of treatment of triangular fibrocartilage complex tears by arthroscopic debridement. *J Hand Surg Am*. 1996;21:406.
38. Hulsizer D, Weiss AP, Akelman E. Ulna-shortening osteotomy after failed arthroscopic debridement of the triangular fibrocartilage complex. *J Hand Surg Am*. 1997;22:694.
39. Hermansdorfer JD, Kleinman WB. Management of chronic peripheral tears of the triangular fibrocartilage complex. *J Hand Surg Am*. 1991; 16:340.
40. Corso SJ, Savoie FH, Geissler WB, et al. Arthroscopic repair of peripheral avulsions of the triangular fibrocartilage complex of the wrist: a multicenter study. *Arthroscopy*. 1997;13:78.
41. Millants P, De Smet L, Van Ransbeeck H. Outcome study of arthroscopic suturing of ulnar avulsions of the triangular fibrocartilage complex of the wrist. *Chir Main*. 2002;21:298.
42. Degreef I, Welters H, Milants P, et al. Disability and function after arthroscopic repair of ulnar avulsions of the triangular fibrocartilage complex of the wrist. *Acta Orthop Belg*. 2005;71:289.
43. Estrella EP, Hung LK, Ho PC, et al. Arthroscopic repair of triangular fibrocartilage complex tears. *Arthroscopy*. 2007;23:729.
44. Shih JT, Lee HM, Tan CM. Early isolated triangular fibrocartilage complex tears: management by arthroscopic repair. *J Trauma*. 2002; 53:922.
45. Baek GH, Chung MS, Lee YH, et al. Ulnar shortening osteotomy in idiopathic ulnar impaction syndrome. *J Bone Joint Surg Am*. 2005; 87:2649.
46. Bernstein MA, Nagle DJ, Martinez A, et al. A comparison of combined arthroscopic triangular fibrocartilage complex debridement and arthroscopic wafer distal ulna resection versus arthroscopic triangular fibrocartilage complex debridement and ulnar shortening osteotomy for ulnocarpal abutment syndrome. *Arthroscopy*. 2004;20:392.

SUGGESTED READING

Kleinman WB. Stability of the distal radioulnar joint: biomechanics, pathophysiology, physical diagnosis, and restoration of function what we have learned in 25 years. *J Hand Surg Am*. 2007;32:1086-1106.

CHAPTER

22

Triangular Fibrocartilage Débridement and Arthroscopically Assisted Ulnar Shortening

Daniel J. Nagle

A tear of the triangular fibrocartilage complex (TFCC) is one of the most frequent causes of ulnar wrist pain. Ulnar-sided wrist pain associated with a TFCC tear in the presence of an ulnar-neutral or ulnar-plus variance constitutes an ulnar abutment syndrome. Successful treatment of an ulnar abutment syndrome requires débridement of the TFCC tear and ulnar shortening.

ANATOMY

The triangular fibrocartilage is the primary stabilizer of the distal radioulnar joint. It attaches radially on the distal lip of the sigmoid notch. Ulnarly, the triangular fibrocartilage inserts at the base of the ulnar styloid by means of a continuation of the dorsal and palmar radioulnar ligaments and the fibers of the ligamentum subcruentum (Fig. 22-1).[1,2]

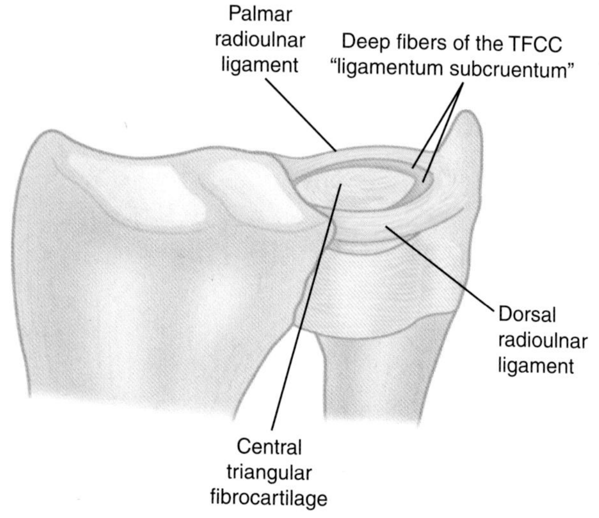

FIGURE 22-1 Triangular fibrocartilage anatomy.

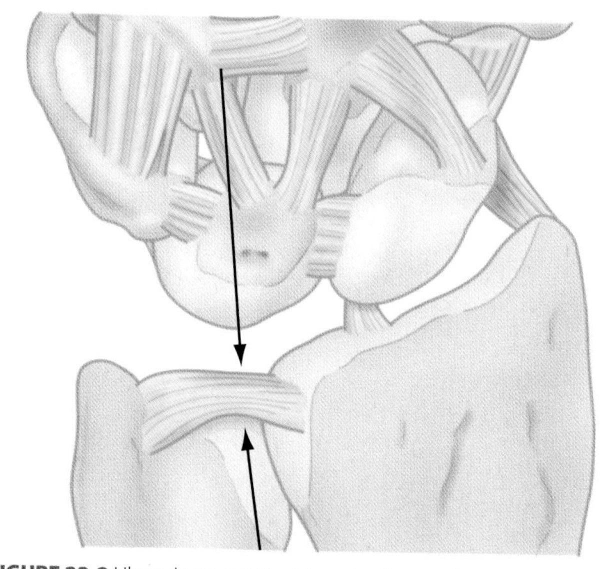

FIGURE 22-2 Ulnar abutment. The triangular fibrocartilage complex is compressed between the proximal ulnar lunate and the distal ulnar head.

A patient with an ulnar abutment syndrome typically presents with a central tear of the TFCC. Chondromalacia can be seen at the ulnar aspect of the lunate and the distal radial surface of the ulnar head. Ulnocarpal synovitis is usually present (Fig. 22-2).

PATIENT EVALUATION

History

Tears of the triangular fibrocartilage are typically the result of a fall on the outstretched upper extremity. The ulna is driven distally and compresses the TFCC between itself and the lunate, producing a central or radial tear of the articular disk. This same mechanism can result in lunatotriquetral tears and peripheral TFCC tears, neither of which is discussed further here.

Forceful ulnar deviation, as observed in racquet sports and golf, can lead to TFCC tears. The combination of ulnar axial load and torque can be sufficient to tear the triangular fibrocartilage. Gymnastics, with its significant axial loading of the wrists, can also lead to a TFCC tear.

At least 50% of intra-articular distal radius fractures are associated with tears of the triangular fibrocartilage. However, many of these remain asymptomatic and require no treatment.

An ulnar abutment syndrome can develop as a result of settling of a distal radial fracture fragment. The radial collapse leads to a relative lengthening of the ulna. Palmer and colleagues[2] demonstrated an increase in the ulnocarpal load with increasing ulnar variance.

Repetitive axial loading of the wrist in a patient with an ulnar-zero or ulnar-plus variance can lead to an attritional tear of the triangular fibrocartilage and ulnar abutment syndrome.

Physical Examination

Ulnocarpal palpation can give some insight into the condition of the TFCC. The synovitis associated with a TFCC tear can render simple palpation of the ulnocarpal joint uncomfortable.

The ulnocarpal compression test (Fig. 22-3) is particularly helpful in assessing the patient with a suspected ulnar abutment syndrome. In this test, the patient sits in front of the examiner with the wrist in supination. The wrist is simultaneously ulnarly deviated and axially loaded while the forearm is supinated and pronated. The patient with an ulnar abutment syndrome experiences pain at the ulnocarpal joint, with or without popping and grinding, during this maneuver.

A variation of the ulnocarpal compression test is the Lester press test (Fig. 22-4).[3] In this test, the patient sits in a chair with sturdy arms and lifts himself or herself off the chair seat. Pain at the ulnocarpal joint is considered pathognomonic for a TFCC tear.

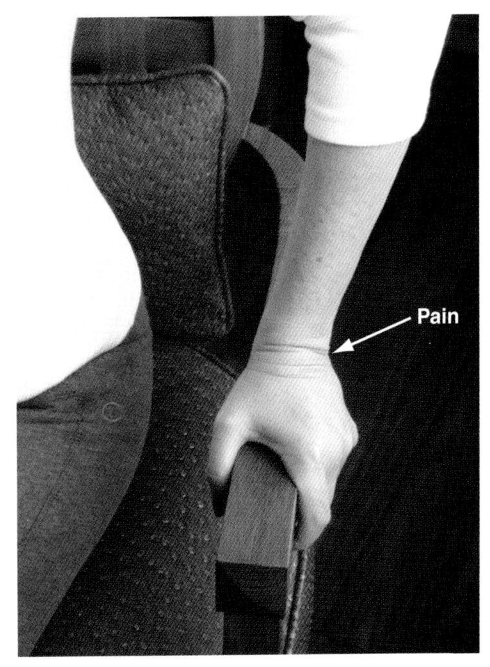

FIGURE 22-4 The Lester press test.

Diagnostic Imaging

The radiographic evaluation of a patient with an ulnar abutment should include a standard wrist series and a Palmer 90 × 90 view (Fig. 22-5). The Palmer 90 × 90 view places the forearm in neutral rotation while the elbow is flexed to 90 degrees and the shoulder is abducted to 90 degrees.[4] The ulnar variance is calculated from this view. An ulnar abutment can be suspected in a patient with an ulnar-zero or ulnar-minus variance. The ulnar aspect of the lunate should be carefully examined for subchondral cysts.

Magnetic resonance imaging (MRI) should be considered when evaluating the patient for ulnar abutment. MRI demonstrates increased signal in the lunate on T2 images (Fig. 22-6), corresponding to a cyst or intraosseous edema. The triangular fibrocartilage

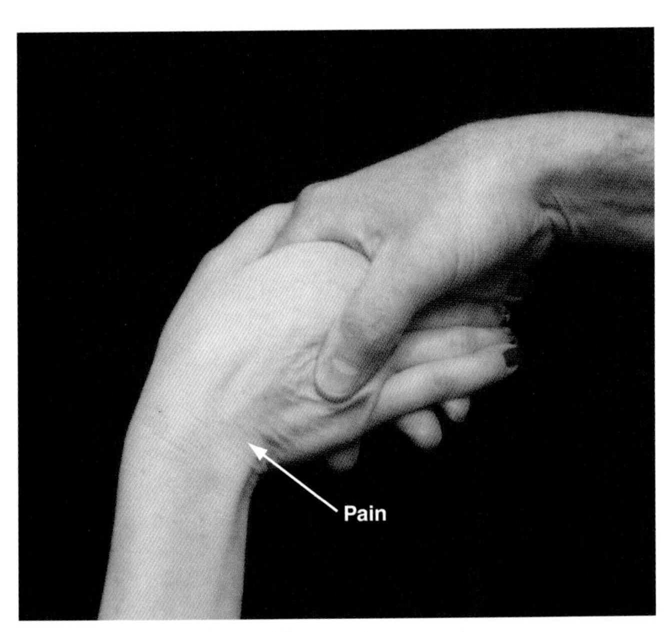

FIGURE 22-3 Ulnocarpal compression test.

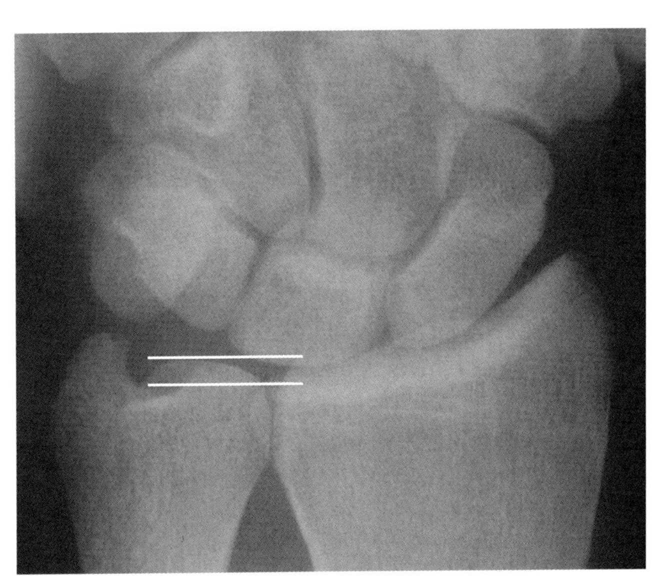

FIGURE 22-5 Ulnar plus variance noted on a Palmer 90 × 90 view.

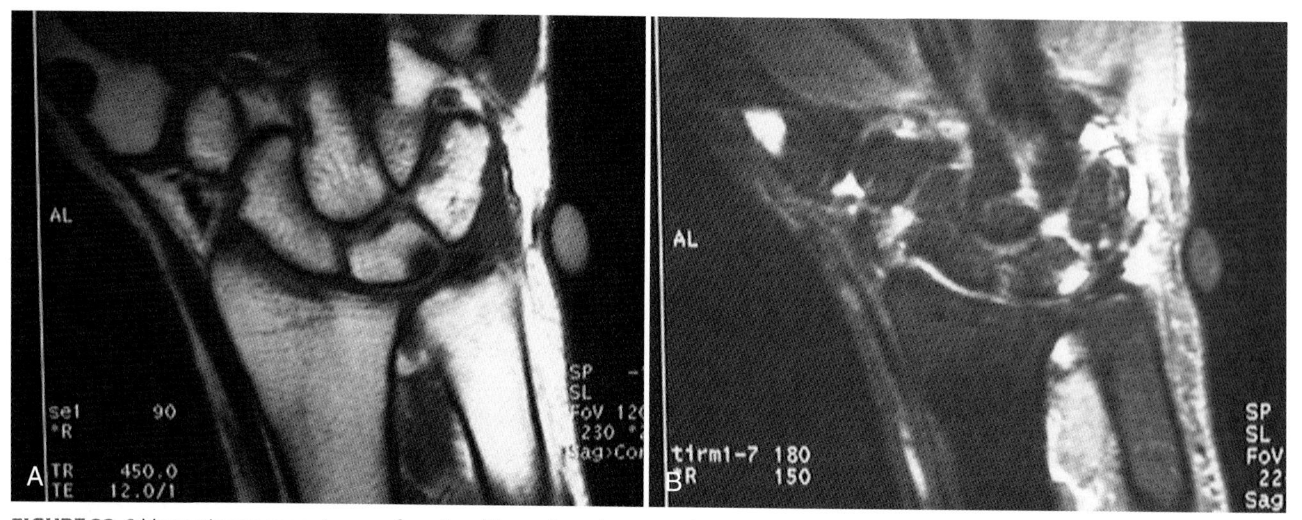

FIGURE 22-6 Magnetic resonance image of a wrist with an ulnar abutment demonstrating the change in signal at the ulnar proximal lunate on T1-weighted and T2-weighted images.

can also be evaluated on the MRI images. Whether a magnetic resonance (MR) arthrogram is needed is a function of the MR resolution. The accuracy of lower-resolution MR is increased with the addition of an intra-articular gadolinium injection.

TREATMENT

Nonoperative Management

Immobilization of the involved wrist with a Munster splint or a long arm cast for 4 weeks, combined with a course of nonsteroidal anti-inflammatory medications, can be helpful in patients who present acutely. A TFCC tear that is exacerbated by specific activities occasionally responds to activity modification.

Indications

The failure of nonoperative treatment (splinting, rest, nonsteroidal anti-inflammatory medications, activity modification and therapy) leads the surgeon and patient to choose surgical treatment.

Preoperative Planning

Preoperative evaluation should include radiographs of the wrist, comprising a wrist series and a 90 × 90 view, as described by Andrew Palmer.[2] An MRI study, with or without an arthrogram, can also be helpful.

The patient must be informed that an arthroscopically assisted ulnar shortening may not be possible if there is laxity of the ulnocarpal ligaments, a peripheral TFCC tear, or a lunatotriquetral laxity. The amount of shortening should be calculated preoperatively. Arthroscopically assisted ulnar shortening is indicated if the ulnar-plus variance is less than 4 mm.

Positioning

The patient is placed in the supine position. A pneumatic tourniquet it is placed on the proximal arm. The patient's involved extremity is prepared and draped in the usual fashion. The wrist is distracted with a commercially available wrist traction device.

Arthroscopic Technique

Triangular Fibrocartilage Complex Débridement: Mechanical

The standard 3-4 and 4-5 or 6-R wrist arthroscopy portals are used for TFCC débridement. These portals should be wide enough to permit the easy passage of instruments. A thorough and systematic examination of the radiocarpal, ulnocarpal, and midcarpal joints should be performed before débriding of the TFCC, as associated intrinsic and extrinsic ligament injury, articular derangement, or synovial pathology could affect the treatment plan. Ulnocarpal synovectomy should be performed to ensure clear visualization of that joint. The initial débridement of the radial, the palmar, and a portion of the dorsal aspect of the TFCC tear is accomplished with an arthroscope in the 3-4 portal while the instruments enter through the 4-5 portal. Small joint punches (straight and angled), graspers, mini-banana blades, and mini-hook knives are used to débride the TFCC. The suction punch is particularly useful. Care should be taken not to injure the overhanging lunate and triquetrum.

After the radial and palmar aspects of the TFCC have been débrided, the arthroscope is moved to the 4-5 portal. The débridement of the ulnar aspect of the triangular fibrocartilage is accomplished with passage of the instruments through the 3-4 portal. Three points must be kept in mind during débridement of the ulnar aspect of the TFCC. The first is to avoid injuring the attachment of the triangular fibrocartilage on its insertion at the base of the ulnar styloid. The second is to avoid injuring the dorsal or palmar radioulnar ligaments. If the ulnar attachment of the TFCC is transected or the dorsal and palmar radioulnar ligaments are injured, distal radioulnar joint instability will result. The third point is to avoid scuffing the articular surfaces while passing the cutting or grasping instruments from the 3-4 portal across the radiocarpal joint and into the ulnocarpal joint.

The dorsal aspect of the TFCC tear usually can be débrided through the 3-4 and 4-5 portals. Occasionally, the instruments

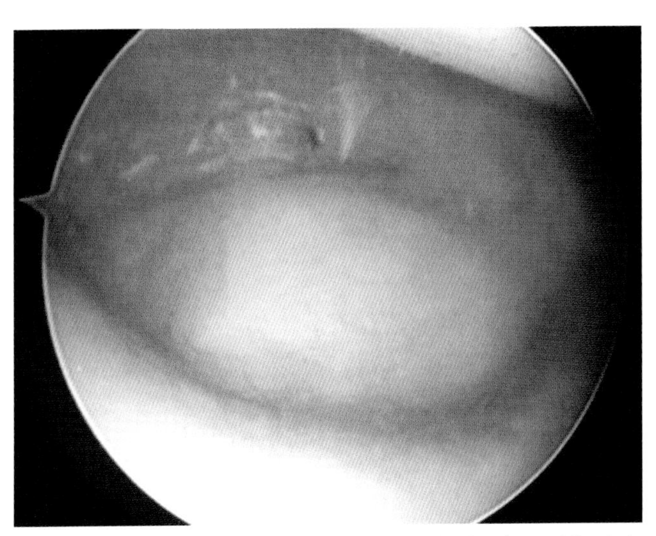

FIGURE 22-7 The triangular fibrocartilage complex has been débrided back to a stable edge. The ulnar head is visible.

need to be passed through the 6-U portal while the arthroscope is placed in the 3-4 portal. Injury to the dorsal sensory branch of the ulnar nerve is avoided when using the 6-U portal with a longitudinal portal incision and blunt dissection to reach the ulnocarpal joint capsule.

After the TFCC has been débrided with the punches and knives, the rough edges of the débrided TFCC are smoothed with the full radius cutters. The 2.0-mm cutters are small but relatively ineffective, whereas the 2.9-mm cutters are effective but must be controlled to avoid collateral damage to the adjacent articular surfaces.

The end point of TFCC débridement is reached when the ulnar head is visible through the TFCC and a stable TFCC perimeter is created (Fig. 22-7). Typically, a central defect measuring at least 1 cm in diameter is created.

Triangular Fibrocartilage Complex Débridement: Laser and Radiofrequency Technique

Mechanical débridement of the triangular fibrocartilage has been successful, although it can be challenging, particularly in regard to débridement of the ulnar and dorsal aspects of the triangular fibrocartilage tear. There are two potential problems with mechanical TFCC débridement. First, the passage of the instruments across the radiocarpal joint places those joints at risk for scuffing. Second, the proximity of the arthroscope to the operative site (TFCC) can distort the operator's perception of the ulnocarpal joint.

The technique of laser-assisted triangular fibrocartilage débridement is similar to that of mechanical débridement of the triangular fibrocartilage, except that the arthroscope can be left in the 3-4 portal while the laser probe is kept in the 4-5 portal. The laser is set to 1.4 to 1.6 joules at a frequency of 15 pulses per second. With the help of a side-firing 70-degree laser tip, the triangular fibrocartilage can be very rapidly and precisely débrided. The 70-degree laser tip permits ablation of the radial and palmar portions of the TFCC tear, as well as the ulnar and dorsal components. There is no need to bring the laser probe in through the 3-4 portal.

Radiofrequency devices have become increasing popular for TFCC débridement because of their small probe size and relatively low cost. The technique is similar to that used for laser-assisted TFCC débridement. Monopolar and bipolar radiofrequency devices are currently in use. The instrument settings vary with the device. Monopolar probes have a theoretical disadvantage in that the energy imparted to the TFCC flows through the adjacent tissue in the direction of the grounding pad. This could lead to tissue damage beyond the TFCC. The flow of irrigation fluid must be sufficient to cool the joint when radiofrequency devices are used.

Arthroscopic Ulnar Shortening Technique

Arthroscopic ulnar shortening is accomplished by placing the arthroscope in the 3-4 portal and introducing the instruments

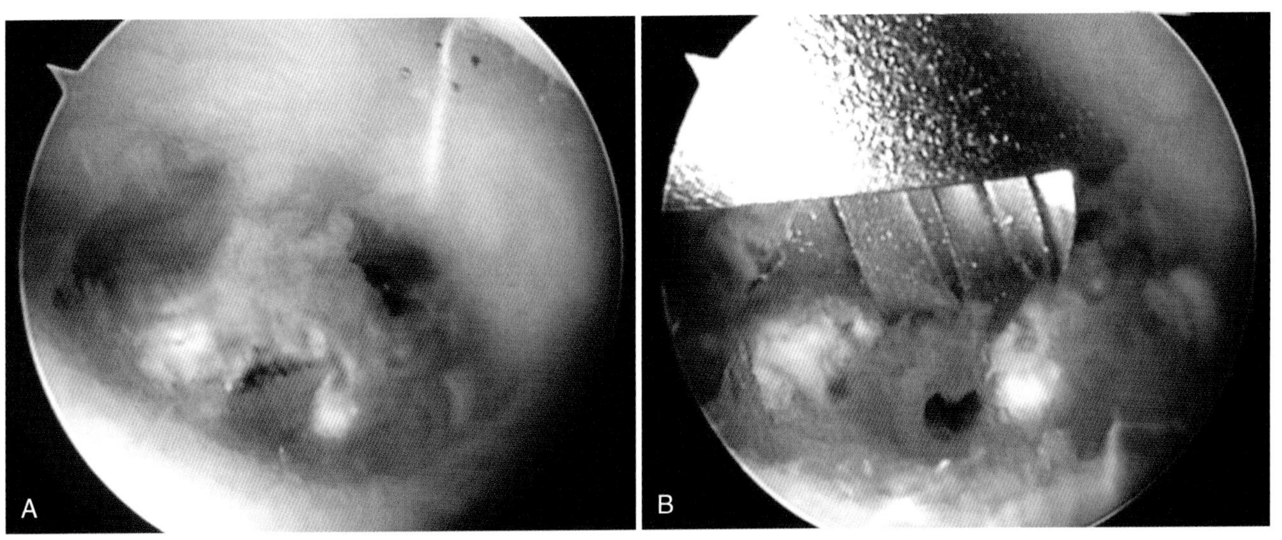

FIGURE 22-8 A, The hyaline cartilage of the ulnar seat has been débrided with the laser. **B,** The subchondral bone is being débrided using the barrel abrader.

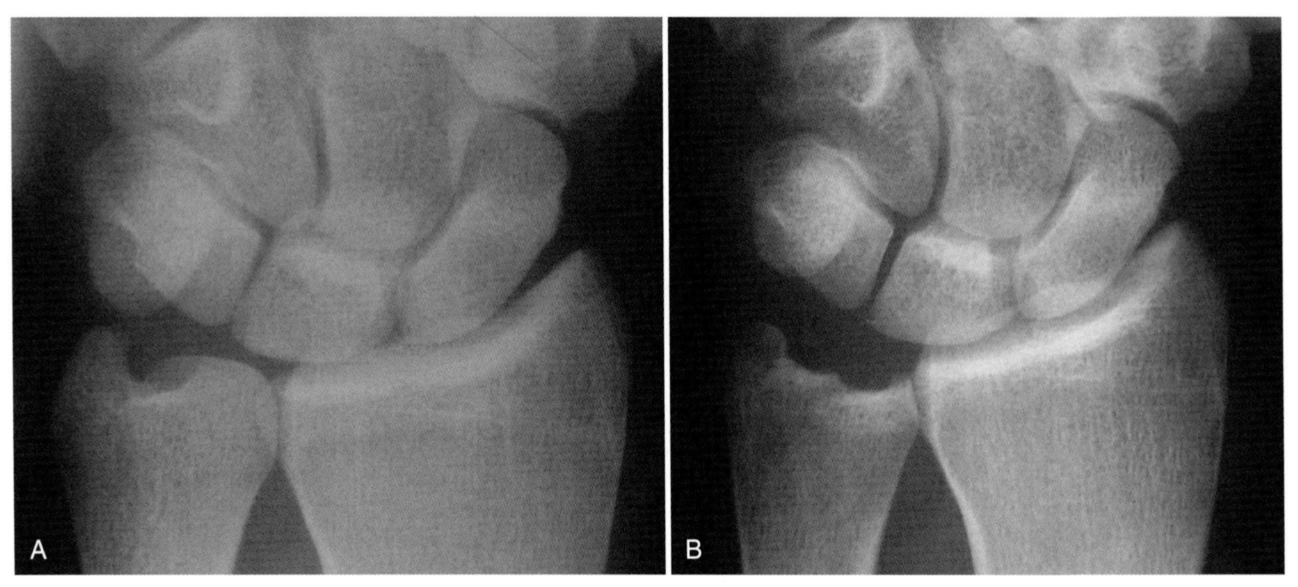

FIGURE 22-9 A, Preoperative radiograph. **B,** Preoperative radiograph.

through the 4-5 portal. Occasionally, the 6-U portal can be used, as can the distal radioulnar joint portal. Although the holmium: yttrium-aluminum-garnet (Ho:YAG) laser is very useful for ulnar shortening, the barrel abrader can be used alone or in combination with the laser. If the Ho:YAG laser is used, it is introduced through the 4-5 portal, and the cartilage and subchondral bone of the ulnar seat of the distal ulna are rapidly vaporized (Fig. 22-8A). The laser becomes less efficient after the trabeculae of the distal ulna are visible. At that point, the 2.9-mm barrel abrader is brought in to finish the shortening (Fig. 22-8B). It is important to avoid injury to the sigmoid notch, and frequent fluoroscopic monitoring of the amount of bone resected is mandatory. Care must be taken to fully supinate and pronate the wrist to adequately débride the ulnar head. All instruments are removed at the end of the procedure, and the wrist is ulnarly deviated, axially loaded, supinated, and pronated to be sure no clicking or popping can be heard. If any clicking or popping emanates from the area of the surgery, further ulnar resection may be required. The goal of the surgery is to create an ulnar-minus variance of 2 mm (Fig. 22-9). Any irregularities of the remaining distal ulna should be minimized. Small irregularities, however, have a tendency to flatten out with the passage of time.

PEARLS & PITFALLS

- Arthroscopically assisted ulnar shortening should not be combined with other procedures that require postoperative wrist immobilization, because early mobilization is critical after an ulnar shortening.
- The 4-5 and 6-R portals should be placed just distal to the distal surface of the TFCC, because distal placement of the portals can lead to scuffing of the lunate and triquetrum. The surgeon should be mindful of the presence of the dorsal branch of the ulnar nerve. This nerve is at risk during the creation of all ulnar portals.
- Injury to the underlying tendons and nerves can be avoided by creating portals using a no. 15 blade held gently against skin, which is moved beneath the blade. Small, transverse incisions in Langer's lines, closed with a subcuticular Prolene, produce a superior cosmetic result. After the skin is cut, blunt dissection with a Hartmann hemostat should be used to dissect through the subcutaneous tissue and penetrate the wrist joint capsule. The curve of the Hartmann hemostat follows the palmar tilt of the distal radius.
- The 1.9-mm arthroscopes are perfectly suited to wrist arthroscopy. Their small size lessens the likelihood of scuffing of the wrist joint articular surfaces.
- Débridement of the TFCC tear must be performed carefully to avoid injury to the peripheral attachments of the TFCC and the dorsal and palmar radioulnar ligaments. Overaggressive débridement can lead to distal radioulnar joint instability.
- A systematic approach to excision of ulnar head is critical. The assistant must take the wrist from full supination to full pronation while the operator maintains the arthroscope in the 3-4 portal and the instruments in the ulnar portals. The ulnar head is débrided as it is presented to the surgeon by the assistant during rotation of the distal radioulnar joint.
- Rehabilitation of the patient is essential to the ultimate success of the procedure. The wrist should not be loaded for at least 4 to 6 weeks.

Postoperative Management

Postoperative care of these patients includes the application of a volar splint, followed by early range of motion. Early range of motion is critical, because it leads to a more supple scar and a better range of motion.

Wounds are closed using subcuticular sutures of 4-0 Prolene; the sutures are removed after 2 weeks. Strengthening exercises can be started at 6 weeks if needed. Premature resumption of heavy lifting or repetitive activities will lead to ulnocarpal synovitis. The patient is instructed to avoid heavy lifting for 3 months.

Typically, patients are able to return to unrestricted activities in 12 weeks, although they may experience some discomfort for 6 to 12 months.

CONCLUSIONS

The results of arthroscopic débridement of traumatic triangular fibrocartilage tears have been very good.[5,6] However, Minami and colleagues[7] found that degenerative tears (Palmer type 2) have a less favorable prognosis because of their associated ulnar wrist pathology. Our results[8] and those reported by Osterman[9] and Palmer[10] suggest that arthroscopically assisted ulnar shortening in properly selected patients provides excellent or good results in more than 80% of cases.

REFERENCES

1. Kleinman WB. Stability of the distal radioulnar joint: biomechanics, pathophysiology, physical diagnosis, and restoration of function. What we have learned in 25 years. *J Hand Surg Am*. 2007;32:1086-1106.
2. Palmer AK, Glisson RR, Werner FW. Relationship between ulnar variance and triangular fibrocartilage complex thickness. *J Hand Surg Am*. 1984;9:681-682.
3. Lester B, Halbrecht J, Levy IM, Gaudinez R. "Press test" for office diagnosis of triangular fibrocartilage complex tears of the wrist. *Ann Plast Surg*. 1995;35:41-45.
4. Palmer AK, Glisson RR, Werner FW. Ulnar variance determination. *J Hand Surg Am*. 1982;7:376-379
5. Husby T, Haugstvedt JR. Long-term results after arthroscopic resection of lesions of the triangular fibrocartilage complex. *Scand J Plast Reconstr Surg Hand Surg*. 2001;35:79-83.
6. Infanger M, Grimm D. Meniscus and discus lesions of triangular fibrocartilage complex (TFCC): treatment by laser-assisted wrist arthroscopy. *J Plast Reconstr Aesthet Surg*. 2009;62:466-471.
7. Minami A, Ishikawa J, Suenaga N, Kasashima T. Clinical results of treatment of triangular fibrocartilage complex tears by arthroscopic debridement. *J Hand Surg Am*. 1996;21:406-411.
8. Nagle DJ, Bernstein MA. Laser-assisted arthroscopic ulnar shortening. *Arthroscopy*. 2002;18:1046-1051.
9. Osterman AL. Arthroscopic debridement of triangular fibrocartilage complex tears. *Arthroscopy*. 1990;6:120-124.
10. Wnorowski DC, Palmer AK, Werner FW, Fortino MD. Anatomic and biomechanical analysis of the arthroscopic wafer procedure. *Arthroscopy*. 1992;8:204-212.

CHAPTER

23

Arthroscopic Excision of Dorsal Ganglions

A. Lee Osterman • Scott Edwards

Arthroscopic dorsal wrist ganglion resection offers several theoretical advantages over open techniques, including improved recovery, better joint visualization, lower complication and recurrence rates, and more satisfying cosmetic results. Initial outcomes after arthroscopic resection of dorsal wrist ganglia have been favorable.[1-3] Although arthroscopic resection of dorsal wrist ganglion cysts is a procedure that is becoming more accepted, several questions remain unanswered. Based on a critical view of the sparse literature on the subject and on clinical observations, this chapter attempts to clarify the ambiguity surrounding arthroscopic dorsal wrist ganglion resection and to determine whether this is a useful technique to add to the arsenal or a triumph of technology over reason.

ANATOMY

Intra-articular Cystic Stalks

In the current literature, the exact roles of intra-articular cystic stalks are somewhat vague. Earlier reports implied, but did not specifically state, that identification and surgical excision of the stalk are paramount when standard arthroscopic techniques are used for ganglion excision. However, the presence of this important structure has been variably reported in the literature. Osterman and Raphael[1] identified a stalk in two thirds of their patients undergoing arthroscopic ganglion excision. Although one third of their patients had no identifiable stalk, ganglions were successfully excised with no recurrences. Other studies have reported a stalk incidence as low as 10%.[2-4] Despite vastly different reports on stalk identification, the importance of such pathology must be questioned. Rather than a cystic stalk, Edwards and Johansen[4] described intra-articular cystic material and redundant capsular tissue in most of their patients with ganglion cysts. This finding, which was more consistently evident than the stalk, was the focus of their resection.

The intra-articular limitations of arthroscopic viewing may explain the paucity of stalk identification. The radiocarpal and midcarpal joints are separated by the extrinsic capsular ligaments. At this separation, the dorsal capsular reflection is adherent to the interosseous scapholunate ligament. It is possible for a ganglion stalk to travel toward the scapholunate ligament within the substance of the dorsal capsular reflection, rather than through the radiocarpal or midcarpal spaces, and the stalk may never be visualized by arthroscopy. Certain observations during arthroscopic resections may support this theory. On several occasions, extravasations of cystic fluid were observed during débridement of the dorsal capsular reflection between the radiocarpal and midcarpal joints when stalks had not been visualized in either compartment. In other words, the stalk might have been hidden within the dorsal capsular extrinsic ligaments.

Intra-articular Associations

The dorsal ganglion may be an overt sign of intra-articular pathology. Povlsen and Peckett[5] found intra-articular abnormalities in 75% of patients with painful ganglia. They concluded that, like the popliteal cyst in the knee, the dorsal ganglion was a marker of joint abnormality. Osterman and Raphael[1] found abnormalities in 42% of their cases, predominately findings at the scapholunate ligament (24%), the triangular fibrocartilage (8%), and the lunatotriquetral ligament (3%) and significant chondromalacia. Despite the fact that only the ganglion was treated, wrist pain resolved in all cases. Edwards and Johansen[4] elaborated on this notion by showing that most ganglia are associated with type II and III scapholunate and type III lunatotriquetral laxity (Table 23-1). Although it is reasonable to propose that increased intercarpal laxity may contribute to ganglion formation, the actual significance is unclear, given that the natural incidence of these ligamentous laxities in the general population is not known.

TABLE 23-1 Classification of Intracarpal Instability

Grade	Description
I	Attenuation and/or hemorrhage of interosseous ligament as observed from the radiocarpal joint. No incongruence of carpal alignment in midcarpal space.
II	Attenuation and/or hemorrhage of interosseous ligament as observed from the radiocarpal joint. Incongruence and/or step-off as observed from midcarpal space. A slight gap (<2 mm) between carpals may be present.
III	Incongruence and/or step-off of carpal alignment are observed in the radiocarpal and midcarpal spaces. The width of a 2-mm probe may be passed through the gap between carpals.
IV	Incongruence and/or step-off of carpal alignment are observed in the radiocarpal and midcarpal spaces. Gross instability occurs with manipulation. A 2.7-mm arthroscope may be passed through the gap between carpals.

Adapted from Geissler WB, Freeland AE, Savoie FH, et al. Intracarpal soft-tissue lesions associated with an intra-articular fracture of the distal end of the radius. J Bone Joint Surg Am. *1996;78:357-365.*

PATIENT EVALUATION

History and Physical Examination

The first question to answer when a patient presents with a mass is whether it is a cyst or a tumor. Many elements of the history and physical examination are not conclusive. Occurrence, progression, size, shape, texture, presence or absence of pain, and association with traumatic or repetitive activities provide little more than suggestions either way. One element of history, however, can be quite helpful in determining whether the lesion is cystic. Cysts and tumors get larger, but only cysts get smaller. There are rare exceptions to this rule, such as some vascular tumors that involute over a period of months to years, but cysts can decrease in size as quickly as overnight. On physical examination, transillumination can be helpful to differentiate a cyst from a tumor. This is performed by holding a penlight up against the lesion. A cystic lesion allows the light to transmit through its fluid medium, whereas the solid tissue of a tumor prevents any propagation of light.

Occasionally, cysts may herald a more dubious underlying pathology, such as a scapholunate ligament injury. The history and physical examination should focus on any recent or remote trauma. Often, patients have incompetent scapholunate ligaments that remain clinically unapparent until the manifestation of an associated ganglion cyst. Palpation of the dorsal portion of the scapholunate ligament, a positive Watson scaphoid shift test, or a positive straight finger resistance test may suggest scapholunate ligament pathology. Cysts may resemble other pathologies, such as gouty tophus, tenosynovitis, and rheumatoid pannus. A careful history and physical examination should suffice to differentiate these conditions.

Diagnostic Imaging

MRI and ultrasonography remain the imaging modalities most commonly used to differentiate fluid-filled cysts from solid tumors. Although both perform this task with equal reliability, MRI may suggest an etiology of a solid tumor, whereas ultrasonography cannot. Nevertheless, there has been a shift toward ultrasonography as the preferred technique, given its lesser comparable cost. Very small ganglions, although clinically significant, can be readily overlooked by both types of imaging. Surgeons should keep a high index of suspicion for these lesions even if the face of a negative reading.

TREATMENT

Nonoperative Management

Although there is no consensus about the best nonoperative treatment for ganglion cysts, restriction of wrist activity seems to be well accepted. The efficacy of anti-inflammatory medications is more controversial. Some believe that reducing inflammation is helpful for patients with painful cysts, whereas others believe that these medications may make the cystic fluid less viscous and possibly more likely to spontaneously decompress. Neither belief has been substantiated in the literature. Needle aspiration seems to be relatively safe for dorsal ganglion cysts, but volar ganglions place neurovascular structures at particular risk with blind aspiration. Patients need to understand that recurrences after aspiration can be high. In summary, nonoperative treatments for dorsal ganglion cysts are unpredictable, and the evidence to support such measures is largely anecdotal. However, most surgeons attempt a trial of nonoperative treatment before committing the patient to surgical excision.

Indications and Contraindications

Indications and contraindications for arthroscopic dorsal wrist ganglion resection are still evolving. Ho and colleagues[2] reported two recurrences after resection of ganglia originating from the midcarpal joint. They concluded that arthroscopic resection was not indicated for cysts originating from the midcarpal joint. Many would agree that most dorsal wrist ganglia originate from the scapholunate interval. Given the capsular limitation in the wrist, this interval is only partially visualized from the radiocarpal joint. One study[4] observed that cysts communicated with the midcarpal joint in 75% of cases. In the same report, 25% of cysts were accessed exclusively through the midcarpal joint, which suggests that evaluation of the midcarpal joint is mandatory for successful resection. Whereas most cysts may be resected successfully through an isolated radiocarpal portal, some require supplemental débridement from the midcarpal joint.

Regarding recurrent cysts, one group of investigators suggested that recurrent cysts after previous open surgical excision should be considered a contraindication for arthroscopic resection.[6] Appropriate concerns are the risk of injury to the extensor tendons because of their potential displacement by the scar from the previous surgery. For this reason, most studies have identified recurrence as an exclusion criterion. One significant exception was a series in which 15% of the patients had recurrent ganglia, and outcomes were comparable to those of primary cyst resections. Based on this experience, the authors stated that arthroscopic resection of recurrent cysts is not contraindicated. In fact, it may be helpful in identifying a potential cause of the recurrence. Studies have identified intra-articular abnormalities such as ligament tears, excessive intercarpal laxities, chondromalacia, and triangular fibrocartilage tears as being associated with ganglion cysts.[1,4] It is unclear whether such findings contribute to cystic development, but, to the degree that they have a role, arthroscopy is more effective than open excision at identifying and addressing these abnormalities. Given a recurrent cyst, an arthroscopic evaluation may identify a partial scapholunate ligament tear that could be débrided, thereby lowering the probability of further recurrence. An open technique may not identify the cause as easily and therefore may doom the recurrent excision to another recurrence.

Cosmetic reasons sometime drive decisions to pursue any endoscopic technique. Although an open incision across the dorsum of the wrist may not seem excessive to a surgeon, the patient may have another perspective. One study reported a very high postoperative satisfaction rate, despite the fact that 17% of the patients were asymptomatic preoperatively and opted surgery for cosmetic reasons.[4] There has been no similar report for open resections. The implication is that it would be reasonable to offer arthroscopic ganglion resections for patients who are primarily interested in the cosmetic appearance of their hands.

Arthroscopic Technique

Before excision of a dorsal wrist ganglion, a tourniquet is placed as a precaution, and it is inflated in the event that intra-articular bleeding obscures visualization. While the patient's arm is suspended in a traction tower with 5 to 10 pounds of traction applied, a 6-R or 6-U portal is created as a visualization portal. The more radial 3-4 or 4-5 portal is avoided at this time, to prevent inadvertent decompression of the cyst. After the 2.7-mm arthroscopic camera is directed toward the dorsal compartment of the wrist, the capsule adjacent to the scapholunate ligament can be visualized. Occasionally, a sessile or pedunculated protrusion into the joint can be seen in the area where the extrinsic capsule joins the distal portion of the dorsal scapholunate ligament. This capsular reflection serves as part of the barrier between the radiocarpal and midcarpal joints, and the protrusion located here has been termed the cystic stalk (Fig. 23-1). More often, the surgeon may be impressed with the amount of synovitis and redundant capsule in this area instead of an actual stalk.

A common technique for arthroscopic ganglionectomy is to place the shaver through the cystic sac, because it often resides directly over the usual 3-4 portal. This action decompresses the cyst and may obscure any presence of an intra-articular stalk. Some think that this has some therapeutic benefit, whereas critics of the procedure argue that arthroscopic excisions are nothing more than glorified aspirations. We recommend a method that attempts to avoid decompressing the cyst with the shaver before excision, so as to observe the possibility of an undisturbed cystic stalk and its path elsewhere outside the radiocarpal joint. The working portal is created adjacent to the immediate area of the cyst, rather than directly over the 3-4 portal. This modified working portal is usually just distal and sometimes slightly radial to the actual 3-4 portal. A 2.9-mm, full-radius shaver is introduced through this portal, and every effort is made to avoid decompressing the cyst with simple introduction of the shaver.

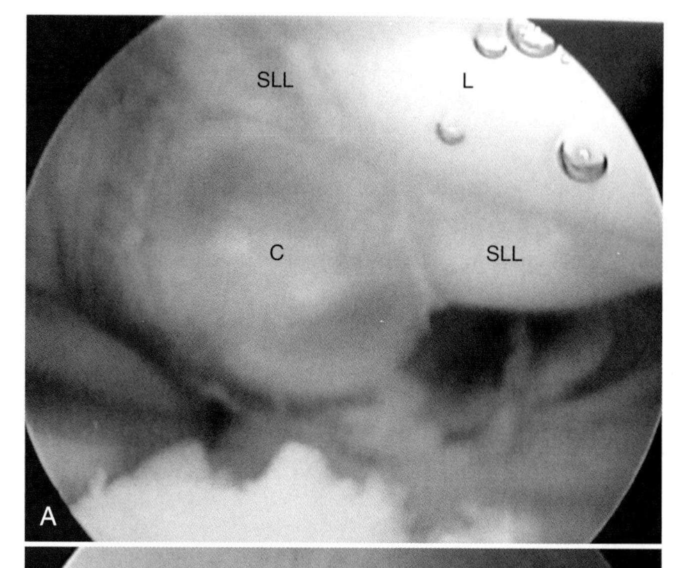

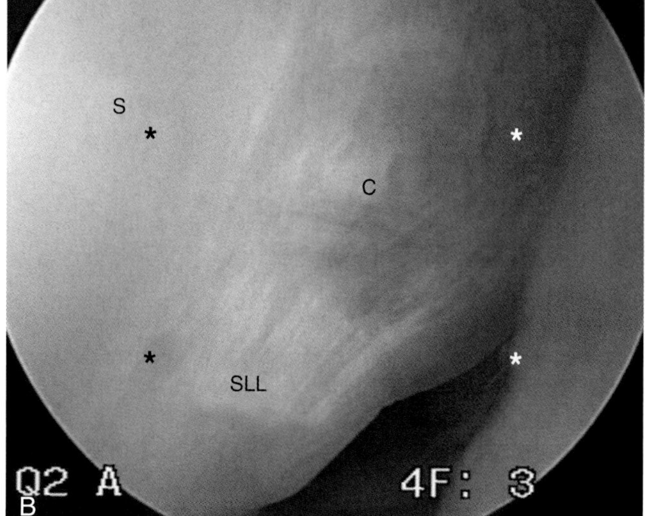

FIGURE 23-1 Cystic stalks. **A,** Pedunculated. **B,** Sessile. C, cyst; L, lunate; SLL, scapholunate ligament.

Although the procedure implies that the cyst is removed by the arthroscope, this is often not the case. The arthroscopy procedure disrupts the communication between the cyst and the joint, leaving behind a deflated sac that cannot re-inflate. Eventually, the empty sac is resorbed. Recurrences can happen only if another cyst is generated.

The focus of the resection begins at the site of the ganglion stalk or redundant capsular material, if identified. This billowing, redundant material appears different from typical reactive synovitis. Although its exact significance is unclear, it seems to be continuous with the capsule that lies adjacent to the cyst. With this landmark, surgeons may confidently begin the capsulotomy. If neither structure is identified, the débridement begins adjacent to the dorsal scapholunate ligament and distal capsular reflection. Commonly, the cyst travels within the capsular reflection as it communicates with the scapholunate joint. Care should be taken to keep the blade of the shaver away from the scapholunate ligament at all times. On initial débridement of the capsular reflection, occasionally a flash of viscous cystic fluid may be visual-

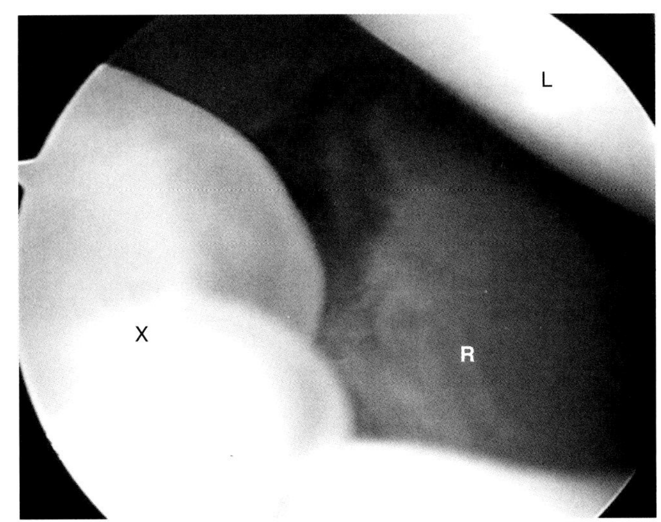

FIGURE 23-2 Complete capsulotomy communicating with the extra-articular space. Notice the visualization of the extensor tendons.

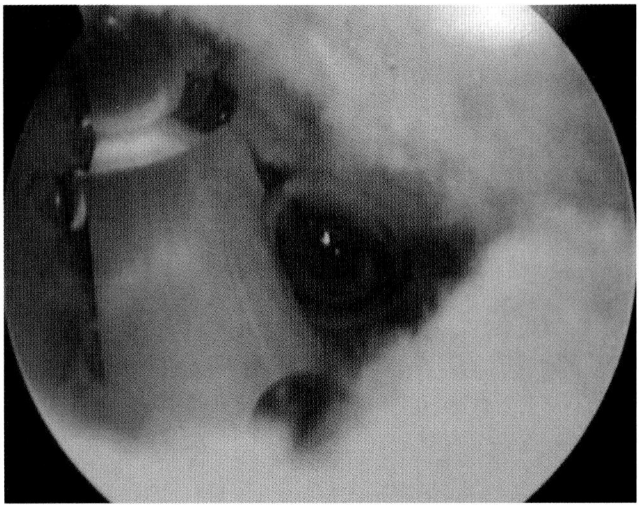

FIGURE 23-3 Redundant capsule and diffuse cystic material. There is no defined cystic stalk. C, cyst; L, lunate, SLL, scapholunate ligament.

ized escaping into the joint. Débridement continues until approximately 1 cm of capsule has been removed.

A common mistake is to make the capsulotomy too small, which is easy to do under magnification. The 2.9-mm shaver is helpful as a reference in gauging the size of the capsulotomy. Another common mistake is to create an incomplete capsulotomy that fails to communicate with the extra-articular space. We advise direct visualization of the extensor tendons to verify that a complete capsulotomy has been performed (Fig. 23-2). Removal of the cystic sac is not necessary, because it often resorbs over time after it is detached from its origin at the joint. If the cyst is particularly large, resorption may take some time, and patients may complain about residual prominence on the dorsum of the hand. Removal of the truncated sac may be performed by pulling it out of the 3-4 portal with a hemostat. Because this is a blind maneuver and the risk of neuroma formation is relatively high, we think that, if removal of the cystic sac is elected, it should be done arthroscopically from inside the joint, provided that the surgeon is comfortable with the technique. Careful extensor tenosynovectomy may be performed at the same time with the shaver, if desired.

To remedy this situation, the arthroscopic camera is introduced through an ulnar midcarpal portal, and a similar capsulotomy is performed adjacent to the scapholunate interval through the radial midcarpal portal. Often, during débridement from the midcarpal joint, a fenestration is created between the midcarpal and radiocarpal joint through the capsular reflection. On removal of the arthroscopic equipment, the wrist is palpated again to ensure that the cyst has been completely excised. This can be difficult, especially if there is fluid extravasation, if substantial amounts of adipose tissue obscure the cyst, or if a very small cyst is present before resection.

Some surgeons close each arthroscopic portal with one simple nonabsorbable suture, but others leave them open with no cosmetic detriment. Open arthroscopic wounds can rarely form sinus tracts, as reported in other joints, so we prefer to close these wounds. A sterile wrist dressing is used in all cases. Splinting for 1 week has been advocated by some, but others believe splinting to be unnecessary.

PEARLS & PITFALLS

- If the cyst is decompressed prematurely by introduction of the instruments, the surgeon cannot confirm by palpation whether the cyst was adequately resected or simply decompressed with a "glorified aspiration."
- A cystic stalk seems to be present variably, and its presence appears to have no effect on the outcomes of the resection. Redundant capsular material (Fig. 23-3) has been described and is reported to serve as a more reliable landmark for resection.
- Know what the shaver is cutting. It takes some pressure to cut into the extrinsic ligaments of the wrist, which is necessary for a complete capsulotomy, and that same pressure may easily cut inadvertently into an extensor tendon lying on the other side of the capsule. Even the most experienced arthroscopists should stop frequently and reassess the terrain.
- After the capsulotomy and cyst excision have been completed from the radiocarpal joint, the camera is removed and the dorsal wrist is palpated to determine the efficacy of the débridement. If a portion of the cyst remains, there is some degree of communication between the cyst and the midcarpal joint that has not yet been addressed.

Postoperative Rehabilitation

Immediately postoperatively, digital motion is encouraged; sutures are removed in 7 to 10 days. Very seldom is any supervised therapy required. If there is residual fullness over the ganglion or its portal, the use of an elastomer as a pressure scar modulator may be helpful. Activity is resumed as tolerated, and the patient is advised against forceful loading of the wrist for 4 weeks. The theoretical advantages of a minimally invasive procedure to reliably remove wrist ganglion cysts seem intuitive but have not been validated until recently. Reduced recovery times, less postoperative pain, and quicker returns to work and athletics have been reported.[4,6]

Patients can expect decreased pain and increased function within 6 weeks after surgery. Outcome surveys, often regarded as the most important assessment of patients, have documented considerable improvements in the short and the long term.[4] However, positive short-term outcomes cannot be referenced to open excisions, because there have not been comparable reports dealing with these procedures.

Although an increasing number of studies have demonstrated that arthroscopic ganglion resection is a safe and effective technique with a predictable and easy recovery, there has been only one prospective, randomized study comparing arthroscopic resection with more traditional open techniques.[7] This study evaluated patients at 4 to 8 weeks and again at 1 year postoperatively and could find no difference in outcomes. Most would agree, however, that the true benefits of a minimally invasive arthroscopy would be most profound within the first 4 weeks. No study has compared the two techniques and specifically assessed patient outcome during this defining time. Until this is done, it is difficult to make any meaningful comparisons between arthroscopic and open resections.

RECURRENCES AND COMPLICATIONS

Recurrence rates have been low (0% to 10%) in virtually every report,[1-3] implying that the recurrence rate for arthroscopic resection may be less than that for open excision, which typically has slightly higher recurrence rates. However, most studies had small cohort sizes, selection bias, and poorly defined follow-up, all of which could potentially distort the actual recurrence rates. In four separate studies[3,4,7,8] with a combined cohort of 233 patients undergoing arthroscopic ganglion resection and an average follow-up of 2 years, only seven recurrences were reported. One prospective series[8] comparing arthroscopic and open resection found no statistical difference in recurrence rates (10.7% versus 8.7%, respectively). Based on a critical review of the relevant literature, recurrence rates for open and arthroscopic techniques are similar and should not be the sole determining factor in selecting either technique.

Complications of open ganglion resections have been reported and include neuroma formation and scapholunate ligament laceration. Similar complications for arthroscopic resections have not been reported. Although arthroscopy may prove to be a safer method of excision, other reasons may explain this discrepancy in the literature. First, more reports on open ganglion resections have been published, and, consequently, more complications have been reported with this technique from a statistical standpoint. Second, much of the literature on open ganglion resections is older; the more recent studies do not report the same variety and extent of complications. We may surmise that techniques have improved, making these previously reported complications not as prevalent.

Reactive tenosynovitis may occur after any arthroscopic procedure, although not commonly. Reports of this complication after wrist arthroscopy are rare. One study evaluating the complications of wrist arthroscopy not limited to ganglionectomy reviewed 210 cases and found "extensor tendon irritation" in only 4 cases.[9] There has been only one report of extensor tenosynovitis after arthroscopic ganglion resection; in that series, it occurred in 6% of patients. This higher incidence was attributed to the extensive capsulotomy required during ganglion excision that does not occur during other arthroscopic procedures. In any case, the risk of extensor synovitis should be part of the preoperative discussion with patients.

CONCLUSIONS

A summation of the literature and clinical experience on arthroscopic dorsal wrist ganglion resection has quieted the debate on several issues but still leaves some issues open. First, patients can experience significant increases in function and decreases in pain within 6 weeks after arthroscopic dorsal wrist ganglion resection, and these initial benefits can be expected to be maintained for at least 2 years. Second, the recurrence and complication rates for arthroscopic ganglion resection appear to be comparable to, if not less than, that those reported for open resections. Third, ganglion cysts have a high association with intra-articular abnormalities, but the significance of this finding is unclear. Fourth, despite previous reports, recurrent ganglia and ganglia originating from the midcarpal joint are not contraindications for arthroscopic resection. In fact, assessment of the midcarpal joint is necessary for complete resection of most ganglia. Identification of a discrete stalk is not always necessary for successful resection. Rather, attention should be focused on any cystic material or redundant capsular thickening within the joints and on performing an adequate capsulotomy.

The debate about whether arthroscopic dorsal wrist ganglion resection is preferable to open resection has shifted issues. Concerns of recurrence and long-term efficacy have been put to rest, because they have been determined to be equivalent in the two approaches. The debate has now turned to whether arthroscopic resection offers patients any benefits in terms of decreased pain and increased motion, compared with open resection, in the initial postoperative course. Further comparative investigations specifically focusing on the immediate short term are required to answer this question. At the very least, arthroscopic ganglion resection remains a safe and effective technique to offer patients.

REFERENCES

1. Osterman AL, Raphael J. Arthroscopic resection of dorsal wrist ganglion of the wrist. *Hand Clin*. 1995;11:7-12.
2. Ho PC, Griffiths J, Lo WN, et al. Current treatment of ganglion at the wrist. *J Hand Surg*. 2001;6:49-58.
3. Rizzo M, Berger RA, Steinman SP, Bishop AT. Arthroscopic resection in the management of dorsal wrist ganglion: results with a minimum 2-yr follow-up period. *J Hand Surg*. 2004;29:59-62.
4. Edwards SG, Johansen JA. Prospective outcomes and associations of wrist ganglion cysts resected arthroscopically. *J Hand Surg*. 2009;34:395-400.
5. Povlsen B, Peckett WR. Arthroscopic findings in patients with painful wrist ganglia. *Scand J Plast Reconstr Surg Hand Surg*. 2001;35:323-328.
6. Singh D, Culp R. Arthroscopic ganglion excisions. Presented at the American Society for Surgery of the Hand (ASSH) meeting, 2002. Phoenix, Ariz.
7. Mathoulin C, Hoyos A, Pelaez J. Arthroscopic resection of wrist ganglia. *Hand Surg*. 2004;9:159-164.
8. Kang L, Akelman E, Weiss AP. Arthroscopic versus open dorsal ganglion excision: a prospective, randomized comparison of rate of recurrence and of residual pain. *J Hand Surg*. 2008;33:471-475.
9. Beredjiklian PK, Bozenka DJ, Leung YL, Monaghan BA. Complications of wrist arthroscopy. *J Hand Surg*. 2004;29:406-411.
10. Geissler WB, Freeland AE, Savoie FH, et al. Intracarpal soft-tissue lesions associated with an intra-articular fracture of the distal end of the radius. *J Bone Joint Surg Am*. 1996;78:357-365.

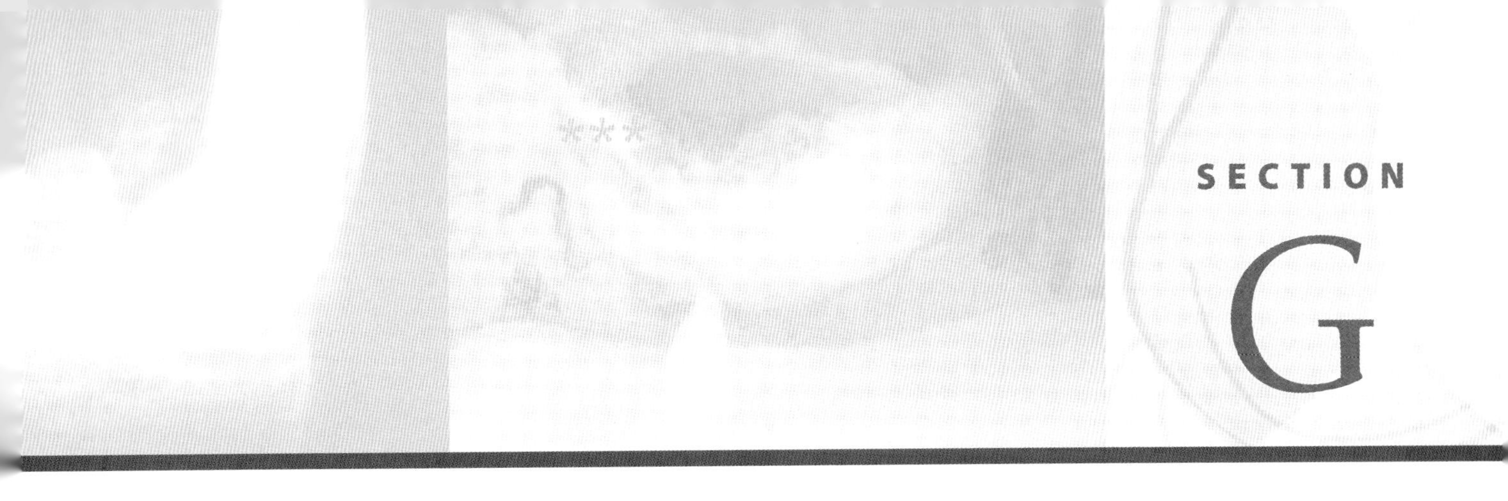

SECTION

G

Advanced Procedures

CHAPTER

24

Lunotriquetral Tears

Michael J. Moskal

After a thorough history, physical examination, and ancillary radiographic imaging, wrist arthroscopy further characterizes a wrist injury to better guide treatment. Arthroscopic evaluation is particularly valuable to examine the anatomy and pathoanatomy of ulnar-sided wrist disorders.[1] Lunotriquetral (LT) interosseous ligament tears may exist in isolation but often are part of a broader spectrum of wrist pathology. The arthroscopic treatment of ulnar-side pathology with LT interosseous ligament tears often includes débridement and synovectomy, repair of chondral injuries and triangular fibrocartilage tears, and LT joint arthroscopic reduction and internal fixation (ARIF).

ANATOMY

The LT interosseous ligament is thicker volarly and dorsally,[2] with a membranous central portion that is not uncommonly torn without resulting in instability; these tears are clinically insignificant. Clinically significant LT instability arises from intrinsic and extrinsic ligamentous injuries.[3-5] Key anatomy for the arthroscopic treatment of LT tears is based on the normal ulnar-sided anatomy. Ulnar-sided stability is imparted from the integrity of the LT ligament[3] in association with the ulnolunate (UL), ulnotriquetral (UT),[3-5] dorsal radiotriquetral, and scaphotriquetral ligaments.[3,4,6] Ulnar wrist forces also pass through the triangular fibrocartilage complex (TFCC) to help stabilize the ulnar carpus and transmit axial forces to the ulna.[7,8] The volar and dorsal aspects of the LT ligament merge with the ulnocarpal extrinsic ligaments volarly and the dorsal radiolunotriquetral ligament dorsally, anchoring the triquetrum.[9] The UL and UT ligaments originate on the volar TFCC and insert on the volar lunate and volar triquetrum, respectively, as well as on the LT ligament.[10-12] Just palmar lies the ulnocapitate ligament, which provides a direct attachment from the ulna to the palmar ulnar ligamentous complex.

Ligament plication has been implemented to manage capitolunate instability.[13] Arthroscopic treatment of LT tears is based on the anatomic and biomechanical contributions of the ulnocarpal ligaments (UL and UT) to LT joint stability. In addition to ARIF of the LT, suture plication augments capsular repair and shortens the ulnocarpal ligaments (reminiscent of ulnar shortening), reducing their contribution to the LT joint to enhance the extrinsic ligament contribution to stability. The ulnocarpal ligaments diverge from their origin on the volar TFCC to insert distally on the triquetrum and lunate in a V formation. Suture plication of the ulnar ligaments closes the V and serves to shorten the ulnar carpal ligaments and augment the palmar capsular tissue of the LT joint.

The TFCC often is a component of more extensive ulnar-sided injuries[14] and does not preclude arthroscopic treatment. Severe LT instability with significant damage to both the dorsal the radiotriquetral and the scaphotriquetral ligament results in volar intercalated segment instability (VISI)[3,4,6]; static instability (VISI) is not readily amenable to complete arthroscopic repair.

PATIENT EVALUATION

History and Physical Examination

Historically, patients may not recall a specific inciting event. Commonly, LT interosseous ligament tears associated with instability result from a single traumatic event, such as a twisting injury or a fall on an outstretched hand with a pronated forearm. The axial and dorsally directed forces result in wrist extension with radial deviation.[15,16] With intercarpal pronation, disruption of the LT interosseous ligament, and associated injury to the disk-triquetral and disk-lunate ligaments, tearing occurs, and LT instability may be greater.

After a general wrist examination, including inspection, palpation, and general range of motion and stability, an examination focused on ulnar-sided pathology is carried out. Patient localization of pain is helpful; diffuse, nonlocalizing pain is not typical of ulnar-sided instability. The dorsal and volar aspects of the

TFCC, the dorsal LT joint, and the extensor carpi ulnaris (ECU) are the main areas to palpate. Depending on the acuteness of the injury, tenderness may or may not be present. Maneuvers to provoke pain caused by excessive unwanted translation of the triquetrum and lunate further elucidate ulnar-sided pain complaints. Although none of the tests is diagnostic in isolation, when performed as part of the comprehensive evaluation, the tests can better characterize pain complaints. Provocative stability maneuvers used to assess the LT joint include LT ballottement (compressing the triquetrum against the lunate), the shuck test as described by Reagan and colleagues,[6] the shear test as described by Kleinman,[17,18] and distal radioulnar translation (to infer stability).[9,19] In addition to ulnar impaction testing, ulnar deviation should be performed with the wrist in flexed, extended, and neutral positions. The stability of the distal radioulnar joint is also assessed. Assessing the patient response to provocative maneuvers and comparing perceived translation with the contralateral wrist are useful.

Diagnostic Imaging

The radiographic evaluation of a painful wrist should start with a minimum of a zero rotation posteroanterior[20,21] view and a true lateral view of the wrist. Comparison views of the contralateral wrist are useful. In these radiographic views and after assessment of the soft tissue shadows, specific osseous relationships should be documented. The focused analysis includes ulnar variance,[22] LT interval, integrity of the subchondral joint surfaces, greater and lesser arc continuity,[23] and radiolunate and scapholunate angles.

The clinical value of advanced radiographic evaluation of the wrist is subject to geographic variability. Magnetic resonance imaging (MRI) with or without the addition of arthrography is beneficial, provided an expert radiologist is available. Variations in the accuracy of MRI and diagnostic arthroscopy may simply be related to skills of the radiologist and the arthroscopic surgeon. In general, a high field magnet with a dedicated extremity helps to optimize spatial resolution.[24] Assessment of the LT joint is variable[25] and should be made in the context of the history and physical examination.

TREATMENT

Indications and Contraindications

The primary contraindication to arthroscopic surgical treatment of LT instability is VISI and severe volar extrinsic ligament tearing. Indications for arthroscopic treatment of static LT instability include isolated LT instability and LT instability in combination with triangular fibrocartilage tears and ulnar impaction.

Conservative Management

Initial treatment for acute LT ligament tears without associated VISI can be short arm cast immobilization with the wrist in neutral position. Steroid injections may be of benefit, based on anecdotal reports.

Surgical Management

With failure of conservative treatment or unstable injuries, arthroscopic treatment of is a reasonable option and includes radiocarpal and midcarpal arthroscopy. The first step is to assess the degree of instability[26] and associated injuries. Partial LT injuries may be treated with débridement alone.[27,28] In 1995, Osterman and Seidman[29] combined débridement with isolated pinning of the LT joint and reported good results. Nonarthroscopic treatment, although not the focus of the chapter, has been described. In a comparison of techniques,[30] subjective results tended to be better for direct repair or reconstruction than for LT fusion.

Arthroscopic Technique

An arthroscopic video system should be positioned to allow a clear view of the monitor by the surgeon and assistant. After the limb is exsanguinated, a traction tower is used, and 8 to 10 pounds of traction is applied through finger traps with the arm strapped to the hand table. The portals used for arthroscopic stabilization include the 3-4, 6-R, volar 6-U, and radial and ulnar midcarpal portals for the arthroscopic capsulodesis and ARIF. Depending on each unique case, the addition of a 4-5 portal as a working or viewing portal can be helpful. The LT joint can be visualized directly from an ulnar portal (6-R or 4-5) to ensure complete, dorsal to palmar visualization of the LT ligament (Fig. 24-1) and débridement as necessary. After identification of pathology and débridement, an ulnar portal at the level of the volar ligaments, volar 6-U, is created after midcarpal assessment and is used for suture passing.

Starting with the arthroscope inserted into the radial midcarpal portal, the surgeon creates an ulnar midcarpal portal for the working portal. The LT joint is assessed for congruency and laxity of the triquetrum. The lunate and triquetrum should be colinear. If the view of the LT joint from the midcarpal radial portal is blocked by a separate lunate facet,[31] the arthroscope is placed in the midcarpal ulnar portal to gain visualization. Under these conditions, the radial articular edge of triquetrum should be aligned with the most ulnar articular edge of the hamate facet of the lunate (Fig. 24-2). The LT joint may be unstable because of excessive laxity while still being congruent. Laxity should be assessed both on triquetral rotation and on separation from the lunate. From the midcarpus, the dorsal portion of the triquetrum is often rotated so that its articular surface is distal to the lunate in an unstable LT joint (Fig. 24-3).

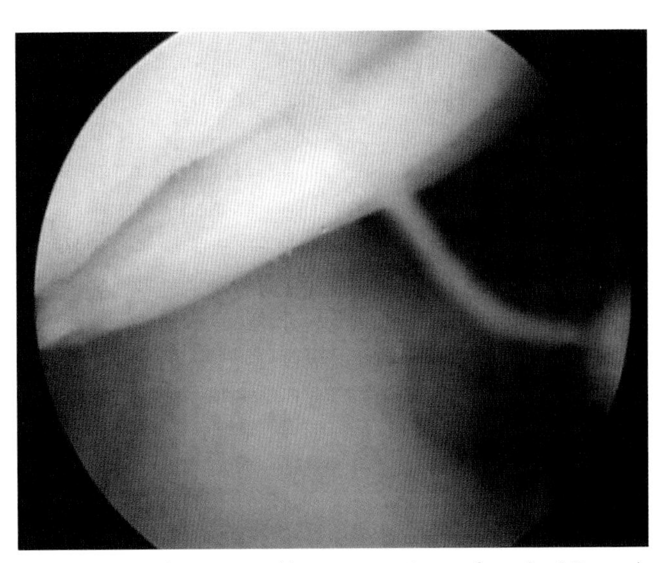

FIGURE 24-1 A lunotriquetral ligament tear is seen from the 6-R portal.

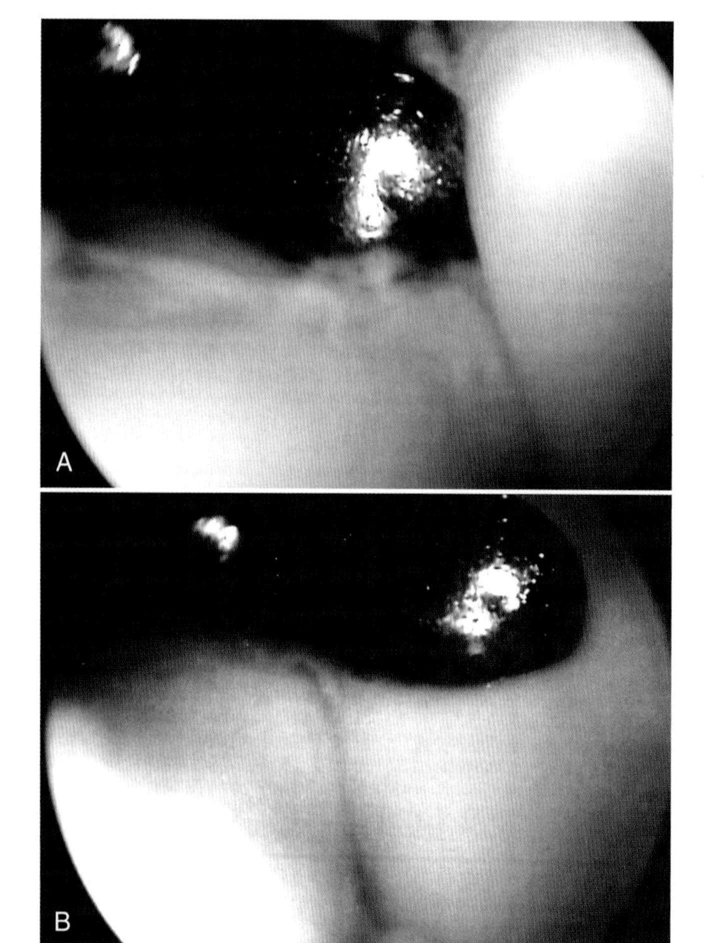

FIGURE 24-2 A, The lunotriquetral joint (triquetrum is right) with a step-off is seen from the ulnar midcarpal portal with a probe inserted from the radial midcarpal portal. **B,** The triquetrum has been reduced, stabilized with Kirschner wires, and made congruent with the lunate *(left).*

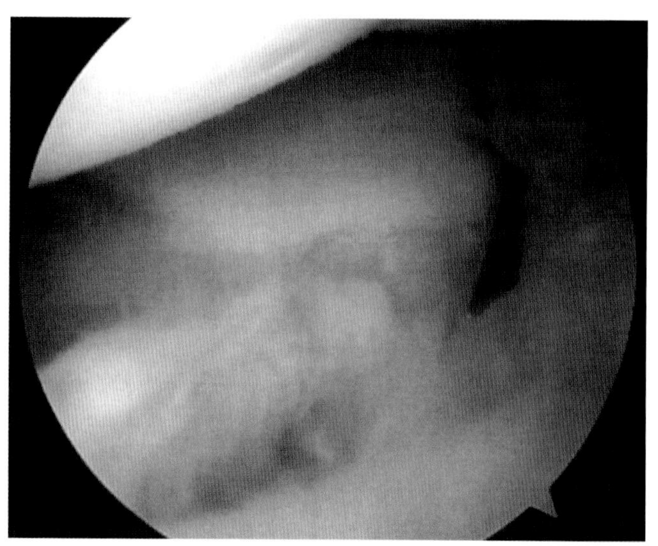

FIGURE 24-4 As viewed from the radial midcarpal portal, the dorsal radiocarpal ligament is avulsed.

The triquetrum can be translated to a reduced state in which the articular surfaces of the triquetrum and lunate are collinear. Further, the triquetrum can be ulnarly translated so as to "gap open" the LT joint. Normal scapholunate joint laxity can be used as a reference. Also, the dorsal radiocarpal and dorsal intercarpal ligaments attached to the lunate and triquetrum may be avulsed (Fig. 24-4) and should be repaired.

After confirmation of LT instability, the arthroscope is placed in the 3-4 portal during ulnocarpal (UL, ulnocapitate, UT) ligament plication. The volar 6-U (v6-U) portal is established. The v6-U portal is similar to the normal 6-U portal, but it is placed just dorsal to the disk-carpal ligaments (Fig. 24-5). Care is taken to avoid injury to the dorsal sensory branches of the ulnar nerve during placement. The UL and UT ligaments are gently débrided to in-

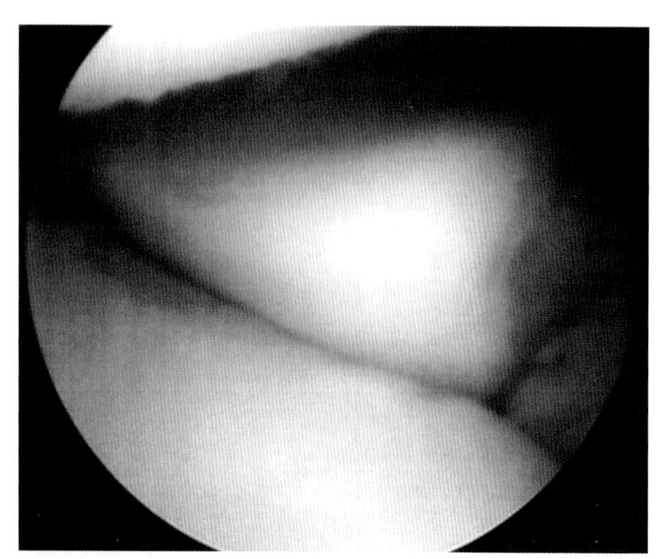

FIGURE 24-3 As seen from the radial midcarpal portal, the dorsal portion of the triquetrum is rotated distally with respect to the dorsal portion of the lunate.

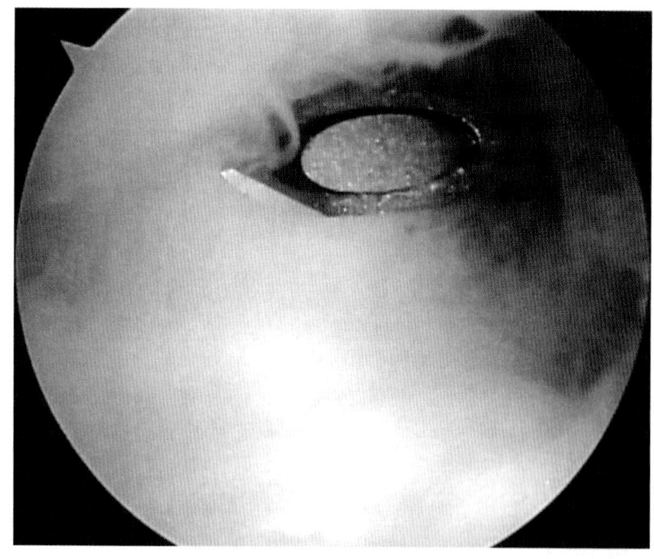

FIGURE 24-5 The spinal needle has entered the radiocarpal joint at the level of the ulnar carpal ligaments. Some fraying of the disk-carpal ligaments is seen and is associated with lunotriquetral ligament injury.

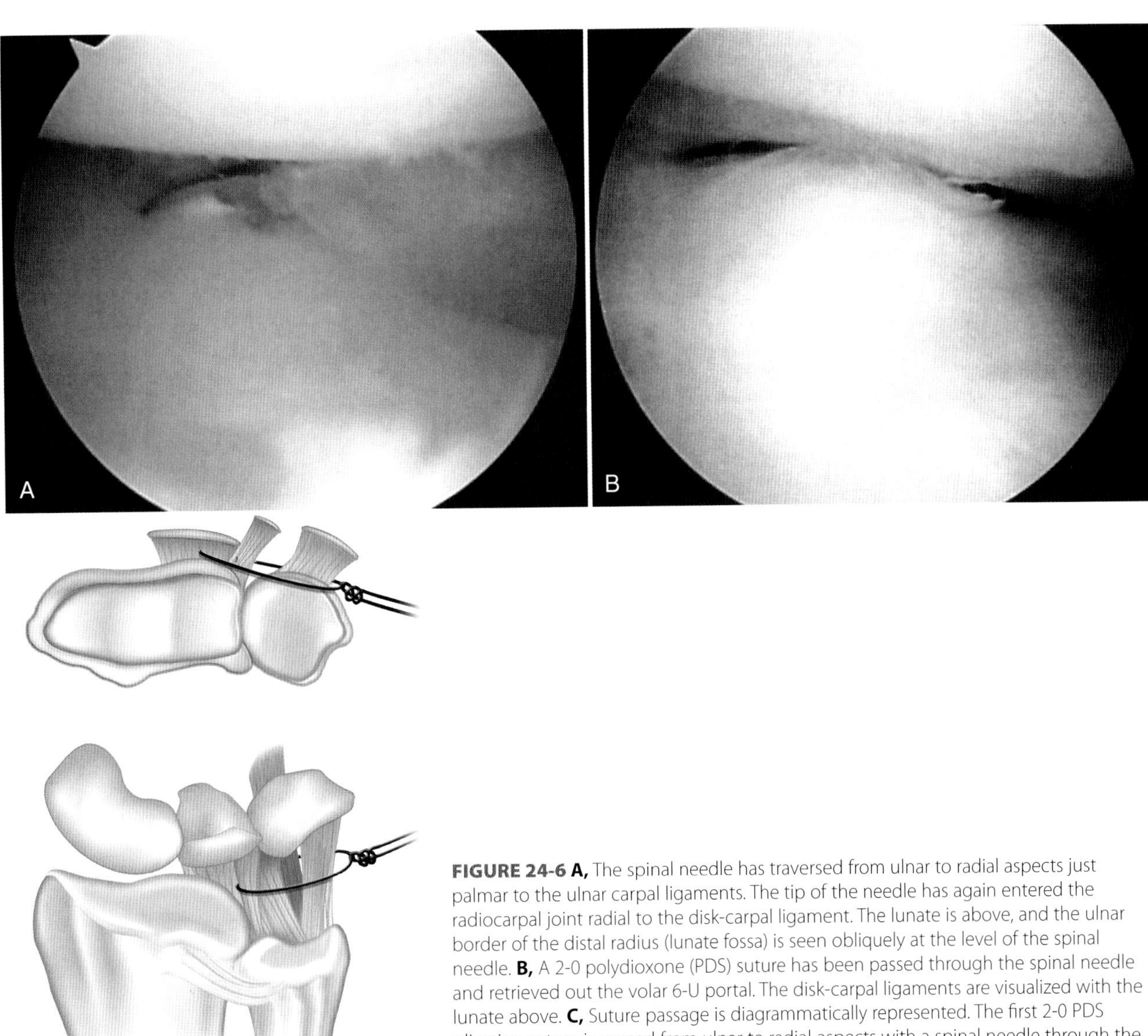

FIGURE 24-6 A, The spinal needle has traversed from ulnar to radial aspects just palmar to the ulnar carpal ligaments. The tip of the needle has again entered the radiocarpal joint radial to the disk-carpal ligament. The lunate is above, and the ulnar border of the distal radius (lunate fossa) is seen obliquely at the level of the spinal needle. **B,** A 2-0 polydioxone (PDS) suture has been passed through the spinal needle and retrieved out the volar 6-U portal. The disk-carpal ligaments are visualized with the lunate above. **C,** Suture passage is diagrammatically represented. The first 2-0 PDS plication suture is passed from ulnar to radial aspects with a spinal needle through the volar 6-U portal and incorporates the ulnocarpal (ulnotriquetral, ulnocapitate, ulnolunate) ligaments.

duce a vascular response. Through the v6-U portal, an 18-gauge spinal needle is passed just volar to the ulnocarpal ligaments and enters the wrist at the radial edge of the UL ligament, just distal to the articular surface of the radius (Fig. 24-6A). A 2-0 polydioxone (PDS) suture is placed through the needle into the joint. The suture is retrieved through the 6-R or the v6-U and tagged as the first plicating suture (see Fig. 24-6B and C). In a similar fashion, the second plicating suture is placed approximately 5 mm distal to the first (Fig. 24-7A), so that the suture loops are parallel to the lunate and triquetrum, and is tagged as the second plicating suture (see Fig. 24-7B and C). Tension on the first stitch often facilitates a second needle passage through the UL and UT ligaments. Adequacy of the plication (tension on the stitch) and its effect on LT interval stability should be assessed after each suture passage. Finally, the spinal needle is passed through the volar aspect of the capsule at the volar-most aspect of the TFCC at the prestyloid recess, as in peripheral repair techniques (Fig. 24-8A). The three sets of sutures are tied at the termination of the procedure, after the LT joint has been congruently reduced and stabilized with Kirschner wires (see Fig. 24-8B).

With the arthroscope in the midcarpal radial portal, a spinal needle can be placed from the ulnar to the radial side across the distal aspect of the LT as a guide for percutaneous Kirschner wire placement with or without concurrent fluoroscopy (Fig. 24-9). After the triquetrum has been reduced through the midcarpal ulnar portal with a probe and traction on the plication sutures, the initial 0.045-inch smooth Kirschner wire is inserted just proximal to the spinal needle and drilled across the LT joint. The second Kirschner wire is placed just proximal to the first (Fig. 24-10). Traction is released after Kirschner wire stabilization, and the forearm is held in neutral rotation while the plication sutures are tied (Fig. 24-11). The Kirschner wires are either cut subcutaneously or bent outside the skin.

In the presence of a peripheral triangular fibrocartilage tear, sutures should be passed after the plication sutures and tied separately in the dorsal incision; central triangular fibrocartilage

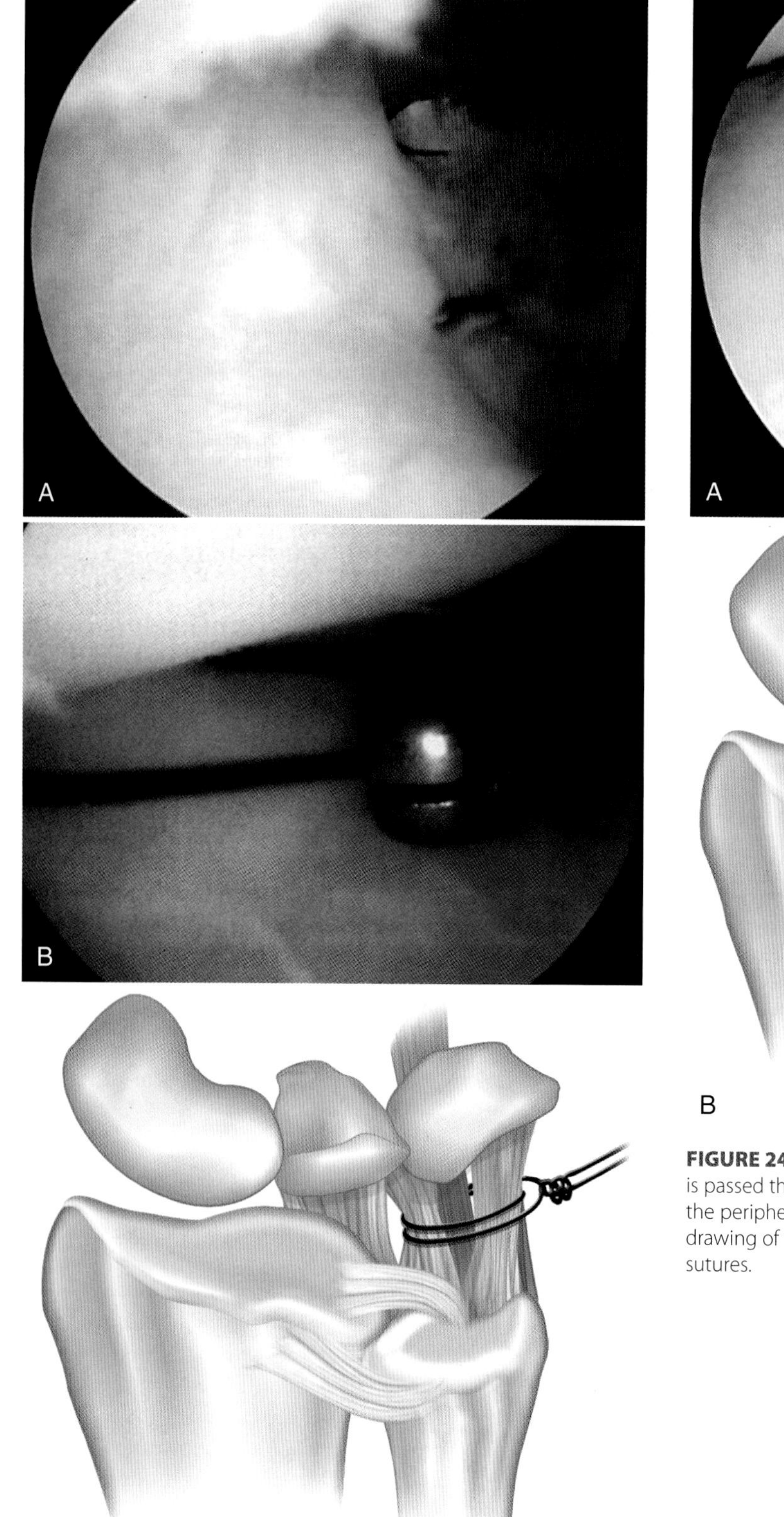

FIGURE 24-7 A, The ulnotriquetral ligament is to the left. The first plicating suture is seen below and to the right (ulnar), exiting ulnarly through the volar 6-U portal. The spinal needle is seen distally as it is ready to be passed for the second plicating suture. **B,** The second 2-0 polydioxone (PDS) plication suture is placed. Tension on the first suture facilitates placement of the second suture, which is placed approximately 5 mm distal to the first suture. **C,** The plication sutures are represented diagrammatically.

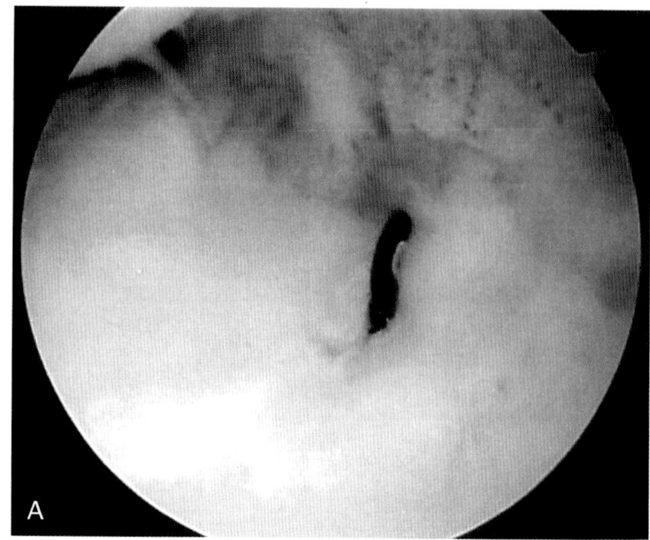

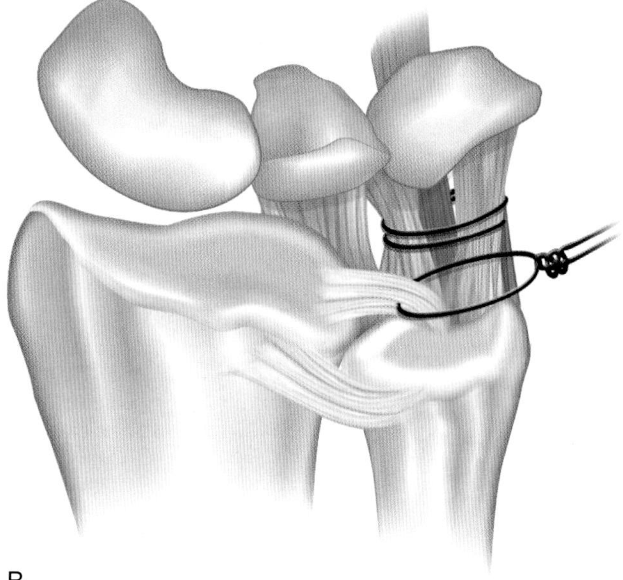

FIGURE 24-8 A, The ulnar capsular tension suture is placed. The suture is passed through the ulnar capsule and through the palmar aspect of the peripheral edge of the fibrocartilage complex (TFCC). **B,** Line drawing of the two plication sutures and the prestyloid and TFCC sutures.

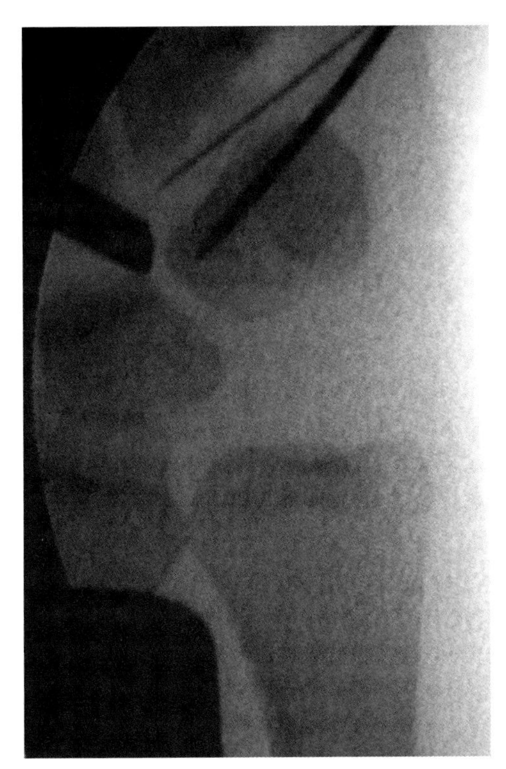

FIGURE 24-9 The viewing portal is in the midcarpal space during arthroscopic reduction and pinning of the lunatotriquetral joint. A needle has been placed into the midcarpal space to act as a guide for Kirschner wire placement.

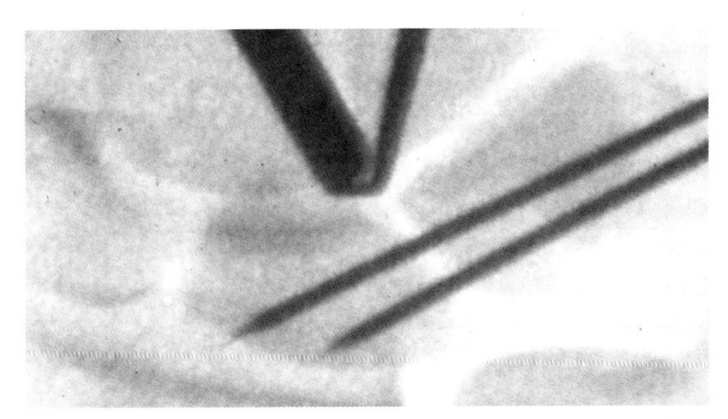

FIGURE 24-10 Two parallel Kirschner wires through the lunotriquetral joint have been passed under direct visualization from the midcarpal joint.

tears can be débrided during the initial débridement. Patients with LT tears often have positive ulnar variance.[32,33] In the presence of ulnar-positive ulnar impaction, an arthroscopic wafer procedure should be considered.

PEARLS & PITFALLS

PEARLS

- Patients who have focal mechanical complaints with a complementary history and physical examination are the best candidates for treatment.
- A spectrum of ulnar-sided pathology including LT ligament tears, chondral injuries, and triangular fibrocartilage tears can be treated concurrently.

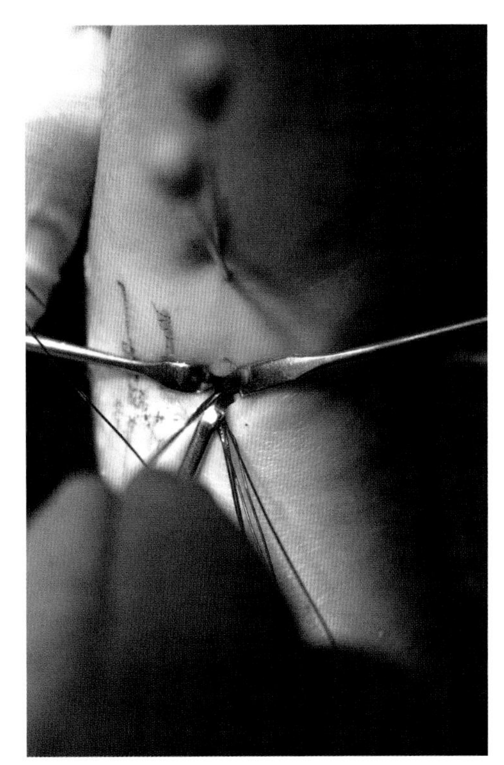

FIGURE 24-11 The sutures and Kirschner wires are in place. Retractors can be used to retract soft tissue and protect the ulnar nerve sensory branches.

PITFALLS

- Clinically insignificant LT tears are common as part of age-related degeneration. MRI findings may or may not be clinically significant.
- Caution should be exercised in patients with diffuse complaints in the absence of correlative mechanical findings.

Postoperative Rehabilitation

After surgery, the patient's extremity is placed into a long arm splint with the elbow flexed at 90 degrees and the forearm and wrist in neutral position. At 2 weeks after surgery, the wounds are assessed and a long cast or a Muenster cast is applied with the forearm and wrist in neutral position. At 6 weeks after surgery, the Kirschner wires are removed and a removable long arm or Muenster splint is used for the ensuing 2 weeks. Supervised therapy at this point includes active and active-assist wrist flexion, extension, pronation, and supination within a painless arc of motion, with progressive motion as tolerated. At 8 weeks after surgery or when motion is almost restored, strengthening exercises are instituted. Return to activities as tolerated typically occurs at approximately 24 weeks after surgery.

CONCLUSIONS

An initial case series of 21 patients were examined retrospectively at a mean of 2 years 6 months (range, 1 week to 5.5 years) after treatment. Seventeen of the patients recalled a specific injury (hyperextension, 12; twisting, 2; unknown, 3), and four described a gradual onset of symptoms without specific recollection of an acute injury. Three patients had additional significant injuries to the affected extremity: elbow dislocation, humeral shaft fracture, and anterior shoulder dislocation. The patients were uniformly experienced tenderness over the LT joint. Provocative tests for LT instability were specifically positive in nine patients and tests for TFCC injury were positive in six. Crepitus was produced with pronosupination or ulnar deviation in 10 patients. The mean preoperative Mayo wrist score was 50, and the mean postoperative score was 88; 19 of 21 patients had excellent and good results, and two had fair results. Three patients had complications including prolonged tenderness along the extensor carpi ulnaris, and one patient had persistent neuritis of the dorsal branches of the ulnar nerve.

Symptomatic LT interosseous ligament tears have been managed by arthroscopic débridement, arthroscopic pinning, ligamentous repair, and intercarpal arthrodesis. Arthroscopic ulnocarpal ligament plication attempts improve the ligamentous checkrein on excessive LT motion, perhaps similar to ulnar shortening procedures. Treatment of LT ligament tears with or without additional ulnar-sided injuries with arthroscopic reduction, pinning, and ligament plication is useful and produces good midterm results.

REFERENCES

1. Kulick M, Chen C, Swearingen P. Determining the diagnostic accuracy of wrist arthroscopy. Paper presented at the annual meeting of the American Society for Surgery of the Hand, 1990, Toronto.
2. Ritt MJ, Bishop AT, Berger RA, et al. Lunotriquetral ligament properties: a comparison of three anatomic subregions. *J Hand Surg Am*. 1998;23: 425-431.
3. Horii E, Gacias-Elias M, An K, et al. A kinematic study of lunatotriquetral dislocations. *J Hand Surg Am*. 1991;16:355-362.
4. Viegas S, Peterson P, Peterson PD, et al. Ulnar-sided perilunate instability: an anatomic and biomechanical study. *J Hand Surg Am*. 1990;15: 268-278.
5. Trumble T, Bour C, Smith R, et al. Kinematics of the ulnar carpus to the volar intercalated segment instability pattern. *J Hand Surg Am*. 1990;15: 384-392.
6. Reagan DS, Linscheid RL, Dobyns JH. Lunotriquetral sprains. *J Hand Surg Am*. 1984;9:502-514.
7. Palmer A, Werner F. Triangular fibrocartilage complex of the wrist: anatomy and function. *J Hand Surg Am*. 1981;6:153-162.
8. Werner F, Palmer A, Fortino M, et al.. Force transmission through the distal ulna: effect of ulnar variance, lunate fossa angulation, and radial and palmar tilt of the distal radius. *J Hand Surg Am*. 1992;17:423-428.
9. Green D. Carpal dislocation and instabilities. In: Green D, ed. *Operative Hand Surgery*. New York, NY: Churchill Livingston; 1988:878-879.
10. Palmer A, Werner F. Biomechanics of the distal radioulnar joint. *Clin Orthop*. 1984;187:26-35.
11. Garcias-Elias M, Domenech-Mateu J. The articular disc of the wrist: limits and relations. *Acta Anat*. 1987;128:51-54.
12. Melone C, Nathan R. Traumatic disruption of the triangular fibrocartilage complex: pathoanatomy. *Clin Orthop*. 1992;275:65-73.
13. Johnson R, Carrera G. Chronic capitolunate instability. *J Bone Joint Surg Am*. 1986;68A:1164-1176.
14. Melone C Jr, Nathan R. Traumatic disruption of the triangular fibrocartilage complex: pathoanatomy. *Clin Orthop*. 1992;275:65-73.
15. Palmer C, Murray P, Snearly W. The mechanism of ulnar sided perilunate instability of the wrist. Paper presented at the 53rd annual meeting of the American Society for Surgery of the Hand, 1998: Minneapolis, MN.
16. Shin AY, Deitch MA, Sachar K, Boyer MI. Ulnar-sided wrist pain: diagnosis and treatment. *Instr Course Lect*. 2005;54:115-128.
17. Kleinman W. Physical examination of lunatotriquetral joint. *Am Soc Surg Hand Corr Newsl*. 1985;51.
18. Kleinman W. Long-term study of chronic scapho-lunate instability treated by scapho-trapezio-trapezoid arthodesis. *J Hand Surg Am*. 1989; 14:429-445.
19. Palmer A. Triangular fibrocartilage complex lesions: a classification. *J Hand Surg Am*. 1989;14:594-606.
20. Palmer A, Glisson R, Werner F. Ulnar variance determination. *J Hand Surg Am*. 1982;7:376-379.
21. Hardy DC, Totty WG, Reinus WR, Gilula L. Posteroanterior wrist radiography: importance of arm positioning. *J Hand Surg Am*. 1987;12: 504-508.
22. Steyers C, Blair W. Measuring ulnar variance: a comparison of techniques. *J Hand Surg Am*. 1989;14:607-612.
23. Gilula L. Carpal injuries: analytic approach and case exercises. *Am J Radiol*. 1979;133:503-517.
24. Tanaka T, Yoshioka H, Ueno T, et al. Comparison between high-resolution MRI with a microscopy coil and arthroscopy in triangular fibrocartilage complex injury. *J Hand Surg Am*. 2006;31:1308-1314.
25. Zanetti M, Saupe N, Nagy L. Role of MR imaging in chronic wrist pain. *Eur Radiol* 2007;17:927-938.
26. Geissler WB, Freeland AE, Savoie FH, et al. Intracarpal soft-tissue lesions associated with an intra-articular fracture of the distal end of the radius. *J Bone Joint Surg Am*. 1996;78:357-365.
27. Weiss AP, Sachar K, Glowacki KA. Arthroscopic debridement alone for intercarpal ligament tears. *J Hand Surg Am*. 1997;22:344-349.
28. Ruch DS, Poehling GG. Arthroscopic management of partial scapholunate and lunotriquetral injuries of the wrist. *J Hand Surg Am*. 1996;21: 412-417.
29. Osterman AL, Seidman GD. The role of arthroscopy in the treatment of lunatotriquetral ligament injuries. *Hand Clin*. 1995;11:41-50.
30. Shin AY, Weinstein LP, Berger RA, Bishop AT. Treatment of isolated injuries of the lunotriquetral ligament: a comparison of arthrodesis, ligament reconstruction and ligament repair. *J Bone Joint Surg Br*. 2001;83: 1023-1028.
31. Viegas S, Wagner K, Patterson R, et al. Medial (hamate) facet of the lunate. *J Hand Surg Am*. 1990;15:564-571.
32. Pin P, Young V, Gilula L, et al. Management of chronic lunatotriquetral ligament tears. *J Hand Surg Am*. 1989;14:77-83.
33. Osterman A, Sidman G. The role of arthroscopy in the treatment of lunatotriquetral ligament injuries. *Hand Clin*. 1995;11:41-50.

SUGGESTED READING

Osterman AL, Bora FW, Martin E: Arthroscopic debridement of the triangular fibrocartilage complex tears. *Arthroscopy*. 1990;6:120-4.

Wnorowski DC, Palmer AK, Werner FW, Fortuno BS. Anatomic and biomechanical analysis of the arthroscopic wafer procedure. *Arthroscopy*. 1992;8:204-12.

CHAPTER
25

Midcarpal Instability

David J. Slutsky

The concept of midcarpal instability (MCI) has unfolded over many years. It represents several distinct clinical entities that differ in their cause and direction of subluxation but share the common characteristic of abnormal force transmission at the midcarpal joint. Lichtman and Wroten consolidated the various forms into intrinsic and extrinsic types. The intrinsic types consist of palmar MCI (PMCI), dorsal MCI (DMCI), and combined forms.[1] There are no arthroscopic findings that are characteristic of MCI, but wrist arthroscopy allows one to examine the chondral surfaces for abnormal wear and has a role in treatment for milder forms of MCI. Extrinsic MCI, as described by Taleisnik and Watson, is caused by a dorsally malunited distal radius fracture.[2] This lesion is typically treated by a distal radius osteotomy to restore the normal palmar tilt and falls outside the scope of this discussion.

ANATOMY

The palmar arcuate ligament complex comprises a radial arm, which is confluent with and distal to the radioscaphocapitate ligament, and an ulnar arm, the triquetrohamate-capitate ligament (TCL) (Fig. 25-1). In the normal situation, the proximal carpal row moves smoothly, from a flexed position when the wrist is in radial deviation to extension when the wrist is in ulnar deviation. This is possible because of the progressive tightening effect of the arcuate ligament as it stretches out to length, incrementally pulling the midcarpal row into extension, and the carpal bone geometry, which causes the triquetrum to translate dorsally along the helicoidal facet of the hamate. If the arcuate ligament is attenuated, this synchronous motion is lost.[3]

Studies by Trumble and colleagues[4] and Viegas and coworkers[5] showed that sectioning of the TCL or the dorsal radiocarpal ligament (DRCL), also known as the dorsal radiotriquetral ligament, could produce a volar intercalated segmental instability (VISI) deformity and simulate PMCI. Lichtman and colleagues showed in vivo that tightening the DRCL alone can stabilize the proximal carpal row and eliminate the clunk of PMCI, emphasizing the potential importance of dorsal ligament laxity in the pathogenesis of this disorder.[6] Lichtman believed that PMCI is caused by laxity of the TCL and DRCL, which allows an excessive palmar sag of the heads of the capitate and hamate at the midcarpal joint. This produces a VISI pattern of the proximal row in the nonstressed wrist. This sag results in a loss of joint contact across the midcarpal joint, which manifests clinically as a loss of the smooth transition of the proximal row from flexion to extension as the wrist deviates ulnarward. The proximal carpal row stays in a flexed position until the terminal extent of ulnar deviation, when the helicoidal shape of the hamate facet suddenly forces the triquetrum to move dorsally. This snaps the lunate, and subsequently the scaphoid, into extension, causing a sudden reversal of the VISI. This sudden proximal row extension is responsible for the painful and rapid catch-up clunk that occurs. As the wrist moves back to neutral position, the triquetrum translates down the hamate facet, allowing the proximal row to drop back into VISI while the distal row again settles palmarly into its slightly subluxated starting point (Fig. 25-2).

The dorsal pattern of MCI has not been studied as extensively. It appears that laxity of the radial arm of the palmar arcuate ligament permits the capitate and hamate to translate dorsally to an excessive degree, especially with ulnar deviation of the wrist.[7,8] In the palmar and dorsal patterns, the proximal row always moves into extension, and the distal row translates dorsally with ulnar deviation. It is the timing and force of this movement that differentiates the two patterns. In PMCI, the distal carpal row starts out in palmar subluxation with the wrist in neutral position. As the wrist moves into ulnar deviation, the subluxation suddenly corrects. In DMCI, the wrist starts out in a reduced position in neutral. Dorsal subluxation of the distal row then occurs with ulnar deviation. In either case, the instability is caused primarily by laxity of the selected extrinsic carpal ligaments that

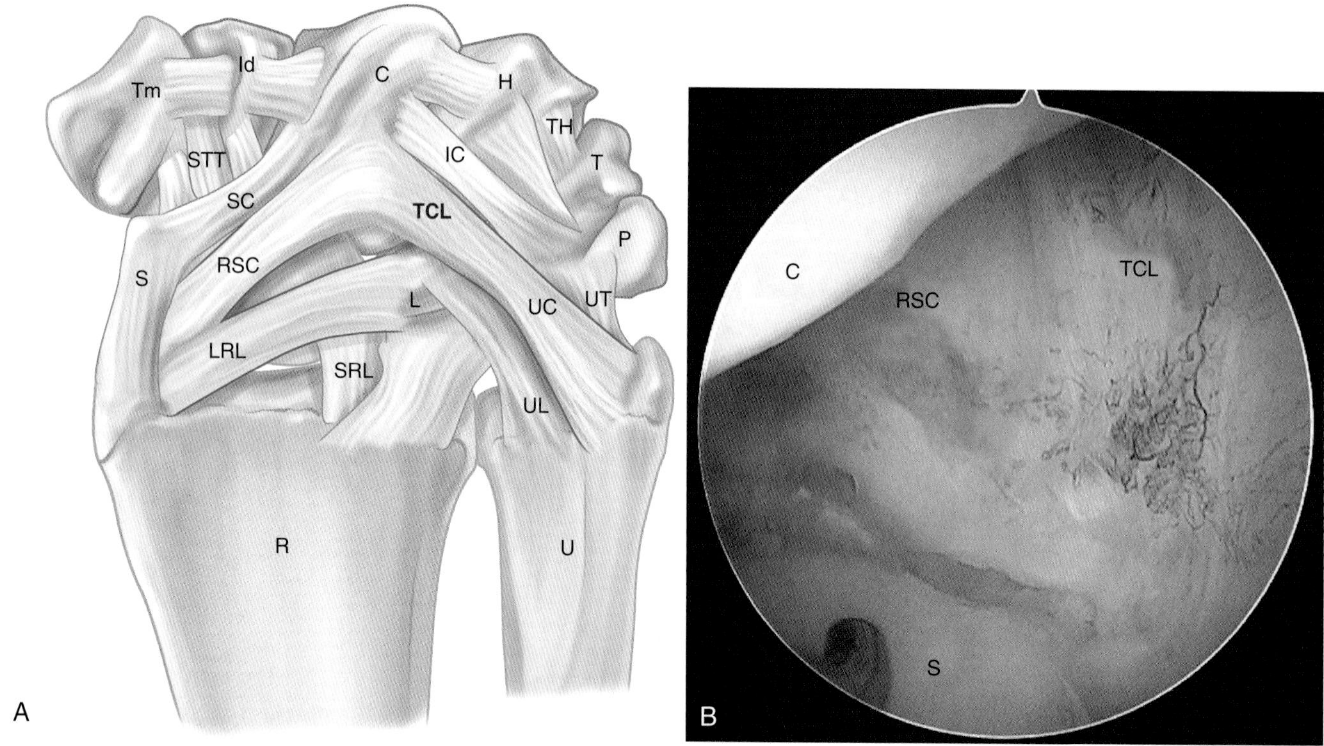

FIGURE 25-1 A, Line drawing of the volar ligaments. *Ligaments:* TCL, triquetrohamate-capitate ligament; RSC, radioscaphoid ligament; LRL, long radiolunate ligament; SRL, short radiolunate ligament; UL, ulnolunate ligament; UC, ulnocapitate ligament; UT, ulnotriquetral ligament; SC, scaphocapitate ligament; STT, scaphotrapezial trapezoidal ligament; TH, triquetrohamate ligament; IC, intercarpal ligament. *Bones:* R, radius; U, ulna; S, scaphoid; L, lunate; C, capitate; T, triquetrum; H, hamate; P, pisiform; Tm, trapezium; Td, trapezoid. **B,** Arthroscopic view of the arcuate ligament from the midcarpal ulnar portal. C, capitate; RSC, radioscaphocapitate ligament; S, scaphoid; TCL, triquetrohamate-capitate ligament.

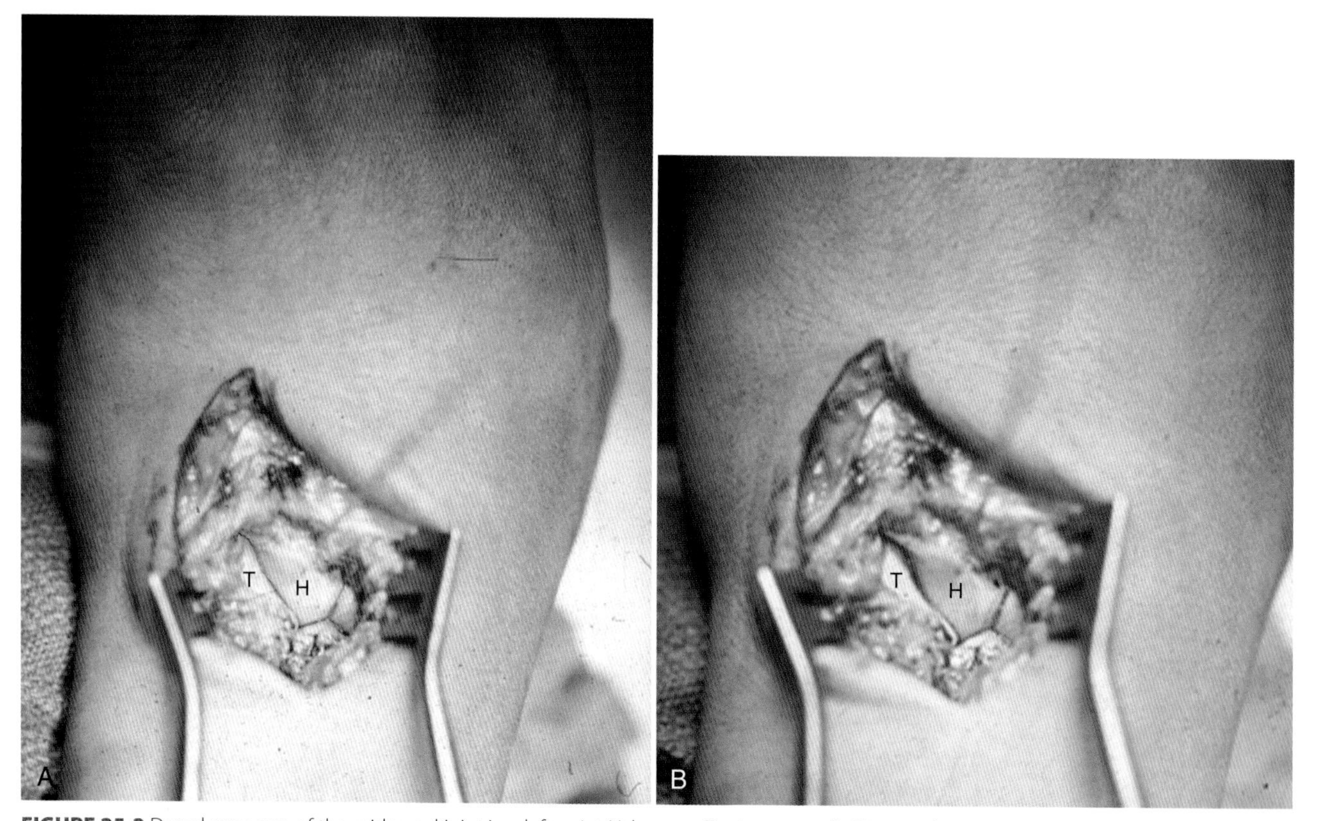

FIGURE 25-2 Dorsal exposure of the midcarpal joint in a left wrist. H, hamate, T, triquetrum. **A,** Triquetrohamate joint with the proximal row reduced. **B,** Subluxed triquetrohamate joint with volar sag of the proximal row. H, hamate, T, triquetrum. *(Courtesy of David J. Slutsky, MD, Torrance, California.)*

support the proximal row, which prevents them from controlling the complex kinematic relationships among the articular surfaces across the midcarpal joint.

PATIENT EVALUATION

History and Physical Examination

In PMCI, the patient presents with a history of clunking of the wrist. Patients can often reproduce the clunk on both sides, because generalized ligamentous laxity frequently coexists. The patient may have a trivial injury that accentuates this normal laxity, resulting in a painful clunk. On physical examination, close inspection reveals a sag of the midcarpal joint with the wrist in radial deviation, which is reduced with active or passive ulnar deviation (Fig. 25-3). The clunk may be reproduced by performing the midcarpal shift test.[3] This test is performed by placing the patient's wrist in neutral position with the forearm in pronation. A palmar force is then applied to the hand at the level of the distal capitate. The wrist is simultaneously loaded and deviated ulnarly. The test result is positive if a painful clunk occurs that reproduces the patient's symptoms.

In DMCI, a history of an extension injury may be present. Patients complain of post-traumatic chronic pain, weakness, and wrist clicking. Tight grasping, especially in supination, aggravates the symptoms. The physical examination also reveals palmar sagging of the ulnar wrist. A dorsal capitate displacement test is performed by applying dorsal pressure to the scaphoid tuberosity while longitudinal traction and flexion are applied to the wrist. There is an associated painful click as the lunate is abruptly shifted dorsally and ulnarly.

Diagnostic Imaging

Static radiographs are typically normal but occasionally reveal a mild VISI pattern with the wrist in the neutral position. Arthrograms are normal unless there are associated intracarpal or triangular fibrocartilage complex tears. Magnetic resonance imaging findings are nonspecific. Videofluoroscopy provides the hallmarks for diagnosis of this condition. With normal wrist kinematics, the proximal carpal row rotates synchronously from flexion to extension as ulnar deviation of the wrist is achieved. With PMCI, the proximal row maintains a volar-flexed position until terminal ulnar deviation is reached, at which time it suddenly snaps into extension (see MCI video).

In dynamic DMCI, the radiographs are usually normal. In chronic cases, they often show a VISI pattern (Fig. 25-4). The capitolunate displacement test shows dorsal subluxation of the proximal carpal row in addition to dorsal subluxation of

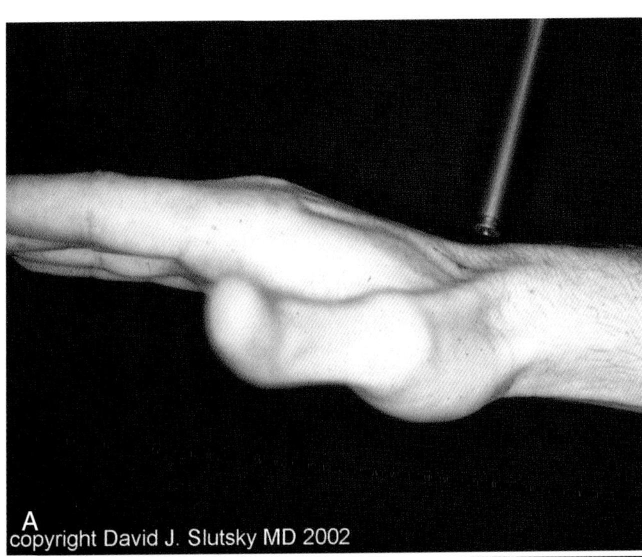

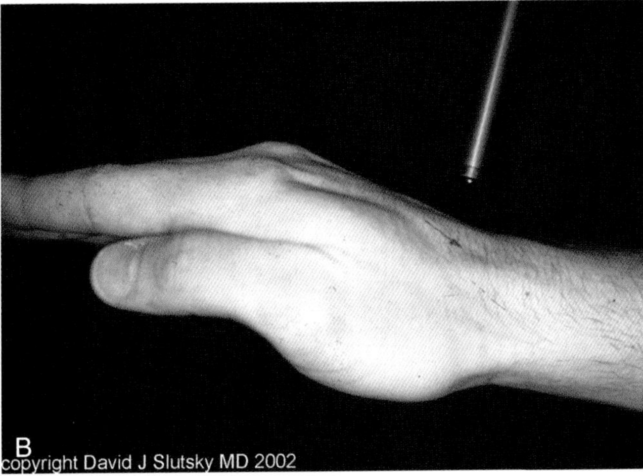

FIGURE 25-3 Palmar midcarpal instability. **A,** Notice the sag in the midcarpal joint with the wrist in radial deviation. **B,** The carpus is reduced in ulnar deviation and the sag disappears. *(Courtesy of David J. Slutsky, MD, Torrance, California.)*

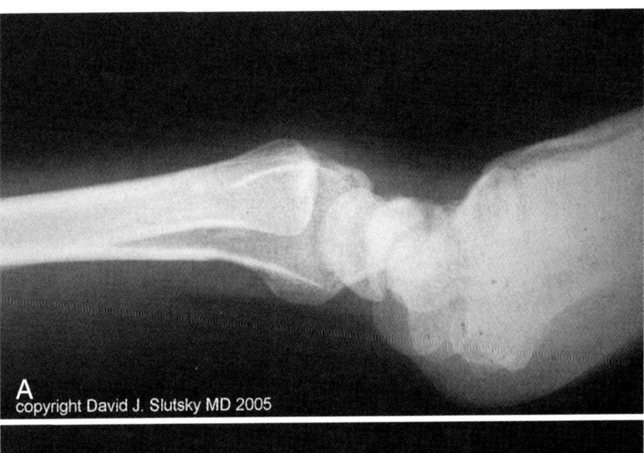

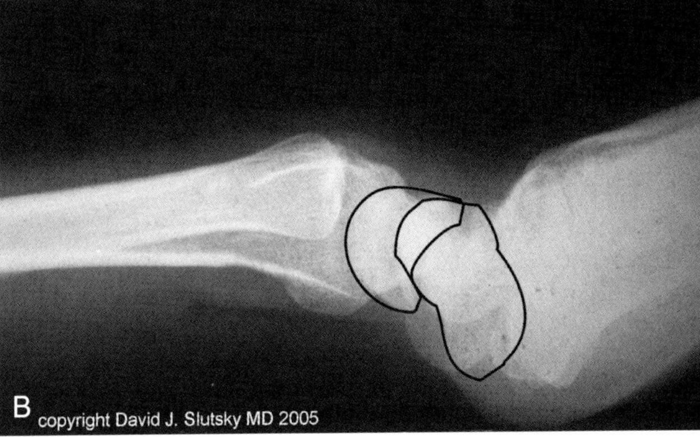

FIGURE 25-4 Volar intercalated segmental instability. **A,** Lateral radiograph shows volar tilting of the lunate and extension of the scaphoid. **B,** The same view is shown with the lunate and scaphoid outlined for clarity. *(Courtesy of David J. Slutsky, MD, Torrance, California.)*

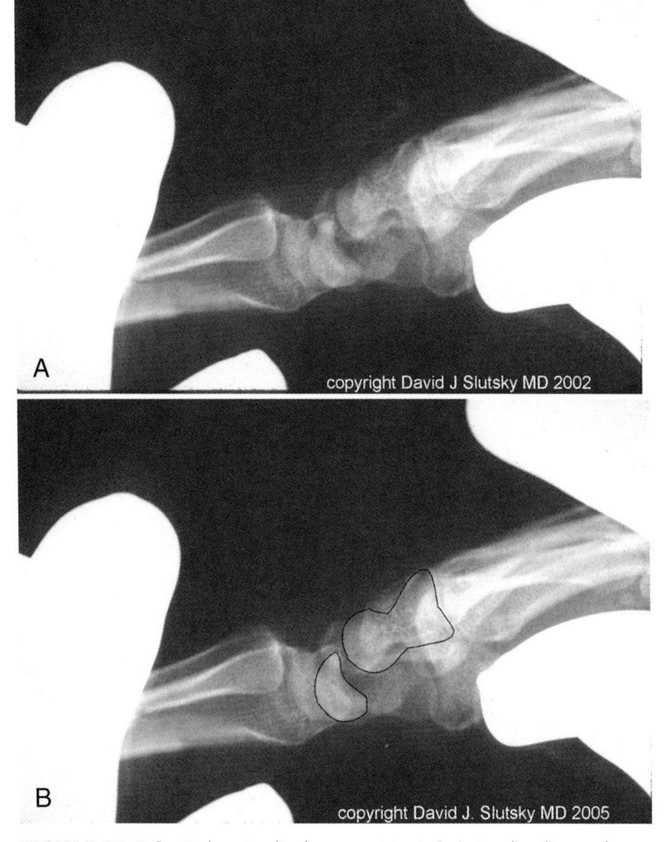

FIGURE 25-5 Capitolunate displacement test. **A,** Lateral radiograph demonstrates dorsal subluxation of the capitate on the lunate. **B,** The same view is shown with the lunate and capitate outlined for clarity. *(Courtesy of David J. Slutsky, MD, Torrance, California.)*

the capitate from the lunate (Fig. 25-5).[9] This effect led Louis and colleagues to coin the term *capitolunate instability pattern* (i.e., CLIP wrist).[10]

Nonoperative Management

Nonsurgical treatment consists of activity modification, nonsteroidal anti-inflammatory medication (NSAIDs), and splinting.[11] Various pisiform support splints have been described. They are based on the observation that application of dorsally directed pressure under the pisiform reduces the carpal sag along with the VISI position of the carpal row. Applying this principle, a three-point dynamic splint may maintain the reduction while permitting wrist motion in milder cases (Fig. 25-6). The splint may be worn full time for 6 to 8 weeks to reduce the midcarpal synovitis and then as needed.

Lichtman and Wroten observed that active co-contraction of the extensor carpi ulnaris, flexor carpi ulnaris, and hypothenar muscles can reduce the sagging of the midcarpal joint. Some patients can eliminate the catch-up clunk by contracting these muscles before ulnar deviation of the wrist. Patients are taught this isometric muscle contraction as a part of the therapy program.[1] However, definitive treatment of this condition ultimately requires surgical treatment.

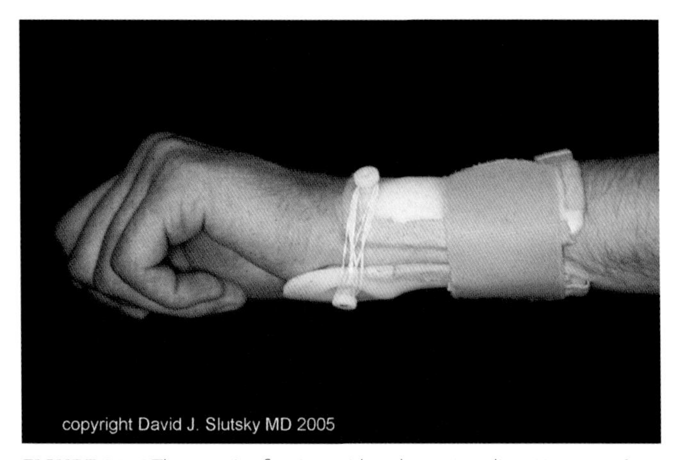

FIGURE 25-6 Three-point fixation with a dynamic splint. *(Courtesy of David J. Slutsky, MD, Torrance, California.)*

TREATMENT

Indications and Contraindications

Arthroscopy is indicated in MCI to rule out associated intercarpal ligament pathology and to inspect the midcarpal joint to assess for chondral damage. Milder forms of PMCI can be treated with a thermal capsulorrhaphy.

A variety of open soft tissue procedures have been generally ineffective for severe forms of MCI[12,13]; hence, arthroscopic treatment should be approached with caution.

Arthroscopic Technique

Arthroscopic Capsular Shrinkage

Although thermal capsular shrinkage has not enjoyed great success in the shoulder, its role in the treatment of wrist disorders remains promising. Thermal energy unwinds the collagen triple helix in capsular and ligamentous structures, with subsequent healing in a shortened or tightened position. The temperature required to achieve the effect is about 70 to 80 degrees; to avoid tissue ablation, the temperature should not exceed 100 degrees. Tissue repair occurs by vascular invasion and fibroblastic activity. In vitro, capsular tissue has been shown to shrink by 9% to 50%, depending on the probe and the type of tissue. After shrinkage, collagen stiffness is reduced to approximately 20% of normal; it returns to normal by about 2 months.[14] This concept has led to the use of these techniques as a treatment option for MCI of the wrist.

The patient is placed in a supine position on the operating table. After exsanguination of the limb, the tourniquet is inflated to 250 mm Hg. A 2.7-mm, 30-degree angle arthroscope, along with a fiberoptic light source and camera setup, are used. Some type of diathermy unit is used to create the thermal shrinkage. Large-bore outflow cannulas are desirable to provide rapid joint irrigation and minimize the risk of chondral damage through heat necrosis. With the use of a tower, 10 pounds of traction is applied to the index and long fingers. The radiocarpal joint is inflated 1 cm distal to Lister's tubercle at the 3-4 portal, and the 2.7-mm arthroscope is introduced. Outflow is established

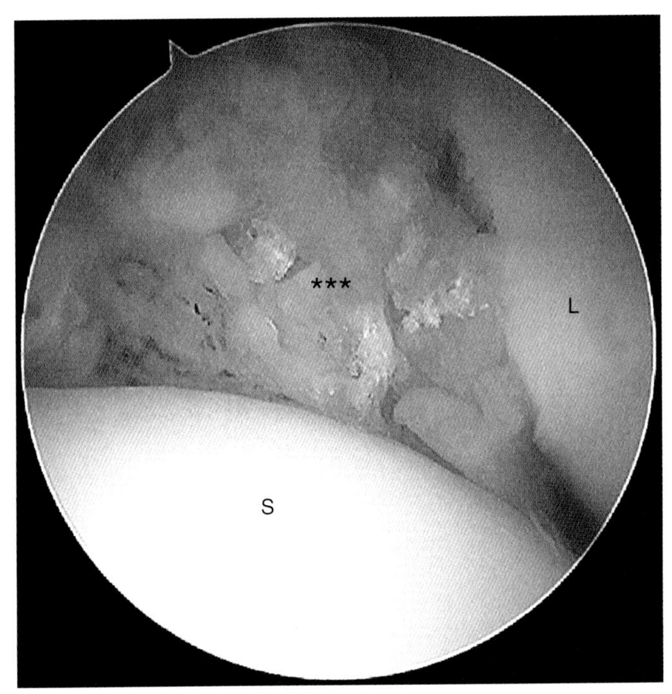

FIGURE 25-7 A, Shrinkage of the arcuate ligament *(asterisks)* as viewed from the midcarpal radial portal. L, lunate; S, scaphoid. *(Courtesy of David J. Slutsky, MD, Torrance, California.)*

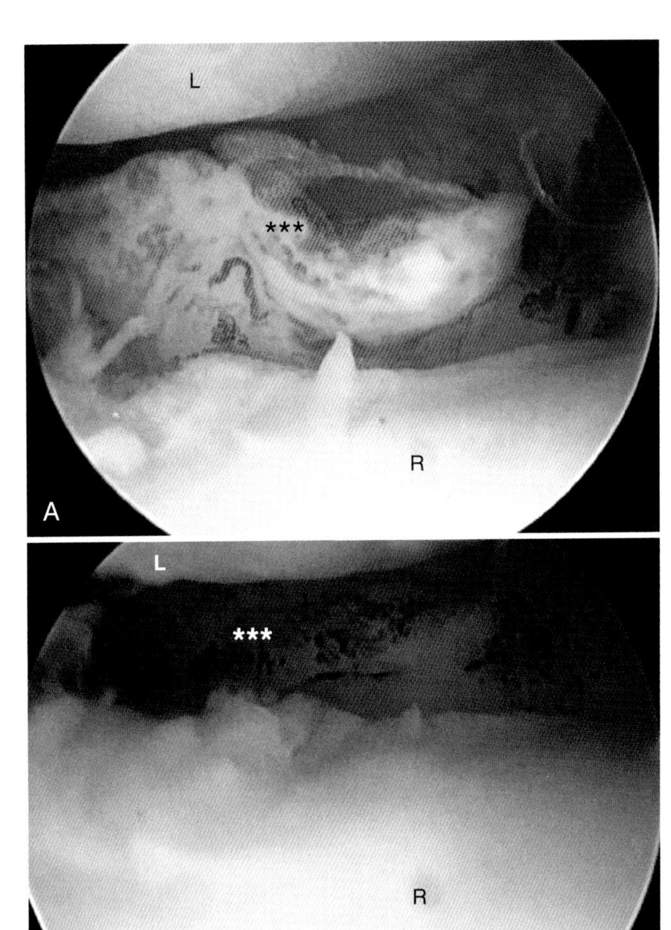

FIGURE 25-8 A, View of a dorsal radiocarpal ligament tear *(asterisks)* from the volar radial portal. **B,** View of a dorsal radiocarpal ligament tear after shrinkage. L, lunate; R, radius. *(Courtesy of David J. Slutsky, MD, Torrance, California.)*

through the 6-R portal. The standard dorsal portals, including a 3-4 and a 4-5 portal, are used for an arthroscopic survey. Any associated triangular fibrocartilage tears or lunotriquetral ligament tears are identified and treated by débridement or repair. The ulnar extrinsic ligaments are assessed for laxity. If laxity is observed, a 1.5-mm electrothermal probe (Arthrocare, Sunnyvale, CA; or Oratec, Menlo Park, CA) is introduced through the 6-R portal. The ulnolunate and ulnotriquetral ligaments are painted with the probe using a stripe technique, leaving sections of untouched ligament in between. The correction of any associated VISI deformity is assessed with a combination of arthroscopy and fluoroscopy.

A midcarpal radial portal is then established. The scapholunate and lunotriquetral joints are inspected and probed for laxity. The TCL is identified as it runs obliquely from the triquetrum, across the proximal corner of the hamate, to the palmar neck of the capitate. A midcarpal ulnar portal is established and used for introduction of the thermal probe. The TCL is then shrunk while the tension is again adjusted with correction of any VISI deformity (Fig. 25-7).

A volar radial portal is established by making a 2-cm longitudinal incision in the proximal wrist crease, exposing the flexor carpi radialis tendon sheath. The sheath is divided, and the tendon is retracted ulnarly. The radiocarpal joint space is identified with a 22-gauge needle, and the joint is inflated with saline. A blunt trocar and cannula are introduced through the floor of the flexor carpi radialis sheath, which overlies the interligamentous sulcus between the radioscaphocapitate ligament and the long radiolunate ligament. A 2.7-mm, 30-degree arthroscope is inserted through the cannula. The DRCL can be seen ulnar to the 3-4 portal and underneath the lunate. If laxity is present, the electrothermal probe is introduced through the 3-4 and 4-5 portals and used to shrink the DRCL (Fig. 25-8). The tension of the DRCL can be adjusted by correcting any VISI deformity with a Kirschner wire in the lunate under fluoroscopic control. At the end of the procedure, 0.045-mm Kirschner wires are used to pin the triquetrum to the capitate and hamate in a neutral and reduced position.

Arthroscopic Findings

There are no arthroscopic findings that are diagnostic of MCI. Inspection of the radiocarpal joint may reveal a nonspecific synovitis. I have seen an associated tear of the DRCL (see Fig. 25-8). In this case, an arthroscopic DRCL repair failed to correct the MCI.[15] Inspection of the midcarpal row may demonstrate erosive lesions along the triquetrum (Fig. 25-9) and the hamate, or both. Laxity of the lunotriquetral ligament may be seen though this is not invariable. Midcarpal arthroscopy may reveal laxity of the TCL (Fig. 25-10).

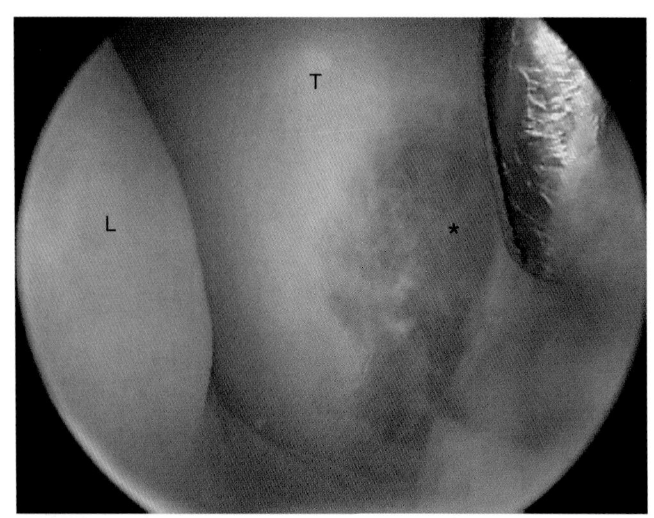

FIGURE 25-9 Erosion of the triquetrum *(asterisk)* is seen from the midcarpal ulnar portal. L, lunate; T, triquetrum. *(Courtesy of David J. Slutsky, MD, Torrance, California.)*

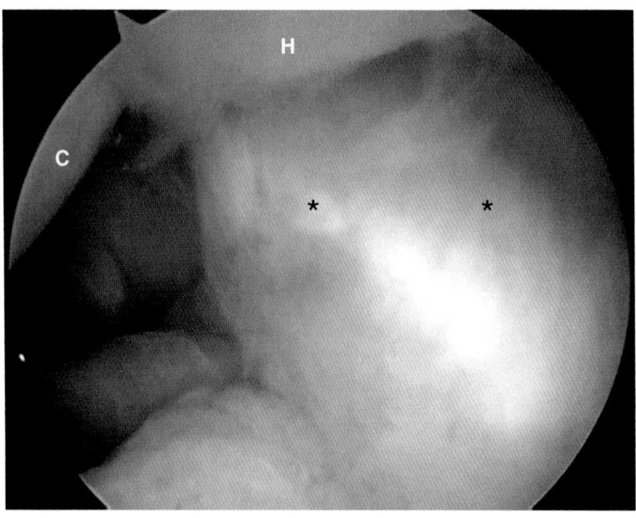

FIGURE 25-10 Laxity of the triquetrohamate-capitate ligament *(asterisks)*. C, capitate; H, hamate. *(Courtesy of David J. Slutsky, MD, Torrance, California.)*

PEARLS & PITFALLS

PEARLS

- Examine the opposite wrist for MCI.
- Examine for a painful midcarpal clunk.
- Videofluoroscopy demonstrates loss of the normal synchronous motion from physiologic dorsal intercalated segmental instability to VISI.
- Perform arthroscopy to assess and treat any associated intercarpal ligament pathology.
- Perform capsular shrinkage for milder forms of MCI.

PITFALLS

- Use rapid fluid irrigation to prevent thermal chondral damage during shrinkage.
- Perform a scaphoid shift test to differentiate the wrist clunk from scapholunate instability.
- A fixed VISI seen on radiography results from other causes.
- No arthroscopic findings are characteristic of MCI.
- Severe MCI is treated with open methods.

Postoperative Rehabilitation

After arthroscopic shrinkage, the patient is placed in a short arm cast. The cast and Kirschner wires are removed at 4 weeks, after which home range of motion exercises and gradual strengthening are introduced.

CONCLUSIONS

There is a paucity of literature on the use of arthroscopy for MCI. In 2003, Lichtman and associates reported their experience of five patients who underwent an arthroscopic capsular shrinkage.[6] The average age was 33 years (range, 29 to 57 years). Follow-up averaged 9 months (range, 3 to 18 months). The midcarpal clunk resolved in six of the eight patients with pain resolution. Range of motion decreased by 20% in the flexion/extension plane, whereas grip strengths increased by an average of 15%.

Mason and Hargreaves[16] reported the results of a prospective study of 13 patients (15 wrists) with painful wrist clunking due to PMCI who underwent arthroscopic thermal capsulorrhaphy after at least 6 months of failed conservative treatment. The mean duration of symptoms was 5 years (range, 8 months to 20 years). Preoperatively, patients were evaluated clinically and by fluoroscopic examination, which confirmed a positive ulnar shift test. A thermal probe was applied to the ulnar arm of the arcuate ligament (i.e., the ulnocapitate, ulnotriquetral, and triquetrocapitate ligaments) and to the radial arm (i.e., radioscaphocapitate, long and short radiolunate ligaments, and accessible parts of the dorsal capsule in the radiocarpal and midcarpal joints). Postoperatively, the patients' wrists were splinted for 6 weeks. Patients were evaluated at a mean follow-up of 42 months (range, 14 to 67 months) by means of the ulnar shift test; grip strength; range of motion; the Disabilities of the Arm, Shoulder, and Hand (DASH) questionnaire; and a structured questionnaire that included a question on their ability to pour a heavy kettle without wrist clunking. Complete resolution of symptoms occurred in 4 patients and almost complete resolution in the remaining 11 patients. Functional improvement was confirmed by an improvement in the mean DASH score from 34 (range, 13-67; SD 16) preoperatively to 12 (range, 0-48; SD 14) at final follow-up. The ulnar shift test was negative in 12 of 14 wrists that were available for examination. Wrist movement was reduced by a mean of 16 degrees in flexion and 10 degrees in extension in 9 wrists compared with the opposite side, but there was no reduction in grip strength.

REFERENCES

1. Lichtman DM, Wroten ES. Understanding midcarpal instability. *J Hand Surg Am.* 2006;31:491-498.
2. Taleisnik J, Watson HK. Midcarpal instability caused by malunited fractures of the distal radius. *J Hand Surg Am.* 1984;9:350-357.
3. Lichtman DM, Schneider JR, Swafford AR, Mack GR. Ulnar midcarpal instability: clinical and laboratory analysis. *J Hand Surg Am.* 1981;6:515-523.
4. Trumble TE, Bour CJ, Smith RJ, Glisson RR. Kinematics of the ulnar carpus related to the volar intercalated segment instability pattern. *J Hand Surg Am.* 1990;15:384-392.
5. Viegas SF, Patterson RM, Peterson PD, et al. Ulnar-sided perilunate instability: an anatomic and biomechanic study. *J Hand Surg Am.* 1990;15:268-278.
6. Lichtman DM, Culp RW, Joshi A. Palmar midcarpal instability. In: McGinty E, ed. *Operative Arthroscopy*. 3rd ed. Philadelphia, PA: Lippincott Williams & Wilkins; 2003:737-742.

7. Johnson RP, Carrera GF. Chronic capitolunate instability. *J Bone Joint Surg Am*. 1986;68:1164-1176.
8. Apergis EP. The unstable capitolunate and radiolunate joints as a source of wrist pain in young women. *J Hand Surg Br*. 1996;21:501-506.
9. White SJ, Louis DS, Braunstein EM, et al. Capitate-lunate instability: recognition by manipulation under fluoroscopy. *AJR Am J Roentgenol*. 1984;143:361-364.
10. Louis DS, Hankin FM, Greene TL. Chronic capitolunate instability. *J Bone Joint Surg Am*. 1987;69:950-951.
11. Lichtman DM, Gaenslen ES, Pollock GR. Midcarpal and proximal carpal instabilities. In: Lichtman DM, Alexander AH, ed. *The Wrist and Its Disorders*. Philadelphia, PA: WB Saunders; 1997:316-328.
12. Goldfarb CA, Stern PJ, Kiefhaber TR. Palmar midcarpal instability: the results of treatment with 4-corner arthrodesis. *J Hand Surg Am*. 2004; 29:258-263.
13. Lichtman DM, Bruckner JD, Culp RW, Alexander CE. Palmar midcarpal instability: results of surgical reconstruction. *J Hand Surg Am*. 1993;18: 307-315.
14. Medvecky MJ, Ong BC, Rokito AS, Sherman OH. Thermal capsular shrinkage: basic science and clinical applications. *Arthroscopy*. 2001; 17:624-635.
15. Slutsky D. Arthroscopic repair of dorsoradiocarpal ligament tears. *J Arthrosc Rel Surg*. 2005;21:1486e1-186e8.
16. Mason WT, Hargreaves DG. Arthroscopic thermal capsulorrhaphy for palmar midcarpal instability. *J Hand Surg Eur*. 2007;32:411-416.

SUGGESTED READING

Lichtman DE, Culp RW, Wroten ES, Slutsky DJ. The role of arthroscopy in midcarpal instability. In: Slutsky DJ, Nagle DJ, eds. *Wrist and Hand Arthroscopy: A Practical Approach*. Philadelphia, PA: Elsevier; 2007.

CHAPTER 26

Displaced Intra-articular Distal Radius Fractures

William B. Geissler

Wrist arthroscopy is a valuable adjunct in the management of complex, displaced intra-articular fractures of the distal radius. The displaced articular surface of the distal radius may be viewed under bright light and magnified conditions with the wrist arthroscope, circumstances that are not available with open arthrotomy. Rotation of fracture fragments can be easily viewed arthroscopically but it is difficult to detect by fluoroscopy. Fracture hematoma and intra-articular loose bodies, which are difficult to detect fluoroscopically, can be arthroscopically lavaged, which may improve the patients' final range of motion and prognosis.

Intra-articular soft tissue lesions, which are associated with intra-articular fractures of the distal radius and which may affect the final prognosis, are easily detected and managed at the same time as fractures. The additional soft tissue pathology can have an important impact on the patient's prognosis and may provide an explanation for why some patients continue to complain of pain postoperatively despite postoperative radiographs that show anatomic reduction of the fracture. Patients frequently continue to complain of ulnar-sided wrist pain postoperatively, which may be caused by an associated injury to the triangular fibrocartilage complex.

Arthroscopic techniques used in the management of displaced intra-articular fractures of the distal radius are described in this chapter. Using wrist arthroscopy in the management of intra-articular distal radius fractures can improve reduction to the articular surface and detect and manage associated soft tissue lesions. With practice, using wrist arthroscopy as an adjunct minimizes operative time and improves the intra-articular reduction. Combining wrist arthroscopy to anatomically reduce the articular surface of the radius with volar plate fixation allows anatomic restoration of the joint surface and stable fixation that enables early range of motion.

PATIENT EVALUATION

Diagnostic Imaging

Standard posteroanterior, oblique, and lateral radiographs are obtained when the patient sustains a displaced intra-articular fracture of the distal radius. Radiographs of the patient's forearm should be included to assess additional injuries proximal to the radius that may involve the operative joint.

Displaced intra-articular fractures of the distal radius are a unique subset of distal radius fractures. These fractures are traditionally unstable and not amenable to traditional methods of closed manipulation and casting. It is important when evaluating a radiograph of a distal radius fracture to understand fracture patterns that may be unstable and require internal fixation. Lafontaine describes several radiographic features that signify unstable fractures of the distal radius.[1] They include dorsal comminution with more than 20 degrees of dorsal tilt, extensive dorsal comminution, an associated ulnar styloid fracture, and significant intra-articular involvement in patients older than 60 years. Additional radiographic parameters include extensive dorsal comminution volar to the midaxle line of the distal radius and initial shortening greater than 4 mm of the distal radius compared with the ulna.

Displaced intra-articular fractures of the distal radius that involve the distal radioulnar joint significantly affect the final prognosis. It is important to reconstruct the bony anatomy of the lesser sigmoid notch of the distal radius to decrease the patient's symptoms with pronation and supination of the forearm. Evaluation with computed tomography (CT) may help to identify any fracture lines that involve the distal radioulnar joint and may be helpful in surgical planning.

Arthroscopic management can further delineate these fracture lines and any associated soft tissue injuries that may involve the distal radioulnar joint and particularly the pathology of the triangular fibrocartilage complex.

Assessment of Associated Soft Tissue Injuries

Several studies have found a high incidence of intra-articular soft tissue injuries associated with displaced intra-articular fractures of the distal radius. Mohanti and Kar[2] and Fontes and colleagues,[3] in two separate wrist arthrography studies, identified a high incidence of injury to the triangular fibrocartilage complex associated with fractures of the distal radius.[2,3] Mohanti and Kar reported a 45% incidence of tears to the triangular fibrocartilage complex in 60 patients.[2] In a similar study, Fontes and coworkers found a 66% incidence of tears of the triangular fibrocartilage complex among 58 patients.[3]

Other arthroscopic studies have demonstrated a high incidence of injury to the triangular fibrocartilage complex. Geissler and colleagues reported their experience with 60 patients with displaced intra-articular fractures of the distal radius.[4] In the series, 49% of the patients had a tear of the triangular fibrocartilage complex, most of which were peripheral and reparable. Injury to the scapholunate interosseous ligament was identified in 32%, and tears of the lunotriquetral interosseous ligament were reported in 15% of the patients.[4] Landau and coworkers, in a similar arthroscopic study of 50 patients, found tears of the triangular fibrocartilage complex were the most common type and occurred in 78% of patients.[5] Tears of the scapholunate interosseous ligament were identified in 54%, and tears of the lunotriquetral interosseous ligament were found in only 16% of the patients. In an arthroscopic study, Hanker reported that tears of the triangular fibrocartilage complex were present in 55% of the 65 patients in his series.[6] Common in all three studies were injuries of the triangular fibrocartilage complex in which ulnar-sided pathology was most commonly associated with displaced intra-articular fractures of the distal radius.

Geissler and associates described an arthroscopic classification of interosseus ligament injuries based on their experience with the arthroscopic management of intra-articular distal radius fractures.[4] They observed that a spectrum of interosseous ligament injury occurred. The interosseous ligament stretches and attenuates, and it eventually tears from a volar to dorsal direction from increased rotation between the carpal bones. The classification of carpal instability is based arthroscopic observation of the interosseous ligament from the radiocarpal and midcarpal spaces, and it evaluates injuries to the scapholunate and lunotriquetral interosseous ligaments (Table 26-1).

In the Geissler classification, grade I injuries have a loss of the normal concave appearance between the carpal bones as the interosseous ligament attenuates and becomes convex, which can be seen with the arthroscope in the radiocarpal space. Hemorrhage may be seen within the ligament in acute injuries, such as a fracture. In the midcarpal space, the interval between the carpal bones is congruent, and there is no step-off.

In Geissler grade II injuries, the interosseous ligament continues to attenuate and becomes convex as seen from the radiocarpal space. There is no gap between the carpal bones when viewed with the arthroscope in the radiocarpal space. In the midcarpal space, an interval between the carpal bones is no longer congruent, and a step-off exists. In scapholunate instability, palmar flexion of the scaphoid, compared with the lunate, can be seen arthroscopically. The dorsal lip of the lunate is distal in relation to the lunate. In lunotriquetral instability, increased translation is seen through the triquetrum and lunate when palpated with a probe.

In Geissler grade III injuries, the interosseous ligament starts to tear, usually in a volar to dorsal direction, and a gap is seen between the involved carpal bones and the radiocarpal space. The probe can be used to separate the involved carpal bones in the radiocarpal space. In the midcarpal space, a 2-mm probe may be placed between the carpal bones and twisted. A portion of the interosseous ligament is still intact, and complete disruption of the interosseous ligament is not observed.

In Geissler grade IV injuries, the interosseous ligament is completely detached and disrupted. The drive-through sign occurs when the arthroscope may be freely passed through the radiocarpal space and the torn interosseous ligament into the midcarpal space.

TREATMENT

Management of Carpal Instability

Geissler grade I injuries are consistent with a typical wrist sprain, and these tears respond to a short period of immobilization. Geissler grade II and III injuries may be easily arthroscopically

TABLE 26-1 Geissler Arthroscopic Classification of Carpal Instability

Grade	Description	Management
I	Attenuation or hemorrhage of the interosseous ligament is seen from the radiocarpal joint. There is no incongruence of carpal alignment in the midcarpal space.	Immobilization
II	Attenuation or hemorrhage of interosseous ligament is seen from the radiocarpal joint. Incongruence or step-off is seen from the midcarpal space. A slight gap (less than width of a probe) between the carpal bones may be present.	Arthroscopic reduction and pinning
III	Incongruence or step-off of carpal alignment is seen in the radiocarpal and midcarpal spaces. The probe may be passed through the gap between the carpal bones.	Arthroscopic or open reduction and pinning
IV	Incongruence or step-off of carpal alignment is seen in the radiocarpal and midcarpal spaces. Gross instability with manipulation is identified. A 2.7-mm arthroscope may be passed through the gap between the carpal bones.	Open reduction and repair

reduced and stabilized in an acute situation. Anatomic reduction of the carpal interval is best viewed with the arthroscope in the midcarpal space opposite to the tear. For example, correction of the rotation to scapholunate instability is best viewed with the arthroscope in the ulnar midcarpal portal. For lunotriquetral instability, the reduction is best viewed with the arthroscope in the radial midcarpal portal. The carpal interval is reduced, and Kirschner wires are placed across the involved interval in oscillation mode to protect the cutaneous nerves. Geissler grade IV injuries have complete detachment of the interosseous ligament, and open repair is recommended for the best prognosis in acute situations.

Arthroscopic Techniques

A patient who sustains a fracture of the distal radius usually presents with a swollen wrist. Because of the swelling, it is usually difficult to palpate the extensor tendon landmarks traditionally used for arthroscopy. However, the bony landmarks are usually easily palpated, and they include the bases of the metacarpals, the ulnar head, and the dorsal lip of the radius.[7]

The wrist is suspended in a traditional traction tower. The standard 3-4 portal is made between the third and fourth dorsal extensor compartments. The 3-4 portal is made in line with the radial border of the long finger when the extensor tendons cannot be palpated. I recommend placing an 18-gauge needle into the proposed location of the 3-4 portal before committing to a skin incision. The arthroscope may be placed within the fracture itself if the portal is placed too proximal or can injure the articular cartilage of the carpus if the portal is placed too distally. After the precise location of the portal is determined, the portal is made on the skin against the surgeon's thumb with the tip of a no. 11 blade. In this manner, the possibility of injury to the dorsal sensory cutaneous branches is decreased. Blunt dissection is continued with a hemostat to the level of the joint capsule, and the arthroscope is then reduced with a blunt trocar inserted into the 3-4 portal.

Intra-articular fractures of the distal radius are usually associated with abundant fracture hematoma and debris.[8] Thorough irrigation of the fracture hematoma is required to evaluate the fracture fragments and to improve the field of view to judge rotation to the fracture fragments. Inflow may be provided through the wrist arthroscopic cannula or through a 14-gauge needle inserted into the 6-U portal. The small cannula used in wrist arthroscopy does not allow much space between the cannula itself and the arthroscope to allow fluid irrigation into the wrist joint. Because of this, separate inflow through the 6-U portal is recommended. Outflow is provided through the arthroscopic cannula with, intervenous extension tubing that drains into a basin on the hand table so the fluid does not go into the surgeon's lap or onto the floor. Separate inflow and outflow cannulas limit fluid extravasation into the soft tissues.

The 4-5 or 6-R working portal may be used to remove debris and hematoma to improve visualization. The 4-5 working portal is made in line with the midaxis of the ring metacarpal when the extensor tendons cannot be palpated. The 6-R portal may be made just radial to the extensor carpi radialis tendon. Similarly to making the 3-4 portal, an 18-gauge needle should be inserted into the proposed location and viewed arthroscopically before committing to a skin incision.

The ideal timing for arthroscopically assisted reduction of intra-articular distal radius fractures is usually between 3 and 10 days.[9] Other attempts at arthroscopic fixation may result in troublesome bleeding, which may obscure visualization. Fractures more than 10 days old may be difficult to disimpact and mobilized percutaneously.

Indications and Operative Setup

Intra-articular fractures of the distal radius without extensive metaphysial comminution are best for arthroscopically assisted management.[10] They include radial styloid fractures, die-punch fractures, and three- and four-part fractures.

With popularity of volar plating, arthroscopy has become a useful adjunct in the management of distal radius fractures with comminution. The fracture is stabilized by a volar plate, and the joint capsule is not incised. The articular reduction is provisionally stabilized with Kirschner wires as viewed fluoroscopically. The wrist is then suspended in a traction tower, and articular reduction may be fine-tuned arthroscopically. The distal screws are then inserted into the plate to stabilize the fracture after the articular reduction is judged to be anatomic. Associated soft tissue injuries may be detected and managed at the same time. Comminuted intra-articular fractures of the distal radius may be stabilized by several modalities, including Kirschner wires, cannulated screws, headless screws, plate fixation, and external fixation. Arthroscopy may be used as an adjunct with any of these modalities.

Large joint instrumentation is not appropriate for wrist arthroscopy. Small joint instrumentation is essential for arthroscopically assisted reduction of intra-articular distal radius fractures. The small joint scope is approximately 2.7 mm in diameter, and even smaller arthroscopes may be used. A small joint shaver (≤3.5 mm) is mandatory to clear fracture hematoma and debris to improve visualization. An oscillating drill is useful when inserting Kirschner wires for visualization and stabilization to prevent injury to the dorsal cutaneous nerves that surround the wrist.

A traction tower is very useful in arthroscopic management of distal radius fractures. The traction tower allows the surgeon to flex, extend, and radial and ulnar deviate the wrist to facilitate reduction of the fracture fragments while maintaining constant traction for visualization. Previous towers suspended the wrist using a traction bar and extended the forearm and hand, which made simultaneous fluoroscopic evaluation of the reduction very difficult. A newer traction tower design allows the surgeon to simultaneously arthroscopically reduce the intra-articular fracture of the distal radius and monitor the reduction fluoroscopically. The traction bar is uniquely placed at the side of the wrist rather than at the center, so it does not block fluoroscopic visualization. The wrist can be manipulated in traction to help reduce the fracture fragments. The tower may be flexed to allow the surgeon to perform wrist arthroscopy in the vertical or horizontal plane, depending on the surgeon's preference. If a traction tower is not available, the wrist may be suspended with finger traps in a shoulder holder or over the end of a hand table. A small bump may be placed in the volar aspect of the wrist to help maintain slight wrist flexion when weights are being used over the end of the hand table.

Injuries Treated Arthroscopically

Radial Styloid Fractures

An isolated fracture of the radial styloid is an ideal fracture pattern to manage arthroscopically, particularly if the surgeon is just beginning to gain experience in arthroscopic management of wrist fractures. The simplest of several techniques is to advance two guidewires under fluoroscopic guidance into the tip of the radial styloid fragment but not across the fracture site. A small incision is made to insert the guidewires through a soft tissue protector or insert the guidewires with an oscillating drill to limit injury to the cutaneous nerves. The position of the guidewires into the radial styloid fragment is evaluated with fluoroscopy.

The wrist is then suspended in the traction tower, and standard portals were made. The radiocarpal space is cleared of hematoma and fracture debris to help facilitate visualization, particularly to judge rotation of the radial styloid fragment. The arthroscope is then transferred to the 6-R or 4-5 portal to view the reduction of the radial styloid fragment by looking across the wrist. It is much easier to assess rotation of the fracture fragment by looking across the wrist joint. The previously placed guidewires are used as joysticks, and the fracture is manipulated under direct observation and anatomically reduced back to the radial shaft. A trocar inserted into the 3-4 protal can aid reduction of the radial styloid fragment and control rotation.

The guidewire is advanced across the fracture site into the radial shaft after the fracture reduction is judged to be anatomic. The articular reduction and the position of the guidewires are evaluated with fluoroscopy. Initially, Kirschner wires were used alone. Headless screws are now recommended to stabilize the fracture because they provide good stability while decreasing soft tissue irritation and the likelihood of pin track infections compared with Kirschner wires. Headless screws may allow earlier range of motion.

Alternatively, closed reduction and percutaneous stabilization of the radial styloid fragment are performed under fluoroscopic guidance, and guidewires are advanced across the fracture site. The fracture is suspended in the traction tower, and the fracture hematoma is débrided. The arthroscope is then placed in the 4-5 or 6-R portal, and the arthroscopist looks across the wrist to evaluate the articular reduction. If the fracture fragment is rotated, the guidewires may be backed out of the shaft, leaving them only in the radial styloid fragment to use as joysticks to again reduce the fracture and then advanced across the fracture site.

Radial styloid fractures have a high incidence of associated injury to the scapholunate interosseous ligament. The zone of injury may pass through the fracture and continue distally through the scapholunate interosseous ligament. After reduction of the fracture, the scapholunate interosseous ligament is evaluated from the radiocarpal and midcarpal spaces.

Three-Part Fractures without Metaphysial Comminution

Displaced three-part fractures involve radial styloid and lunate facet fracture fragments (Fig. 26-1). The radial styloid fragment usually can be reduced by closed manipulation (Fig. 26-2). The radial styloid fragment is reduced and provisionally stabilized with Kirschner wires inserted by an oscillating drill, thereby stabilizing the styloid fragment back to the radial shaft. The wrist is then suspended in a traction tower, and the fracture debris and hematoma are evacuated (Figs. 26-3 to 26-5). The reduced radial styloid fragment may be used as a landmark to reduce the depressed lunate facet fracture fragment (Fig. 26-6). The arthroscope is placed in the 3-4 portal, and an 18-gauge needle is placed percutaneously into the radiocarpal space over the depressed lunate facet fragment. A large Kirschner wire may then be placed about 2 cm proximal to the previously placed 18-gauge

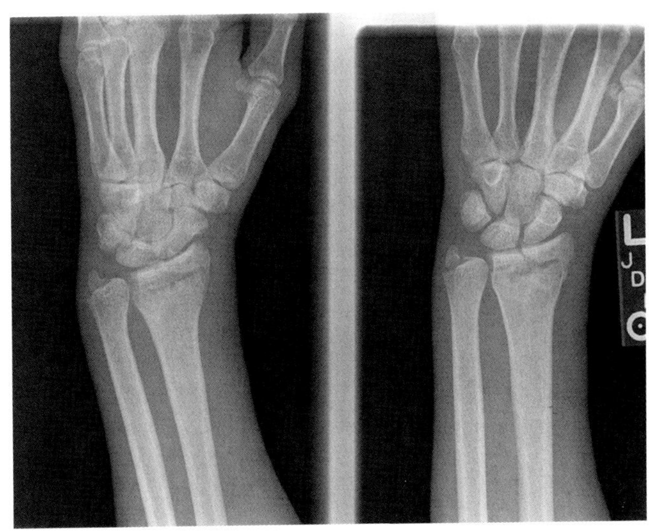

FIGURE 26-1 Posteroanterior radiographs show a three-part intra-articular fracture of the distal radius on the associated base of the ulnar styloid fragment.

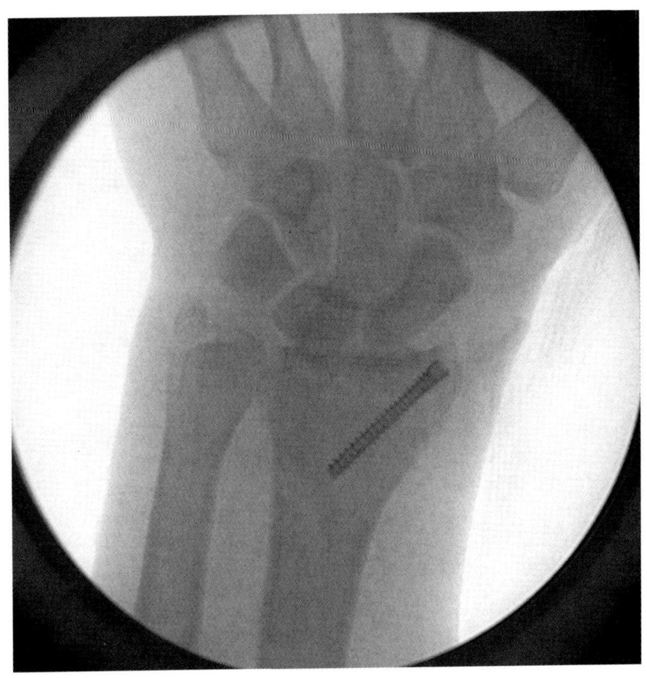

FIGURE 26-2 The radial styloid is closed reduced, and a headless cannulated screw is inserted to support the fracture fragment.

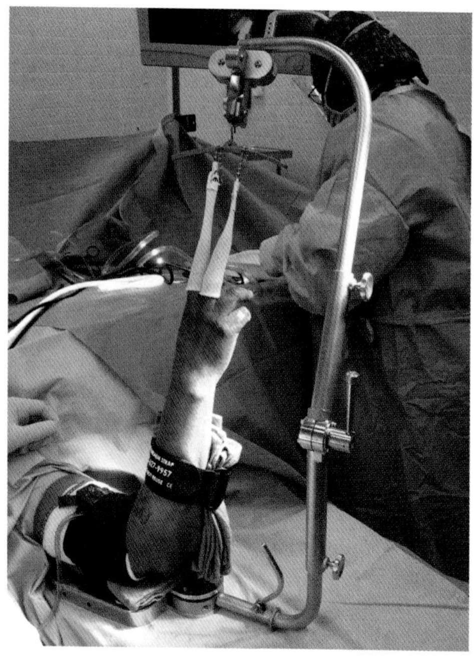

FIGURE 26-3 The wrist is suspended in the Acumed traction tower (Hillsboro, OR).

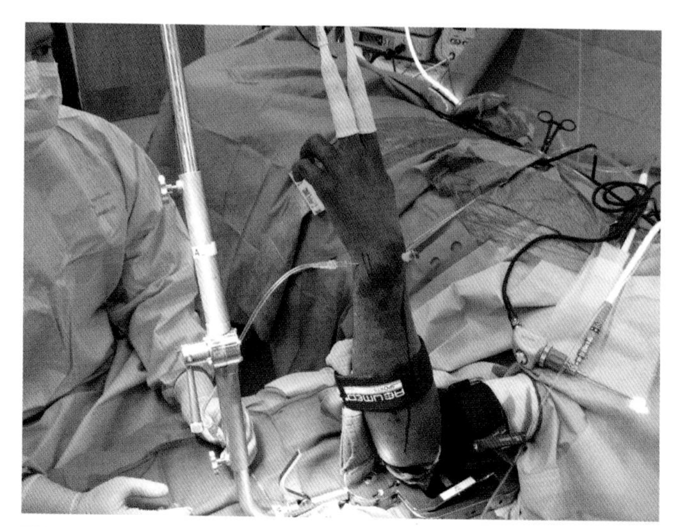

FIGURE 26-4 Patients with fractures of the distal radius usually present with swollen wrists. It is useful to identify the proposed portal with an 18-gauge needle before committing to a skin incision.

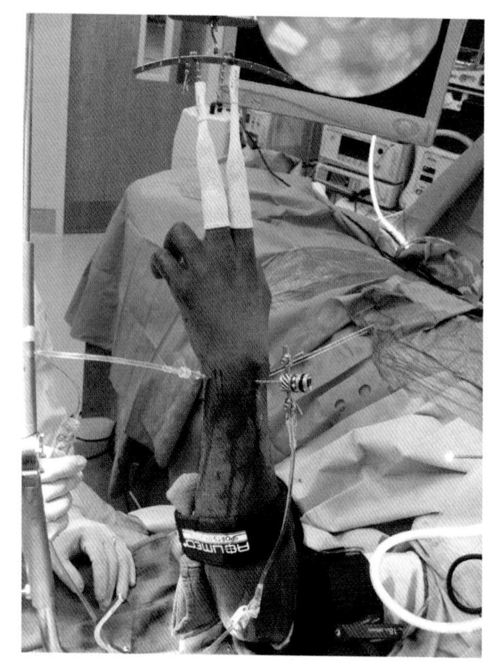

FIGURE 26-5 Washing out the fracture hematoma and debris can improve visualization. A separate inflow is provided through a needle through the 6-U portal, and outflow is provided through an extension through the arthroscopic cannula.

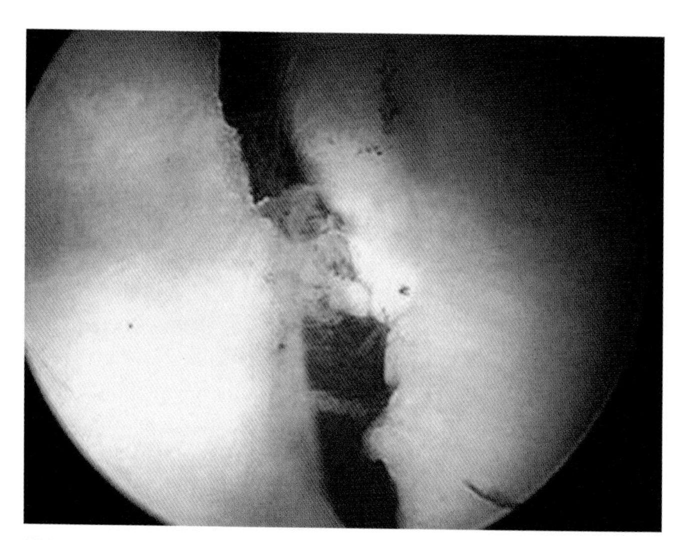

FIGURE 26-6 The depressed lunate facet fragment is identified with the arthroscope in the 3-4 portal.

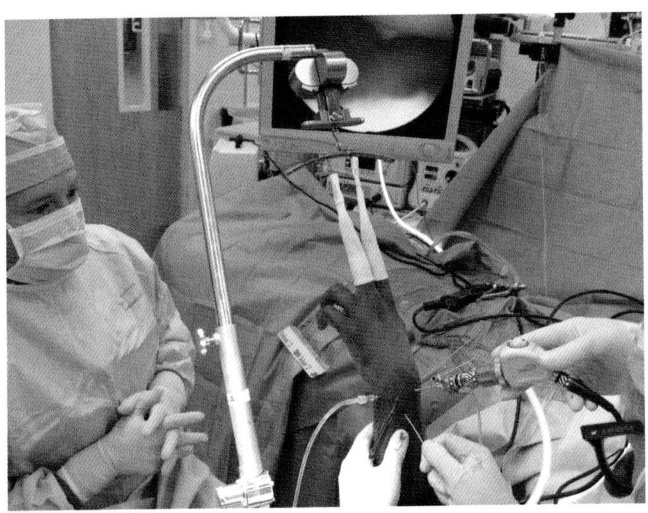

FIGURE 26-7 With the arthroscope in the 3-4 portal, the depressed fragment is percutaneously elevated with a large Kirschner wire inserted approximately 2 cm proximal to the fracture, and it is elevated as viewed arthroscopically.

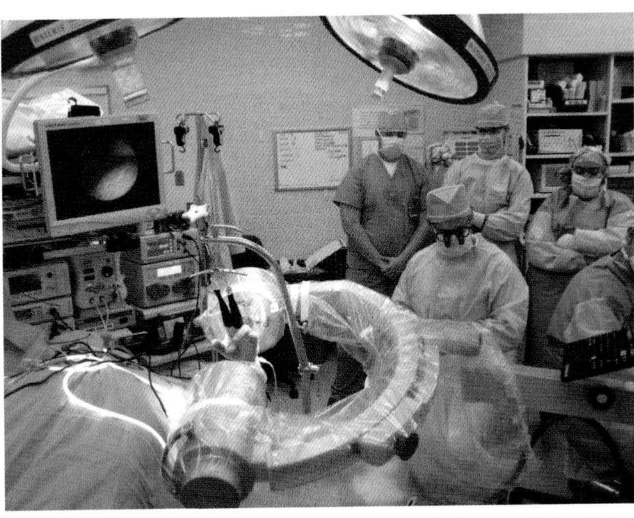

FIGURE 26-9 The Acumed wrist traction tower (Hillsboro, OR) is mini-C-arm friendly. The Orthoscan C-arm (Phoenix, AZ) is brought in to confirm the articular reduction to the lunate facet and position of the guidewires.

needle, and it is used to elevate the depressed lunate facet fragment (Fig. 26-7). A bone tenaculum can further reduce the fracture gap between the fragments. Guidewires are placed transversely from the radial styloid just beneath the articular surface into the lunate facet fragment after the fracture fragments are anatomically reduced, as confirmed arthroscopically (Figs. 26-8 to 26-10). If a dorsal die-punch fragment is present, it is important to aim the transverse wires dorsally to capture and stabilize this dorsal fragment.

After placement of the transverse guidewires, the forearm is pronated and supinated to ensure the guidewires have not violated the distal radioulnar joint. Headless cannulated screws may then be placed over the guidewires to stabilize the radial styloid fragment and the impacted lunate facet fragment. Typically, one

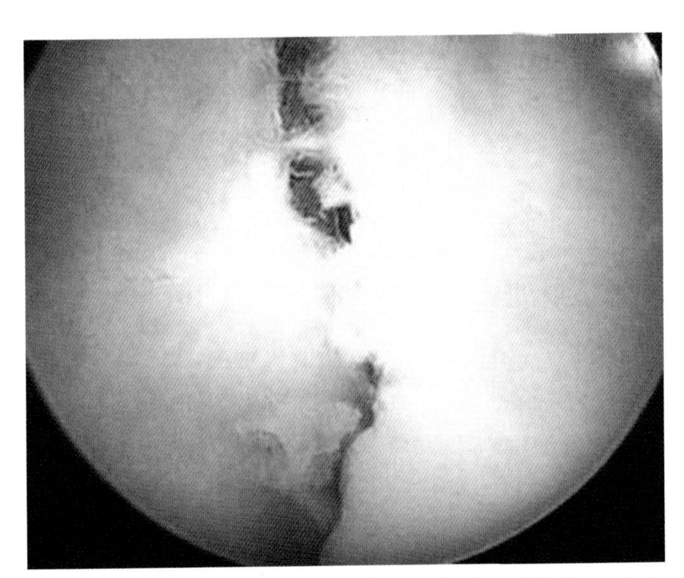

FIGURE 26-8 The arthroscopic view shows reduction of the impacted lunate facet fragment. After the fragment is elevated, transverse guidewires are placed through the radial styloid into the impacted lunate facet fragment.

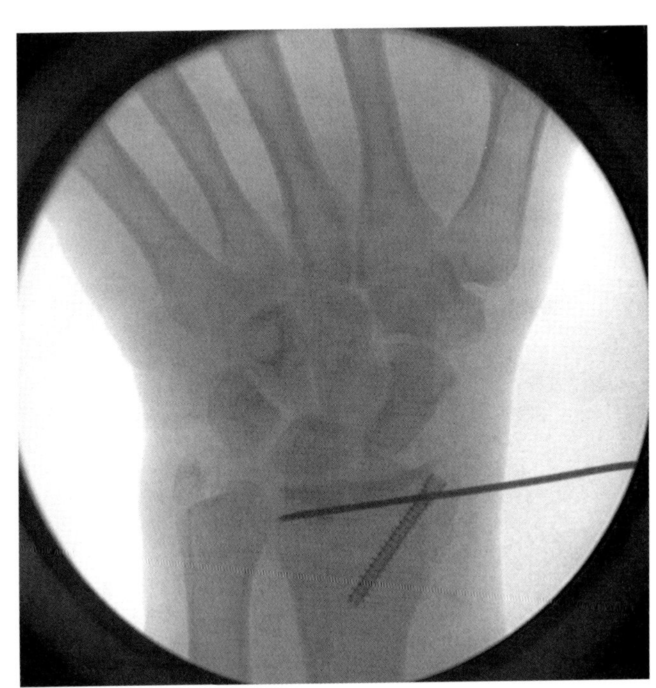

FIGURE 26-10 The fluoroscopic view confirms anatomic reduction to the articular surface and ideal placement of the guidewires volar and dorsal to the previous hemi-screw inserted into the radial styloid.

headless screw is used to stabilize the radial styloid fragment (Figs. 26-11 and 26-12). One or two headless screws placed volar and dorsal to the radial styloid screw may then be placed to stabilize the lunate facet fragment. Further stabilization of the lunate facet fragment may be performed by adding bone graft through a small incision placed between the fourth and fifth dorsal compartments to avoid late settling of the fracture fragments. Cancellous allograft bone chips or bone substitutes may be used.

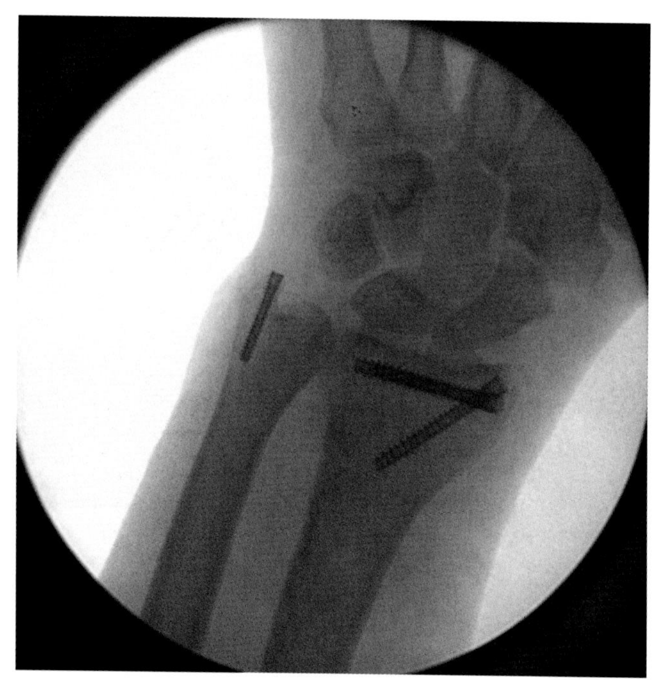

FIGURE 26-11 The postoperative fluoroscopic view shows anatomic reduction to the articular surface and ideal placement of the headless cannulated screws. The articular disk had lost its tension when palpated, and no peripheral tear was identified. In this instance, a micro-Acutrak (Acumed, Hillsboro, OR) was placed through the ulnar styloid fragment.

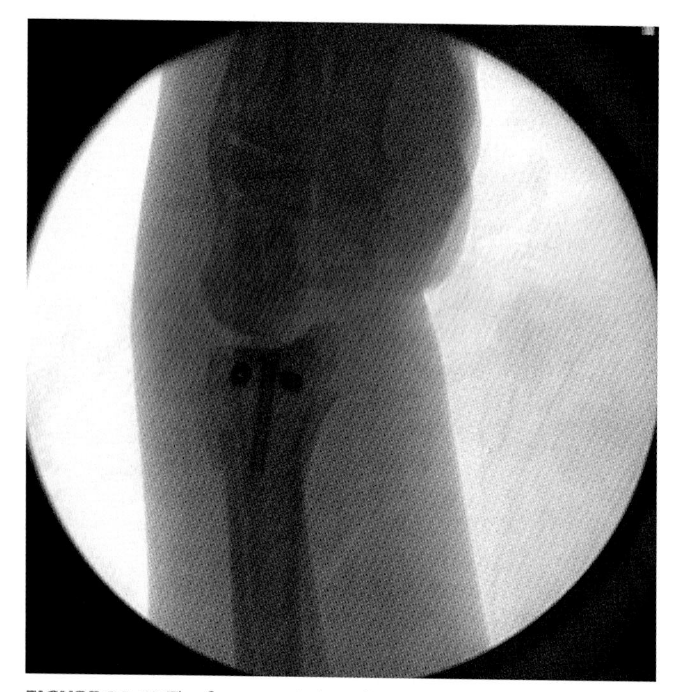

FIGURE 26-12 The fluoroscopic lateral view confirms anatomic reduction to the articular surface, with headless screws placed anteroposterior to the radial styloid screw.

Three- and Four-Part Fractures with Metaphysial Comminution

A combination of open surgery and adjunctive wrist arthroscopy is used for three-part and four-part fractures with metaphysial comminution. A standard volar approach is made to the distal radius over the radial side of the flexor carpi radialis tendon. The flexor pollicis longus tendon is identified and retracted to protect the median nerve, and the pronator quadratus is released from the radial border of the distal radius. The brachioradialis may be further released from the radial styloid to facilitate fracture reduction. The joint capsule is not opened. The fracture is provisionally reduced and stabilized with a volar plate. The first screw is placed in the offset hole in the volar plate to stabilize the plate to the radial shaft. The articular reduction is manipulated as anatomically as possible as viewed by fluoroscopy, and Kirschner wires to the plate provide provisional stabilization.

The wrist is then suspended in the traction tower, and the articular reduction is viewed arthroscopically. If the articular reduction is not anatomic, the pins are removed from the plate, and the reduction is fine-tuned under arthroscopic visualization. After the reduction is judged to be anatomic arthroscopically, the pins are placed back through the plate to provide provisional stabilization to the fracture fragments. The wrist must be solidly flexed in the traction tower to help reduce the distal radius to the plate and prevent a gap. A nonlocking distal screw is initially placed in the distal aspect of the plate to further reduce the fracture fragments to the plate so there is no gap. The remaining distal screws are inserted, and the reduction is viewed fluoroscopically and arthroscopically. In distal dorsal lip fragments, arthroscopy is useful to judge stability as the distal screws are being inserted, and they can be seen stabilizing the dorsal distal fragments. Dorsal lip fragments are best seen with the arthroscope in the 6-R portal or through a volar radial portal between the radial scaphocapitate and long radial lunate ligament.

In four-part fractures, the lunate facet is divided into volar and dorsal fragments (Figs. 26-13 and 26-14). The volar ulnar fragment is reduced under direct observation through the volar approach, reducing it back to the shaft into the radial styloid fragment, and it is provisionally pinned (Fig. 26-15). The volar distal radius plate is used to provisionally stabilize the radial styloid and volar ulnar fragments (Figs. 26-16 and 26-17). The wrist is then suspended in the traction tower. With the arthroscope in the 6-R portal, the dorsal lunate fragment is visualized and percutaneously elevated (Fig. 26-18). After the articular surface is anatomic as seen arthroscopically, the provisional fixation is advanced from volar to dorsal aspects to provisionally stabilize the dorsal fragment (Figs. 26-19 and 26-20). The distal screws are then placed in the volar plate (Figs. 26-20 and 26-21).

Volar plate stabilization using wrist arthroscopy as an adjunct to view the articular reduction is preferred if metaphysial comminution is present. This produces a very stable construct and enables early range of motion and rehabilitation compared with the use of Kirschner wires or headless screws alone. Late settling of the fracture fragments is likely to be seen with volar plate stabilization compared with percutaneous Kirschner wires or cannulated screws.

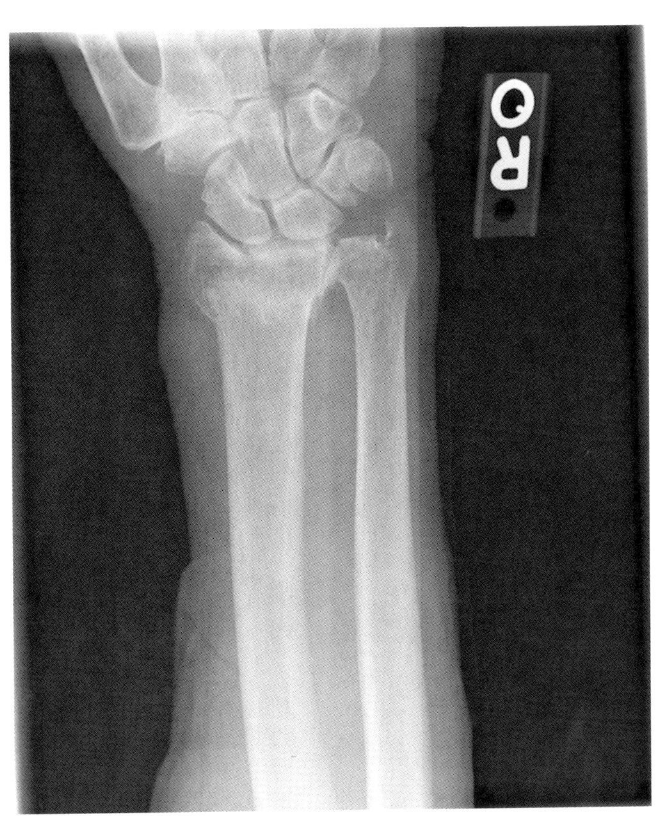

FIGURE 26-13 The posteroanterior radiograph shows a displaced intra-articular fracture of the distal radius with radial shortening.

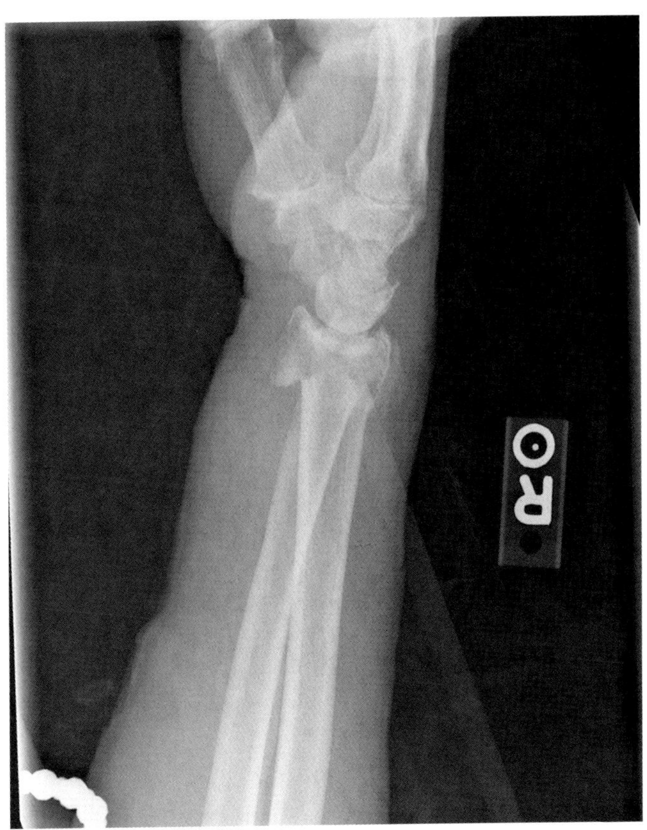

FIGURE 26-14 The lateral view demonstrates a four-part fracture of the distal radius with a displaced volar ulnar fragment. This fracture cannot be closed reduced and requires open reduction and stabilization.

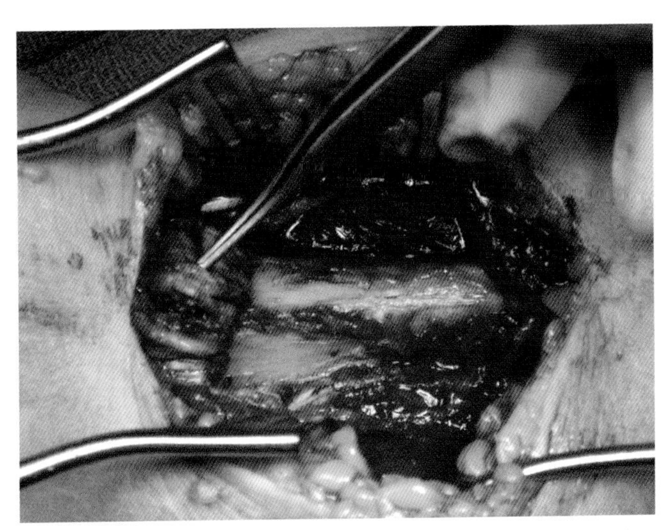

FIGURE 26-15 The intraoperative view shows reduction of the radial styloid and the volar ulnar fragment back to the radial shaft.

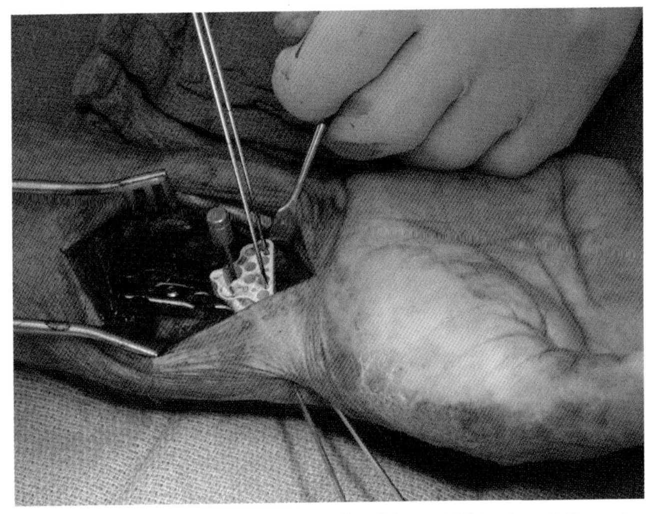

FIGURE 26-16 The Acu-Loc (Acumed, Hillsboro, OR) is placed through the volar incision. The fracture is provisionally stabilized with Kirschner wires placed through the radial styloid and the plate to support the articular surface reduction.

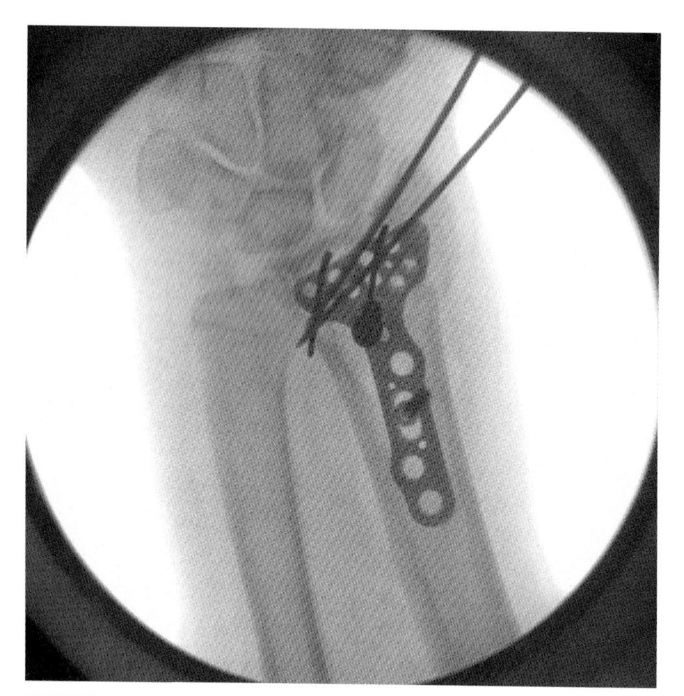

FIGURE 26-17 The fluoroscopic view demonstrates the provisional articular reduction to the distal radius.

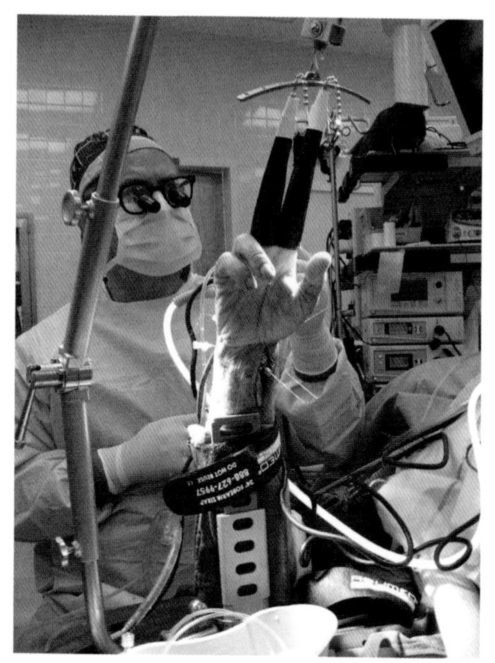

FIGURE 26-18 The wrist is suspended in the Acumed wrist traction tower (Hillsboro, OR), and articular reduction is evaluated. The tower gives full exposure to the volar aspects of the wrist so the Kirschner wires can be removed and replaced if the articular surface reduction is not satisfactory.

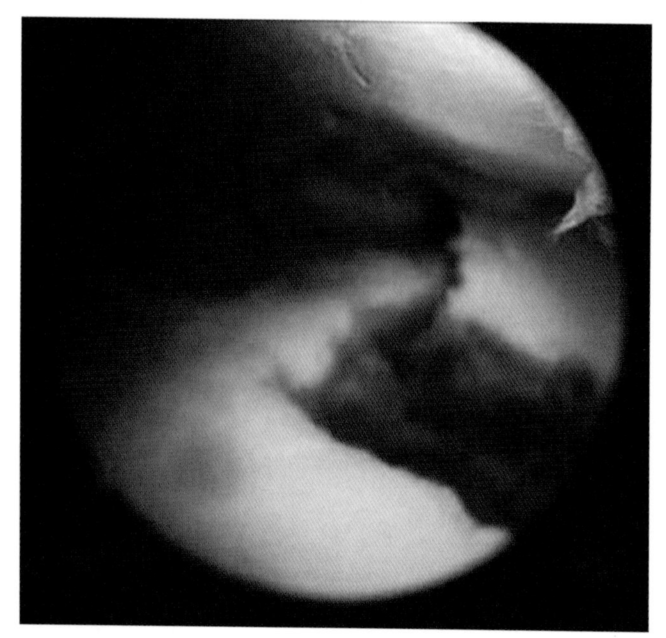

FIGURE 26-19 The arthroscopic view with the arthroscope in the 6-R portal shows displacement of the dorsal ulnar fragment.

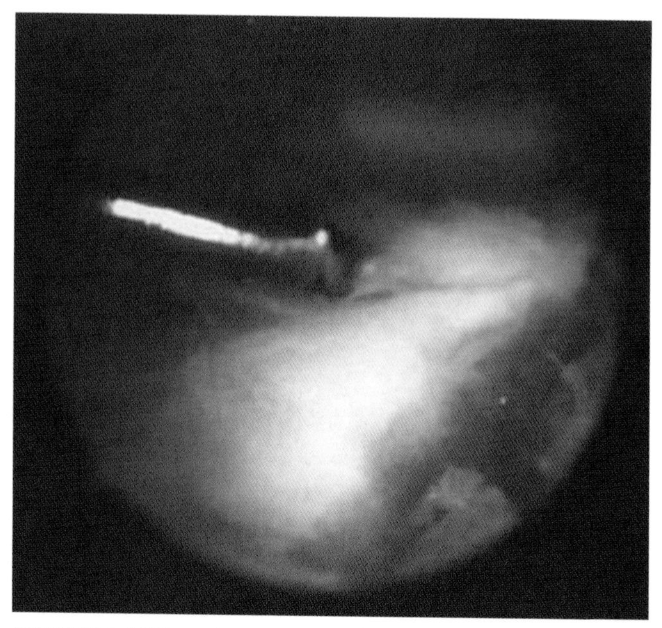

FIGURE 26-20 The arthroscopic view shows reduction of the dorsal ulnar fragment back to the volar ulnar fragment as viewed with the arthroscope in the 6-R portal.

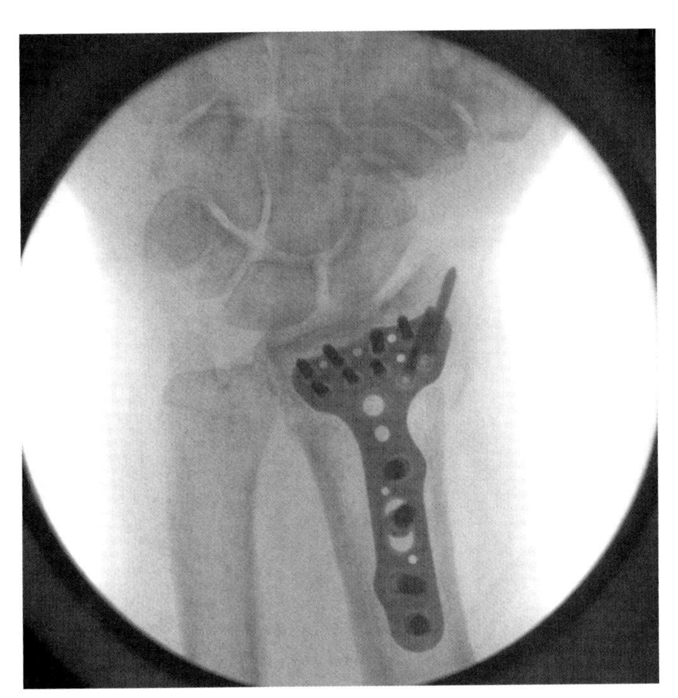

FIGURE 26-21 The posteroanterior fluoroscopic view shows placement of the Acu-Loc plate and anatomic restoration to the articular surface.

Information gained from arthroscopic evaluation of the wrist after stabilization of the distal radius fracture provides some rationale about when to stabilize an associated ulnar styloid fragment (Fig. 26-22), although recommendations about the timing are controversial. After anatomic reduction of a distal radius fracture, the tension of the articular disk is palpated with a probe. The arthroscope is placed in the 3-4 portal, the probe is inserted through the 6-R portal, and the tension of the disk is evaluated. Most fibers of the triangular fibrocartilage complex are still attached to the base of the ulnar and not to the displaced ulnar styloid fragment when there is good tension on the articular disk when it is palpated. A peripheral tear of the triangular fibrocartilage complex is suspected if there is loss of tension on the disk when palpated. A peripheral tear often is covered with hematoma or synovitis, and the hematoma must be débrided to obtain direct visualization of the periphery of the articular disk.

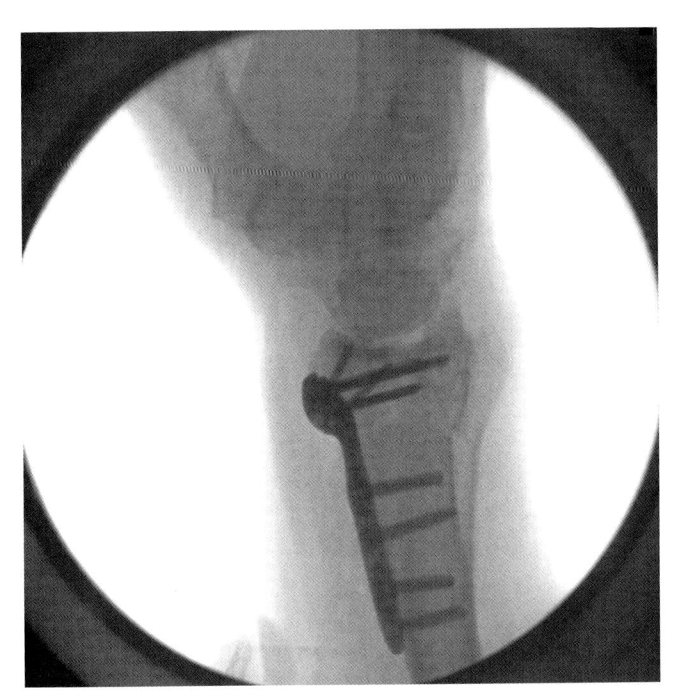

FIGURE 26-22 The lateral fluoroscopic view confirms anatomic reduction to the articular surface and reduction of the volar and dorsal lunate facet fracture fragments.

When detected, a peripheral tear is repaired arthroscopically. Stabilization of a large ulnar styloid fragment is considered when there is loss of tension on the articular disk and no peripheral ulnar tear of the articular disk is identified. In this instance, most fibers of the articular disk are attached to the ulnar styloid fragment. The incision is made in the interval between the extensor carpi ulnaris and flexor carpi ulnaris, and blunt dissection is carried down to protect the dorsal sensory branch of the ulnar nerve, which runs along the volar aspect of the incision. The ulnar styloid fragment is anatomically reduced and may be stabilized with a tension band, Kirschner wire, or preferably, a small headless cannulated screw.

PEARLS & PITFALLS

- Precise portal placement is mandatory in wrist arthroscopy.
- For a swollen wrist, the external landmarks usually can be palpated to help in portal placement. The 3-4 portal is made in line with the radial border of the long finger; the 4-5 portal is in line with the midaxis of the ring finger; and the 6-R portal is just radial to the extensor carpi ulnaris tendon.
- Place a needle into a portal location before committing to a skin incision.
- Wash out fracture hematoma and debris to improve visualization.
- It is easier to judge rotation of a fracture fragment by looking across the wrist from the fragment. A radial styloid fragment is best visualized with the arthroscope in the 6-R portal, and depressed lunate facet fragments are best visualized with the arthroscope in the 3-4 portal.
- Be wary of the cutaneous sensory nerves about the wrist. Insert guidewires through a small incision, a trocar, or in oscillation mode.
- Combining wrist arthroscopy with volar plating for fractures with extensive metaphysial involvement allows anatomic restoration of the joint surface and produces good stability, which enables an early range-of-motion program.

OUTCOMES

Wrist arthroscopy takes advantage of its ability to view the articular surface under bright light and magnified conditions. Two millimeters of articular displacement has become an established criterion for congruency of the distal radius over the past several years. Knirk and Jupiter demonstrated the importance of an articular reduction of the distal radius within 2 mm or less.[11] Patients whose articular reduction was greater than 2 mm at the final follow-up visit demonstrated significantly higher incidences of degenerative changes within their wrists. Bradway and Amadio reported similar findings.[12]

Fernandez and Geissler reported their series of 40 patients and observed that the critical threshold might be 1 mm or less.[13] They reported that the complication rate was substantially lower when the articular reduction was 1 mm or less. Trumble and colleagues, in their review of 52 intra-articular distal radius fractures, found that the factors that most strongly correlated with a successful outcome included the amount of residual radial shortening and articular incongruence.[14]

Edwards and colleagues described the advantage of viewing intra-articular reduction by wrist arthroscopy compared with monitoring by fluoroscopy alone.[15] In their series of 15 patients who underwent arthroscopic evaluation of the articular surface after reduction and stabilization under fluoroscopic guidance, 33% of patients still had an articular step-off of 1 mm or more. Frequently, the fracture fragment was rotated. They found that wrist arthroscopy was particularly useful in judging rotation of the fracture fragments, a situation that is not readily identifiable under fluoroscopy alone. It is easy to judge rotation of the fracture fragment by looking across the wrist. For example, to judge rotation of a radial styloid fragment, it is best to place the arthroscope in the 4-5 or 6-R portal. Similarly, to view reduction of a lunate facet fragment, it is best to place the arthroscope in the 3-4 portal to view reduction of the die-punch fragment. Fractures of the dorsal lip may be viewed with the arthroscope in the 6-R portal or the volar portal.

The literature is sparse regarding the results of arthroscopically assisted fixation of displaced intra-articular fractures of the distal radius. Stewart and coworkers compared 12 open and 12 arthroscopically assisted reductions of comminuted AO type C fractures of the distal radius.[16] The arthroscopically treated group had five excellent results, six good results, and one fair result. The open group had no excellent results. The investigators found that the arthroscopic group had increased range of motion compared with the group that underwent open stabilization for similar fracture patterns.

Doi and colleagues reported a similar comparison of 38 patients who underwent arthroscopically assisted fixation or open reduction and fixation.[17] They reported results similar to those of earlier studies, and they observed that the arthroscopic group had improved range of motion compared with the group that underwent open stabilization.

Ruch and coworkers compared 15 patients who underwent arthroscopically assisted reduction and 15 patients who underwent closed reduction and external fixation.[18] Of the 15 patients who underwent arthroscopic reduction, 10 patients had a tear of the triangular fibrocartilage complex, seven of which were peripheral and were stabilized. No patients in the arthroscopic group had any signs of instability of the distal radioulnar joint at the final follow-up visit. In contrast, 4 of the 15 patients who were managed by external fixation alone continued to complain about instability of the distal radioulnar joint. These patients potentially had a peripheral tear of the triangular fibrocartilage complex at the time of fracture that was not repaired.

Geissler and coworkers reported the results of 33 patients who underwent arthroscopically assisted reduction of extra-articular distal radius fractures.[10] In their series, 25 patients had anatomic reduction of the articular surface, and 8 patients had a 1-mm step-off. They analyzed the results based on associated soft tissue injuries and found that a Geissler grade II injury of the scapholunate interosseous ligament did not affect the final prognosis. However, for patients with a Geissler grade III or IV tear and an AO type C fracture, the final result was significantly affected by the soft tissue injury.

CONCLUSIONS

Wrist arthroscopy has proved to be a valuable adjunct in the management of intra-articular distal radius fractures. Wrist arthroscopy allows visualization of the articular reduction under bright light and magnified conditions. Wrist arthroscopy combined with volar plating enables precise reduction of the articular surface, stabilization of the volar plate, and early range of motion. The importance of anatomic restoration of the articular surface has been confirmed by several studies.[11,12,14] Arthroscopic lavage of fracture hematoma and debris also can improve the patient's final range of motion. Studies by Stewart and associates[16] and Doi and colleagues[17] showed improved range of motion in patients who underwent arthroscopic reduction compared with those who underwent open reduction alone.

Wrist arthroscopy enables detection and management of the soft tissue injuries that frequently are associated with intra-articular fractures of the distal radius.[2-6,18,19] Arthroscopic findings can establish the grade of severity of the injury and determine the type of surgical management needed for these soft tissue injuries.

It is much easier to manage an acute soft tissue lesion with a better prognosis than to undertake reconstruction of a chronic injury. Tears of the triangular fibrocartilage complex are the most common type of soft tissue injury associated with fractures of the distal radius.[20] This may explain why some patients continue to complain of persistent ulnar-sided wrist pain despite an anatomic articular reduction seen on plain radiographs.

Wrist arthroscopy can help the surgeon in determining when and when not to stabilize a displaced large ulnar styloid fragment. When the articular disk is lax after restoration of the articular distal radius surface and no peripheral tear of the articular disk is identified, consideration should be given to stabilization of a large ulnar styloid fragment.

REFERENCES

1. Lafontaine M, Hardy D, Delince P. Stability assessment of distal radius fractures. *Injury*. 1989;20:208-210.
2. Mohanti RC, Kar N. Study of triangular fibrocartilage of the wrist joint in Colles fracture. *Injury*. 1979;11:311-324.
3. Fontes D, Lenoble E, DeSomer B, et al. Lesions ligamentaires associus aux fractures distales du radius. *Ann Chir Main*. 1992;11:119-125.
4. Geissler WB, Freeland AE, Savoie FH, et al. Carpal instability associated with intraarticular distal radius fractures. In: Proceedings of the American Academy Orthopedic Surgeons Annual Meeting. 1993; San Francisco, CA.
5. Lindau T. Treatment of injuries to the ulnar side of the wrist occurring with distal radial fractures. *Hand Clin*. 2005;21:417-425.
6. Hanker GJ. Wrist arthroscopy in distal radius fractures. In: Proceedings of the Arthroscopy Association North America Annual Meeting, 1993; Albuquerque, NM.
7. Geissler WB, Savoie FH. Arthroscopic techniques of the wrist. *Mediguide Orthop*. 1992;11:1-8.
8. Geissler WB. Arthroscopically assisted reduction of intra-articular fractures of the distal radius. *Hand Clin*. 1995;11:19-29.

9. Geissler WB. Intraarticular distal radius fractures: the role of arthroscopy? *Hand Clin*. 2005;21:407-416.
10. Geissler WB, Freeland AE. Arthroscopically assisted reduction of intraarticular distal radial fractures. *Clin Orthop Relat Res*. 1996;(327):125-134.
11. Knirk JL, Jupiter JB. Intra-articular fractures of the distal end of the radius in young adults. *J Bone Joint Surg Am*. 1986;68:647-658.
12. Bradway JK, Amadio PC, Cooney WP. Open reduction and internal fixation of displaced comminuted intra-articular fractures of the distal end of the radius. *J Bone Joint Surg Am*. 1989;71:839-847.
13. Fernandez DL, Geissler WB. Treatment of displaced articular fractures of the radius. *J Hand Surg*. 1991;16:375-384.
14. Trumble TE, Schmitt SR, Vedder NB. Fractures affecting functional outcome of displaced intra-articular distal radius fractures. *J Hand Surg Am*. 1994;19:325-340.
15. Edwards CC III, Harasztic J, McGillivary GR, Gutow AP. Intra-articular distal radius fractures: arthroscopic assessment of radiographically assisted reduction. *J Hand Surg Am*. 2001;26:1036-1041.
16. Stewart NJ, Berger RA. Comparison study of arthroscopic as open reduction of comminuted distal radius fractures. Presented at the 53rd Annual Meeting of the American Society for Surgery of the Hand (Programs and Abstracts), January 11, 1998; Scottsdale, AZ.
17. Doi K, Hattori T, Otsuka K, et al. Intra-articular fractures of the distal aspect of the radius arthroscopically assisted reduction compared with open reduction and internal fixation. *J Bone Joint Surg Am*. 1999;81:1093-1110.
18. Ruch DS, Vallee J, Poehling GG, et al. Arthroscopic reduction versus fluoroscopic reduction of intra-articular distal radius fractures. *Arthroscopy*. 2004;20:225-230.
19. Mudgal CS, Jones WA. Scapholunate diastasis: a component of fractures of the distal radius. *J Hand Surg Br*. 1990;15:503-505.
20. Hollingworth R, Morris J. The importance of the ulnar side of the wrist in fractures of the distal end of the radius. *Injury*. 1976;7:263.

CHAPTER

27

Acute Scaphoid Fractures in Nonunions

William B. Geissler

The scaphoid is the most frequently fractured bone in the carpus and accounts for approximately 70% of all carpal fractures.[1] This fracture typically occurs in young men between the ages of 15 and 30 years.[2] A scaphoid fracture is a common athletic injury, occurring most often in contact sports, particularly in football and basketball players. It is estimated that 1 of 100 college football players will sustain a fracture of the scaphoid.[3] Commonly, an injured athlete continues to compete and eventually presents to the treating physician after the season is over with a scaphoid nonunion.

Acute nondisplaced fractures of the scaphoid have traditionally been managed with cast immobilization.[4,5] Nondisplaced scaphoid fractures usually heal in 8 to 12 weeks when immobilized in long arm or short arm spica casts.[4-6] Although cast immobilization is successful in up to 85% to 90% of cases, it must be asked what the cost is to the patient, particularly the athlete, who may not be able to tolerate a lengthy course of immobilization during the season or while actively training.[4-6] Prolonged immobilization may lead to muscle atrophy, disuse osteopenia, joint contracture, and financial hardship. Until the fracture unites, the athlete may be inactive for 6 months or longer.

The duration of cast immobilization varies dramatically according to the fracture site. A fracture of the scaphoid tubercle may be healed within a period of 6 weeks, whereas a fracture of the waist of the scaphoid may require immobilization for 3 months or longer. A fracture of the proximal third of the scaphoid may take 5 months or longer to heal with a cast because of the vascularity of the scaphoid.[7] This may result in loss of an athletic scholarship or loss of employment.

Displaced scaphoids have a reported nonunion rate of up to 50%.[2] Factors that decrease the prognosis for healing include the amount of displacement, associated carpal ligament instability, and delayed presentation (>4 to 6 weeks).[1] Traditionally, acute displaced fractures of the scaphoid and scaphoid nonunions have been managed by open reduction and internal fixation.[1,2,8-16] Complications associated with open reduction fixation include avascular necrosis, carpal instability, donor site pain, infection, screw protrusion, and reflex sympathetic dystrophy resulting from the significant soft tissue dissection that is required.[4,17] The most commonly reported complication in one series was hypertrophic scarring.[2] Although jigs have been designed to assist an open reduction, they frequently are difficult to apply and may necessitate further extensive surgical dissection.[18]

Wrist arthroscopy has revolutionized the practice of orthopedics by allowing the surgeon to examine and treat intra-articular abnormalities of the wrist joint under bright light and magnification.[19] The scaphoid is well visualized from the radiocarpal and midcarpal spaces. Whipple is credited with being the first surgeon to attempt arthroscopic management of scaphoid fractures.[19] His preliminary work set the stage for the current concepts and treatment by arthroscopy of these common fractures.

Fractures of the scaphoid are best visualized with the arthroscope in the midcarpal space. Fractures of the proximal pole of the scaphoid are best seen with the arthroscope in the ulnar midcarpal portal, and fractures of the waist are best visualized with the arthroscope in the radial midcarpal portal. Arthroscopic reduction of scaphoid fractures allows direct visualization and reduction of the scaphoid as the guidewires and percutaneous screws are being inserted. Associated soft tissue injuries that may occur with a fracture of the scaphoid can be arthroscopically detected and managed at the same sitting.

The indications and techniques of arthroscopic management of acute scaphoid fractures and selected nonunions are reviewed in this chapter. Arthroscopic stabilization provides direct visualization of the fracture reduction, screw insertion, and limited surgical dissection, which may allow for a greater range of motion and earlier return to competition or employment.

PATIENT EVALUATION

Diagnostic Imaging

Posteroanterior and lateral radiographs are mandatory to assess displacement, alignment, and angulation of a scaphoid fracture. Semisupinated and pronated views can demonstrate the proximal and distal poles of the scaphoid. It is often helpful to place the wrist in ulnar deviation, which extends the scaphoid in a posteroanterior view for detection of fracture displacement. A nondisplaced fracture of the scaphoid will not become apparent on radiographs for several weeks after injury. It is important to mobilize the patient who presents with snuffbox tenderness until the pain has resolved or until a diagnosis has been confirmed radiographically.

Computed tomography (CT) parallel to the longitudinal axis of the scaphoid is useful to evaluate displacement, angulation, and healing when further information is required to assess the fracture. The patient is placed prone with the arms extended overhead and the wrist radially deviated to obtain longitudinal access to the scaphoid. Coronal CT slices are obtained with supination of the forearm to a neutral position. CT evaluation is particularly helpful when nonoperative management of scaphoid fractures is selected, because it can be difficult to judge healing of the scaphoid by plain radiography. This is particularly important when returning an athlete back to contact sports. One advantage of operative fixation is that the screw acts as an internal splint to stabilize the fracture, and the exact timing of return to competition is less critical compared with nonoperative management.

TREATMENT

Indications

Arthroscopic fixation may be performed for acute nondisplaced fractures of the scaphoid and acute displaced fractures of the scaphoid that are reducible. For acute nondisplaced fractures, the risks and benefits of arthroscopic stabilization compared with cast immobilization must be discussed with the patient so that an informed decision can be made by the patient and associated family members. For acute fractures of the scaphoid that are reducible, the fracture may be reduced by manipulation of the wrist in a traction tower or by joysticks inserted into the proximal and distal poles of the scaphoid, with the reduction viewed with the arthroscope in the midcarpal space.

Arthroscopic stabilization of selected scaphoid nonunions may be performed. Slade and Geissler published their radiographic classification of scaphoid nonunions (Table 27-1).[20]

- Type I fractures are the result of a delayed presentation (4 to 12 weeks after injury).
- In type II injuries, a fibrous union is present. A minimal fracture line may be seen on plain radiographs. The lunate is not rotated, and there is no humpback deformity.
- In type III injuries, minimal sclerosis is seen at the fracture site. Sclerosis is less than 1 mm long, the lunate is not rotated, and no humpback deformity is seen.
- In type IV injuries, cystic formation is present. The cystic formation is between 1 and 5 mm in diameter. No humpback deformity or rotation of the lunate is seen on plain radiographs.

TABLE 27-1 Slade-Geissler Classification of Scaphoid Nonunions

Type	Description
I	Delayed presentation at 4-12 wk
II	Fibrous union, minimal fracture line
III	Minimal sclerosis < 1 mm
IV	Cystic formation, 1-5 mm
V	Humpback deformity with > 5-mm cystic change
VI	Wrist arthrosis

- In type V injuries, the cystic changes are larger than 5 mm in diameter, and rotation of the lunate has occurred, resulting in a humpback deformity as seen with plain radiography or CT. The lunate has rotated to a position of dorsal intercalated segment instability (DISI).
- In type VI injuries, secondary degenerative changes are present, with spurring along the radial border of the scaphoid and peaking of the radial styloid (i.e., scaphoid nonunion advanced collapse [SNAC]).

Arthroscopic stabilization of selected scaphoid nonunions is indicated in fracture types I through IV. After a humpback deformity occurs, arthroscopic stabilization is not recommended, and open reduction is needed to correct the humpback deformity and the DISI rotation of the lunate.

Arthroscopic Techniques

Various arthroscopically assisted and percutaneous techniques for fractures of the scaphoid have been described in the literature.[21-32] Haddad and Goddard[24] popularized the volar approach, and the dorsal approach was popularized by Slade and colleagues.[26] Geissler and Slade described a technique in which the starting point of the guidewire and the eventual screw insertion are determined arthroscopically, which limits guesswork concerning the insertion point.[32]

Volar Percutaneous Approach

In the volar percutaneous technique that was popularized by Haddad and Goddard, the patient is placed supine with the thumb suspended in a Chinese finger trap.[24] Placing the thumb under suspension allows ulnar deviation of the wrist, which improves access to the distal pole of the scaphoid. Under fluoroscopic guidance, a longitudinal, 0.5-cm skin incision is made over the most distal radial aspect of the scaphoid. Blunt dissection is used to expose the distal pole of the scaphoid. The cutaneous nerves must be protected when using this technique.

A percutaneous guidewire is introduced into the scaphoid trapezial joint and advanced proximally and dorsally across the fracture site. The position of the guidewire is easily checked in the anteroposterior, oblique, and lateral planes by rotating the forearm under fluoroscopy. This provides an almost 360-degree view of the position of the guidewire within the scaphoid. The length of the guidewire within the scaphoid is determined by placing a second guidewire next to the initial one and measuring the difference between the two. A drill is inserted through the soft tissue protector, and the scaphoid is reamed. A headless cannulated screw is then placed over the guidewire. A second guidewire may be useful to prevent rotation of the fracture fragments while the screw is being inserted.

Haddad and Goddard reported their initial results in a pilot study of 15 patients with acute fractures of the scaphoid.[24] Union was achieved in all patients within an average of 57 days (range, 38 to 71 days). With this percutaneous technique, the range of motion after union was equal to that of the contralateral limb, and grip strength averaged 90% at 3 months. The patients were able to return to sedentary work within 4 days and to manual work within 5 weeks.

This technique is fairly simple and straightforward, and it requires minimal specialized equipment. The disadvantage is the possibility that the screw may be placed slightly oblique to the midwaist fracture line in the scaphoid.

Dorsal Percutaneous Approach

Slade and coworkers popularized the dorsal percutaneous approach.[26,27] This technique has become popular because it involves limited surgical dissection and allows arthroscopic evaluation and reduction of the scaphoid fracture. The patient is placed in the supine position on the table with the arm extended. Several towels are placed under the elbow to support the forearm parallel to the floor. The wrist is then flexed and pronated under fluoroscopy until the distal and proximal poles of the scaphoid are aligned to form a perfect cylinder. Continuous fluoroscopy is recommended as the wrist is flexed to obtain a true ring sign as the proximal and distal poles are aligned.

Under fluoroscopy, a 14-gauge needle is placed percutaneously in the center of the ring sign and parallel to the fluoroscopy beam. A guidewire is then inserted through the 14-gauge needle and driven across the central axis of the scaphoid from dorsal to volar until the end of the guidewire comes into contact with the distal scaphoid cortex. The position of the guidewire is then evaluated under fluoroscopy in the posteroanterior, oblique, and lateral planes while the wrist is maintained in flexion. The wrist must not be extended at this time, because doing so may bend the guidewire. A second guidewire is placed parallel to the first so that it touches the proximal pole of the scaphoid, and the difference in the lengths of the two guidewires is measured to determine the length of the screw. Use of a screw 4 mm shorter than what is measured is recommended.

The primary guidewire is advanced volarly through a portion of the trapezium and along the radial side of the thumb metacarpal until it exits the skin on the volar aspect of the hand. The wire continues to be advanced volarly until it is flush with the proximal pole of the scaphoid dorsally and the wrist is extended.

The wrist is suspended in a traction tower, and the radiocarpal and midcarpal spaces are arthroscopically evaluated. The radiocarpal space is evaluated for associated soft tissue injuries. The reduction of the scaphoid is best seen with the arthroscope in the midcarpal space. After the reduction of the scaphoid fracture is considered satisfactory, the primary guidewire is advanced back dorsally and proximally with the wrist flexed. A portion of the guidewire should be left extending out of the volar and dorsal aspects of the wrist; if the guidewire breaks, it is easy to remove. Blunt dissection is continued around the guidewire dorsally to minimize the risk of soft tissue injuries, particularly injury to the extensor tendons as the scaphoid is reamed and the screw is inserted over the guidewire. Through a soft tissue protector, the scaphoid is drilled over the guidewire, and a headless cannulated screw is inserted.

The dorsal approach has the advantage that the screw can be inserted down the central axis of the scaphoid. This allows compression directly across the fracture site, compared with the more oblique orientation of the screw when the volar technique is used. The concern with the dorsal percutaneous approach is that the wrist is hyperflexed; this may displace the scaphoid fracture to create a humpback deformity if it is unstable. The reduction of the scaphoid should be evaluated with the arthroscope in the midcarpal space when this technique is used to ensure that the fracture is not hyperflexed.

Geissler Technique for Arthroscopic Reduction

The advantage of using my arthroscopic technique for reduction of acute scaphoid fractures and certain scaphoid nonunions[33] is that the starting point for the guidewire is viewed directly through the arthroscope, and there is no guesswork concerning the insertion point and the location of the headless cannulated screw. I think this is a simpler approach than the dorsal percutaneous approach with the ring sign. The wrist is not hyperflexed, which could distract the scaphoid fracture and cause a humpback deformity.

Using the Geissler technique, the wrist is initially suspended in a wrist traction tower (Acumed, Hillsboro, OR) (Fig. 27-1). The arthroscope is initially placed in the 3-4 portal to evaluate any associated soft tissue injuries that may occur with a scaphoid fracture. After evaluation and treatment of the soft tissue injuries, the arthroscope is transferred into the 6-R portal. The wrist is flexed ap-

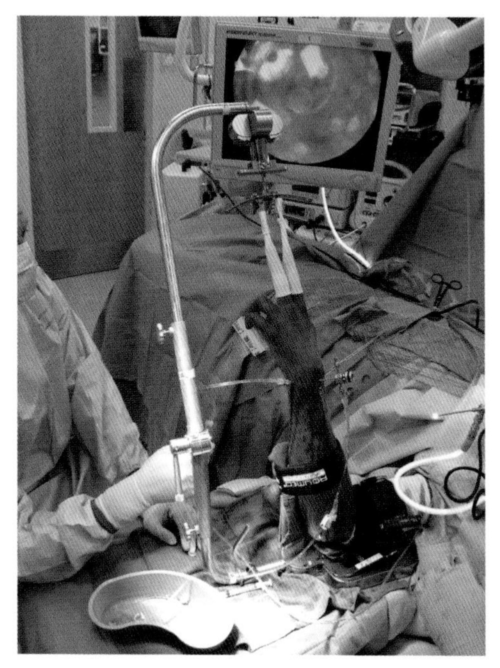

FIGURE 27-1 The wrist is suspended in 30 degrees of flexion in the Acumed wrist traction tower.

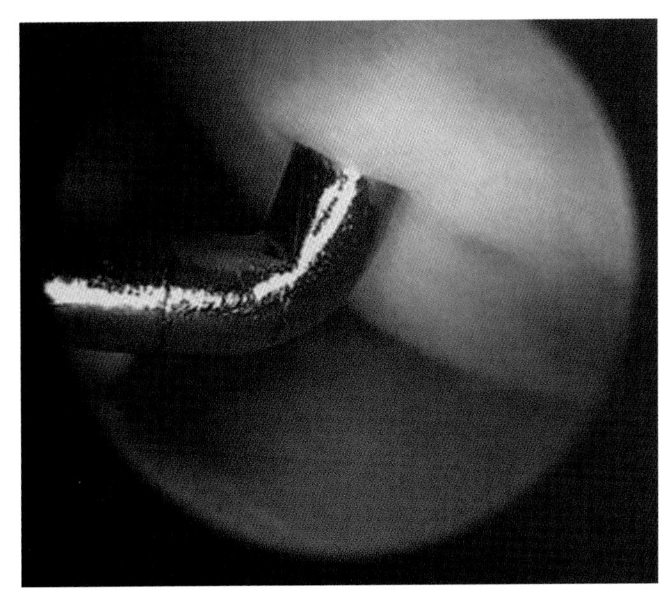

FIGURE 27-2 After arthroscopic evaluation of the wrist with the arthroscope in the diagnostic 3-4 portal, the it is switched to the 6-R portal, and the junction of the scapholunate interosseous ligament to the proximal pole of the scaphoid is palpated with a probe.

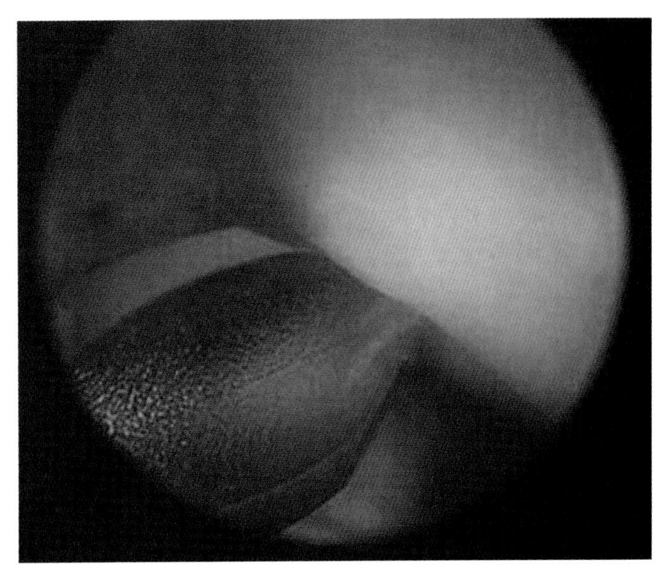

FIGURE 27-4 Arthroscopic confirmation of the 14-gauge needle is obtained as it impales the proximal pole of the scaphoid at the junction of the scapholunate interosseous ligament.

proximately 30 degrees in the traction tower. A 14-gauge needle is inserted through the 3-4 portal, and the junction of the scapholunate interosseous ligament as it inserts onto the proximal pole of the scaphoid is palpated. The junction of the scapholunate interosseous ligament onto the scaphoid along the middle third is the ideal starting point for the screw (Fig. 27-2). A 14-gauge needle is advanced and impaled into the proximal pole of the scaphoid at the insertion of the scapholunate interosseous ligament (Figs. 27-3 and 27-4).

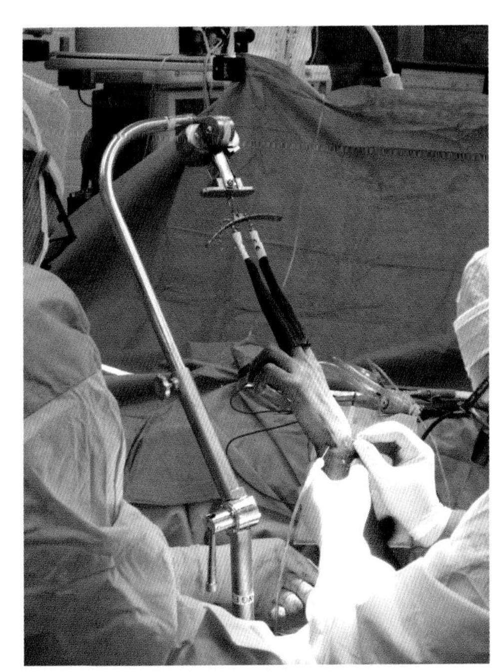

FIGURE 27-3 A 14-gauge needle is inserted through the 3-4 portal at the junction of the scapholunate interosseous ligament to the proximal pole of the scaphoid.

Occasionally, some dorsal synovitis blocks visualization of the starting point and may need to be débrided.

The traction tower is then flexed, and the starting point of the needle is evaluated under fluoroscopy (Figs. 27-5 and 27-6). With this technique, the starting point is consistently determined to be at the most proximal pole of the scaphoid. The needle is simply aimed toward the thumb under fluoroscopy, and a guidewire is advanced through the needle down the central axis of the scaphoid to abut the distal pole. The position of the guidewire is checked in the posteroanterior, oblique, and lateral planes under fluoroscopy by rotating the forearm in the traction tower (Figs. 27-7 and 27-8). The fluoroscopic image is not hindered by the support beam

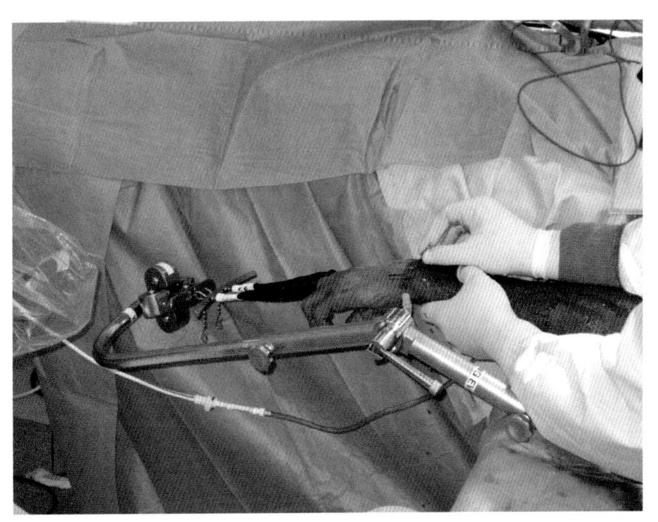

FIGURE 27-5 The Acumed wrist traction tower is flexed, and fluoroscopic confirmation of the ideal starting point is obtained.

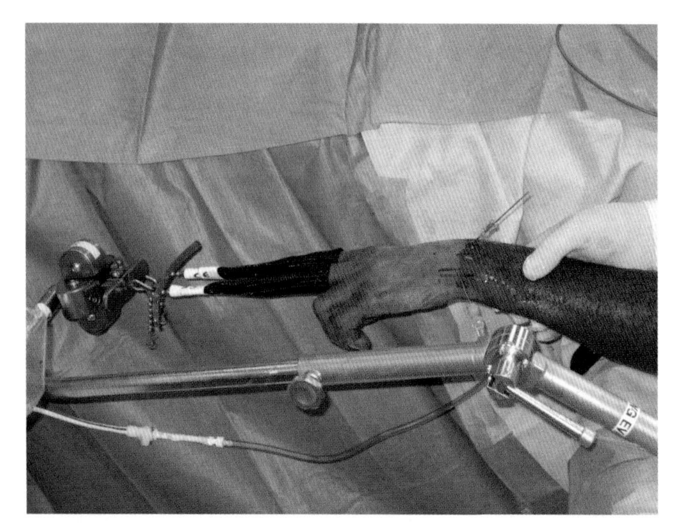

FIGURE 27-6 From the starting point, the needle is aimed toward the thumb, and a guidewire is advanced down the central axis of the scaphoid.

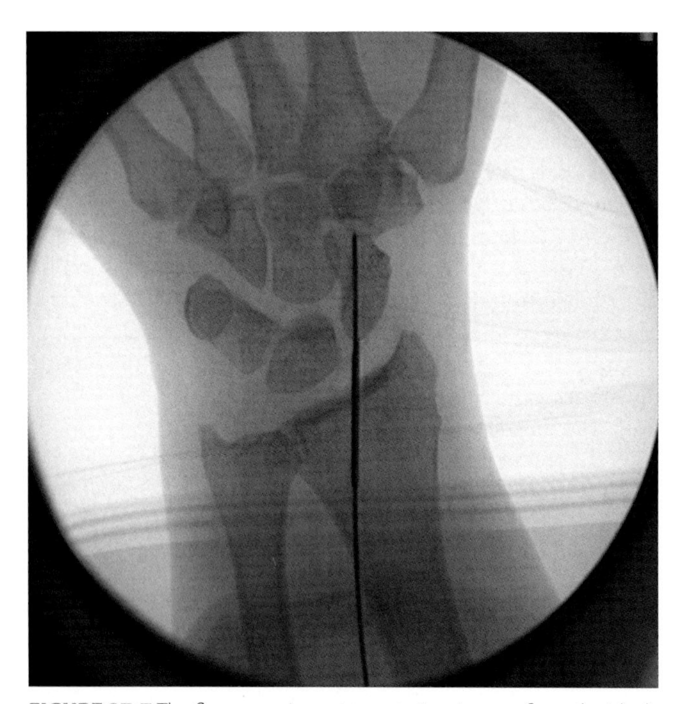

FIGURE 27-7 The fluoroscopic posteroanterior view confirms the ideal starting point of the guidewire and placement of the wire down the central axis of the scaphoid.

of the tower, which is off to the side rather than in the central axis. A second guidewire is advanced against the proximal pole of the scaphoid, and the length of the screw is determined by the difference of the two guidewires. A screw at least 4 mm shorter than this measurement is recommended.

The reduction of the scaphoid is evaluated with the arthroscope in the radial and ulnar midcarpal portals. If reduction is unsatisfactory, the guidewire is advanced volarly across the wrist but still within the distal pole of the scaphoid. An additional Kirschner wire may be placed in the proximal pole of the scaphoid. These wires may be used as joysticks to further reduce the fracture anatomically under direct view with the arthroscope in

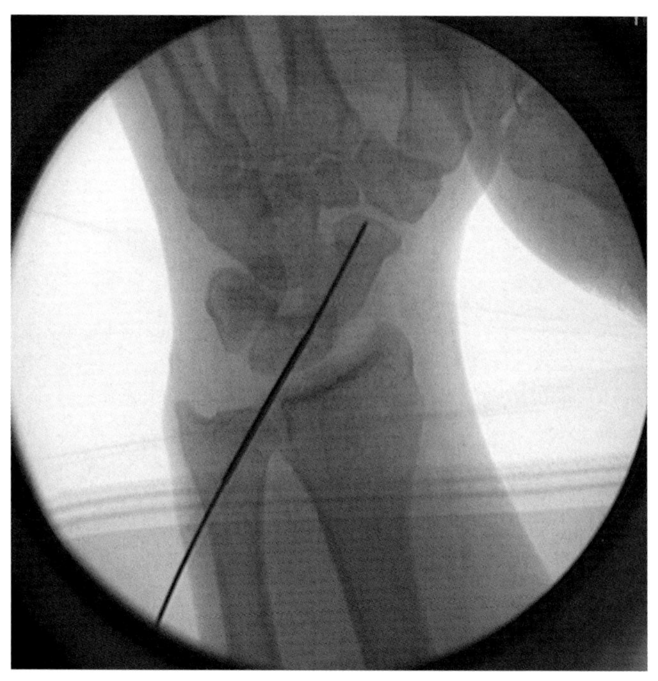

FIGURE 27-8 The fluoroscopic oblique view confirms ideal placement of the guidewire down the central axis of the scaphoid.

the midcarpal portal. It helps to manipulate the wrist in the traction tower, usually with the wrist in extension, which further reduces the fracture. After the fracture is judged to be satisfactory, the guidewire is advanced proximally into the proximal pole of the scaphoid. The scaphoid is then reamed with the cannulated drill (Fig. 27-9).

In cases of acute fractures or stable fibrous nonunions, demineralized bone matrix (DBM) is not used, and a headless cannulated screw is inserted over the guidewire (Fig. 27-10). The position of the screw is checked in the posteroanterior, oblique, and lateral planes under fluoroscopy with the wrist stabilized by the traction

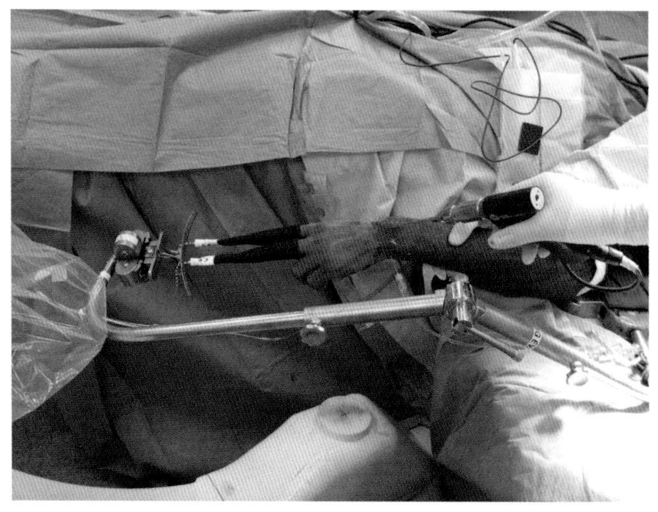

FIGURE 27-9 After the length of the screw has been determined, the guidewire is advanced out the volar aspect of the wrist, and the scaphoid is reamed with a cannulated drill.

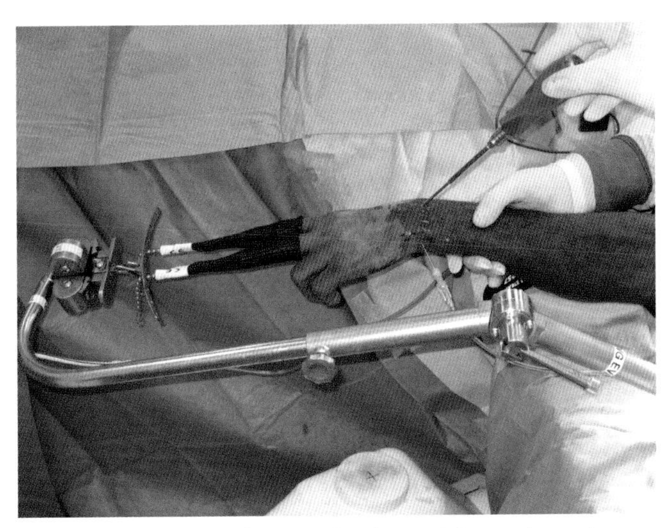

FIGURE 27-10 The headless cannulated screw is inserted over the guidewire and down the central axis of the scaphoid.

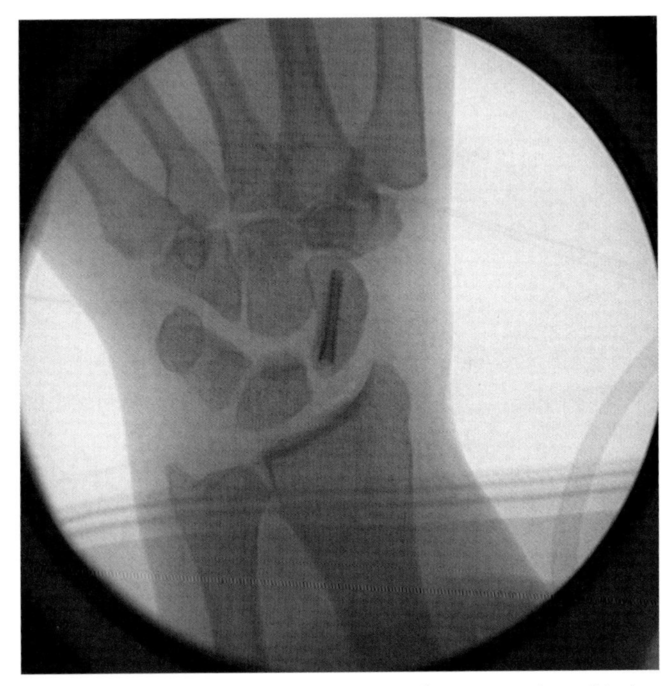

FIGURE 27-11 On the posteroanterior view, fluoroscopy shows ideal placement of the screw and reduction of the scaphoid.

tower (Figs. 27-11 and 27-12). The wrist is again evaluated from the radiocarpal and midcarpal spaces. It is important to check from the radiocarpal space that the headless screw is inserted into the scaphoid and is not protruding, which may injure the articular cartilage of the scaphoid facet and the distal radius. The final reduction of the scaphoid fracture may be viewed with the arthroscope in the midcarpal space (Figs. 27-13 and 27-14).

Scaphoid Nonunions

Geissler and Slade described their use of Slade's dorsal percutaneous fixation technique in 15 patients with stable fibrous nonunion of the scaphoid.[32] Their series included 12 horizontal oblique fractures, 1 transverse fracture, and 2 proximal pole fractures. The average time between presentation and surgery was 8 months. All patients underwent percutaneous dorsal fixation with a headless cannulated screw and no accessory bone grafting procedure, and all fractures healed in an average time of 3 months. Eight of the 15 patients underwent CT evaluation to further document healing. The patients had excellent range of motion at their final follow-up visit because of minimal surgical dissection. Twelve of the 15 patients had excellent results according to the modified Mayo wrist scale. Dorsal percutaneous fixation without bone grafting is recommended for patients with a stable fibrous nonunion who have no signs of hump-

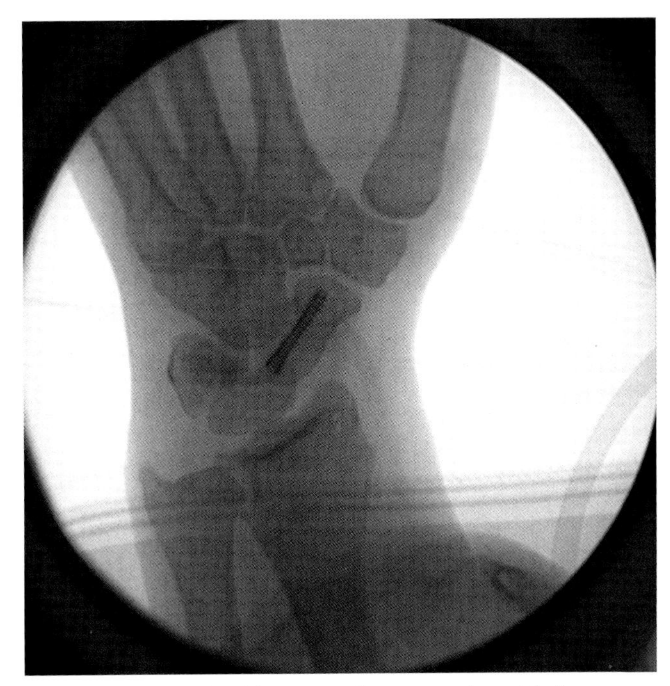

FIGURE 27-12 On the oblique view, fluoroscopy shows ideal placement of the headless cannulated screw.

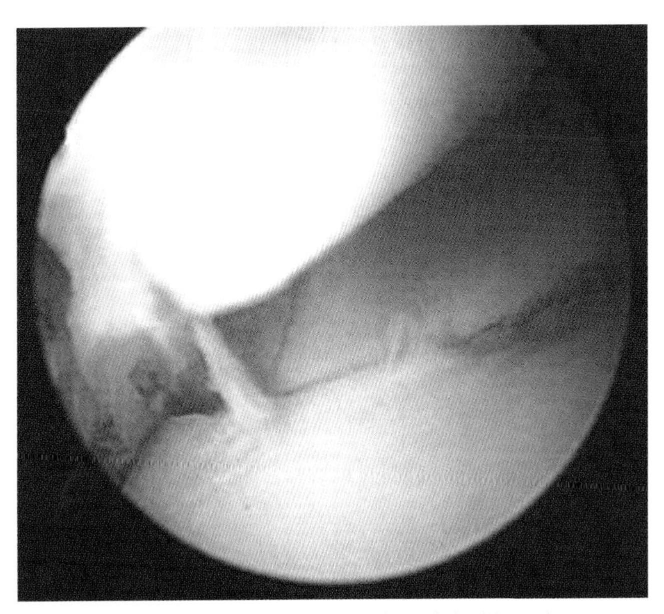

FIGURE 27-13 The arthroscopic view in the radial midcarpal space confirms good compression of the scaphoid fracture and anatomic reduction with no rotation.

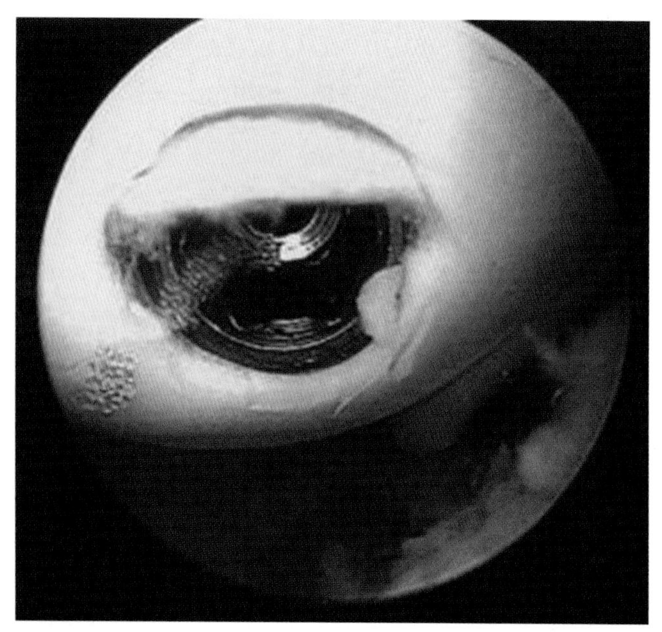

FIGURE 27-14 The arthroscopic view from the 3-4 portal confirms screw placement in the scaphoid.

back deformity and do not have extensive sclerosis of the fracture site. The scaphoid nonunion classification scheme proposed by Slade and Geissler was used to include patients with type I through III scaphoid nonunions in the study, with a 100% success rate.

For patients who have cystic scaphoid nonunions without a humpback deformity, percutaneous cancellous bone grafting or injection of DMB may be used. Applying Geissler's technique, the scaphoid is reamed through a soft tissue protector.[33] A bone biopsy needle is filled with DBM putty. The needle is placed over the guidewire from dorsal to proximal and inserted through the drill hole directly into the nonunion site. The guidewire is then retracted distally out of the proximal pole of the scaphoid while still remaining in the distal pole of the scaphoid. DBM is injected through the bone biopsy needle directly into the central hole of the scaphoid at the nonunion site. The guidewire is advanced back through the bone biopsy needle from volar to dorsal. In this manner, the guidewire passes back through the original reamed hole of the proximal pole of the scaphoid and out dorsally, protruding from the skin. The needle is then removed, and a headless cannulated screw is inserted over the guidewire across the scaphoid nonunion. The radiocarpal and midcarpal spaces are re-evaluated arthroscopically to confirm reduction and placement of the screw.

I described a technique of arthroscopic reduction of cystic scaphoid nonunions without humpback deformity using DBM putty.[33] In this technique, 1 mL of DBM (Accell, Irving, CA) is injected percutaneously into the nonunion site of the scaphoid. According to the Slade and Geissler classification, the series was composed of type IV cystic scaphoid nonunions. In 14 of the 15 patients, the scaphoid nonunion healed after use of this technique. Arthroscopic evaluation of the wrist from the radiocarpal and midcarpal spaces showed no extravasation of the DBM into the joint.

PEARLS & PITFALLS

- Clear arthroscopic visualization of the proximal pole of the scaphoid is mandatory. Any dorsal synovitis that may obscure visualization should be shaved.
- The starting point for the guidewire is the junction of the scapholunate interosseous ligament at the proximal pole of the scaphoid.
- Reduction of the scaphoid fracture should be visualized with the arthroscope in the midcarpal space.
- The position of the guidewire must be checked in posteroanterior, oblique, and lateral planes before reaming and insertion of the headless screw.
- A second guidewire may help to protect against rotation of the fracture fragments as the headless cannulated screw is being inserted.
- The position of the screw inserted in the scaphoid must be checked with the arthroscope in the radiocarpal space to ensure that it is not prominent.
- Final reduction of the scaphoid after screw insertion should be checked with the arthroscope in the midcarpal space.

CONCLUSIONS

Fractures of the scaphoid are a common athletic injury, especially in young men.[34,35] Although most nondisplaced fractures of the scaphoid heal with cast immobilization, nonunion rates of 10% to 15% have been reported. Union rates of 100% for acute fractures of the scaphoid managed by percutaneous arthroscopically assisted fixation have been consistently reported in the literature.

Although cast immobilization is effective, it has certain disadvantages, including muscle atrophy, joint contracture, and stiffness. For this reason, arthroscopic fixation of acute scaphoid fractures, particularly in athletes, is recommended after the advantages and disadvantages of the procedure have been discussed with the patient and the family. This approach can allow the patient to return quickly to the workforce or to competition. Arthroscopic fixation of scaphoid fractures allows limited surgical dissection, which may result in improved range of motion, and enables detection and management of associated soft tissue injuries, which may result from the scaphoid fracture.

Arthroscopically assisted fixation has been beneficial in treating type I through type IV scaphoid nonunions by the classification scheme of Slade and Geissler.[36] In patients with a stable fibrous nonunion, stabilization with a screw alone has been effective. In patients with cystic changes, arthroscopic stabilization and percutaneous injection of DBM into the nonunion site has been successful.[33] Percutaneous bone grafting may be another option.

Compared with previously described percutaneous fluoroscopic techniques, arthroscopic fixation limits the guesswork concerning the exact location of the starting point of the screw. The guidewire starting point is at the most proximal pole of the scaphoid, at the junction of the scapholunate interosseous ligament. It is reproducible, as confirmed under fluoroscopy. The wrist is not hyperflexed, because such movement may flex the fracture fragment into a humpback deformity. Dorsal insertion of the screw enables central placement down the axis of the scaphoid. Early arthroscopic evaluation allows detection and management of associated soft tissue injuries (Figs. 27-15 to 27-18).

Neither arthroscopic nor percutaneous techniques are indicated for patients who have a severe humpback deformity, which is not correctable, or for those with advanced arthrosis of the radiocarpal joint (i.e., SNAC).[37]

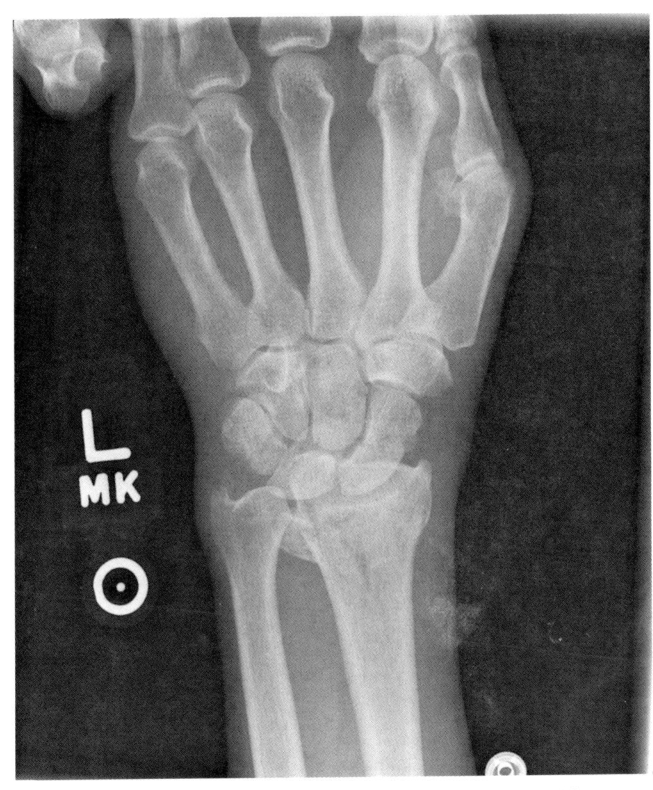

FIGURE 27-15 The posteroanterior radiograph of a 42-year-old man shows a combined distal radius and scaphoid fracture.

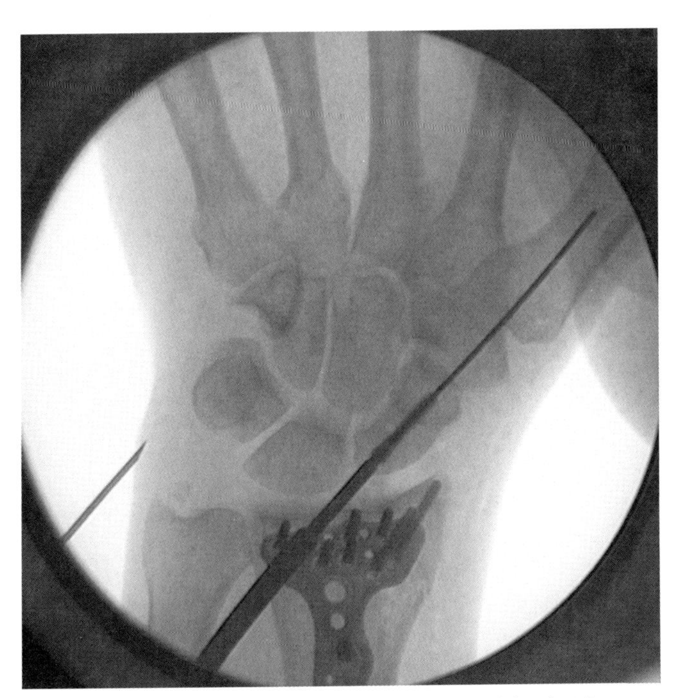

FIGURE 27-16 The distal radius fracture has been stabilized with an Acumed distal radius plate through the volar approach. After the distal radius fracture is stabilized, the scaphoid is arthroscopically reduced by the technique previously described.

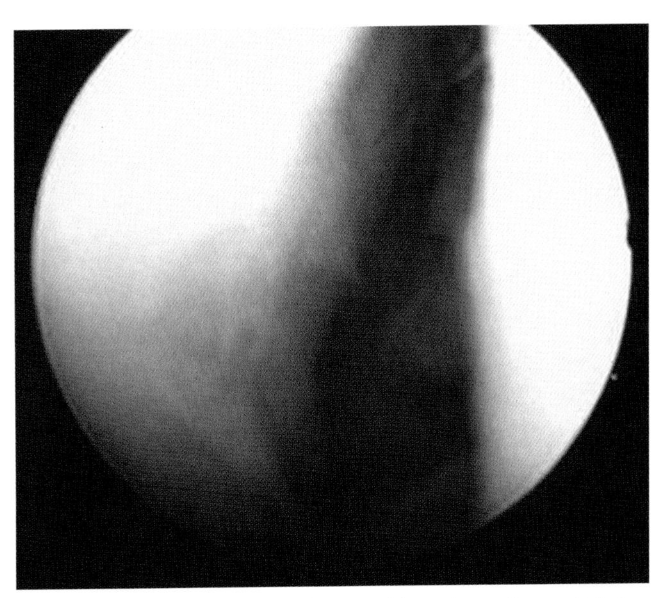

FIGURE 27-17 Arthroscopic evaluation of the wrist confirms a Geissler grade III tear to the scapholunate interosseous ligament. This was not apparent on plain radiographs.

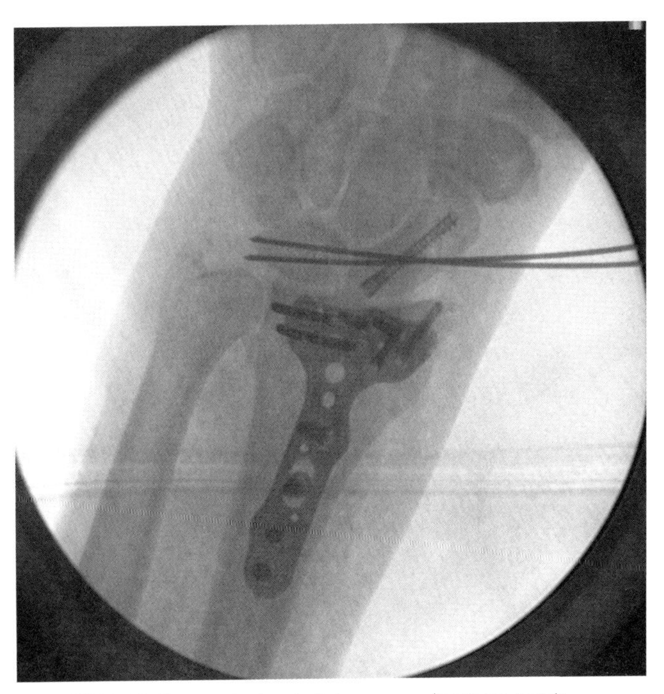

FIGURE 27-18 The scapholunate interosseous ligament tear is arthroscopically reduced and percutaneously stabilized with Kirschner wires after reduction of the distal radius and scaphoid fractures.

REFERENCES

1. Gelberman RH, Wolock BS, Siegel DB. Current concepts review: fractures and nonunions of the carpal scaphoid. *J Bone Joint Surg Am*. 1989; 71:1560-1565.
2. Cooney WP, Dobyns JH, Linscheid RL. Fractures of the scaphoid: a rational approach to management. *Clin Orthop*. 1980;(149):90-97.
3. Rettig AC, Ryan RO, Stone JA. Epidemiology of hand injuries in sports. In: Strickland JW, Rettig AC, eds. *Hand Injuries in Athletes*. Philadelphia, PA: WB Saunders; 1992:37-48.
4. Gellman H, Caputo RJ, Carter V, et al. Comparison of short and long thumb spica casts for non-displaced fractures of the carpal scaphoid. *J Bone Joint Surg Am*. 1989;71:354-357.

5. Kaneshiro SA, Failla JM, Tashman S. Scaphoid fracture displacement with forearm rotation in a short arm thumb spica cast. *J Hand Surg*. 1989;71:354-357.
6. Skirven T, Trope J. Complications of immobilization. *Hand Clin*. 1994; 10:53-61.
7. Gelberman RH, Menon J. The vascularity of the scaphoid bone. *J Hand Surg*. 1980;5:508-513.
8. Rettig AC, Weidenbener EJ, Gloyeske R. Alternative management of mid-third scaphoid fractures in the athlete. *Am J Sports Med*. 1994; 22:711-714.
9. DeMaagd RL, Engber WD. Retrograde Herbert screw fixation for treatment of proximal pole scaphoid nonunions. *J Hand Surg*. 1989;14: 996-1003.
10. Filan SL, Herbert TJ. Herbert screw fixation of scaphoid fractures. *J Bone Joint Surg Br*. 1996;78:519-529.
11. Herbert TJ, Fisher WE. Management of the fractured scaphoid using a new bone screw. *J Bone Joint Surg Am*. 1984;66:114-123.
12. O'Brien L, Herbert TJ. Internal fixation of acute scaphoid fractures: a new approach to treatment. *Aust N Z J Surg*. 1985;55:387-389.
13. Rettig ME, Raskin KB. Retrograde compression screw fixation of acute proximal pole scaphoid fractures. *J Hand Surg*. 1999;24:1206-1210.
14. Russe O. Fracture of the carpal navicular: diagnosis, nonoperative treatment and operative treatment. *J Bone Joint Surg Am*. 1960;42:759.
15. Toby EB, Butler TE, McCormack TJ, et al. A comparison of fixation screws for the scaphoid during application of cyclic bending loads. *J Bone Joint Surg Am*. 1997;79:1190-1197.
16. Trumble TE, Clarke T, Kreder HJ. Nonunion of the scaphoid: treatment with cannulated screws compared with treatment with Herbert screws. *J Bone Joint Surg Am*. 1996;78:1829-1837.
17. Garcia-Elias M, Vall A, Salo JM, et al. Carpal alignment after different surgical approaches to the scaphoid: a comparative study. *J Hand Surg*. 1988;13:604-612.
18. Adams BD, Blair WF, Regan DS, et al. Technical factors related to Herbert screw fixation. *J Hand Surg Am*. 1988;13:893-899.
19. Whipple TL. The role of arthroscopy in the treatment of intraarticular wrist fractures. *Hand Clin*. 1995;11:13-18.
20. Slade JF, Merrell GA, Geissler WB. Fixation of acute and selected nonunion scaphoid fractures. In: Geissler WB, ed. *Wrist Arthroscopy*. New York, NY: Springer; 2005:112-124.
21. Geissler WB. Arthroscopic assisted fixation of fractures of the scaphoid. *Atlas Hand Clin*. 2003;8:37-56.
22. Geissler WB, Hammit MD. Arthroscopic aided fixation of scaphoid fractures. *Hand Clin*. 2001;17:575-588.
23. Cosio MQ, Camp RA. Percutaneous pinning of symptomatic scaphoid nonunions. *J Hand Surg*. 1986;11:350-355.
24. Haddad FS, Goddard NJ. Acute percutaneous scaphoid fixation: a pilot study. *J Bone Joint Surg Br*. 1998;80:95-99.
25. Shin A, Bond A, McBride M, et al. Acute screw fixation versus cast immobilization for stable scaphoid fractures: a prospective randomized study. Paper presented at the annual meeting of the American Society Surgery for the Hand, October 5-7, 2000, Seattle, WA.
26. Slade JF III, Grauer JN, Mahoney JD. Arthroscopic reduction and percutaneous fixation of scaphoid fractures with a novel dorsal technique. *Orthop Clin North Am*. 2000;30:247-261.
27. Slade JF III, Jaskwhich J. Percutaneous fixation of scaphoid fractures. *Hand Clin*. 2001;17:553-574.
28. Taras JS, Sweet S, Shum W, et al. Percutaneous and arthroscopic screw fixation of scaphoid fractures in the athlete. *Hand Clin*. 1999;15: 467-473.
29. Slade JF III, Grauer JN. Dorsal percutaneous repair of scaphoid fractures with arthroscopic guidance. *Atlas Hand Clin*. 2001;6:307-323.
30. Wozasek GE, Moser KD. Percutaneous screw fixation of fractures of the scaphoid. *J Bone Joint Surg Br*. 1991;73:138-142.
31. Kamineni S, Lavy CBD. Percutaneous fixation of scaphoid fractures: an anatomic study. *J Hand Surg*. 1999;24:85-88.
32. Geissler WB, Slade JF. Arthroscopic fixation of scaphoid nonunions without bone grafting. Paper presented at the 33rd Annual Meeting of the American Society Surgery of the Hand, September 2002. Phoenix, AZ.
33. Geissler WB. Arthroscopic fixation of cystic scaphoid nonunions with DBM. Paper presented at the annual meeting of the American Association Hand Surgery, January 2006. Tucson, AZ.
34. Geissler WB. Carpal fractures in athletes. *Clin Sports Med*. 2001;20: 167-188.
35. Rettig AC, Kollias SC. Internal fixation of acute stable scaphoid fractures in the athlete. *Am J Sports Med*. 1996;24:182-186.
36. Geissler WB. *Wrist Arthroscopy*. New York, NY: Springer; 2005.
37. Fernandez DL. Anterior bone grafting and conventional lag screw fixation to treat scaphoid nonunions. *J Hand Surg Am*. 1990;15:140-147.

CHAPTER

28

Carpal, Metacarpal, and Phalangeal Fractures

Phani K. Dantuluri • Sidney M. Jacoby • Randall W. Culp • A. Lee Osterman

Carpal, metacarpal, and phalangeal fractures are among the most common injuries treated by hand surgeons. Historical data suggest that 10% of all fractures occur in the metacarpals and phalanges and that 80% of all hand fractures involve the tubular bones.[1-3] Until the early 20th century, most carpal and hand fractures were treated nonoperatively. Even today, fractures that are nondisplaced or minimally displaced may be viewed as stable and treated conservatively or with closed reduced and cast immobilization. Unstable fractures require surgical fixation to maintain length, alignment, and rotation. Other options for fixation include percutaneous pinning, external fixation, traditional open reduction and internal fixation, and arthroscopically assisted reduction and internal fixation (AARIF).

HISTORICAL BACKGROUND

Arthroscopic surgery of the wrist and hand is a rapidly evolving discipline. Since Chen first reported on diagnostic arthroscopy of the wrist and finger joints in 1979 with the Watanabe no. 24 arthroscope, techniques for small joint arthroscopy have developed at a rapid pace.[4] Current indications include the diagnosis and treatment of numerous wrist disorders, including fractures, soft tissue pathology, and arthritis. Arthroscopy of small joints, including the metacarpophalangeal (MCP) and interphalangeal (IP) joints, has lagged compared with the phenomenal interest generated by wrist arthroscopy. Badia theorized that minimal reporting in the literature and lack of direct teaching of this technique have contributed to the limited use of this potentially useful technology.[5]

In 1995, more than 15 years after Chen's classic article, Ryu and Fagan described their experience treating the ulnar collateral ligament Stener lesion in eight thumbs with success.[6] Arthroscopic reduction was achieved by reducing the lesion until the avulsed ligament sat juxtaposed to its insertion site on the proximal phalanx. After the reduction was performed, the ligament ends were débrided, and the joint was pinned. The results were excellent, with range of motion and strength comparable to those of the unaffected contralateral thumb.

In 1999, Rozmaryn and Wei presented a paper detailing the technical aspects of MCP arthroscopy, with general references to the potential use of this technique in treating juxta-articular and intra-articular fractures.[7] In the same year, Slade and Gutow published a review article on arthroscopy of the MCP joint.[8] They offered detailed technical explanations and emphasized that small joint arthroscopy requires specialized instruments and a thorough knowledge of the anatomy within these specialized joints. In 2006, Badia reported encouraging results treating bony gamekeeper's thumb with AARIF.[9]

ANATOMY

Because of the relatively small working space in the MCP and IP joints, knowledge of normal wrist and hand anatomy, accurate portal placement, and appropriately sized instrumentation are key to successful small joint arthroscopy. Fracture fixation of small joints presents unique challenges that test the skills necessary to successfully restore articular congruity in AARIF.

The MCP joint is composed of several structures, including the osseous metacarpal head, the proximal phalangeal base, and soft tissue restraints, which include the stout volar plate, collateral ligaments, and a relatively thin and flimsy dorsal capsule. Strong extensor tendons run dorsal to the dorsal capsule and are held in check by capsular fibers and the sagittal bands. On either side of the joint are the insertions of the intrinsic muscles on the extensor mechanism. The digital neurovascular bundles rest volar to the joint, along with the flexor tendons; the terminal branches of the dorsal sensory nerves are less predictably centered over the dorsum of the joint.

PATIENT EVALUATION

History and Physical Examination

As with any patient who presents with wrist or hand pain after an acute injury, a detailed history and physical examination are essential before surgical intervention is considered. Preoperative assessment of surgical candidates typically focuses on the condition of the digit, particularly the ability to fully flex and extend it. Patients with small joint injuries typically present with tenderness and swelling about the joint. Any suspicious laceration or cut in the region of the injured joint should heighten suspicion for an open articular fracture. Rotational malalignment is often associated with displaced articular fragments and indicates unstable fracture patterns.

Particular attention should be paid to patients with frail or "rice paper" skin, such as those with chronic disease and those receiving steroids.[10] If small joint arthroscopy is performed on these patients, special care should be taken to limit traction forces across the joint to prevent significant disruption of the skin surface.

Diagnostic Imaging

Plain radiographs provide most of the information necessary to diagnose lesions of the MCP joints. Special views, including oblique and Brewerton views to evaluate the metacarpal head, may be useful adjuncts to traditional posteroanterior and lateral radiographs. Computed tomographic (CT) scans aligned in the sagittal plane can help to define the step-off of intra-articular fractures, and bone scans can help to identify increased activity in the metacarpal head, which suggests possible osteochondral defects.[8]

TREATMENT

Indications and Contraindications

AARIF is an excellent choice for juxta-articular fractures of the carpometacarpal (CMC) and MCP joints of the thumb and digits, because these small joint injuries require anatomic reduction to prevent post-traumatic arthritis. As Slade and Gutow pointed out in their 1999 article describing arthroscopic techniques for MCP joint fixation, minimal surgical manipulation of the soft tissue envelope and preservation of the blood supply during operative exposure are indispensable for obtaining an optimal result.[8] AARIF preserves vascular blood supply to bony fragments by minimizing dissection of the soft tissue envelope surrounding the joints of the hand. Open surgery of tissues surrounding these small joints may contribute to collateral ligament and flexor tendon scarring and shortening, which ultimately limit tendon excursion and lead to stiffness and suboptimal results.[11]

A example of a fracture pattern amenable to AARIF is the simple two-part fracture with displacement greater than 1 mm involving the metacarpal head or base of the proximal phalanx.[10] Other excellent indications for AARIF are for reduction of an avulsion fracture with a rotated fragment from the collateral ligament insertion and for treatment of die-punch articular fractures of the proximal phalangeal base. AARIF enables the surgeon to use the arthroscope to clearly visualize articular reduction with a probe or Kirschner wire and to visualize subsequent percutaneous fixation.[5] In pediatric cases, Salter-Harris type III physeal fractures may be reduced and secured without additional injury to the growth plate with the use of AARIF.

Slade and colleagues presented their results using AARIF in 1998 at the Annual Meeting of the Arthroscopy Association of North America (AANA). This study documented fewer complications and improved final range of motion when fractures were treated with AARIF compared with the results of standard open reduction.[12]

Contraindications to the use of AARIF for MCP and proximal IP fractures are poor soft tissue coverage, open fractures, and active cellulitis.[10] Fractures with three or more fragments, comminution, or associated diaphyseal extension that cannot be easily reduced through percutaneous means are also disqualified for AARIF, because these fractures are better treated with standard open approaches.

Conservative Management

Most acute traumatic injuries involving the MCP and proximal IP joints can be managed conservatively with a trial of splint or cast immobilization. Fractures that result in rotational malalignment, an inability to fully extend the digits, or intra-articular displacement are best treated by some form of operative intervention, because nonoperative care may lead to long-term disability, such as pain, stiffness, or post-traumatic arthritis. As the surgeon becomes more adept at small joint arthroscopy, acute indications may evolve due to more accurate assessment of the extent of injury and more precise treatment.[5]

Arthroscopic Technique

Instruments

Specialized small joint instruments are necessary for arthroscopy of small joints. Adequately sized cameras, cannulas, shavers, punches, graspers, radiofrequency ablation probes, and wire drivers are among the instruments commonly used in AARIF of CMC, MCP, and proximal IP joints. Ideally, a 1.9-mm, 30-degree arthroscope is used in conjunction with a 2.2-mm cannula. Instruments and shavers between 2.0 and 2.5 mm wide can pass easily into the joint.

Inflow may be provided through a gravity system using a pinch pump and small joint tubing or the camera itself and a standard arthroscopy pump set to maintain a pressure between 50 and 80 mm Hg. The small radius of the inflow cannulas requires higher pressures to ensure adequate irrigation.[8]

Adequate traction is vital for all joints, particularly those as small as the CMC, MCP, and proximal IP joints. Several commercial traction devices are available to adequately distract the joint and provide traction with the assistance of sterile, disposable plastic finger traps (Fig. 28-1). A mini-fluoroscope is essential to help localize the joint space, assess fracture reduction, and visualize fixation. Standard small hand instruments are also necessary, including a wire driver, mini-curettes, mini-fragment screws, and a power drill for final implant seeding.

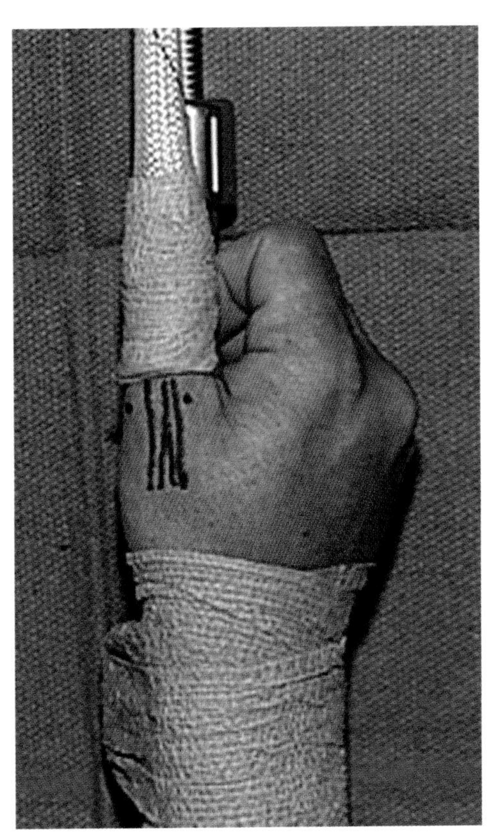

FIGURE 28-1 Standard small joint arthroscopy setup with Chinese finger traps suspending the thumb.

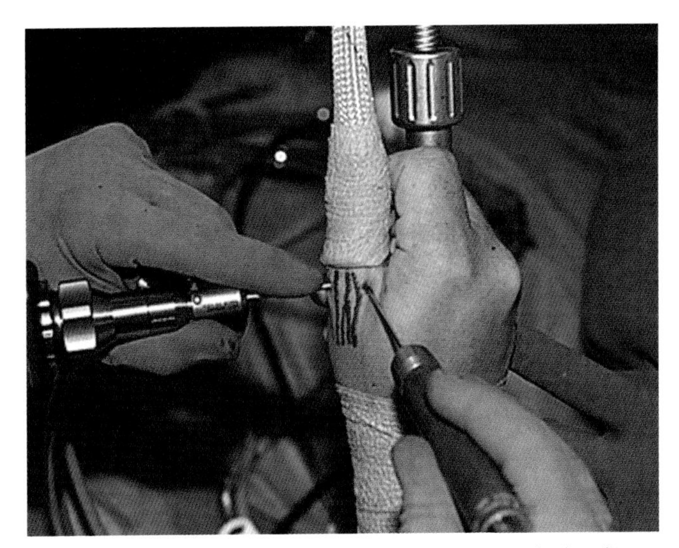

FIGURE 28-2 Coban wrap was used to set and maintain the hand in the proper position.

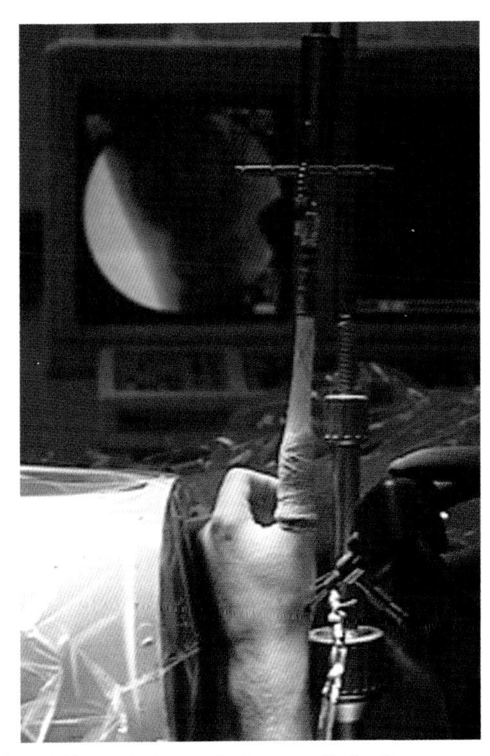

FIGURE 28-3 The typical setup is shown, with the C-arm appropriately positioned adjacent to the traction tower but away from the surgeon, providing unobstructed access to the joint of interest.

Types of Injuries Treated Arthroscopically

We espouse a systematic approach for small joint arthroscopy and fracture fixation that is reproducible and efficient. As with most surgical procedures, surgeons who employ a consistent algorithm may quickly gain proficiency while integrating a new technique into their practice. We present a broad overview of AARIF of small joint fractures and offer additional insight into specific small joint fracture patterns.

The patient is placed supine on the operating table, and a tourniquet is placed on the upper arm and preset to 250 mm Hg. General or regional anesthesia is appropriate for AARIF, as long as adequate sedation is achieved to allow painless elevation of the tourniquet for the necessary period. The affected arm is positioned on a radiolucent arm table, and the surgeon is positioned at the cephalic side of the arm. With the use of a Chinese finger trap, 5 pounds of longitudinal traction is typically applied to the thumb or affected digit, with the possibility of increasing traction to as much as 10 or 12 pounds. Care is taken to place the operative finger in the line of axis of traction, with the other two surrounding digits providing rotational control.[10] Coban is used to wrap the wrist in place against the wrist tower, and it provides additional stabilization for the thumb or digits if the finger trap is loose fitting (Fig. 28-2). A mini–C-arm fluoroscopy machine is positioned parallel to the table, out of the way of the operating surgeon (Fig. 28-3).

After elevation of the tourniquet, the joint of interest is localized with an 18-gauge needle. The skin is incised with a no. 11 blade, and care is taken to remain superficial so as not to incise too deeply and injure branches of the dorsal sensory nerves. We prefer to bluntly insert the trocar and arthroscopic camera with one smooth stroke, thereby achieving a "suction seal" with the portal. Alternatively, a small, curved clamp can be inserted through the joint capsule before inserting the arthroscope. With either method, the trocar must be introduced into the joint in an atraumatic fashion.

Small joints of the hand offer minimal joint spaces, and considerable iatrogenic injury may be caused if care is not taken. In recently traumatized hands, excessive swelling may obscure superficial landmarks, and the surgeon should not hesitate to use C-arm fluoroscopy to assist in localization.[10] We agree with Badia, who described an orderly evaluation of the joint beginning with one collateral ligament, followed by assessment of the volar plate and evaluation of the contralateral collateral ligament. This is followed with evaluation of the dorsal capsule and extensor mechanism and examination of the articular surface of the proximal phalanx and metacarpal head.[5] After the particular pathology has been identified and addressed, the arthroscope is removed, and the portals are closed with nylon sutures.

Thumb Carpometacarpal Injuries

Intra-articular fractures of the CMC joint of the thumb represent a subset of injuries amenable to AARIF. In the case of the thumb CMC joint, the base of the first metacarpal is identified and palpated. The incision for the 1-R (radial) portal is placed just volar to the abductor pollicis longus (APL) tendon, and the incision for the 1-U (ulnar) portal is made just ulnar to the extensor pollicis brevis (EPB) tendon (Figs. 28-4 and 28-5). Before the skin incision is made, the CMC joint is distended by injection of 2 mL of normal saline. A 1.9-mm arthroscope is atraumatically introduced into the joint at the 1-R portal, and under direct visualization, the working portal or 1-U portal is established in a similar fashion. Viewing and working portals are interchanged to ensure complete visualization of the critical ligamentous structures, including the dorsoradial, posterior oblique, ulnar collateral, and anterior oblique ligaments.

After the thumb CMC joint has been entered, it is often necessary to débride synovitis and fracture hematoma debris with an arthroscopic shaver (Fig. 28-6). A systematic approach is used to visualize critical structures such as the anterior oblique ligament and fracture fragments such as those seen in intra-articular fractures of the thumb metacarpal, including the

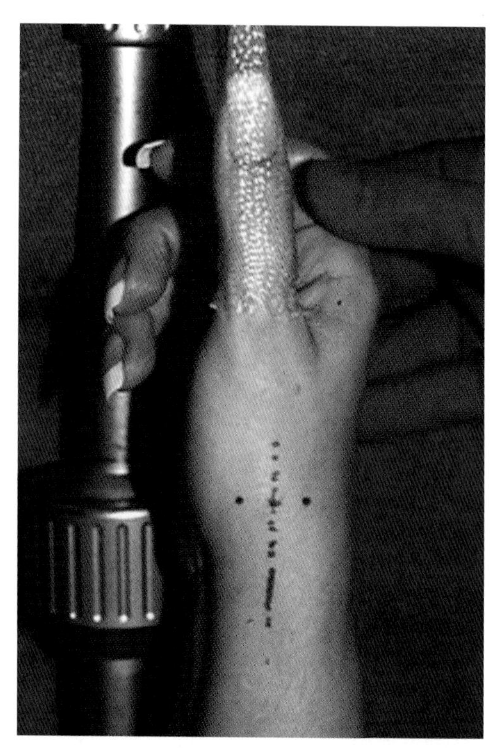

FIGURE 28-5 The clinical photograph shows superficial portal markings at the 1-R and 1-U intervals.

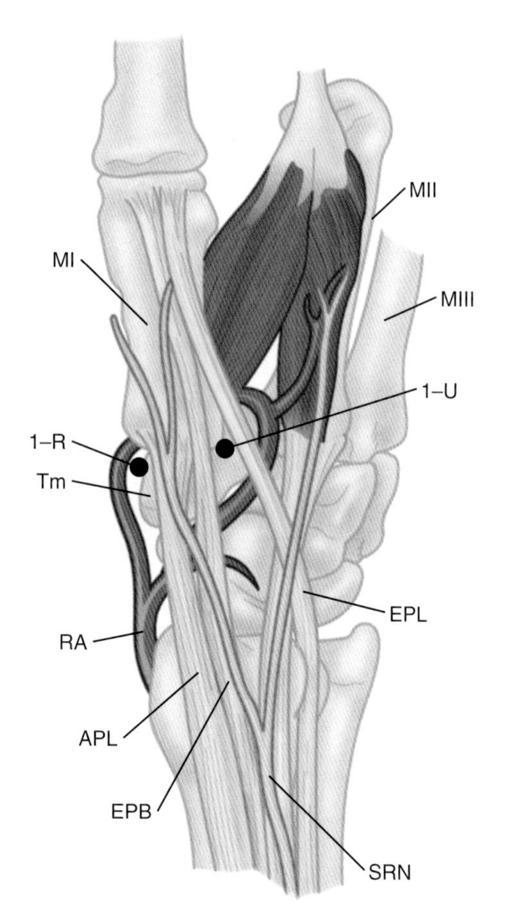

FIGURE 28-4 The incision for the 1-R (radial) portal is placed just volar to the abductor pollicis longus (APL) tendon, whereas the incision for the 1-U (ulnar) portal is made just ulnar to the extensor pollicis brevis (EPB) tendon.

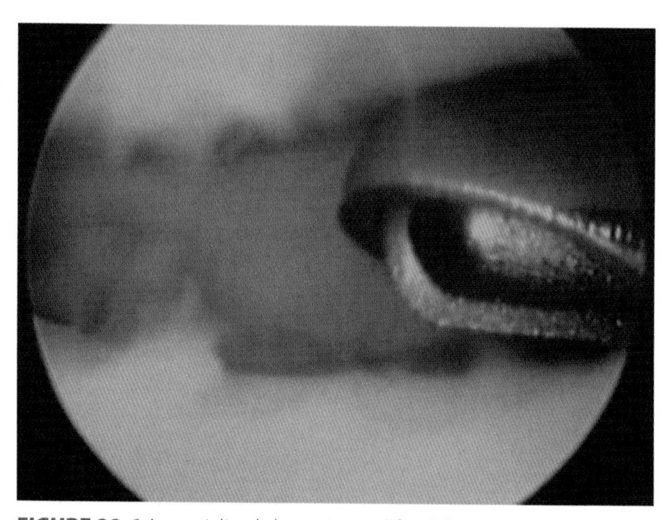

FIGURE 28-6 A specialized shaver is used for débriding synovitis within the small joint to improve fracture visualization.

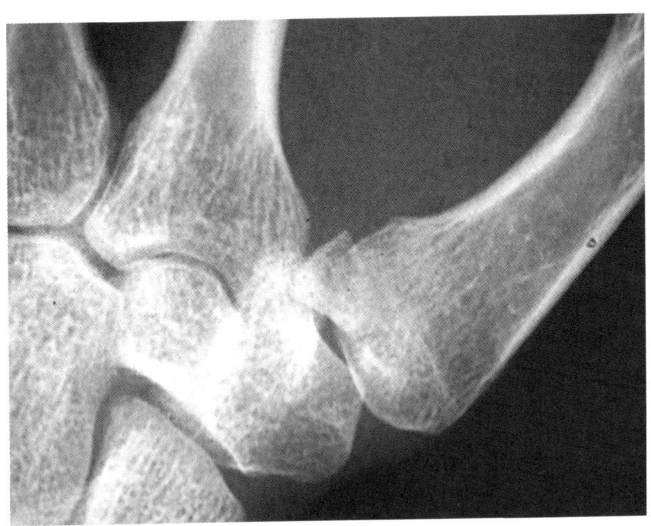

FIGURE 28-7 The radiograph demonstrates the characteristic appearance of a Bennett fracture, the most common fracture pattern at the base of the thumb metacarpal. This fracture is intra-articular, begins at the ulnar base of the thumb metacarpal, and is rotated in supination by the pull of the abductor pollicis longus (APL).

more common Bennett's fracture and the less common Rolando variant (Fig. 28-7).

After the joint surfaces have been probed and examined, a blunt probe or trocar is used to manipulate fracture fragments into acceptable position (Fig. 28-8). If the fracture fragment is relatively small (<40% of the articular surface), Kirschner wires may be used to transfix the fragment and provide adequate fixation (Fig. 28-9). For larger fragments, a cannulated screw system may be used. However, we have found it essential to ensure rotational control with a second Kirschner wire fixation before the cannulated screw is inserted over the first Kirschner wire. We introduce the Kirschner wire just up to the fracture site, while holding the fracture fragment with a probe before transfixing the fracture with the Kirschner wire. After fixation is obtained, the arthroscope may be used to verify anatomic reduction and to ensure proper position of the Kirschner wire or screw.

Trapezial Fractures

Fractures of the trapezium are rare, comprising less than 5% of all small bone fractures. These injuries occur when the trapezial body of an adducted thumb is forced onto the articular surface of the carpal bone. Forced radial deviation of the thumb may result in small avulsion fractures caused by capsular strain (Fig. 28-10). Portals are created as previously described for CMC arthroscopy, albeit slightly more proximal, so that the scaphotrapeziotrapezoid (STT) joint may be evaluated. After débridement and evacuation of hematoma to ensure adequate visualization, the fracture fragments are manipulated into position with a probe or Kirschner wire. A 0.035- or 0.045-inch Kirschner wire is useful for this purpose, and it can be used as a joystick to reduce and pin the fragments. Alternatively, one or two fixation screws may be used. Most cannulated screw systems come in a variety of sizes and may be inserted over a 0.035- or 0.045-inch Kirschner wire.

After the fracture has been adequately reduced, the guidewire is inserted as nearly perpendicular to the fracture plane as possible. A second guidewire is inserted to maintain rotational control and fixation during application of the cannulated screw. After proper screw length is measured and chosen, the appropriate screw is inserted over the guidewire, and the fracture is visualized as the screw is inserted. C-arm fluoroscopy is

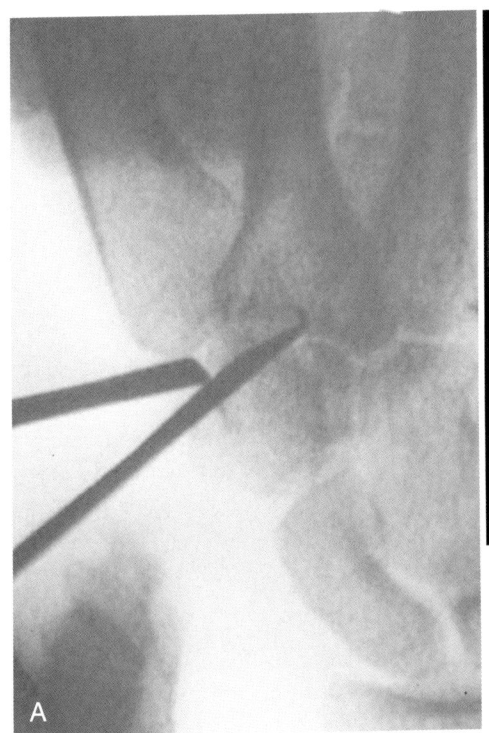

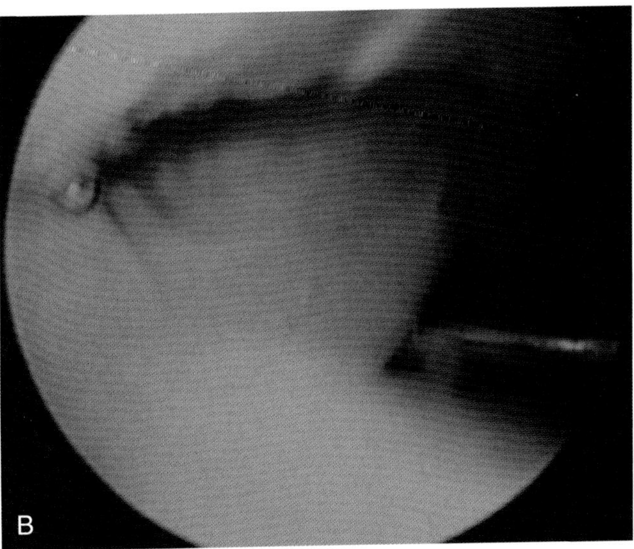

FIGURE 28-8 A, The fluoroscopic image shows probe holding the volar fracture fragment in good position. **B,** The arthroscopic view verifies the anatomic reduction of an intra-articular Bennet fracture. The probe is holding the reduction before Kirschner wire fixation.

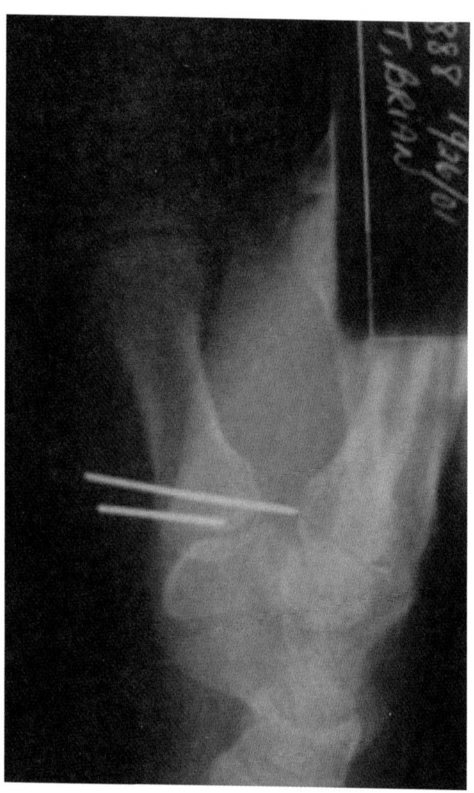

FIGURE 28-9 The postoperative radiograph demonstrates percutaneous fixation of a Bennett fracture in an excellent position.

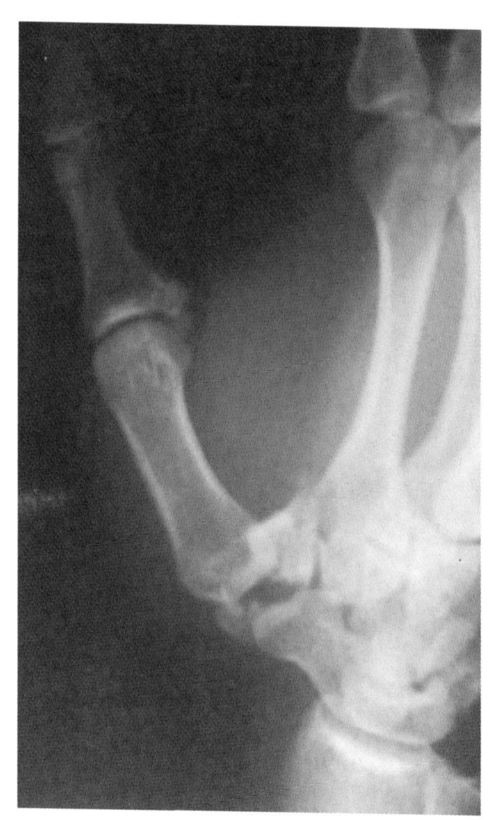

FIGURE 28-10 The radiograph demonstrates a displaced fracture of the trapezium.

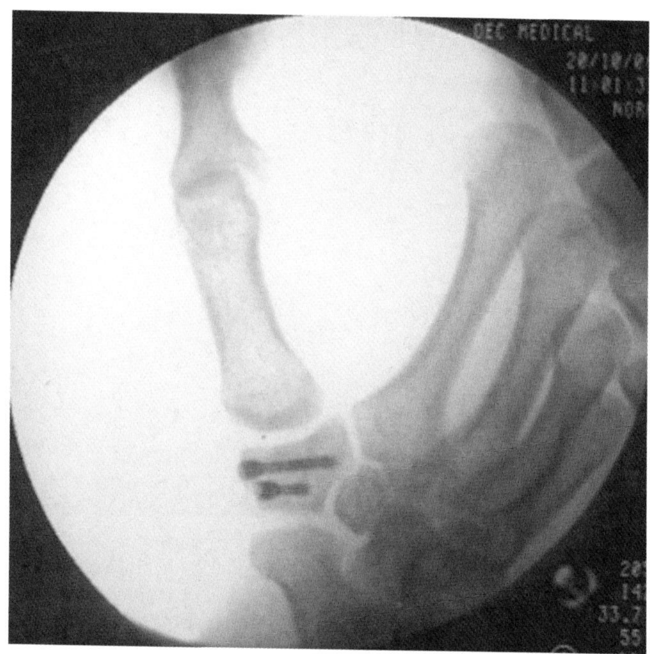

FIGURE 28-11 The final fluoroscopic image reveals two cannulated screws that provide fixation of a trapezial fracture and restoration of the thumb's carpometacarpal joint congruity.

useful during fixation and final reduction. Final fluoroscopic pictures are taken after stability has been confirmed, and the joint is taken through a final range of motion (Fig. 28-11). The topic of carpal bone fixation is addressed more thoroughly elsewhere in this text, but the principles are similar to those discussed here.

Thumb and Digital Metacarpophalangeal Injuries

After the patient is positioned and the thumb is suspended as previously described, the principles for thumb MCP AARIF are quite similar to those for CMC arthroscopy and are exemplified by a thumb radial collateral ligament avulsion fracture (Fig. 28-12). The portals for MCP arthroscopy are simple, because they lie on either side of the visible extensor tendon (Fig. 28-13). The interval between the metacarpal head and the proximal phalanx is narrow, and the joint space is localized with an 18-gauge needle before a nick incision of the skin. The arthroscope is introduced at the same angle, and thorough joint inspection is performed along with synovectomy and débridement of fracture hematoma. Fracture reduction is achieved with the use of a probe, and a Kirschner wire is inserted in a perfect position to maintain anatomic reduction (Figs. 28-14 and 28-15). For thumb MCP injuries, we use a short arm thumb spica splint in extension to protect the joint during the initial postoperative period.

Digital MCP injuries may include fractures of the metacarpal head or the base of the proximal phalanx with or without intra-articular extension. Other fracture patterns include die-punch fractures with impaction of the joint surface, which may complicate fracture reduction. Intra-articular fractures at the base of the index proximal phalanx exhibit disruption of the normal contour and loss of the normal *sourcil*, a French term meaning "eyebrow"

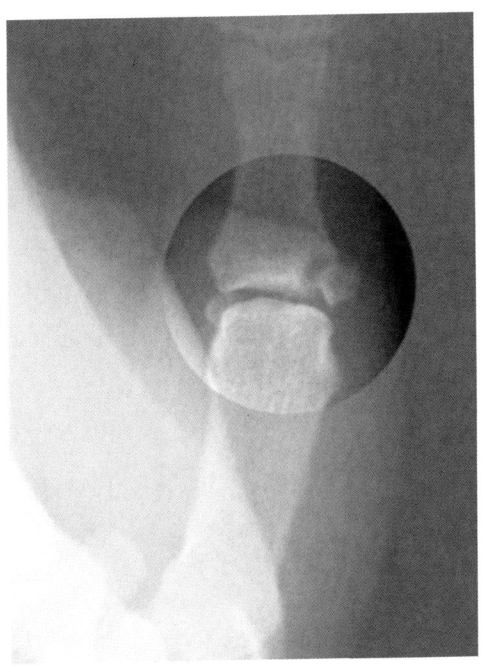

FIGURE 28-12 The posteroanterior radiograph demonstrates a radial collateral ligament avulsion fracture at the base of the proximal phalanx of the thumb.

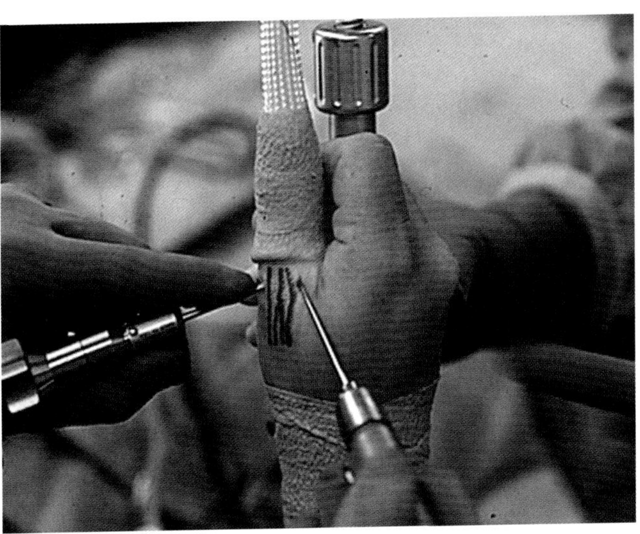

FIGURE 28-13 Standard portals are seen on either side of the visible extensor tendon (i.e., confluence of the extensor pollicis longus [EPL] and extensor pollicis brevis [EPB]) with the arthroscopic camera in the 1-R portal and the shaver in the 1-U portal.

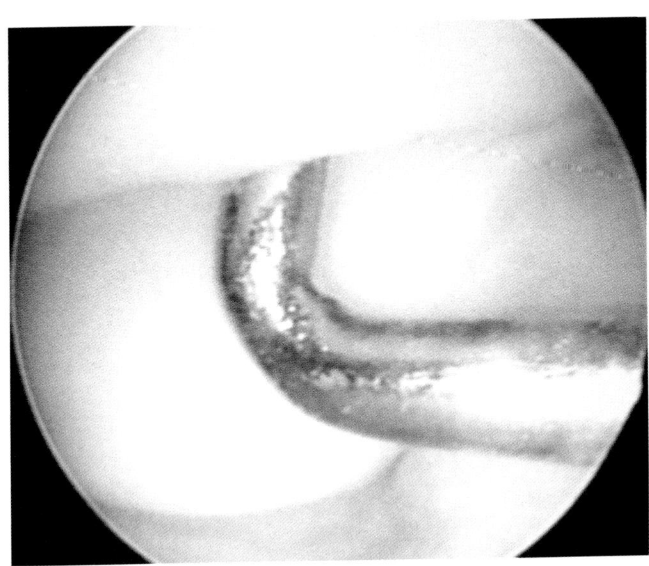

FIGURE 28-14 The arthroscopic view shows anatomic fixation of a radial collateral ligament avulsion fracture.

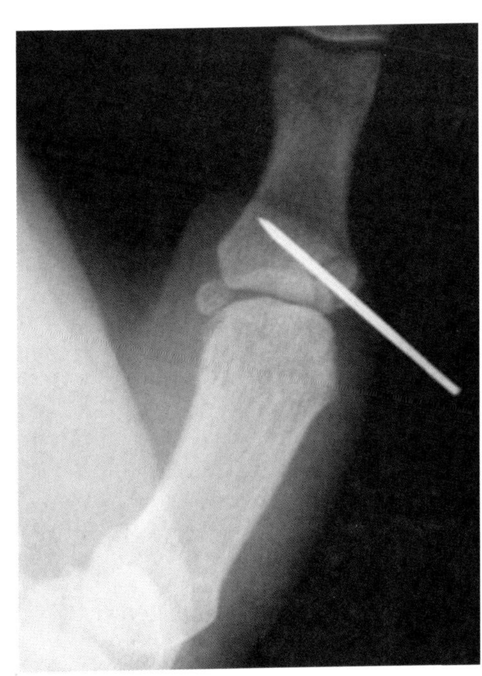

FIGURE 28-15 The postoperative radiograph shows fixation of a radial collateral ligament avulsion fracture with a percutaneous Kirschner wire.

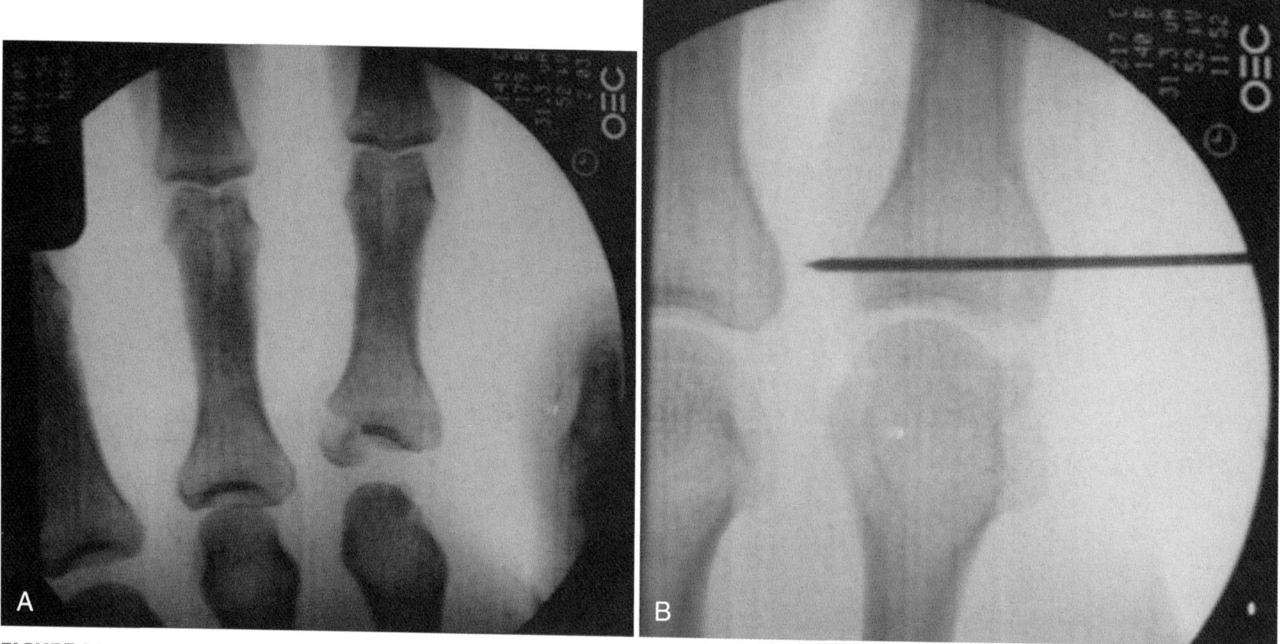

FIGURE 28-16 A, An intra-articular fracture occurred at the base of the proximal phalanx. The typical curvature, or *sourcil*, is lost with this fracture. **B,** The view after reduction shows the index proximal phalanx with restoration of the normal contour at the base.

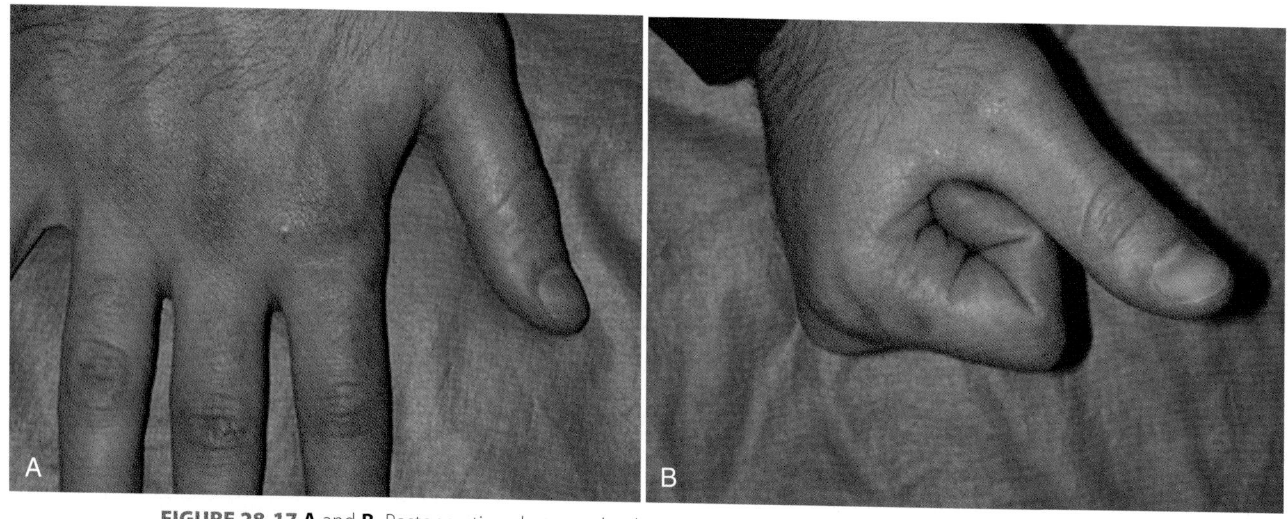

FIGURE 28-17 A and **B,** Postoperative photographs show well-healed surgical scars with full range of motion.

(Fig. 28-16A). After arthroscopic reduction and pinning, the final fluoroscopic images and postoperative radiographs demonstrate excellent alignment, fixation, and healing (see Fig. 28-16B). Postoperative photographs show barely perceptible but well-healed surgical scars and a full range of motion (Fig. 28-17).

Intra-articular fractures with impaction, known as die-punch fractures, require a more delicate approach to fixation. A probe is used to gently disimpact the depressed fragment. Care must be taken not to disengage the fragment, thereby destabilizing it and creating a loose body in the joint. A percutaneous Kirschner wire can be used to fine tune the reduction while the probe is used to reduce the fragment. Definitive fixation is achieved with a subcutaneous buttress pin. Additional pins may be required to hold the fixation.

A displaced fracture of the metacarpal head is shown in Figure 28-18. Preoperative CT in the coronal and sagittal planes provides additional insight into the degree of displacement of the fracture and visualization of the intra-articular component, which is not fully appreciated on plain radiographs (Fig. 28-19). AARIF allows superior visualization of the metacarpal fracture component and the adequacy of reduction after pinning. Postoperative radiographs demonstrate excellent alignment and anatomic re-

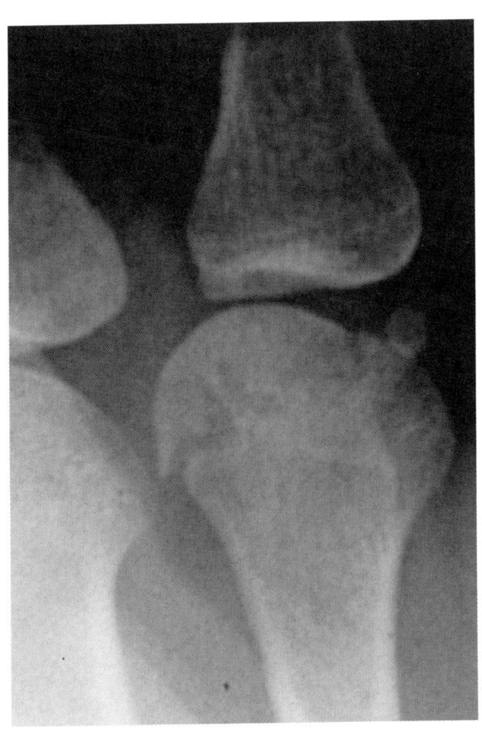

FIGURE 28-18 The radiograph demonstrates a metacarpal head fracture with intra-articular involvement.

duction with no intra-articular step-off or deformity (Fig. 28-20). Final clinical pictures show full motion with no evidence of lag or rotational malalignment (Fig. 28-21). Restoration of joint congruity minimizes the likelihood of future post-traumatic arthrosis in patients treated with AARIF.

PEARLS & PITFALLS

PEARLS

- When inserting the trocar into the joint, use a steady, smooth stroke to create a "suction seal" effect. Use of a curved hemostat to open the capsule is often unnecessary if the joint is entered smoothly. Avoiding the use of a hemostat ensures a tight fit of the arthroscope into the portal.
- When attempting to capture a disengaged fragment, introduce the Kirschner wire up to the fracture site while holding it steadily in place with a probe. After the fracture is anatomically reduced, drive the Kirschner wire through the fragment for definitive fixation.
- If screw fixation is chosen, an additional Kirschner wire is necessary to maintain reduction and rotation control while engaging the fracture fragment with the screw.
- For large fracture fragments, use a fracture reduction clamp to assist with rotational control before attempting to pin the fracture fragment with a Kirschner wire.
- For die-punch fractures with impaction, use a probe in the joint to reduce the fracture while simultaneously manipulating the impacted fragment with a percutaneous Kirschner wire.

PITFALLS

- Ensure that all necessary arthroscopic equipment is available and that C-arm fluoroscopy is positioned appropriately before beginning the procedure.
- Portal placement is key. Care should be taken to raise the skin to the blade so as not to incise too deeply and possibly injure the radial artery and dorsal sensory nerves.
- When manipulating fracture fragments, particularly impacted fractures, avoid destabilizing the fragment so as not to create a loose body or chondral defect.

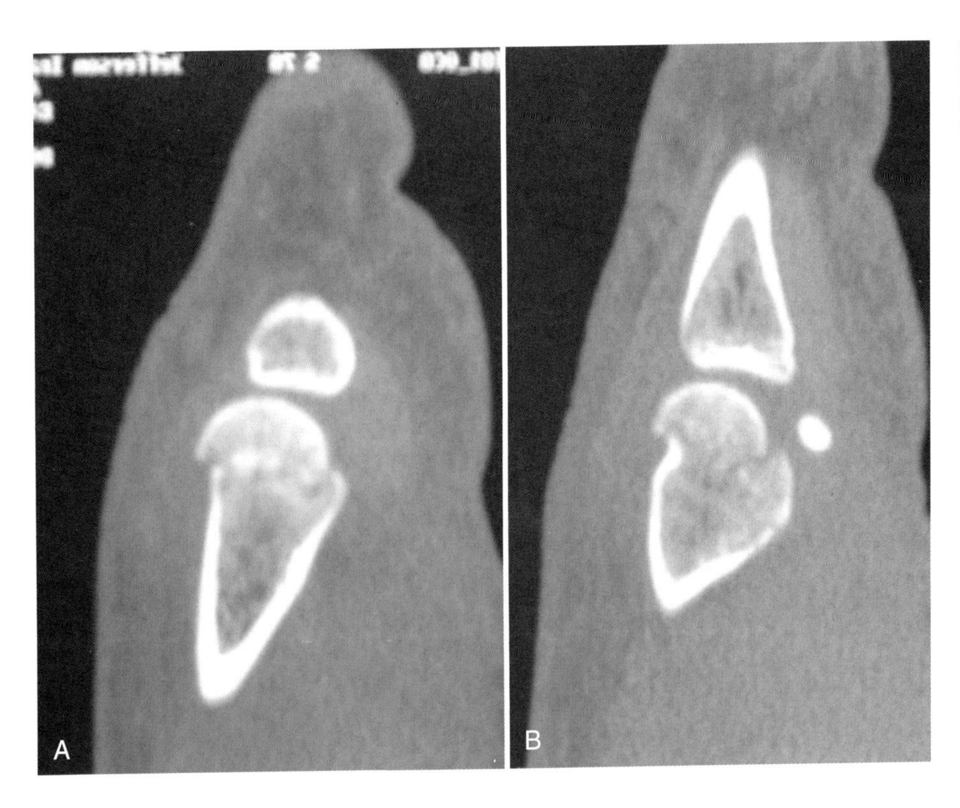

FIGURE 28-19 Coronal (**A**) and sagittal (**B**) images reveal the degree of displacement and articular involvement of a metacarpal head fracture.

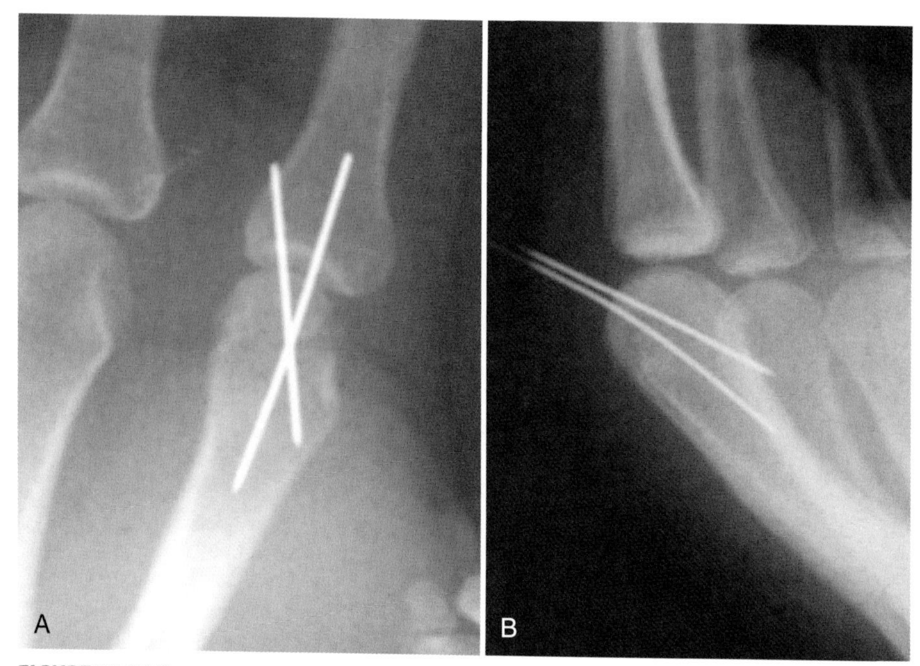

FIGURE 28-20 Postoperative posteroanterior (**A**) and lateral (**B**) radiographs demonstrate excellent alignment and fixation of an intra-articular metacarpal head fracture.

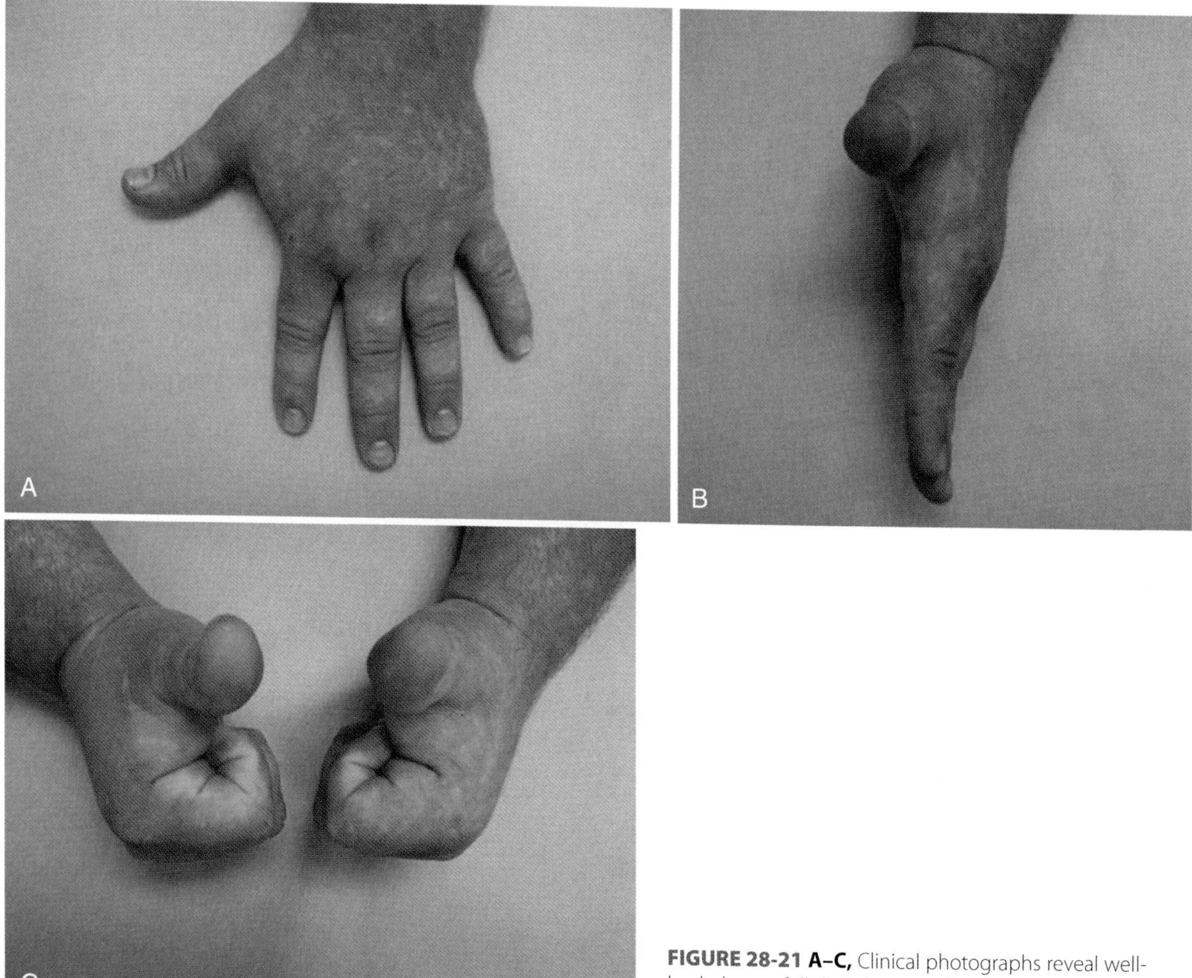

FIGURE 28-21 A–C, Clinical photographs reveal well-healed scars, full digital range of motion, and no evidence of extensor lag or rotational malalignment.

Postoperative Rehabilitation

Therapy after minimally invasive surgery in general and after AARIF in particular is one of the principal advantages of this technique. AARIF of small joints offers the benefit of minimal capsular, collateral ligament, and tendon scarring. Consequently, there is faster recovery of the full digital range of motion.[9]

The usual postoperative protocol involves a short arm thumb spica splint for MCP or CMC arthroscopy and a dorsal MCP block splint in flexion for digital MCP arthroscopy. Splinting in the "safe position" allows the collateral ligaments to heal in their most taut position to prevent loss of motion. The IP joints are left free. Sutures are removed 7 to 10 days postoperatively, and Kirschner wires are removed at approximately 4 weeks. Complications are rarely encountered but may include pin tract infection, Kirschner wire migration, and digital stiffness. Formal occupational therapy is initiated if necessary, but most patients are able to follow a home exercise program.

OUTCOMES

In one of the only known studies comparing AARIF with the standard open approach, Slade and Gutow reviewed the outcomes of 14 consecutive patients with displaced fractures of the MCP joint treated with AARIF.[8] All of the patients presented with closed injuries, and all digits of the hand were represented: six thumbs, two index fingers, two long fingers, three ring fingers, and one small finger. The operating time for AARIF averaged 1.8 hours. The final range of motion for the MCP joint averaged 81 degrees, and the total final range of motion for the proximal IP joint averaged 98.8 degrees. There was only one complication, a loss of reduction that required a second AARIF, which ultimately resulted in a successful outcome. The average time before return to work or unrestricted athletic activities was compared with that of a matched set of similar injuries treated with a standard open technique at the same institution. AARIF patients had greater final motion and earlier return of motion than their counterparts who were treated with an open approach.

For 23 patients, we used AARIF for the treatment of small joint fractures involving CMC and MCP joints, with follow-up ranging from 12 to 71 months. Final total active motion (TAM) and quality of fracture reduction were used as the end points. Eighty-nine percent of patients achieved good or excellent results, with TAM averaging 90% of the contralateral side. There were no extensor tendon complications and only one case of pin tract infection, which resolved with oral antibiotic therapy.

CONCLUSIONS

The general benefits of arthroscopy are well known. Specific advantages of small joint arthroscopy include smaller incisions with less dissection and preservation of the stabilizing dorsal capsule, collateral ligaments, and tendons in the hand. Small joint arthroscopy allows direct visualization and palpation of chondral defects and synovial tissue and assessment of concurrent intercarpal ligament injuries and instability. Arthroscopic assessment of fracture reduction is also superior to fluoroscopy as used in standard open cases because of its ability to magnify and brightly illuminate the fracture reduction. Other benefits associated with a minimally invasive approach to the small bones of the hand are lower morbidity, expedited recovery, improved motion, and greater patient satisfaction. With such powerful capabilities, AARIF may one day be considered the gold standard for the diagnosis and treatment of small joint pathology.

In the future, the indications for AARIF may expand include proximal IP joint injuries. Controlled studies may compare the efficacy of this technique with others, such as closed reduction and percutaneous pinning or open reduction and internal fixation.

REFERENCES

1. Green DP, Rowland SA, Hotchkiss RN. Fractures and dislocations in the hand. In: *Operative Hand Surgery*. New York, NY: Churchill Livingstone; 1991.
2. Kelsey JL, Pastides H, Kreiger N, et al. *Upper Extremity Disorders: A Survey of Their Frequency and Cost in the United States*. St. Louis, MO: CV Mosby; 1980:1-71.
3. Emmett JE, Breck LW. A review and analysis of 11,000 fractures seen in a private practice of orthopaedic surgery, 1937-1956. *J Bone Joint Surg Am*. 1958;40:1169-1175.
4. Chen YC. Arthroscopy of the wrist and finger joints. *Orthop Clin North Am*. 1979;10:723-733.
5. Badia A. Arthroscopy of the trapeziometacarpal and metacarpophalangeal joints. *J Hand Surg Am*. 2007;32:707-724.
6. Ryu J, Fagan R. Arthroscopic treatment of acute complete thumb metacarpophalangeal ulnar collateral ligament tears. *J Hand Surg Am*. 1995;20:1037-1042.
7. Rozmaryn LM, Wei N. Metacarpophalangeal arthroscopy. *Arthroscopy*. 1999;15:333-337.
8. Slade JF III, Gutow AP. Arthroscopy of the metacarpophalangeal joint. *Hand Clin*. 1999;15:501-527.
9. Badia A. Arthroscopic reduction and internal fixation of bony gamekeepers thumb. *Orthopaedics*. 2006;29:675-678.
10. Barbieri RA. Arthroscopic treatment of metacarpophalangeal joint fractures in the hand. In: Capo J, Tan V, eds. *Atlas of Minimally Invasive Hand and Wrist Surgery*. New York, NY: Informa Healthcare; 2008:235-238.
11. Woods GL. Troublesome shaft fractures of the proximal phalanx. *Hand Clin*. 1988;4:75-85.
12. Slade JF III, Cappelino A, Ansah P. The efficacy of arthroscopic treatment of intra-articular fractures of the small joints of the hand. Paper presented at the 17th Annual Meeting of the Arthroscopy Association of North America, 1998. Orlando, FL.

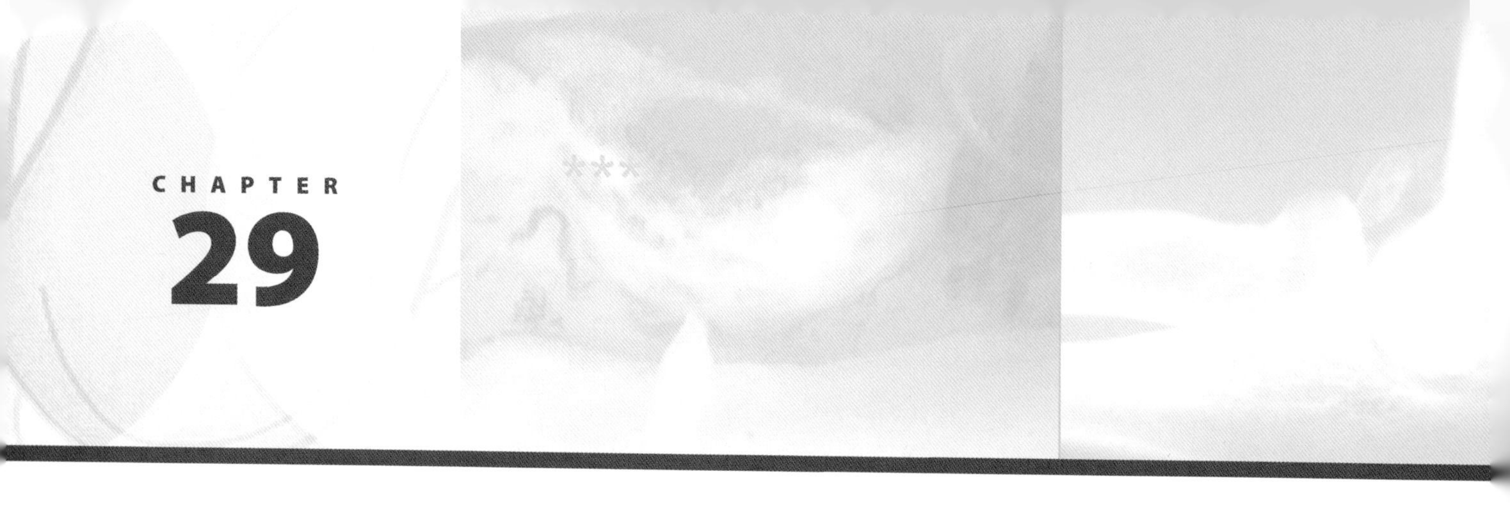

Wrist Arthritis:
Arthroscopic Synovectomy, Abrasion Chondroplasty, and Radial Styloidectomy of the Wrist

Kevin Plancher ● Eric J. Balaguer

The wrist, with its many articular surfaces, is a crucial anatomic link between the hand and forearm. When afflicted by arthritis and conditions limiting the range of motion, the wrist greatly affects the daily lives of patients. The advent of arthroscopy has revolutionized the practice of orthopedic and hand surgeons. Newer techniques and significant application of wrist and small joint arthroscopy can be attributed to many pioneers.[1,2]

Wrist arthroscopy has provided a tool with which to examine and treat intra-articular abnormalities. Early results for arthroscopic synovectomy of the wrist showed that it reduced pain and swelling and improved joint function.[3-6] The transitory or permanent effects depend mainly on the activities of the patient and underlying cause of arthritis. Abrasion chondroplasty of the wrist has not been described at length, but it is known that "repair cartilage" (i.e., fibrocartilage) replaces articular cartilage, as demonstrated in several canine models.[7] Abrasion chondroplasty appears to have a therapeutic role in patients with proximal pole hamate arthrosis or radiocarpal arthrosis. Preliminary results of this procedure have been excellent.[8-10] This chapter surveys the indications and techniques for arthroscopic synovectomy, abrasion chondroplasty, and radial styloidectomy.

ANATOMY AND PHYSIOLOGY

The anatomy of the wrist joint is probably the most complex of all the joints in the body. The wrist is a collection of many bones and joints, which allow the use of our hands in many different ways. The wrist must be extremely mobile to give hands a full range of motion. At the same time, the wrist must provide the strength for gripping heavy objects.

Fifteen bones form connections from the end of the forearm to the hand. The wrist itself contains eight carpal bones. These bones are grouped in two rows across the wrist. Beginning with the thumb side of the wrist, the proximal row of carpal bones is made up of the scaphoid, lunate, and triquetrum. The distal row is made up of the trapezium, trapezoid, capitate, hamate, and pisiform bones. One reason that the wrist is so complicated is because every small carpal bone forms a joint with the bone next to it. The wrist joint is composed of many small joints.

Articular cartilage is the material that covers the ends of the bones of any joint. Articular cartilage can be up to one fourth of an inch thick in the large, weight-bearing joints. It is thinner in joints such as the wrist that do not support much weight. Articular cartilage is white and shiny, and it has a rubbery consistency. It is slippery, which allows the joint surfaces to slide against one another without causing damage.

Articular cartilage absorbs shock and provides an extremely smooth surface to facilitate motion. Articular cartilage exists almost everywhere that two bony surfaces move against one another, or articulate. In the wrist, articular cartilage covers the sides of all the carpals and the ends of the bones that connect from the forearm to the fingers.

Matrix metalloproteinases and proinflammatory cytokines (e.g., interleukin-1) are important mediators of cartilage destruction in patients with primary osteoarthritis. Interleukin-1 increases the synthesis of matrix metalloproteinases and thereby plays an important role in osteoarthritis.

During the initial stages of osteoarthritis, the superficial layers of the articular cartilage fibrillate and crack. As degeneration progresses, deep layers become involved, resulting in erosions that produce bare subchondral bone. Denatured type II collagen is found in abundance in osteoarthritic articular cartilage, with decreased water content and decreased ratio of chondroitin sulfate to keratan sulfate constituents. In chronic injuries of the scapholunate ligament and in scaphoid nonunions, osteoarthritis starts in the radioscaphoid joint and progresses to the capitolunate joint. The radiolunate joint remains unaffected during the early stages.

Rheumatoid arthritis is a progressive inflammatory disease characterized by synovitis and joint destruction. Synovial cell proliferation results in pannus formation and fibrosis, which cause erosion of cartilage and bone. Cytokines, prostanoids, and proteolytic enzymes mediate this process. A cell-mediated immune response to an unidentified antigen appears essential in the pathogenesis of rheumatoid arthritis. Proinflammatory cytokines, such as interleukin-1 and tumor necrosis factor α, and T-cell initiation are the central mediators in rheumatoid arthritis.

In gouty arthritis, allantoin, the enzyme uricase that breaks down uric acid into a more soluble product, is deficient, resulting in tissue deposition of crystalline forms of uric acid. Although hyperuricemia is a risk factor for the development of gout, the exact relationship between hyperuricemia and acute gout is unclear. Acute gouty arthritis can occur in the presence of normal serum uric acid concentrations. Conversely, many patients with hyperuricemia may never develop gouty arthritis.

Secondary osteoarthritis resulting from previous trauma to the carpal bones or ligaments results in abnormal joint reaction forces with each movement of the wrist, causing misdirected forces that lead to some combination of loading forces. This process produces degeneration of the articular cartilage, resulting in radiocarpal arthritis, selective intercarpal arthritis, or pancarpal arthritis, depending on the initial injury and subsequent healing.

Scaphoid fractures can result in osteoarthritis by three mechanisms:

1. If the fracture results in nonunion, abnormal movement occurs between the fragments, leading to an abnormal distribution of forces across the wrist and resulting in early degeneration of the radioscaphoid joint.
2. In a malunion, the height of the scaphoid may be reduced, and the range of motion in one or more planes may be restricted, resulting in increased strain and leading to osteoarthritic changes over time.
3. Scaphoid fractures resulting in avascular necrosis of the proximal pole can lead to collapse and degeneration of the radioscaphoid joint, which may involve the lunate and then the entire wrist.

Kienböck disease results in lunatomalacia. The weakened lunate is subjected to a nutcracker effect between the prominent radius and the capitate head, causing progressive collapse. In its final stages, Kienböck disease leads to osteoarthritis in the radiolunate joint.

PATIENT EVALUATION

History and Physical Examination

The predominant symptom of osteoarthritis is pain. Pain that is usually aggravated during the extremes of movement in the early stages gradually worsens to involve the full available range of motion. The range of motion may gradually deteriorate, and the osteoarthritis progresses. In severe cases, the wrist has no movement, resulting in stiffness.

Deformity is another feature of wrist arthritis. This is common in rheumatoid arthritis, in which deformity may be complicated by associated subluxation of the radiocarpal and inferior radioulnar joints. Swelling of the wrist, one of the most common manifestations of rheumatoid arthritis, may occur because of synovial thickening.

Because the wrist stabilizes the hand for functioning, pain and deformity may result in weakness of the hand grip. Wrist deformity and instability reduce support for the hand to grasp, impairing dexterity, whereas stiffness and the inability to extend the wrist deprive the fingers of the tenodesis effect.

Classic rheumatoid wrist arthritis begins with radial deviation of the wrist, resulting in ulnar head prominence. This progresses to supination and ulnar translation of the carpus, leading to volar subluxation of the radiocarpal joint. Crepitus in the wrist becomes more apparent as joint disease progresses.

Diagnostic Imaging

The radiographic evaluation system we use for wrist arthritis is the Outerbridge classification of cartilage defects (Fig. 29-1). We have found that with an appropriate clinical history, dedicated articular cartilage imaging has a sensitivity and specificity reaching the 95% confidence interval. This tool has been confirmed by arthroscopic findings and clinical correlations. However, Haims and colleagues think that magnetic resonance imaging (MRI) of the wrist (41 indirect MR arthrograms and 45 unenhanced [nonarthrographic] MR images) was not adequately sensitive or accurate for diagnosing cartilage defects in the distal radius, scaphoid, lunate, or triquetrum, as demonstrated by correlating MRI with arthroscopic findings.[11] In cases of synovitis and ulnar-sided pathology, MRI results are a strong indicator of which areas need to be addressed with the arthroscope. Cartilage defects are often confirmed after diagnostic arthroscopy is completed.

Arthroscopic abrasion arthroplasty, subchondral drilling, and microfracture can be performed for focal chondral defects in patients with moderate degenerative wrist arthritis or when plain radiographs indicate vascular necrosis. MRI is a sensitive method for excluding the diagnosis of avascular necrosis and for evaluating the extent to which fibrocartilaginous repair tissue has formed postoperatively. These methods have been demonstrated for knee pathology, and we have established the same protocols for wrist defects.[11,12]

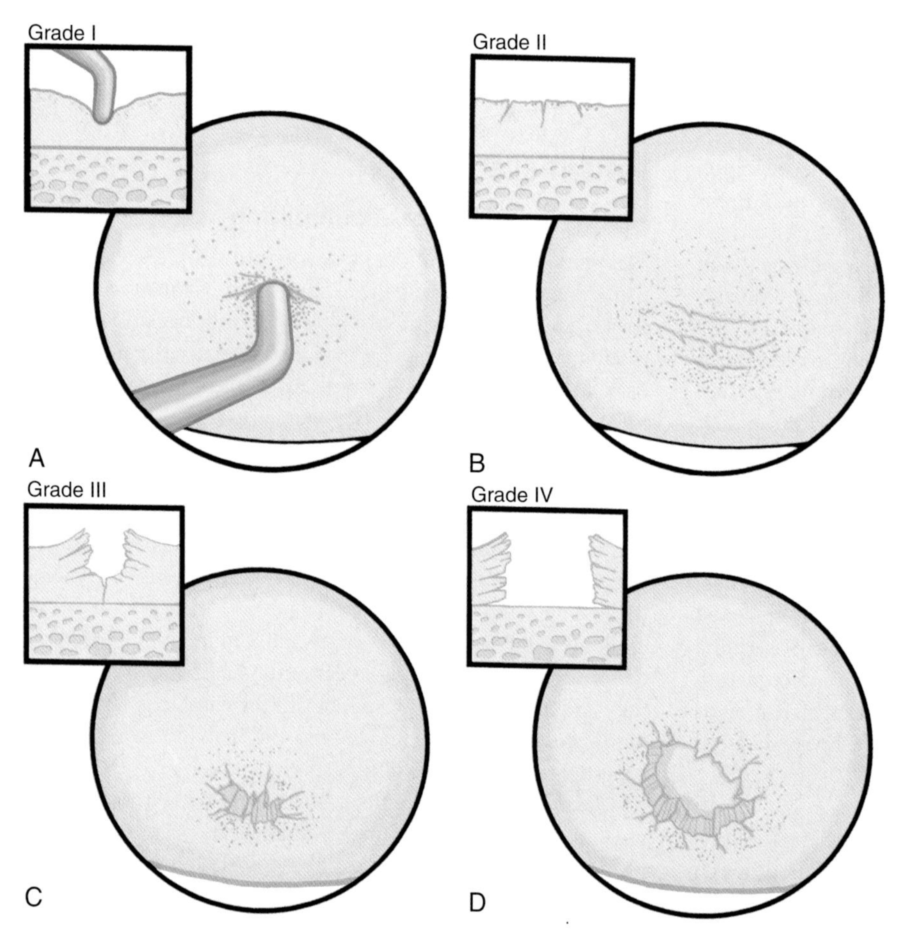

FIGURE 29-1 The Outerbridge classification of articular cartilage lesions: grade 0, normal cartilage; grade I, superficial softening; grade II, fibrillation; grade III, fissuring; grade IV, loss of all cartilage layers and exposure of subchondral bone.

TREATMENT

Indications and Contraindications

Arthroscopic synovectomy provides effective treatment of patients with rheumatoid arthritis, juvenile rheumatoid arthritis, systemic lupus erythematosus, and postinfectious arthritis.[3-5] Patients with post-traumatic joint contractures and septic arthritis of the wrist after failed systemic antibiotics and lavage also benefit from arthroscopic synovectomy. For rheumatoid patients, we follow the protocol established by Adolfsson.[5] We treat those who with persistent joint synovitis have failed to respond to pharmacologic treatment for more than 6 months and who present with radiographic changes of grade 0, I, or II according to the staging system by Larsen and colleagues.[13] For nonrheumatoid patients, the radiographic classification system used to evaluate the progression of disease is the Outerbridge classification system, which was originally developed for chondromalacia patellae.[14] Patients with early presentation of systemic lupus erythematosus or reactive arthritis (bacterial or viral) and those with osteoarthritis with nominal radiographic changes and florid synovitis are also considered candidates for wrist synovectomy. Patients after intra-articular fractures or multiple previous wrist interventions also benefit from capsular release, removal of adhesions, and synovectomy.

Abrasion chondroplasty is effective in patients with proximal pole hamate arthrosis, which is a cause of ulnar-sided pain in wrists loaded during ulnar deviation; it is particularly effective in those with a type II lunate defect. When the arthrosis in this area is advanced and subchondral bone is exposed (Outerbridge grade IV), we follow the recommendation of Yao and coworkers: excision of the proximal pole.[15] Lunate morphology plays a key role in this condition. The type II lunate and its medial facet during contact loading of the proximal pole of the hamate can lead to arthritis, with a reported occurrence of 44% for type II lunates but only 2% for type I lunates.[9,15-21] Patients with this condition may have concomitant injuries that require treatment, such as triangular fibrocartilage complex (TFCC) tears, lunotriquetral interosseous ligament tears,[9] ulnar impaction, and radial-sided pathology. A TFCC injury is almost always noted in the absence of any other structural problem when synovitis is noted on the ulnar side of the wrist.

Patients who require extensive open wrist procedures are not candidates for arthroscopic synovectomy. MRI in conjunction with clinical assessment of the patient aids decision making. Abrasion arthroplasty is contraindicated for patients with active rheumatoid disease, those who are medically unfit, and patients with active infections not located in the wrist.

TREATMENT

Conservative Treatment

Nonoperative measures for wrist arthritis are primarily aimed at relieving pain in the wrist. Rest in the form of splinting with removable thermoplastic splints may be useful during exacerbations. However, overuse of splinting may result in a poor outcome as a result of wrist stiffness and weakness produced by immobilization. The wrist is usually maintained in neutral or slight dorsiflexion, which is the functional position for the wrist.

Nonsteroidal anti-inflammatory drugs can control inflammation, thereby reducing synovitis and swelling. They are most useful in inflammatory arthritis. Antirheumatism medications, including systemic steroids, methotrexate, and anti–tumor necrosis factor, help patients with rheumatoid arthritis. Allopurinol may be useful in patients with gouty arthritis of the wrist.

Steroid injections, with or without local anesthetic into the joint, may be performed, but the results are equivocal. Methylprednisolone acetate injection into the wrist may play a role in treating a degenerate triangular fibrocartilage. When combined with a local anesthetic, local steroid injections may aid in the diagnosis, but we have found the effect to be transient, and repeated injections may be needed.

Surgical Treatment

Surgery for wrist arthritis depends on the severity and the extent of arthritis in the wrist. In the earliest stages, when the problems are mainly caused by carpal instability (i.e., prearthritic stage), the aim of the surgery is to rectify the anatomic position and to correct the carpal instability to prevent degeneration of the wrist. In the late stages of severe wrist arthritis, a partial or total wrist arthrodesis or an arthroplasty may be contemplated. In the intermediate stages, when the patient has well-established arthritis but a well-preserved range of motion, no standard treatment has been established. The available options are wrist arthroscopic débridement and wrist denervation.

Traditional Arthroscopic Technique

Arthroscopic wrist procedures are most useful as diagnostic tools, but they are occasionally used as therapeutic procedures. An arthroscopic wrist procedure is done to examine the joint articular surfaces, and it is useful for synovial biopsy, removal of loose bodies, and wrist débridement in patients with early-stage arthritis. Arthroscopy is most accurate for diagnosing degenerate triangular fibrocartilage lesions.

Arthroscopic synovectomy has become a well-described procedure.[15] Aggressive arthroscopic débridement, including radial styloidectomy and partial resection of the scaphoid, has been reported. Resection of the lunate in patients with Kienböck disease may be performed arthroscopically. In the distal radioulnar joint, arthroscopy can be used for débridement of the TFCC and for a modified Darrach procedure that involves distal ulna resection. Arthroscopic reconstructive procedures have been described for repair of the lunate-triquetrum ligament and ulnocarpal ligament complex and for capsular placation. Arthroscopic wrist portals are described in Table 29-1.

Arthroscopic Synovectomy and Abrasion Chondroplasty

General or regional anesthesia is preferred. The patient is supine on the operating table with the shoulder along the edge of the table. A tourniquet is placed above the elbow and inflated to 250 mm Hg. The shoulder is abducted 70 to 90 degrees, and the forearm is suspended vertically by finger traps from an articulating arm attached to the operating table, and traction of 10 pounds is applied to help open the joint (Fig. 29-2).

We tend to use the long and index finger, but in rheumatoid patients with delicate skin, all digits may be placed in the finger traps to distribute the traction load. A sling with 7 to 10 pounds of weight is placed over the tourniquet to provide downward countertraction and distraction of the wrist joint. A 2.5-mm arthroscope is used with a 30-degree viewing angle. A short bridge arthroscope (lever arm of 100 mm) allows better control. The wrist is examined, and landmarks are palpated.

The 3-4 portal is established in the soft spot 1 cm distal to Lister's tubercle (Fig. 29-3). An 18-gauge needle is inserted first and angled 10 degrees volar to be parallel to the joint surface, thereby decreasing the risk of articular damage. The wrist is then distended with 5 to 7 mL of saline solution. A vertical stab incision

TABLE 29-1 Arthroscopic Wrist Portals

Dorsal Portals	Technique	Comment
1-2	Inserted in the extreme dorsum of the snuffbox just radial to the extensor pollicis longus tendon to avoid the radial artery	Gives access to the radial styloid, scaphoid, lunate, and articular surface of the distal radius
3-4	1 cm distal to Lister's tubercle, between the tendons of the third and fourth compartment	Main working portal; gives a wide range of movement and view
4-5	Between the common extensor fourth compartment and extensor indices in the fifth compartment	Main working portal
6-R	Located distal to the ulna head and radial to the extensor carpi ulnaris tendon; established with a needle under direct vision through the arthroscope, avoiding damage to the triangular fibrocartilage complex	Alternate working portal allows visualization back to radial side of wrist
6-U	Established under direct vision, similar to the 6-R portal; blunt dissection always used to avoid the dorsal branches of the ulnar nerve	Access to the ulnar-sided structures and visualization to radial side of wrist

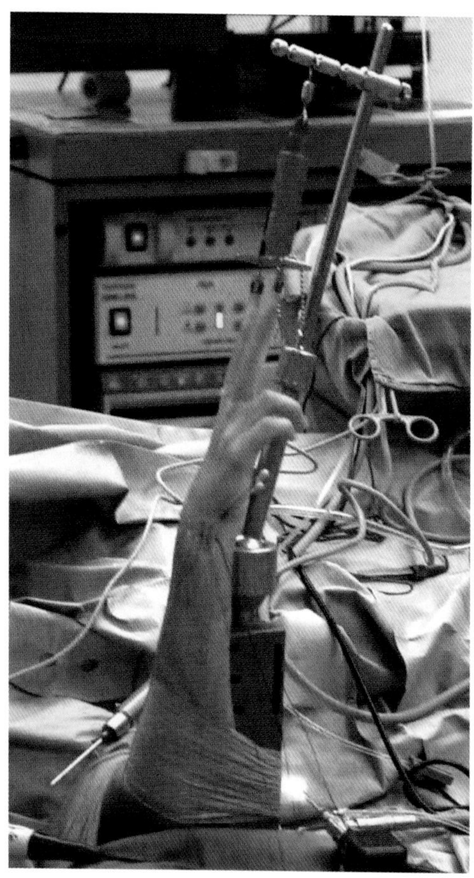

FIGURE 29-2 Wrist arthroscopy setup. The patient's index and long fingers are placed in finger traps. A traction force of 10 pounds is applied to allow better access and mobility inside the wrist joint.

is made with a no. 15 scalpel blade. A blunt trocar is then introduced into the joint. To maintain orientation, the thumb is kept on Lister's tubercle until the arthroscope has been introduced. Inflow of lactated Ringer's solution is gravity fed (i.e., no pump required). Subsequent portals are made with an outside-in technique, in which the needle is introduced in the joint. The 4.5 or maybe 6-R portal is used for a radiocarpal portal. They are identified by use of transillumination and introduction of the needle either radial to the extensor carpi ulnaris tendon or ulnar to the common extensor tendons and distal to the TFCC.

The arthroscopic synovectomy can be carried out with general or regional anesthesia with the forearm suspended in a traction tower device with finger traps. We use the long and index fingers, but for rheumatoid patients with delicate skin, all digits can be placed in the finger traps to distribute the traction load. Traction of 10 to 15 pounds is applied. Passive infusion from an elevated bag of saline solution through a separate inflow cannula or within the scope itself can be used. A 2.7-mm diameter, 30-degree arthroscope is inserted through the 3-4, 4-5, and 6-R working portals for the radiocarpal joint. The 6-U portal is used for outflow. The radial and ulnar midcarpal portals are used to access the midcarpal joint. Efficiency and speed is important to decrease wrist swelling. In cases with severe scaphotrapeziotrapezoid joint arthritis, a separate portal can be established.

All of the inflamed tissue is removed using a motorized shaver system with a 3.5-mm-diameter synovial resector blade and 3.5-mm flexible shaver (Fig. 29-4). We have had good results with thermoregulation, which also decreases bleeding, but are careful not to touch the articular surfaces. Flow must be maintained within the wrist joint when using thermoregulation to avoid heat buildup. It is important to inspect the radial styloid, the radioscapholunate and radioscaphocapitate ligament, ulnar prestyloid recess, and the dorsoulnar region underneath the extensor carpi ulnaris subsheath. Midcarpal space synovitis is often found along the dorsoulnar region, volarly underneath the capitohamate joint, and in the scapho-

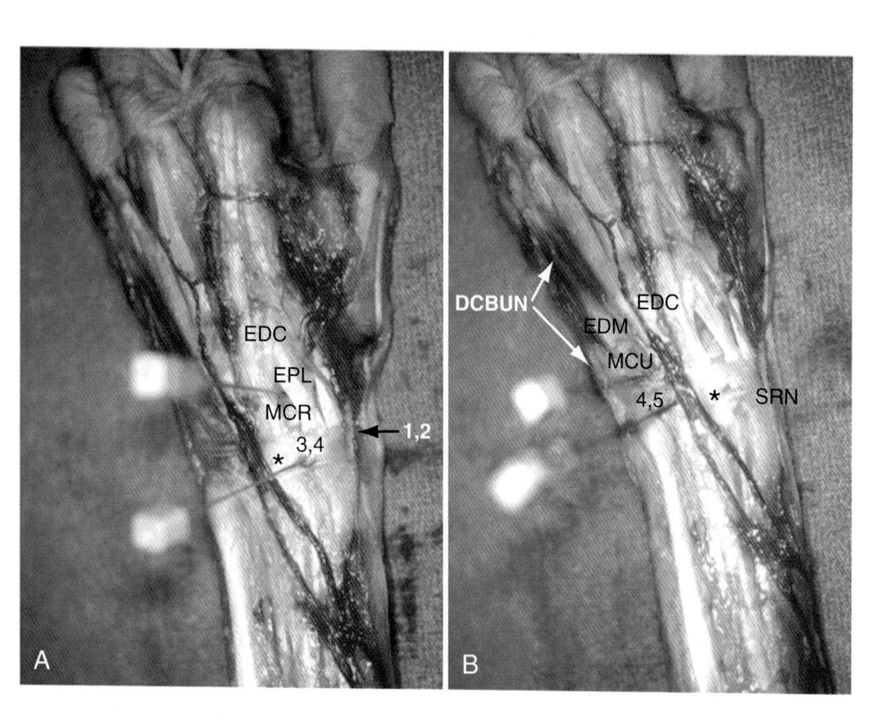

FIGURE 29-3 Dorsal portal anatomy. **A,** Cadaver dissection of the dorsal aspect of a left wrist demonstrates the relative positions of the dorsoradial portals. **B,** Relative positions of the dorsoulnar portals are shown. Asterisk, Lister's tubercle; EDC, extensor digitorum communis; EDM, extensor digiti minimi; EPL, extensor pollicis longus; DCBUN, dorsal cutaneous branch of the ulnar nerve; MCU, midcarpal ulnar portal.

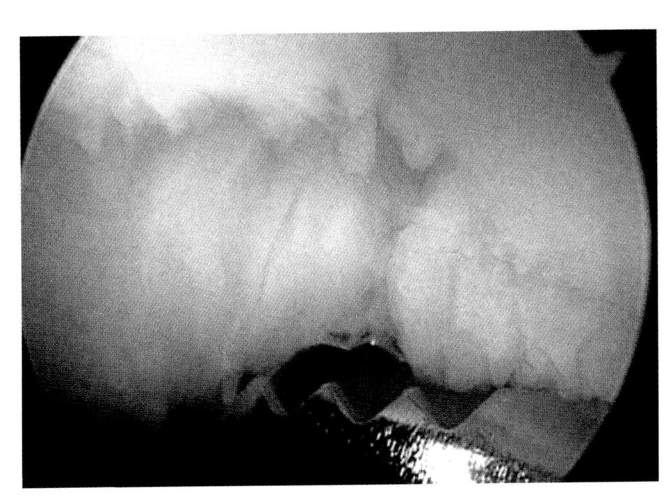

FIGURE 29-4 The rotator shaver is used to perform the synovectomy and remove all fibrillated cartilage.

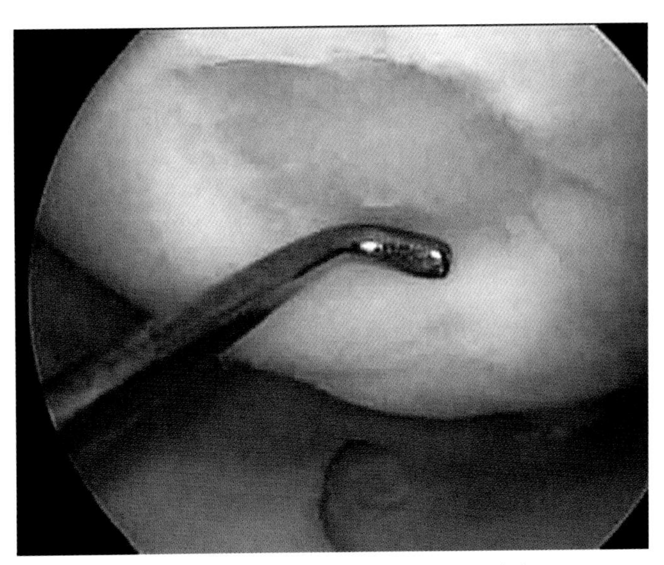

FIGURE 29-5 The chondral lesion is débrided and ready for chondroplasty.

trapeziotrapezoid joint. The distal radioulnar joint is inspected, and this can usually be done through a central defect in the horizontal portion of the TFCC, with synovectomy carried out through the 6-R portal. A separate distal radioulnar joint portal immediately proximal to the TFCC can be used for shaving while viewing through the radiocarpal joint if this defect is not present. Meticulous care must be used at all times to avoid chondral damage to the articular surfaces. Incisions are closed with Dermabond and augmented with Steri-Strips or with subcuticular Monocryl.

The skin incision for the 6-U portal is done with caution to avoid laceration or a painful neuroma of the dorsal sensory branch of the ulnar nerve. Light dressing is placed, and range of motion is tested immediately postoperatively under the supervision of a hand therapists. Radiocarpal arthritis treated with abrasion arthroplasty is carried out as described by Steadman and coworkers for the knee.[10] Working portals in the wrist and the operative setup are established as previously described. Loose bodies are removed while doing the diagnostic part of the wrist arthroscopy. After a focal area of chondral damage is identified, specially designed awls (2.5 and 3.5 mm) are used to make multiple perforations, or microfractures, into the subchondral bone plate (Fig. 29-5). Perforations are made as close together as possible, but not so close that one breaks into another. They usually are approximately 1 to 2 mm apart (Fig. 29-6).

The integrity of the subchondral bone plate should be maintained. The released marrow elements (i.e., mesenchymal stem cells, growth factors, and other healing proteins) form a surgically induced superclot that provides an enriched environment for new tissue formation.[10] The rehabilitation program is crucial to optimize the results of the surgery and early range of motion. Dressings and closure are carried out as previously described.

If indicated, we also perform a radial styloidectomy to alleviate the symptoms of wrist arthritis. The radial styloidectomy can be done arthroscopically.[22]

Arthroscopy aids in visualization to ensure complete resection of the arthritic portion of the styloid without sacrificing the ligamentous support of the wrist. A 3.5-mm burr is used by entering the

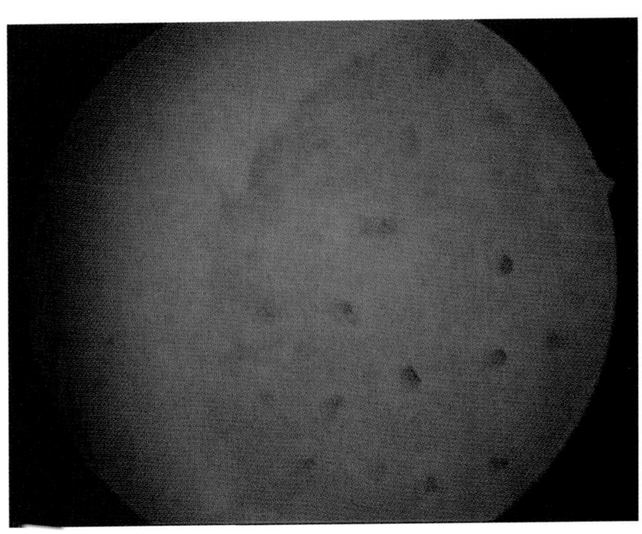

FIGURE 29-6 With the use of specially designed awls, microfractures are created in the subchondral bone 1 to 2 mm apart.

1-2 portal. The diameter of the burr is a good benchmark to gauge the amount of styloid removed, and ideally, this is less than 4 mm. An 18-gauge needle can be introduced into the bone to mark the end point of the styloid resection and verified by fluoroscopy. After we complete the procedure, we remove all debris and lose bodies from the wrist joint using the shaver (Figs. 29-7 and 29-8).

Interpositional arthroplasty on the wrist joint is another adjunct procedure performed by some surgeons. The technique was first attempted in the 1970s with the use of silicone sheets. The result did not last long, and it produced a serious inflammatory reaction in the wrist. More recently, tensor fascia lata allografts have been used for this purpose with good success. This procedure cannot be done arthroscopically. A 3-cm elongation of the 3-4 portal is done. The wrist capsule is opened, and the tensor fascia lata allograft is inserted into the joint. Care must be taken not to overstuff the joint. Long-term results of prospective, randomized studies are not available.

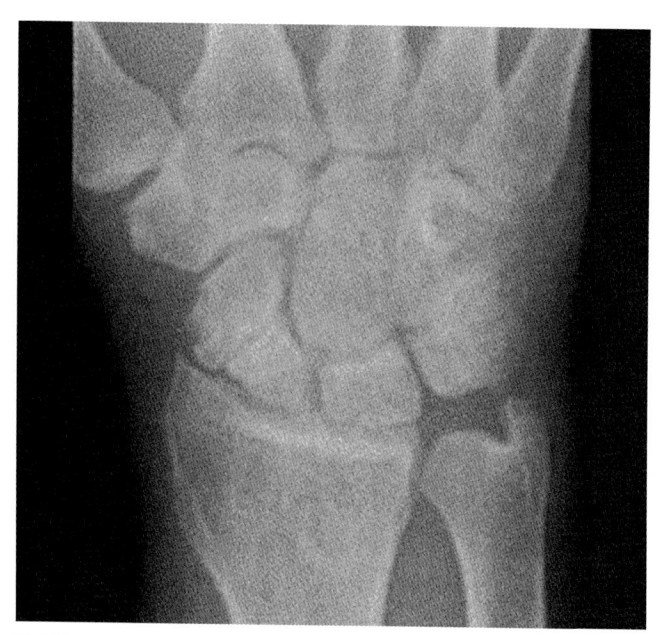

FIGURE 29-7 Radiocarpal arthritis has resulted from a scaphoid nonunion fracture (i.e., SNAC wrist). Penciling of the radial styloid is pathognomonic for this condition.

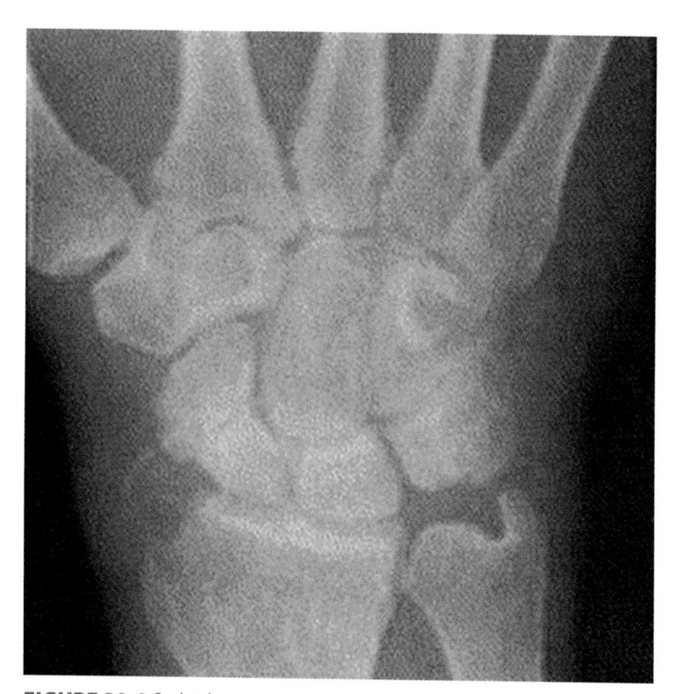

FIGURE 29-8 Styloidectomy is performed. An area of approximately 4 mm was removed from the radial styloid, decompressing the articular surface of the scaphoid and the radius.

Wrist denervation by excising a 1-cm portion of the anterior and posterior interosseous nerve can be performed. We have found, along with studies, that this procedure decreases wrist pain significantly while improving range of motion and grip strength of the hand.[23]

PEARLS & PITFALLS

PEARLS

- When using the traction device, ensure at least 15 pounds of traction to help visualization in an already compromised joint space.
- Remove all loose bodies in the radial carpal and midcarpal joints.
- When performing microfracture or chondroplasty, use commercially available picks, and separate holes to avoid defects. Remove the calcified layer with a curette.

PITFALLS

- Place the arthroscope with a blunt trocar to avoid penetration to the articular cartilage.
- Avoid ligament injury by understanding wrist anatomy.
- Avoid débridement and resection of the radial styloid below the level of the radial scaphocapitate ligament; failure to do so can lead to instability of the wrist.

Postoperative Rehabilitation

Postoperatively, patients are placed in a volar-based short arm splint for 7 to 10 days when a simple arthroscopy is performed, after which patients return for a wound check and suture removal at 2 weeks. Immediate wrist motion is encouraged, along with protection against vigorous activity for 6 weeks.

REFERENCES

1. Ekman EF, Pochling GG. Principles of arthroscopy and wrist arthroscopy equipment. *Hand Clin*. 1994;10:557-566.
2. Gupta R, Bozentka DJ, Osterman AL. Wrist arthroscopy: principles and clinical applications. *J Am Acad Orthop Surg*. 2001;9:200-209.
3. Adolfsson L, Nylander G. Arthroscopic synovectomy of the rheumatoid wrist. *J Hand Surg Br*. 1993;18:92-96.
4. Adolfsson L, Frisen M. Arthroscopic synovectomy of the rheumatoid wrist. A 3.8 year follow-up. *J Hand Surg Br*. 1997;22:711-713.
5. Adolfsson L. Arthroscopic synovectomy in wrist arthritis. *Hand Clin*. 2005;21:527-530.
6. Roth JH, Poehling GG. Arthroscopic "ectomy" surgery of the wrist. *Arthroscopy*. 1990;6:141-147
7. Altman RD, Kates J, Chun LE, et al. Preliminary observations of chondral abrasion in a canine model. *Ann Rheum Dis*. 1992;51:1056-1062.
8. Steadman JR, Briggs KK, Rodrigo JJ, et al. Outcomes of microfractures for traumatic chondral defects of the knee: average 11-year follow-up. *Arthroscopy*. 2003;19:477-484.
9. Harley BJ, Werner FW, Boles SD, Palmer AK. Arthroscopic resection of arthrosis of the proximal hamate: a clinical and biomechanical study. *J Hand Surg Am*. 2004;29:661-667.
10. Steadman JR, Rodkey WG, Rodrigo JJ. Microfracture: surgical technique and rehabilitation to treat chondral defects. *Clin Orthop Relat Res*. 2001;(391 Suppl):S362-S369.
11. Haims AH, Moore AE, Schweitzer ME, et al. MRI in the diagnosis of cartilage injury in the wrist. *AJR Am J Roentgenol*. 2004;182:1267-1270.
12. Amrami KK, Askari KS, Pagnano MW, Sundaram M. Radiologic case study. Abrasion chondroplasty mimicking avascular necrosis. *Orthopedics*. 2002;25:1018, 1107-1108.
13. Larsen A, Dale K, Eek M. Radiographic evaluation of rheumatoid arthritis and related conditions by standard reference films. *Acta Radiol Diagn (Stockh)*. 1977;18:481-491.
14. Outerbridge RE. The etiology of chondromalacia patellae. *J Bone Joint Surg Br*. 1961;43:752-757.
15. Yao J, Osterman AL. Arthroscopic techniques for wrist arthritis (radial styloidectomy and proximal pole hamate excisions). *Hand Clin*. 2005;21:519-526.
16. Nakamura K, Patterson RM, Moritomo H, Viegas SF. Type I versus type II lunates: ligament anatomy and presence of arthrosis. *J Hand Surg Am*. 2001;26:428-436.

17. Nakamura K, Beppu M, Patterson RM, et al. Motion analysis in two dimensions of radial-ulnar deviation of type I versus type II lunates. *J Hand Surg Am*. 2000;25:877-888.
18. Malik AM, Schweitzer ME, Culp RW, et al. MR imaging of the type II lunate bone: frequency, extent, and associated findings. *AJR Am J Roentgenol*. 1999;173:335-338.
19. Dautel G, Merle M. Chondral lesions of the midcarpal joint. *Arthroscopy*. 1997;13:97-102.
20. Viegas SF, Wagner K, Patterson R, Peterson P. Medial (hamate) facet of the lunate. *J Hand Surg Am*. 1990;15:564-571.
21. Viegas SF. The lunatohamate articulation of the midcarpal joint. *Arthroscopy*. 1990;6:5-10.
22. Yao J, Osterman AL. Arthroscopic techniques for wrist arthritis (radial styloidectomy and proximal pole hamate excisions). *Hand Clin*. 2005;21:519-526.
23. Weinstein LP, Berger RA. Analgesic benefit, functional outcome, and patient satisfaction after partial wrist denervation. *J Hand Surg Am*. 2002;27:833-839.

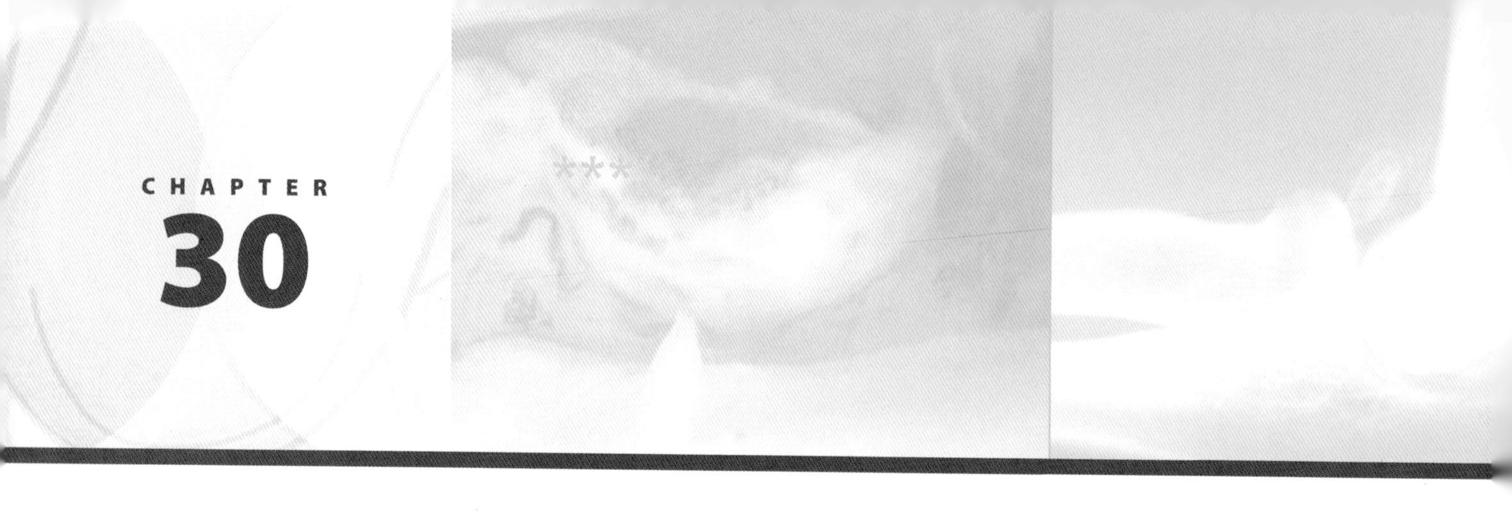

Arthroscopic Proximal Row Carpectomy

Randall W. Culp • Matthew J. Boardman

Proximal row carpectomy (PRC) is a reliable alternative to arthrodesis in the treatment of wrist osteoarthritis. PRC is a motion-preserving salvage procedure that involves excision of the scaphoid, lunate, and triquetrum and converts the complex link joint of the wrist into a simple hinge.[1] The procedure has faced considerable criticism in regard to alteration of the normal anatomy of the wrist joint, impairment of strength and motion, improper redistribution of joint loading, subsequent radiocapitate arthritis, and an unpredictable outcome.[2] Conversely, many investigators have documented satisfactory motion preservation, maintained grip strength, pain relief, and patient satisfaction. Several medium- and long-term follow-up studies have demonstrated that PRC is a reliable procedure with outcomes comparable to those of other reconstructive and salvage procedures of the wrist.[3-17]

ANATOMY

The wrist joint allows complicated interactions among an array of anatomic structures, each playing a role in radiocarpal stability and mobility. A host of factors contribute to the precise mechanism of wrist function, and traumatic disruption of any link in the anatomic chain alters the carpal mechanics, leading to a predictable and progressive degeneration of the joint. Scaphoid pathology is often primarily responsible for the development of wrist arthritis. As articular contact area decreases, load distribution becomes irregular, and shearing occurs.

The proximal row of carpal bones operates as an intercalated segment between the distal radius and the distal carpal row. Proximal row intercarpal ligament disruption leads to wrist instability. Injuries to the scapholunate interosseous ligament and the extrinsic ligamentous complex allow the lunate to extend, creating dorsal intercalated segment instability.[18] The resultant palmar flexion of the scaphoid alters load distribution across the radioscaphoid articulation, increasing contact pressures and eventually leading to degenerative changes.[19] The sequential progression of arthritis that ensues is referred to as scapholunate advanced collapse (SLAC) wrist.[20]

Stage I SLAC wrist involves degeneration between the distal pole of the scaphoid and the radial styloid. In stage II, joint degeneration includes the scaphoid's proximal pole and the entire scaphoid fossa. In the third stage, the capitate drifts proximally between the scaphoid and lunate, and the capitolunate articulation degenerates.

Another form of scaphoid pathology associated with wrist arthritis is that which results from nonunion or malunion after a scaphoid fracture. This arthritic condition also follows a predictable pattern of progression, known as scaphoid nonunion advanced collapse (SNAC).[21] In stage I, incongruity of the distal radioscaphoid articulation leads to degenerative changes that compromise the scaphoid's ability to stabilize the carpal rows. Stage II involves arthrosis of the scaphocapitate articulation. As wrist stability deteriorates in stage III, the capitate migrates proximally, and arthrosis between the capitate head and scapholunate complex results. The radiolunate and proximal scaphoid pole articulations are typically spared even in advanced disease.

PATIENT EVALUATION

History and Physical Examination

Primary osteoarthritis of the wrist is uncommon, because most arthritic conditions of the radiocarpal joint are post-traumatic in nature. The primary diagnoses most often are SLAC wrist occurring after a scapholunate ligament injury and SNAC wrist occurring after a scaphoid nonunion or as a sequela of an intra-articular distal radius fracture. Patients may also present with a remote history of an apparent "wrist sprain" that was neglected.

Middle-aged men, notably laborers, make up much of this patient population. Patients present with a history of a prior injury most likely incurred by a fall onto an outstretched hand or a previous wrist surgery. Although the SLAC wrist is not always symptomatic, the patient typically complains of decreased grip and pinch strength and of activity-related pain, particularly wrist extension and radial deviation.

Physical examination may reveal dorsoradial swelling and tenderness to palpation over the carpus and radial scaphoid articulation, especially in patients with SLAC or SNAC wrist arthrosis. Motion is often diminished and painful, exhibiting considerable crepitus in passive and active ranges.

Physical examination may be facilitated by employing Watson's standard approach to the examination of radial-sided wrist pain.[22] The first maneuver assesses the articular–nonarticular (ANA) junction as the wrist is ulnarly deviated and the junction between the articular and nonarticular cartilage is palpated. Second, the scaphotrapeziotrapezoid (STT) joint is palpated by following the second metacarpal proximally until a space is reached, denoting the STT joint. Third, the dorsal wrist syndrome is ruled out by palpating between the second and fourth dorsal compartments of the wrist. A fourth test is the Watson scaphoid shift, which is performed by attempting to push the scaphoid dorsally from its volar side while passively radially deviating the wrist. A positive test elicits wrist pain as a result of scapholunate injury or ligamentous laxity. The fifth examination maneuver is the finger extension test, in which the wrist is flexed and the fingers are extended against resistance; increased loading of the radiocarpal joint and extensor tendon pressure produce pain.

Diagnostic Imaging

Standard radiographic imaging is all that is necessary to diagnose post-traumatic arthrosis of the wrist. Posteroanterior, lateral, and oblique views of the radiocarpal joint in this patient population reveal joint space narrowing, subchondral sclerosis, and cyst formation in the carpal bones and distal radius.

TREATMENT

Indications and Contraindications

The indications for the standard open PRC are also those that are applied to the arthroscopic technique. They include degenerative conditions of the proximal carpal row, such as SLAC, SNAC, chronic perilunate dislocation, Preiser's disease, and Kienböck's disease. One indication for PRC is complex fracture dislocation of the wrist.[14] The rationale cited by the authors of this 2005 case series[14] was to avoid the disadvantages of arthrodesis while anticipating the likely post-traumatic arthrosis in this patient population. Failed carpal implants, cerebral palsy and spasticity, and reimplantation have also been described as indications for PRC, although we do not recommend the latter groups of patients for an arthroscopic technique.[23]

The relative contraindications to PRC are multicystic carpal disease, preexisting ulnar translocation of the carpus, and degenerative changes of the lunate fossa or capitate head. A 2007 study investigated a method to salvage a PRC for patients with degenerative changes of the head of the capitate. Tang and Imbriglia performed osteochondral resurfacing of the capitate in eight patients undergoing PRC who had a grade II to IV (modified Outerbridge scale) area of capitate chondrosis less than 10 mm in diameter.[24] The results with osteochondral resurfacing compared favorably with published results of conventional PRC in terms of pain relief, employment status, range of motion, and grip strength. Culp and associates[4] and Ferlic and colleagues[25] did not recommend PRC for patients with inflammatory arthropathy because of its high failure rate.

Therapeutic Options

The biomechanical literature has focused on compensatory radiocarpal loading and kinematics after PRC. Blankenhorn and coworkers performed a cadaveric study using computed tomography to assess wrist motion before and after PRC.[26] Their results showed that wrist range of motion after PRC was sufficient for activities of daily living. Flexion and extension motion at the radiocarpal joint after PRC was greater than motion at the radiocarpal and midcarpal joints of the intact wrist, whereas overall wrist motion decreased. After PRC, the normal rotational motion of the capitate head (in the intact wrist midcarpal joint) was altered to a combination of rotation and translation.

More contemporary reports have included Disabilities of the Arm, Shoulder, and Hand (DASH) scores as a measurement of upper extremity disability after PRC. Whereas several Scandinavian studies[17,27-30] with variable follow-up times published DASH scores ranging from 28 to 36, DiDonna and associates reported an average DASH score of 9 in their study of 22 wrists after a minimum follow-up of 10 years.[12]

Cohen and Kozin published their results for a prospective cohort of similar patient groups with wrist osteoarthritis treated with scaphoid excision and four-corner fusion or PRC.[9] Follow-up examination revealed no significant difference in the flexion-extension arc, ulnar deviation, or grip strength between the groups. The investigators also reported pain relief and patient satisfaction to be similar.

Based on combined outcomes from the larger series in the literature, PRC results in approximately 60% of the average flexion-extension arc and 71% of the grip strength of the contralateral wrist.[4,7-9,31-36] The degree of patient satisfaction is high, ranging from 80% to 100%,[7-9,11,13,31-40] and failure rates tend to be low, ranging from 0% to 20%.[4,31,32,34,38] One criticism of PRC is that it causes radiocapitate arthrosis. DiDonna and colleagues observed degeneration of the radiocapitate articulation in 14 of 17 wrists during an average follow-up time of 14 years. Despite the degree of radiographic degenerative changes, there was no significant association between the arthrosis and wrist pain, range of motion, work restrictions, or patient satisfaction.[12]

Arthroscopy has become an increasingly valuable tool in the treatment of wrist pathology. The breadth of treatment options in the wrist surgeon's armamentarium continues to grow, as do advances in the arthroscopic equipment available. The pathologic conditions of the wrist that the arthroscopist is capable of treating include triangular fibrocartilage complex tears, distal radius and carpal fractures, cartilage injuries, and bone resections. There is scant literature available discussing arthroscopic PRC. Although there are no long-term follow-up studies, the short-term studies have described promising results.[5,41-44]

Conservative Management

Nonoperative treatment may begin with activity modification and non-steroidal anti-inflammatory medication. Splinting of the wrist or steroid injections may be used to provide the patient with symptomatic relief, particularly in sedentary and low-demand situations. However, patients are counseled on the predictable course of degeneration in their particular form of wrist arthritis. Although stage I SLAC or SNAC conditions and early radiocarpal degeneration may respond to these measures, a staged approach to treatment is based on the extent of disease, and a late presentation may preclude relief from conservative measures.

Arthroscopic Technique

The patient is placed in the supine position, with the affected upper extremity on a radiolucent hand table. Operative time is usually less than 2 hours, and regional or general anesthesia is adequate for this procedure. A well-padded tourniquet is wrapped around the upper arm, and the wrist is suspended in a traction tower with 10 to 15 pounds applied (Fig. 30-1). The tourniquet is inflated, but additional exsanguination is unnecessary. After distraction is introduced, the dorsal aspect of the wrist is palpated for landmarks, and the portals are made. The 3-4 portal is routinely used as the primary viewing portal.

To perform an arthroscopic PRC, the required instruments include a traction tower, a 2.7-mm arthroscope, a hook probe, a 2.9-mm shaver or radiofrequency tool, a 4.0-mm burr, small osteotomes, pituitary rongeurs, and image intensification equipment.

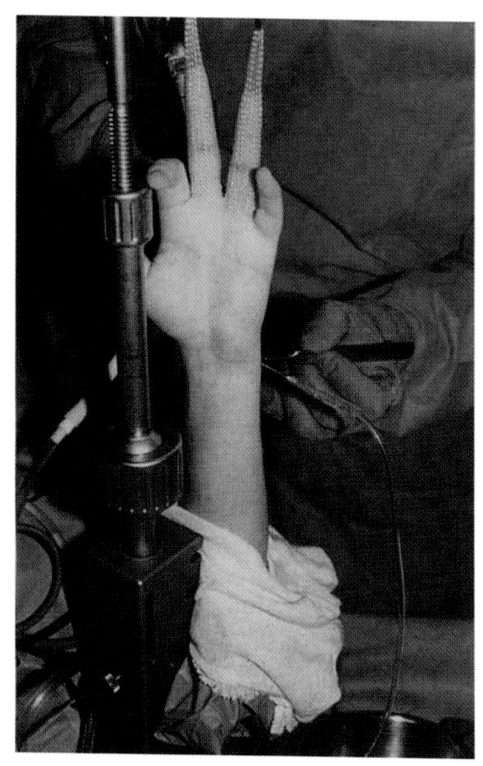

FIGURE 30-1 Standard traction tower with finger traps. An 18-gauge needle in the 6-U portal placed to gravity drainage serves as outflow. *(From Culp RW, Osterman AL, Talsania JS. Arthroscopic proximal row carpectomy.* Tech Hand Up Extrem Soc. *1997;2:116-119.)*

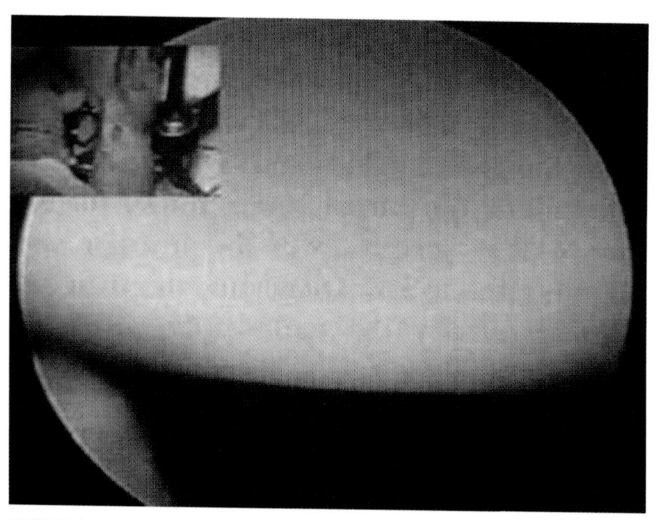

FIGURE 30-2 A healthy-appearing proximal capitate is seen through the midcarpal portal. *(From Culp RW, Osterman AL, Talsania JS. Arthroscopic proximal row carpectomy.* Tech Hand Up Extrem Soc. *1997;2:116-119.)*

The 2.7-mm arthroscope is introduced after the radiocarpal joint is insufflated with saline solution. A 6-R outflow portal is created under direct visualization at the prestyloid recess. Constant intra-articular pressure and flow are maintained with a mechanical pump. The joint is inspected in a routine fashion, with particular attention directed to the lunate fossa of the distal radius. The volar extrinsic ligaments are identified and preserved throughout the procedure—particularly the radioscaphocapitate, because it plays an essential role in stabilizing the new joint and preventing volar dislocation and ulnar translocation of the distal carpal row. The ulnar extrinsic ligaments and triangular fibrocartilage complex are identified as the arthroscope is directed ulnarly.

To assess the integrity of the proximal capitate surface, the midcarpal joint is visualized (Fig. 30-2). If the quality of this cartilaginous surface is questionable, we proceed to an alternative procedure (i.e., four-corner fusion, capitolunate arthrodesis, PRC with interpositional arthroplasty, or wrist arthrodesis). Visualization of the midcarpal joint is performed by establishing a radial midcarpal portal. This location is determined by measuring approximately 1 cm distal to the 3-4 portal.

After the surgeon is satisfied with the status of the cartilaginous surfaces of the proximal capitate and lunate fossa, the first step in performing the PRC is to remove the scapholunate and lunatotriquetral ligaments with a shaver or radiofrequency probe. This step is carried out through the 4-5 portal or the 6-R portal, or both. This is followed by removal of the core of the lunate with a burr (Fig. 30-3). Care is taken not to damage the proximal capitate or lunate fossa, which is accomplished by leaving behind an eggshell rim of the lunate. This remainder of the lunate is then morcellized with a pituitary rongeur under direct vision or image intensification.

The next step is fragmentation of the scaphoid and triquetrum with an osteotome and burr under image intensification and removal of the fragments in a piecemeal fashion with a pituitary rongeur while working through the 3-4 or 4-5 portal (Figs. 30-4 and 30-5). The surgeon can ensure easy removal and greater

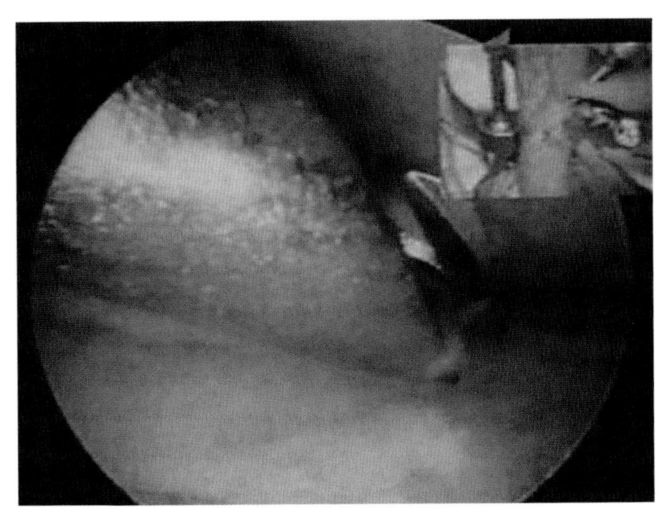

FIGURE 30-3 Large burr removes the center of the lunate, with care taken not to destroy the proximal capitate or the lunate fossa of the radius. *(From Culp RW, Osterman AL, Talsania JS. Arthroscopic proximal row carpectomy.* Tech Hand Up Extrem Soc. *1997;2:116-119.)*

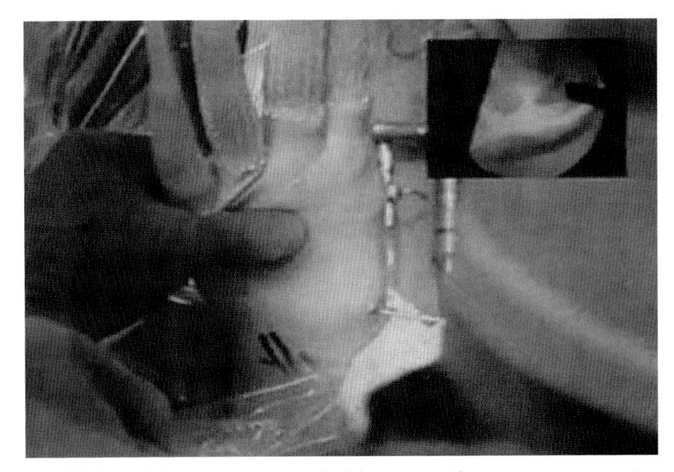

FIGURE 30-4 An osteotome used with x-ray guidance to remove part of the scaphoid and triquetrum. *(From Culp RW, Osterman AL, Talsania JS. Arthroscopic proximal row carpectomy.* Tech Hand Up Extrem Soc. *1997;2: 116-119.)*

protection of the articular cartilage by first coring out and fragmenting these carpal bones.

After the entirety of the proximal carpal row has been removed, the wrist is examined under image intensification (Fig. 30-6). Special attention is paid to the radial styloid area to be sure there is no impingement against the trapezium. Some surgeons recommend a moderate styloidectomy. Although we rarely carry out this aspect of the procedure, it can be done quite easily with the aid of the image intensifier.

If the surgeon chooses, a posterior interosseous neurectomy can be performed through a separate 1.5-cm incision just on the ulnar side of Lister's tubercle. The fourth extensor compartment is opened on its radial side, and with a bipolar electrocautery, 1 cm of the nerve is resected. The fourth compartment is repaired with absorbable suture, and all wounds are closed with a 4-0 nylon monofilament suture.

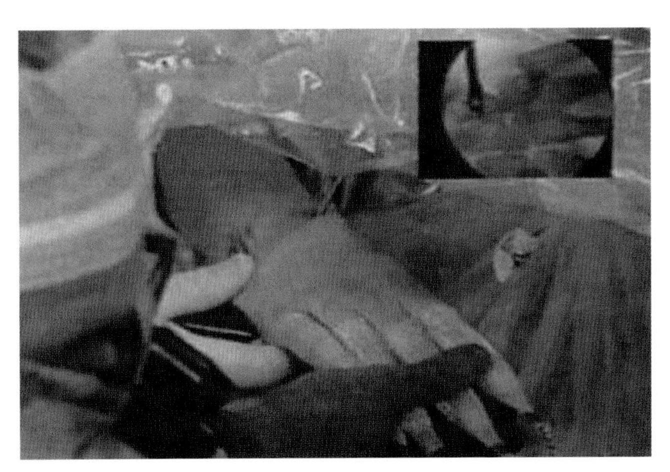

FIGURE 30-5 A pituitary rongeur is used with x-ray guidance to remove the fractionated scaphoid. This procedure can be performed with the wrist suspended in the traction tower on the radiolucent hand table. *(From Culp RW, Osterman AL, Talsania JS. Arthroscopic proximal row carpectomy.* Tech Hand Up Extrem Soc. *1997;2:116-119.)*

PEARLS & PITFALLS

- The midcarpal joint must be visualized to assess the integrity of the proximal surface of the capitate. An alternative procedure should be performed if the cartilaginous surface of the capitate is compromised.
- Preservation of the radioscaphocapitate ligament is an integral part of the procedure. Sacrifice of this ligament destabilizes the new radiocarpal joint.
- Special care must be taken when removing the lunate. We recommend leaving a thin rim of bone behind to be sure the proximal capitate and lunate facet are not damaged during the process.
- Using a burr to core out the carpal bones before removal with a pituitary rongeur facilitates carpectomy and protects the surrounding areas of articular cartilage.

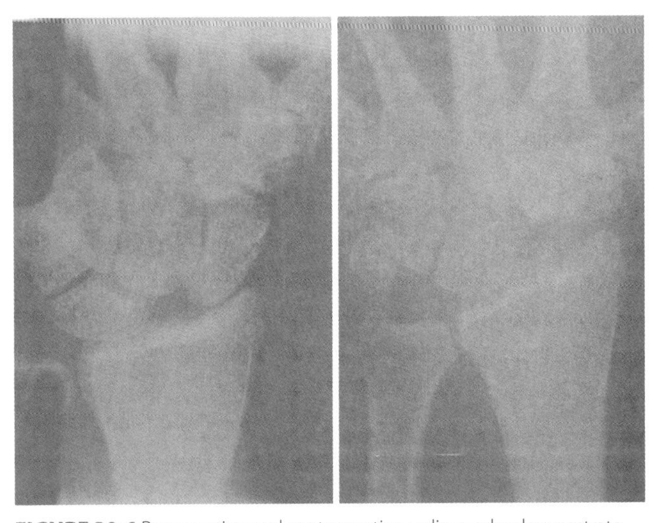

FIGURE 30-6 Preoperative and postoperative radiographs demonstrate scapholunate dissociation and the area after arthroscopic proximal row carpectomy, respectively. *(From Culp RW, Osterman AL, Talsania JS. Arthroscopic proximal row carpectomy.* Tech Hand Up Extrem Soc. *1997;2:116-119.)*

Postoperative Rehabilitation

Initially, patients are placed in a short arm volar plaster splint. Between 7 and 10 days postoperatively, the portal sutures are removed, and immobilization is continued with a short arm thermoplastic splint for an additional 3 weeks. At 4 weeks, the splint is removed and gentle range-of-motion exercises are begun. Strengthening is started approximately 8 weeks after surgery.

COMPLICATIONS

Arthroscopic PRC has several potential complications, and the two most important are highlighted here. Otherwise, the standard possible complications from arthroscopic surgery apply. They include infection and neurovascular embarrassment, which results from use of the osteotomes and may involve the dorsal ulnar sensory, median, and especially the ulnar nerves.

Iatrogenic articular cartilage damage must be avoided, especially at the lunate fossa and proximal capitate. The surgeon must not violate the extrinsic ligaments, particularly the radioscaphocapitate ligament, while excising the proximal carpal row (see Figs. 30-4 and 30-5). This is accomplished by coring out these carpals in such a way that a thin shell of cortical bone is left attached to the volar radiocarpal ligaments.

Compared with the standard open technique, arthroscopic PRC only minimally disrupts the capsuloligamentous structures about the wrist. Theoretically, this would result in less dorsal scar formation, which may lead to dorsal instability. This complication has not occurred in our practice, but if it should become evident, the surgeon should consider concurrent or subsequent electrothermal capsulorrhaphy.

CONCLUSIONS

Although proponents of the standard open approach may cite decreased operative time and less technical difficulty, we think that the arthroscopic method involves less dissection, postoperative pain, and stiffness and shorter recovery time. There is less harm to the dorsal ligamentous structures, which are left almost completely intact, compared with the open technique. The excellent visualization afforded by arthroscopy reduces the likelihood of volar extrinsic ligament damage.

Arthroscopic PRC requires less dissection and therefore leads to potentially less morbidity. However, this technique requires excellent arthroscopic skills. The overall patient satisfaction level has been high, and postoperative pain levels have been low. Patients are pleased with the smaller scars associated with arthroscopy. In our experience, patients who undergo arthroscopic PRC have had functional range of motion, satisfactory grip strength, and acceptable pain relief.

REFERENCES

1. Stamm TT. Excision of the proximal row of the carpus. *Proc R Soc Med.* 1944;38:74-75.
2. Lee RW, Hassan DM. Proximal row carpectomy. In: HK Watson, J Weinzweig, eds. *The Wrist.* Philadelphia, PA: Lippincott Williams & Wilkins; 2001:545-554.
3. Culp RW. Proximal row carpectomy. *Operat Tech Orthop.* 1996;2:69-71.
4. Culp RW, McGuigan FX, Turner MA, et al. Proximal row carpectomy: a multicenter study. *J Hand Surg Am.* 1993;18:19-25.
5. Roth JH, Poehling GG. Arthroscopic "-ectomy" surgery of the wrist. *Arthroscopy J Arthroscop Relat Surg.* 1990;6:141-147.
6. Siegel JM, Ruby LK. A critical look at intercarpal arthrodesis: review of the literature. *J Hand Surg Am.* 1996;21:717-23.
7. Tomaino MM, Delsignore J, Burton RI. Long-term results following proximal row carpectomy. *J Hand Surg Am.* 1994;19:694-703.
8. Wyrick JD, Stern PJ, Kiefhaber TR. Motion-preserving procedures in the treatment of scapholunate advanced collapse wrist: proximal row carpectomy versus four-corner arthrodesis. *J Hand Surg Am.* 1995;20:965-970.
9. Cohen MS, Kozin SH. Degenerative arthritis of the wrist: proximal row carpectomy versus scaphoid excision and four-corner arthrodesis. *J Hand Surg Am.* 2001;26:94-104.
10. Culp RW, Williams CS. Proximal row carpectomy for the treatment of scaphoid nonunion. *Hand Clin.* 2001;17:663-669.
11. Jebson PJ, Hayes EP, Engber WD. Proximal row carpectomy: a minimum 10-year follow-up study. *J Hand Surg Am.* 2003;28:561-569.
12. DiDonna ML, Kiefhaber TR, Stern PJ. Proximal row carpectomy: a study with a minimum of ten years of follow-up. *J Bone Joint Surg Am.* 2004;86:2359-2365.
13. Imbriglia JE. Proximal row carpectomy: technique and long-term results. *Atlas Hand Clin.* 2000;5:101-109.
14. Van Kooten EO, Coster E, Segers MJM, Ritt MJPF. Early proximal row carpectomy after severe carpal trauma. *Injury.* 2005;36:1226-1232.
15. Thomas AA, Rodriguez E, Segalman K. Kienböck's disease in an elderly patient treated with proximal row carpectomy. *J Hand Surg Am.* 2004;29:685-688.
16. Diao E, Andrews A, Beall M. Proximal row carpectomy. *Hand Clin.* 2005;2:553-559.
17. De Smet L, Robijns F, Degreef I. Outcome of proximal row carpectomy. *Scand J Plast Reconstr Surg Hand Surg.* 2006;40:302-306.
18. Linscheid RL, Dobyns JH, Beabout JW, Bryan RS. Traumatic instability of the wrist: diagnosis, classification, and pathomechanics. *J Bone Joint Surg Am.* 1972;54:1612-1632.
19. Burgess RC. The effect of rotatory subluxation of the scaphoid on radioscaphoid contact. *J Hand Surg Am.* 1987;12(pt 1):771-774.
20. Watson HK, Ballet FL. The SLAC wrist: scapholunate advanced collapse pattern of degenerative arthritis. *J Hand Surg Am.* 1984;9:358-365.
21. Vender MI, Watson HK, Wiener BD, Black DM. Degenerative change in symptomatic scaphoid nonunion. *J Hand Surg Am.* 1987;12:514-519.
22. Watson HK, Weinzweig J. Physical examination of the wrist. *Hand Clin.* 1997;13:17-34.
23. Calandruccio JH. Proximal row carpectomy. *J Am Soc Surg Hand.* 2001;2:112-122.
24. Tang P, Imbriglia J. Osteochondral resurfacing (OCRPRC) for capitate chondrosis in proximal row carpectomy. *J Hand Surg Am.* 2007;32:1134-1142.
25. Ferlic DC, Clayton ML, Mills MF. Proximal row carpectomy: review of rheumatoid and non-rheumatoid wrists. *J Hand Surg Am.* 1991;16:420-424.
26. Blankenhorn BD, Pfaeffle HJ, Tang P, et al. Carpal kinematics after proximal row carpectomy. *J Hand Surg Am.* 2007;32:37-46.
27. Nagelvoort R, Kon M, Schuurman A. Proximal row carpectomy: a worthwhile salvage procedure. *Scand J Plast Reconstr Surg Hand Surg.* 2002;36:289-299.
28. Lukas B, Herter F, Englert A, Backer K. Advanced carpal collapse: proximal row carpectomy or midcarpal arthrodesis? *Handchir Mikrochir Plast Chir.* 2003;35:304-309.
29. Streich N, Martini A, Daeke W. Proximal row carpectomy in carpal collapse. *Handchir Mikrochir Plast Chir.* 2003;35:299-303.
30. Trankle M, Sauerbier M, Blum K, et al. Proximal row carpectomy: a motion preserving procedure in the treatment of advanced carpal collapse. *Unfallchirurg.* 2003;106:1010-1015.
31. Jorgensen EC. Proximal row carpectomy: an end-result study of twenty-two cases. *J Bone Joint Surg Am.* 1969;51:1104-1111.
32. Neviaser RJ. Proximal row carpectomy for posttraumatic disorders of the carpus. *J Hand Surg Am.* 1983;8:301-305.
33. Green DP. Proximal row carpectomy. *Hand Clin.* 1987;3:163-168.
34. Imbriglia JE, Broudy AS, Hagberg WC, McKernan D. Proximal row carpectomy: clinical evaluation. *J Hand Surg Am.* 1990;15:426-430.
35. Tomaino MM, Miller RJ, Cole I, Burton RI. Scapholunate advanced collapse wrist: proximal row carpectomy or limited wrist arthrodesis with scaphoid excision? *J Hand Surg Am.* 1994;19:134-142.
36. Krakauer JD, Bishop AT, Cooney WP. Surgical treatment of scapholunate advanced collapse. *J Hand Surg Am.* 1994;19:751-759.

37. Crabbe WA. Excision of the proximal row of the carpus. *J Bone Joint Surg Br*. 1964;46:708-711.
38. Inglis AE, Jones EC. Proximal-row carpectomy for diseases of the proximal row. *J Bone Joint Surg Am*. 1977; 59:460-463.
39. Neviaser RJ. On resection of the proximal carpal row. *Clin Orthop*. 1986;(202):12-15.
40. Begley BW, Engber WD. Proximal row carpectomy in advanced Kienböck's disease. *J Hand Surg Am*. 1994;19:1016-1018.
41. Culp RW, Osterman AL, Talsania JS. Arthroscopic proximal row carpectomy. *Tech Hand Up Extrem Soc*. 1997;2:116-119.
42. Gupta R, Bozentka DJ, Osterman AL. Wrist arthroscopy: principles and clinical applications. *J Am Acad Orthop Surg*. 2001;9:200-209.
43. Nagle DJ. Laser-assisted wrist arthroscopy. *Hand Clin*. 1999;15:495-499.
44. Atik TL, Baratz ME. The role of arthroscopy in wrist arthritis. *Hand Clin*. 1999;15:489-494.

CHAPTER

31

Trapeziometacarpal Arthritis

Julie E. Adams • Scott P. Steinmann

Trapeziometacarpal arthritis is a common condition seen in hand surgery practice. The typical patient is a middle-aged woman who describes the gradual onset of thumb basilar joint discomfort, pain with gripping or pinching, difficulty opening jars, and diminished strength. Treatment options depend on the symptoms, the radiographic stage, and the preferences of the surgeon and patient.

ANATOMY

The anatomy of the thumb basilar joint is complex. This biconcave-convex saddle-shaped joint has minimal bony constraints, permitting a wide arc of mobility and facilitating prehension. The ligamentous structures about the elbow promote stability, and the muscular forces about the thumb confer large forces on the thumb in pinch and grasp.[1] Basilar joint arthritis at the thumb is related to a variety of factors, including age and use, genetics, and hormonal effects. Bettinger and colleagues described the complex ligamentous structure about the trapeziometacarpal joint and 16 ligaments that stabilize the joint.[2] The important anterior oblique (beak) ligament is considered the primary stabilizer of the trapeziometacarpal joint.[3] Bettinger and coworkers described superficial and deep components of the beak ligament.[2] The superficial and deep anterior oblique ligament, the dorsoradial ligament, the posterior oblique ligament, the ulnar collateral ligament, the intermetacarpal ligament, and the dorsal intermetacarpal ligament stabilize the thumb carpometacarpal (CMC) joint; the other nine ligaments stabilize the trapezium.[2] The degree of anterior oblique ligament degeneration corresponded with the extent of arthritis[4] in a cadaveric study. Laxity of the beak ligament may alter the contact pressures and congruity of the joint, leading to joint subluxation and arthritic changes.[5]

PATIENT EVALUATION

History and Physical Examination

The history should include information regarding age, gender, and handedness. Attention should be paid to duration of symptoms, exacerbating and relieving factors, and the nature and location of discomfort. Occupations and avocations should be explored, particularly in relation to symptoms. The patient's prior treatments and response to these should be explored.

Examination may elicit the shoulder sign, in which the CMC joint is subluxated and the metacarpus adducted. The CMC grind test is performed by axial loading and circumduction of the metacarpal on the trapezium. Concomitant or alternative diagnoses should be ruled out; patients may have carpal tunnel syndrome (estimated to coexist in 43% of cases), deQuervain's tendonitis, or hypermobility of the CMC joint.[3,6] The status of the scaphotrapeziotrapeziod (STT) joint and arthritis in this joint should be assessed. Range of motion at the wrist and thumb should be documented, including thumb abduction and opposition (i.e., ability touch the base of the small finger) and metacarpophalangeal (MCP) motion. The MCP joint must be examined in hyperextension, which exacerbates metacarpal adduction. If MCP hyperextension is not addressed during ligament reconstruction, the stresses on the reconstruction may lead to failure. If hyperextension is greater than 30 degrees, the MCP joint should be treated with fusion, capsulodesis, or sesmoidectomy.[7] If hyperextension is less than 30 degrees, the surgeon can consider pinning the MCP joint with a Kirschner wire for 4 to 6 weeks.

Diagnostic Imaging

Radiographs that should be obtained include posteroanterior, lateral, and Bett's views. From plain film radiographs, the extent of disease may be staged according to the system described by

Eaton.[8] However, it is important to consider the patient's radiographic stage and symptoms together. Radiographs often demonstrate severe arthritis in a patient with only minimal symptoms; conversely, some patients have minimal changes on radiographs but are quite symptomatic.

TREATMENT

Indications and Contraindications

Painful first CMC joint arthritis that interferes with activities and has failed nonoperative management is an indication for surgery. Contraindications include active infection.

TREATMENT

Many patients respond to a nonoperative approach. Consideration should be given to activity modification, thumb spica splinting, use of nonsteroidal anti-inflammatory medications, and intra-articular corticosteroid injections. These forms of management are often most helpful in the early stages of the disease.

Eaton divided thumb CMC joint arthritis into stages, which are useful for deciding on treatment options.[8] The stage I joint is essentially radiographically normal but may have slight widening caused by synovitis or effusion. It may be treated by conservative means, such as nonsteroidal anti-inflammatory drugs and immobilization, but some authorities advocate ligament reconstruction, arthroscopy, or metacarpal osteotomy for stage I disease. Stage II disease is characterized by further joint space narrowing, changes with osteophyte formation (<2 mm), and mild to moderate joint subluxation. Stage III disease is characterized by moderate joint subluxation and prominent osteophyte formation (>2 mm), and stage IV is pantrapezial arthritis. Stages II through IV may be treated by arthroscopic or by open partial or complete trapeziectomy, with or without ligament reconstruction and interposition, fusion, or arthroplasty.

Patients with Eaton stage I, II, or III disease may be candidates for arthroscopy to determine the true extent of joint changes. In the early stages, in which the articular cartilage is intact but synovitic changes or ligamentous laxity is present, the pathology may be addressed by débridement and capsular shrinkage of the ligaments. Patients with more apparent changes, such as attenuation of the anterior oblique ligament and partial volar cartilage loss, may be candidates for extension osteotomy or arthroscopic débridement and interposition arthroplasty, whereas those with widespread cartilage loss may do best with arthroscopic débridement and interposition arthroplasty or conversion to an open procedure.[9,10]

Arthroscopic Technique

The technique for arthroscopy of the CMC joint has previously been described.[11,12] The thumb is suspended in traction (Fig. 31-1), and surface landmarks are marked (Fig. 31-2). The joint is penetrated with a needle; fluoroscopy can help to confirm correct entry into the trapeziometacarpal joint rather than the STT joint. After the needle position is confirmed, the joint is insufflated with saline.

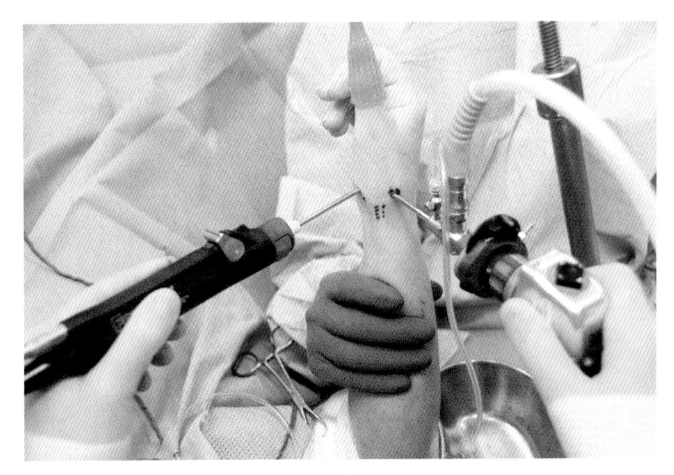

FIGURE 31-1 Arthroscopic setup.

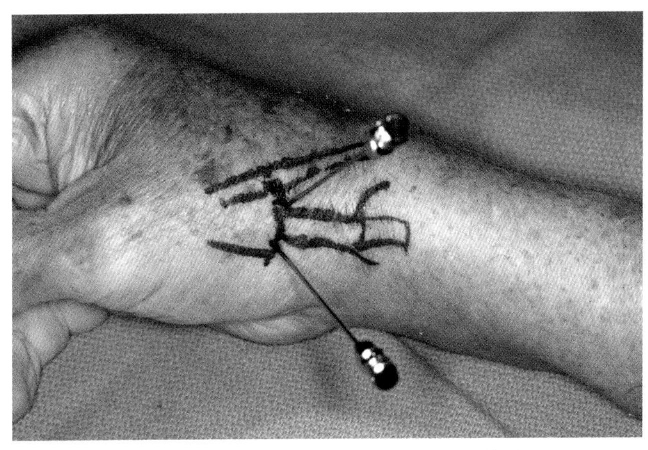

FIGURE 31-2 Surface landmarks are marked.

The 1-R (radial) and the 1-U (ulnar) portals are used (Fig. 31-3). The 1-R portal is made between the abductor pollicis longus and flexor carpi radialis tendons at the CMC joint level. The 1-R portal is useful to examine the dorsal radial, palmar oblique, and ulnar collateral ligaments, and it provides a view of the radial aspect of the joint. It also allows visualization of the intermetacarpal ligament and the distal insertions of the anterior oblique ligament into the first metacarpal (Fig. 31-4).

The 1-U portal is placed just ulnar to the extensor pollicis brevis tendon. This area can have a higher incidence of superficial radial nerve branches crossing the portal site than the 1-R portal area does. The radial artery is only a few millimeters from the ulnar side of the portal. Similar to the procedure used when establishing the 1-R portal, the skin should be carefully incised, and a small hemostat should be used to gently dissect and spread down to the capsular tissue. This helps to avoid traumatic injury to branches of the superficial radial nerve or the radial artery. The 1-U portal tends to enter the joint through the dorsal radial ligament or between the dorsal radial ligament and the palmar oblique ligament, and this portal allows visualization of the anterior oblique and ulnar collateral ligaments (Fig. 31-5). It may also be used as the main working portal for interventions after diagnostic arthroscopy.[11]

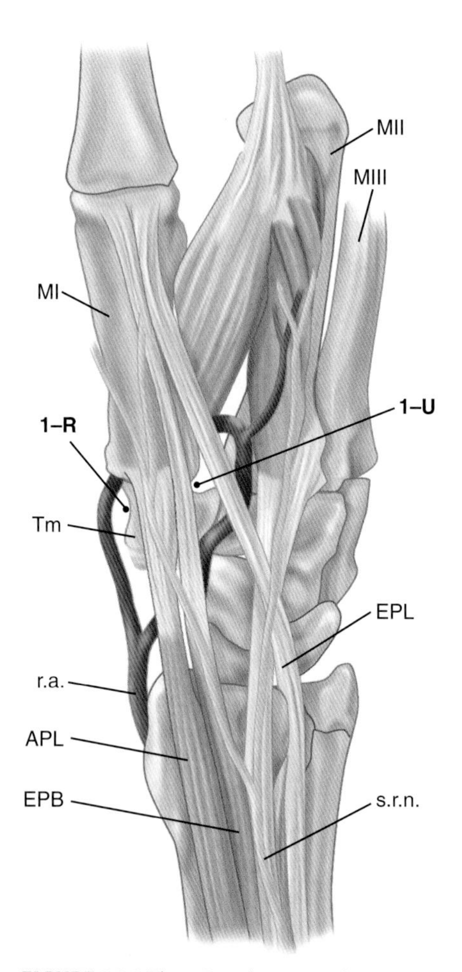

FIGURE 31-3 The 1-R and 1-U portals are used.

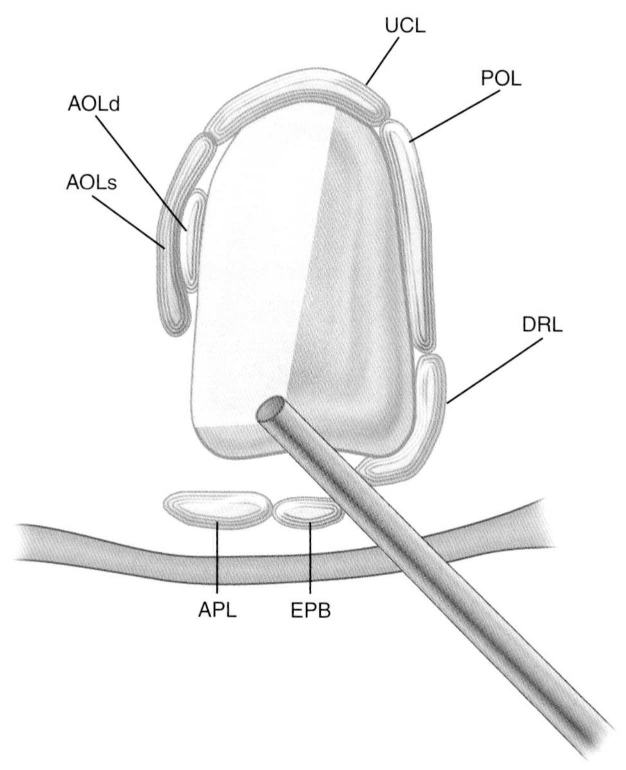

FIGURE 31-5 View from the 1-U portal.

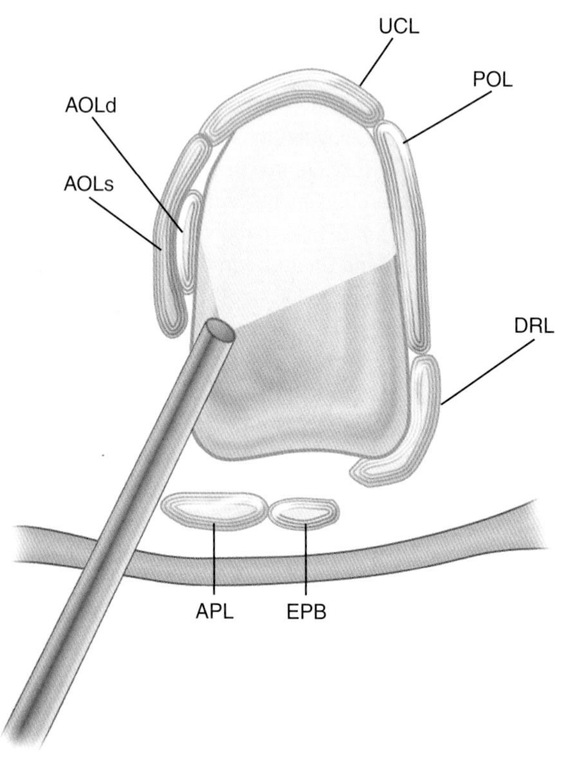

FIGURE 31-4 View from the 1-R portal.

A standard, 2.7-mm wrist arthroscope is used to visualize the CMC joint. The camera and working portal may be switched between the 1-R and 1-U portals as the arthroscopic procedure progresses. After diagnostic arthroscopy, the radiofrequency ablation probe is helpful to débride the joint of soft tissue. Radiofrequency ablation is useful for capsular shrinkage if laxity is present. A 3.5-mm joint shaver may be used to further débride the joint. Visualization is improved by the use of a standard arthroscopic mechanical pump to continuously irrigate the joint with saline. A dedicated outflow cannula is not needed if both working portals are large enough to allow egress of fluid.

If bony work after synovectomy or soft tissue débridement is indicated, a 2.7- or 3.5-mm burr may be used to remove the distal trapezium. Care is taken to remove bony osteophytes from the volar ulnar edge of the joint near the second metacarpal. After initial bony work is done, the arthroscope may be removed and the burring continued under fluoroscopy to ensure adequate removal of bone.

After the bony work has been completed, the interposition material is placed. Some surgeons have used autograft tissue, such as one half of the flexor carpi radialis tendon or the palmaris longus.[12,13] Xenograft, allograft, or manufactured materials may be cut to match the articular surface area of the joint. Several commercial materials have been advocated for this purpose.[14-17] The interposition material is placed into the joint with a small, curved hemostat through a portal.

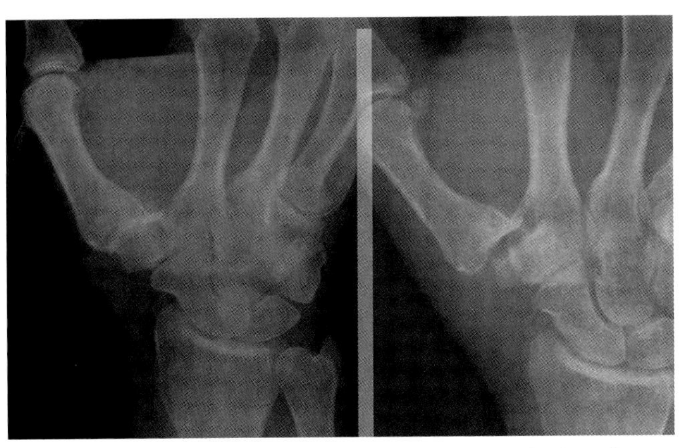

FIGURE 31-6 Preoperative and postoperative radiographs show first carpometacarpal joint arthroscopic débridement and interposition arthroplasty.

PEARLS & PITFALLS

PEARLS

- Traction is applied on the thumb by means of an arthroscopy tower.
- Standard arthroscopic equipment is needed, including a 2.7-mm wrist arthroscope, a 2.7- or 3.5-mm shaver and burr, and a radiofrequency ablator.
- The 1-R (radial) and 1-U (ulnar) portals are used.
- The 1-R portal is located between the abductor pollicis longus and flexor carpi radialis tendons.
- The 1-U portal is located just ulnar to the extensor pollicis brevis.
- Either portal may be started first, and each may be used as a working portal.
- The distal 3 to 4 mm of trapezium is removed, and interposition material is placed.
- The patient is immobilized for a total of 6 weeks in a forearm-based thumb spica splint or cast.

PITFALLS

- When portals are made, care should be taken to avoid injury to branches of the superficial radial nerve and the radial artery by incising through the skin only and then bluntly dissecting to the capsule with a hemostat.
- It is easy to inadvertently enter the CMC joint rather than the STT joint. Fluoroscopy can help to confirm the correct site.
- Care is taken to ensure removal of bony osteophytes from the ulnar aspect of the joint near the second metacarpal.

Postoperative Rehabilitation

The portals are closed, and a thumb spica splint is applied. Radiographs are obtained (Fig. 31-6) and may be compared with subsequent x-ray films in the clinic. Immobilization is continued for a total of 6 weeks.

CONCLUSIONS

Although limited data are available regarding outcomes after arthroscopic first CMC joint procedures, existing series document results similar to those for ligament reconstruction or ligament reconstruction and tendon interposition.[9,10,12,14,17]

REFERENCES

1. Cooney WP 3rd, Chao EY. Biomechanical analysis of static forces in the thumb during hand function. *J Bone Joint Surg Am*. 1977;59:27-36.
2. Bettinger PC, Linscheid RL, Berger RA, et al. An anatomic study of the stabilizing ligaments of the trapezium and trapeziometacarpal joint. *J Hand Surg Am*. 1999;24:786-798.
3. Eaton RG, Littler JW. Ligament reconstruction for the painful thumb carpometacarpal joint. *J Bone Joint Surg Am*. 1973;55:1655-1666.
4. Doerschuk SH, Hicks DG, Chinchilli VM, Pellegrini VD Jr. Histopathology of the palmar beak ligament in trapeziometacarpal osteoarthritis. *J Hand Surg Am*. 1999;24:496-504.
5. Pellegrini VD Jr. Osteoarthritis of the trapeziometacarpal joint: the pathophysiology of articular cartilage degeneration. I. Anatomy and pathology of the aging joint. *J Hand Surg Am*. 1991;16:967-974.
6. Florack TM, Miller RJ, Pellegrini VD, et al. The prevalence of carpal tunnel syndrome in patients with basal joint arthritis of the thumb. *J Hand Surg Am*. 1992;17:624-630.
7. Lourie GM. The role and implementation of metacarpophalangeal joint fusion and capsulodesis: indications and treatment alternatives. *Hand Clin*. 2001;17:255-260.
8. Eaton RG, Glickel SZ, Littler JW. Tendon interposition arthroplasty for degenerative arthritis of the trapeziometacarpal joint of the thumb. *J Hand Surg Am*. 1985;10:645-654.
9. Badia A. Trapeziometacarpal arthroscopy: a classification and treatment algorithm. *Hand Clin*. 2006;22:153-163.
10. Badia A, Khanchandani P. Treatment of early basal joint arthritis using a combined arthroscopic débridement and metacarpal osteotomy. *Tech Hand Up Extrem Surg*. 2007;11:168-173.
11. Berger RA. A technique for arthroscopic evaluation of the first carpometacarpal joint. *J Hand Surg Am*. 1997;22:1077-1080.
12. Menon J. Arthroscopic management of trapeziometacarpal joint arthritis of the thumb. *Arthroscopy*. 1996;12:581-587.
13. Menon J. Arthroscopic evaluation of the first carpometacarpal joint [comment]. *J Hand Surg Am*. 1998;23:757.
14. Adams JE, Merten SM, Steinmann SP. Arthroscopic interposition arthroplasty of the first carpometacarpal joint. *J Hand Surg Eur* 2007;32:268-274.
15. Adams JE, Steinmann SP. Interposition arthroplasty using an acellular dermal matrix scaffold. *Acta Orthop Belg*. 2007;73:319-326.
16. Adams JE, Steinmann SP, Culp RW. Trapezium-sparing options for thumb carpometacarpal joint arthritis. *Am J Orthop*. 2008;37(suppl 1):8-11.
17. Culp RW, Rekant MS. The role of arthroscopy in evaluating and treating trapeziometacarpal disease. *Hand Clin*. 2001;17:315-319.

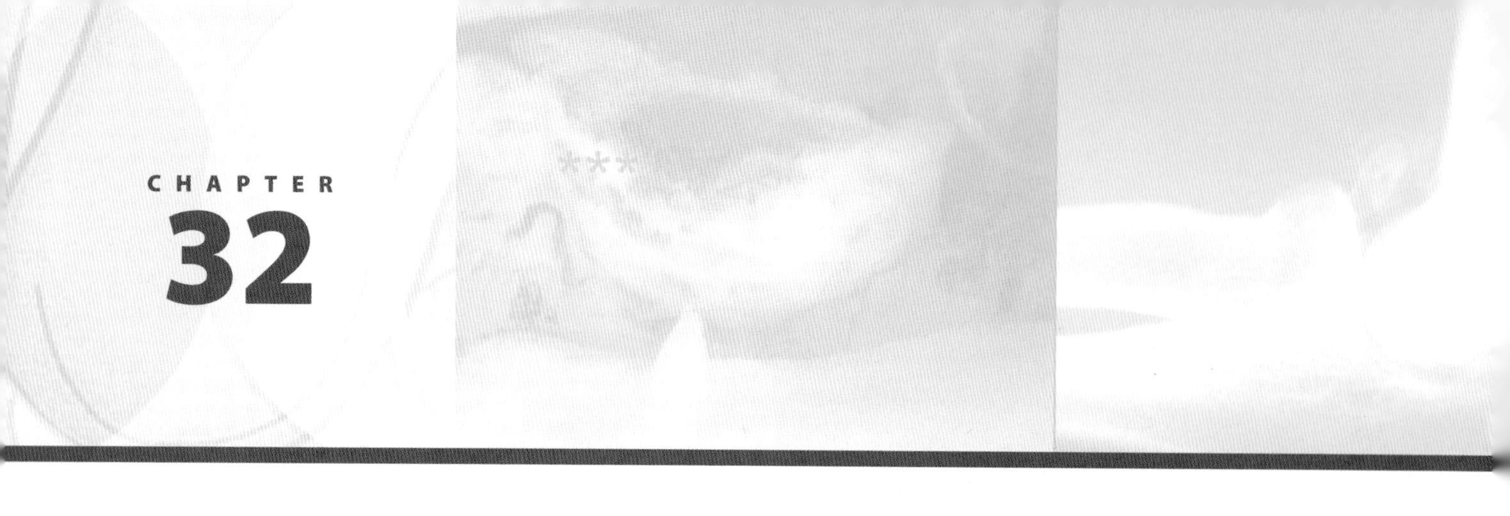

CHAPTER

32

Degenerative Disease of the Metacarpophalangeal and Proximal Interphalangeal Joints

Alejandro Badia

Developments in the early 1970s enabled use of the arthroscope to resolve small joint problems, similar to its application in treating large joint pathology. Despite the availability of this technology for almost 30 years, arthroscopy remains underused for treating small joints. Limited scientific literature regarding techniques and outcomes, poor delineation of the indications, and lack of reports on its benefits have hindered the acceptance and exploitation of small joint arthroscopy.

The concept of small joint arthroscopy was first delineated by Young Chang Chen, who presented a broad treatise on arthroscopy of the wrist and finger joints at a symposium that was later published in the July 1979 issue of *Orthopedic Clinics of North America*.[1] Chen described cadaver arthroscopic anatomy and clinical cases involving the wrist, metacarpophalangeal (MCP) joints, and proximal interphalangeal (PIP) joints of the hand. The thumb trapeziometacarpal joint was not addressed. However, the smaller joint arthroscopy was described using a no. 24 Watanabe arthroscope, which was the precursor of the modern small joint arthroscope and micro-arthroscope.

The first clinical report of MCP joint arthroscopy was not published until 1985, when Vaupel and Andrews described diagnostic and operative arthroscopy of the thumb MCP joint in a professional golfer who had experienced 1 year of pain, swelling, and stiffness in his nondominant thumb.[2] The technique was briefly described, and the clinical indications and results were outlined as a case report.

Arthroscopy of the proximal PIP joint had been mentioned in a cursory fashion in many case reports, beginning as early as 1997 by Richard Berger, but it was not clearly outlined until 2002, when Thomsen and colleagues described the clinical indications and arthroscopic portals in "Arthroscopy of the Proximal Interphalangeal Joints of the Finger," published in the *British Journal of Hand Surgery*.[3] MCP joint and PIP joint arthroscopic techniques have remained little explored by the hand surgery community, and they are virtually unknown among general orthopedic surgeons.

ANATOMY

The MCP and PIP joints are condylar hinge joints with relatively straightforward anatomy. The joint is essentially a box, with the floor represented as the less pliable volar plate and the roof as the thin dorsal capsule covered by the extensor mechanism. On either side are the collateral ligaments, which run in a dorsal to ventral oblique direction and insert distally. The MCP joint, particularly in the thumb, has a better-defined accessory collateral ligament that is located ventrally. The arthroscopic anatomy is less well defined, because the volar plate is covered with capsule and synovium, and the undersurface of the extensor mechanism also cannot be clearly visualized. The collateral ligaments are seen as fibers that pass in the oblique direction. The lateral and medial recesses are seen as deep valleys sitting below the origin of the collateral ligaments. This arthroscopic anatomy is less succinct when significant synovitis is present.

Arthroscopy may be more advantageous within the small joints than the larger joints, because open management is inherently difficult without destabilizing the joint itself. Arthroscopic management of degenerative joint disease in the MCP and PIP joints represents a logical extension of arthroscopic technique.

Degenerative joint disease can be divided into post-traumatic disease, osteoarthritis, and inflammatory arthropathy, such as rheumatoid arthritis. In the MCP and PIP joints, the post-traumatic variant is most common, because these joints are frequently injured. However, rheumatoid arthritis also is a common indication, particularly in the MCP joint, which is a hallmark of rheumatoid disease in the hand. In 2002, Sisato Sekiya of Nagoya Medical School in Japan evaluated arthroscopic rheumatoid synovectomy in the PIP and MCP joints in *Arthroscopy: The Journal of Arthroscopic and Related Surgery*,[4] but a review of degenerative joint disease in the MCP and PIP joints is lacking. This chapter outlines the indications and the operative technique for arthroscopy of these critical joints, addressing acute and chronic pathology.

METACARPOPHALANGEAL JOINT ARTHROSCOPY

Background

Primary indications for MCP arthroscopy include chronic pain, which likely suggests degenerative joint disease of these small joints, and treatment of acute fractures or ligamentous lesions. Although acute indications may be more common for certain joints, such as the frequently injured thumb MCP joint, the chronic degenerative conditions are ideally suited for arthroscopic management, particularly because there are few other treatment options. Implant joint arthroplasty can be considered only in advanced disease and for low-demand patients.

Chen was the first to formally describe the arthroscopic anatomy of the MCP joint[1]; in several case reports, he described the arthroscopic findings and their clinical relevance. He performed 90 arthroscopies in multiple joints encompassing 34 clinical cases and in two amputated arms from November 1973 to August 1978. In 1984, Vaupel and Andrews described a case at the annual meeting of the American Orthopaedic Society for Sports Medicine.[2] A professional golfer presented with a 1-year history of chronic painful synovitis within the thumb MCP joint. Six months after arthroscopic synovectomy and débridement of a small chondral defect, the patient was able to return to his sport and was essentially pain free at a follow-up examination after almost 2-years.. These results were published in the *American Journal of Sports Medicine*, but hand surgeons were not affected by this novel technique.

In 1987, L.L. Wilkes, an orthopedic surgeon, presented the first series of rheumatoid pathology treated by arthroscopic means in the MCP joint.[5] Arthroscopic rheumatoid synovectomy was performed on 13 joints in five patients with chronic rheumatoid arthritis. The patients lacked significant joint deformity, or even ulnar drift, but they did have significant synovitis within the recesses of the collateral ligament origins. Close clinical follow-up for 4 years demonstrated recurrence of pain and suggested that this technique altered progression of disease at the rheumatoid MCP joint only minimally. However, the transient pain relief and minimally invasive nature of the procedure led the investigator to conclude that it was a worthwhile procedure warranting further refinement. This innovative paper was published in the *Journal of the Medical Association of Georgia* but still did not influence the field of hand surgery.

This technique reached a broad audience of hand surgeons in 1994 through publication of a case report in the *Journal of Hand Surgery* (British edition).[6] The patient was a young man who presented with swelling and recurrent locking of the MCP joints of the index and middle fingers bilaterally. This is a typical presentation for hemochromatosis, a rarely seen hematologic condition that is treated with phlebotomy and for which the joint manifestations are poorly understood. Until that time, the treatment of arthropathy was osteotomy, arthroplasty, and occasionally joint arthrodesis. Arthroscopy was an excellent alternative to open surgery, with better visualization of the joint, facilitating treatment of the synovitis, and more rapid recovery aided by its minimally invasive nature. The emphasis of the case report was on the condition itself, and no further recommendations were given beyond the suggestion that arthroscopic surgery was "of value." Probably because the arthroscopic treatment was overshadowed by the unusual pathology being treated, the common clinical application of this technology was still not clear.

In 1995, Ryu and Fagan presented their series on treatment of the ulnar collateral ligament Stener lesion, which offered a common clinical application for this new technology.[7] Their retrospective series study described arthroscopic reduction of Stener lesions in eight thumbs, with an average follow-up period of slightly more than 3 years. The technique involved reduction of the Stener lesion into the joint so that the avulsed ligament was juxtaposed to its insertion site on the base of the proximal phalanx. Previously, the ligament had been sitting outside the adductor aponeurosis and could not heal in appropriate position. After the reduction, the ligament ends were débrided and the joint pinned for stability. On removal of the cast, a brief course of therapy was introduced, and at follow-up no patient reported any pain or functional limitation. Range of motion was excellent, and strength parameters were equal to or greater than those of the thumb on the unaffected side. The only complication was a pin tract infection. These results indicated that an arthroscopic reduction of a Stener lesion could obviate the need for open repair with its inherent complications, such as prolonged recovery, stiffness, and dysesthetic scar. This series represented the first broad clinical indication for arthroscopic management of a small joint lesion. However, there was no mention of bony gamekeeper's lesions and no comparative analysis with the open technique.

The primary benefit of this article was that it was published in a widely read journal and introduced the concept of small joint arthroscopic surgery to the broader hand surgery community. Although the paper was published a decade ago, the technique remains at the periphery, and few clinical series have been published since then.

In April of 1999, Rozmaryn and Wei presented the first paper on the practical aspects of MCP arthroscopy, with amplification of the possible indications and advantages of this still new technique.[8] This was not a clinical series discussing outcomes; rather they addressed the sentiment that the MCP joint is too small for arthroscopic procedures and provided a summary of the broad indications that could be treated with this procedure. They specifically mentioned joint synovectomies, débridement, and biopsies and supported the possibility of collateral ligament débridement and true ligament repair. They also reviewed removal of loose bodies, treatment of osteochondral lesions, management of periarticular lesions, and treatment of articular fractures. Although their article reviewed technical aspects and further delineated anatomic landmarks not discussed since Chen's description 20 years earlier, it had little influence on field of hand surgery. They predicted, however, that the advantages of arthroscopic techniques and the indications would evolve over time.

Later in 1999, Slade and Gutow published a review paper, "Arthroscopy of the Metacarpophalangeal Joint," in *Hand Clinics*.[9] For the first time, a description of the technique was presented, including the surgical procedure, indications, and some typical cases. The investigators touched on complications and their management. They emphasized that small joint arthroscopy required small but resilient instrumentation and good knowledge of the anatomy of these joints. Their experience revealed broad indications for this methodology, although the treatment of degenerative joint disease was not discussed in any depth. Much more detailed surgical techniques were described, mainly regarding the management of intra-articular fractures, with supporting case studies. A challenging and innovative technique was described in which arthroscopy was combined with the application of small bone anchors for reattachment of injured collateral ligaments.

Slade and Gutlow[9] pointed to the advantages of arthroscopy (e.g., rheumatoid synovectomy), as communicated by Patrick Ansah in Heidelberg. Ansah had begun comparing arthroscopic synovectomies and open procedures in joints of rheumatoid patients. In all of his cases, the surgeon and patient were impressed by the diminished postoperative swelling and improved rehabilitation with earlier return to activity provided by arthroscopic treatment. This unpublished series is an early illustration of the benefits of arthroscopic management of small joint degenerative disease. Coincidentally, a rheumatology paper published that same year discussed the use of mini-arthroscopy in MCP joints to stage the inflammatory arthropathy and to assist as a biopsy tool. This paper emphasized its clinical utility in the assessment of synovitis in rheumatoid patients but offered little discussion of the operative technique.[10] The investigators commented that micro-arthroscopy provided the rheumatologist an objective technique for joint evaluation and visual guidance of synovial biopsy with increased accuracy and decreased risk of sampling errors. General anesthesia was not necessary, and the procedure could be done on an outpatient basis.

In 1999, Wei and associates presented a series of 21 arthroscopic synovectomies in patient with recalcitrant rheumatoid arthritis.[11] Although this was predominantly an article describing the technique, the investigators reported that all patients had good short-term and commented that investigation of the utility of this procedure in other types of arthritis and other orthopedic conditions was warranted. They questioned the long-term effect of this procedure on joint preservation and the optimal timing for the operation in rheumatoid patients. We hope that increased use of MCP joint arthroscopy may answer these and many other questions.

Focusing on inflammatory small joint arthropathy, Sekiya and colleagues expanded on previous descriptions by evaluating 21 patients with rheumatoid arthritis in 27 PIP joints and 16 MCP joints.[4] This was one of the earliest clinical descriptions of PIP joint arthroscopy, and it added further information about MCP joint arthroscopic surgery.[4] The study authors found arthroscopic assessment of the articular surface and synovial membrane to be an excellent application of this tool and thought that more accurate biopsies could be taken. They speculated that arthroscopy for the small joints in the hands "will become a standard procedure in the near future."[4] Their study did not assess other types of arthritides.

In 2006, Badia reviewed basal joint and MCP arthroscopy, focusing on the development and indications for these still little-used techniques.[12] Management of degenerative joint disease was discussed in a general fashion, with the conclusion that this is a useful indication, but long-term studies are necessary to determine its place in the hand surgeon's armamentarium.

Patient Evaluation

History and Physical Examination

Patients typically present with a history of persistent pain in the involved joints for a variable period with no response to conservative management (e.g., use of nonsteroidal anti-inflammatory drugs, one or more corticosteroid injections). The degree of swelling depends on chronicity, severity, and whether the arthropathy is an inflammatory arthritis, such as rheumatoid arthritis. The deformity usually is not severe, because arthroscopic treatment is more often used to treat inflammation and pain rather than mechanical deformity. Osteoarthritis manifests as thick joints with bony prominences caused by osteophytes, whereas rheumatoid arthritis typically manifests as boggy swelling on the dorsum of the joint and ligamentous laxity identified on examination.

Diagnostic Imaging

MCP arthritis usually can be seen on plain radiographs. However, early stages may be seen only at the time of arthroscopy, and later analysis of the radiographs may hint at joint widening or soft tissue shadowing due to severe synovitis. Imaging of more advanced osteoarthritis shows narrowing of the MCP joints and small, marginal osteophytes. Rheumatoid involvement of the MCP joints is seen as narrowing of the joint space on posteroanterior views, which is a result of palmar subluxation of the proximal phalanx relative to the metacarpal heads. More advanced disease is indicated by early ulnar drift and erosions of the origins of collateral ligaments. These advanced rheumatoid changes may prompt consideration of arthroplasty, such as silicone interposition arthroplasty, rather than arthroscopic treatment.

Treatment

Indications and Contraindications

Pathology of the MCP joint is relatively common. Although this discussion focuses on management of degenerative joint disease, acute trauma can involve any one of the MCP joints, with the thumb being the most commonly affected. Gamekeeper's or skier's thumb is a frequent injury seen in any hand surgeon's practice. Ryu described arthroscopic management of the classic Stener lesion, and Badia presented a series of bony gamekeeper's thumbs treated solely by arthroscopic means.[13] Acute trauma can also involve the finger MCPs, with ligamentous and articular fractures occasionally seen.

The overuse syndromes may reflect a previously unrecognized acute injury that was not addressed or may be a more chronic type of synovitis of unknown origin. Arthroscopy of the MCP joints can assist in diagnosing the condition and can provide treatment. For example, vague but chronic pain of the index finger MCP joint is often seen in laborers. Initial treatment often consists of corticosteroid injection, but relief is frequently short lived, and pain recurs. Arthroscopic synovectomy and débridement offer a more definitive solution. In this scenario, the surgeon may see a frayed and scarred radial collateral ligament covered by dense synovitis, which often masks the underlying pathology. The surgeon must perform the synovectomy by mechanical means or radiofrequency ablation and must treat the underlying pathology to minimize the chance of recurrent synovitis and pain. This usually involves resection of the redundant capsular and ligamentous tissue, followed by radiofrequency shrinkage to restore some integrity and tautness to the capsuloligamentous complex. Avoidance of thermal injury is key, and the surgeon must be well versed in the use of small joint radiofrequency therapy.

Idiopathic pain, occasionally associated with mild swelling, may be an indication for arthroscopic evaluation. This may occur as a result of unrecognized injury, early osteoarthritis, or idiopathic synovitis. Middle-aged women who present with this type of occult pain and a benign history may have a joint reaction to metabolic changes related to estrogen levels. Steroid injections can help but can lead to acceleration of cartilage and capsular degeneration. The problem is what to do after several injections have provided a short-lived clinical response or incomplete pain relief. Patients should understand that pain often worsens for 1 to 2 days after administration of the corticosteroid before improving. Arthroscopic débridement can avoid joint complications arising from recurrent steroid use and may retard the degenerative process due to synovial resection. Another benefit is that complications are negligible and the recovery rapid.

Early- stage osteoarthritis may not be seen on plain radiographs, and the diagnosis must be based on clinical characteristics. After adequate conservative treatment with nonsteroidal anti-inflammatory drugs or other therapy, the next level of treatment is an intra-articular corticosteroid injection. If symptoms recur despite several injections, arthroscopic débridement becomes the best option short of joint replacement. Open synovectomies are difficult because of poor visualization and limited access to all regions of the joint, and they can produce considerable postoperative stiffness. Although silicone arthroplasty remains the gold standard for treating advanced rheumatoid involvement of the MCP joints, post-traumatic arthrosis and osteoarthritis usually are generally not good indications for silicone implant arthroplasty. Newer metallic nonconstrained MCP joints are better indicated, but arthroscopic débridement is best suited to delay or obviate this procedure. Pyrocarbon implants have a more appropriate modulus of elasticity but are also unpredictable in the long term. Arthroscopy is a good alternative before resorting to these nonconstrained replacement options. The thumb MCP joint should always undergo arthrodesis (instead of arthroplasty) and should be considered for arthroscopic débridement before being declared refractory to treatment.

Inflammatory arthritides, such as rheumatoid arthritis, usually are managed with the newer disease-modifying agents, oral steroids, and in the late stages, replacement arthroplasty if corticosteroid injections are not helpful or ulnar drift becomes pronounced. Occasionally, a mono-articular or pauci-articular form is encountered, and an arthroscopic biopsy may assist in making the diagnosis. Early involvement of these joints may warrant an arthroscopic synovectomy and capsular shrinkage, which may retard the process of joint destruction in response to cytokines. Research must be directed to assessing how arthroscopic synovial resection can alter this destructive inflammatory cascade. Currently, this procedure is best suited for retarding the destructive process in one to two of the most involved joints. Initial results are promising,[4] but long-term results of this procedure have not been reported, and the basic science needs to be better understood.

MCP arthroscopy is contraindicated in cases where attempts at synovectomy would provide only very transient relief. Advanced changes require arthroplasty and patients must understand that arthroscopic débridement and synovectomy can only affect change when the joint anatomy is still relatively preserved. Conversely, early arthritis is optimal as there are little drawbacks due to the minimally invasive nature of the surgery.

Conservative Management

Conservative management of MCP arthrosis is more focal in osteoarthritis and systemic in nature with rheumatoid arthritis. Disease-modifying agents usually benefit the boggy synovitis seen in rheumatoid MCP joints. Persistent pain warrants a corticosteroid injection, and a repeat injection is indicated for patients with a suitable response for a sufficient period, such as 3 months. Repeat injections run the risk of accelerating the articular cartilage loss due to the catabolic nature of steroids.

Conservative therapy can improve or maintain the range of motion and strengthen surrounding muscle-tendon units to stabilize the joint and improve overall function. However, progressive and persistent arthritic symptoms often do not respond to conservative means, and arthroscopy offers a minimally invasive alternative that allows the clinician to recommend surgery much earlier in the course of treatment.

Arthroscopic Technique

A 1.9-mm arthroscope is essential to explore the MCP joint. The 30-degree scope commonly is used by maxillofacial surgeons for temporomandibular pathology. A 2.0-mm shaver typically is the main operative instrument, and small radiofrequency probes are used for ablation and shrinkage. A small joint grabber and a small basket forceps are needed for more aggressive débridement and loose body removal.

For small joint procedures, it is prudent to use local anesthesia and light sedation. Several milliliters of lidocaine are introduced into the joint after the hand is suspended using a single Chinese finger trap on the affected digit and 5 pounds of traction (Fig. 32-1). A

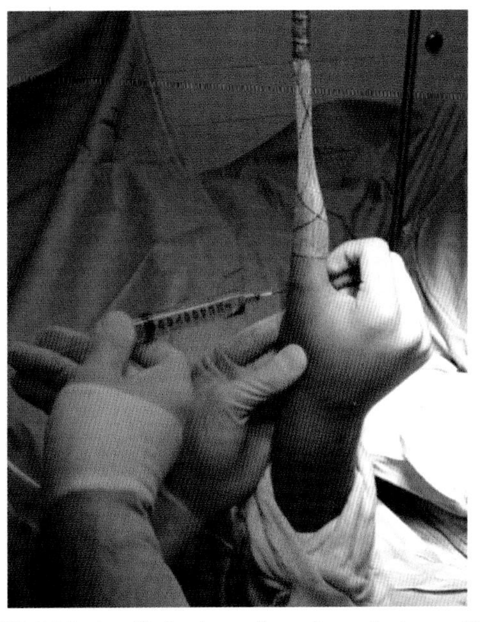

FIGURE 32-1 Joint insufflation is usually performed using an 18-gauge needle that is oriented superiorly to minimize chondral damage and facilitate joint distention.

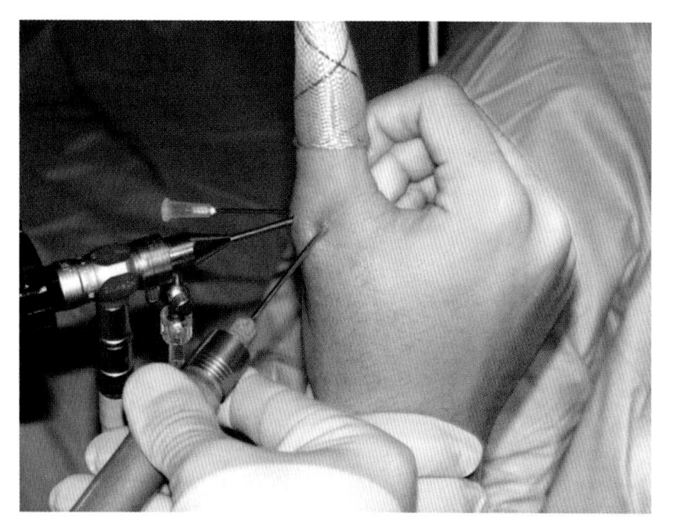

FIGURE 32-2 The arthroscope and 2.9-mm, full-radius shaver are in place, and standard portals are used on either side of the extensor mechanism. Occasionally, an 18-gauge needle is needed for outflow to improve visualization.

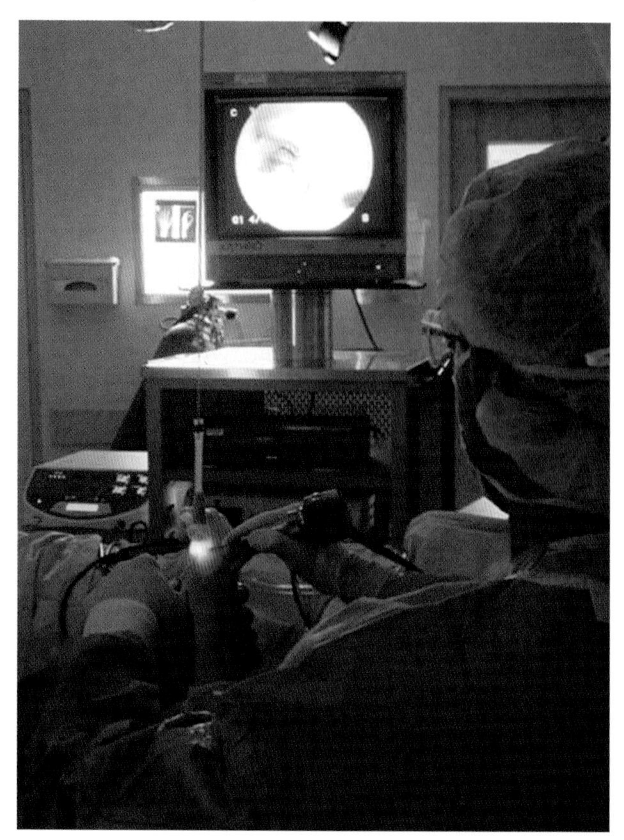

FIGURE 32-3 The arthroscopy setup shows the thumb in traction. The shoulder holder allows good visualization of the monitor in front and access to the joint from all directions without interference.

small piece of gauze is usually tied around junction of the finger trap and skin to minimize chance of slippage. A shoulder holder may be used so that 360-degree access is available for fluoroscopy to guide pinning, but a standard wrist traction tower can be used. Adequate sedation is then achieved to allow elevation of the tourniquet for the necessary period.

The trocar must be introduced into the joint in an atraumatic fashion. These joint spaces are tiny, and considerable iatrogenic injury to the articular cartilage can occur if care is not taken. Even with distraction, the space between metacarpal head and proximal phalanx base is very narrow. The appropriate level and insertion angle can be found by inserting a small, curved clamp after the joint is sufficiently distended with lidocaine or Ringer's solution. The arthroscopic cannula is then introduced at the same angle, and the joint is thoroughly inspected.

The portals lie on either side of the often-palpable extensor tendon, and the surgeon can feel the indentation just underneath the proximal phalanx base. Occasionally, a third portal is used for outflow, and it is placed by palpating the capsule, identifying the interval as seen on the monitor, and then passing an 18-gauge needle (Fig. 32-2).

A synovectomy is initially performed to allow good joint visualization and identification of pathology. This is done with the 2.0-mm, full-radius shaver, revealing the capsule and ligamentous structures (Fig. 32-3). A radiofrequency ablator probe expedites this process but must be used sparingly, because the thin joint capsule and skin can suffer thermal injury.

After synovectomy is performed, the surgeon looks for abnormal anatomy in a methodical fashion to avoid missing a lesion. The surgeon can begin with one collateral ligament and then assess the volar plate, sesamoid bones, contralateral ligament, dorsal capsule, and extensor mechanism. The articular surface of the proximal phalanx and metacarpal head is then assessed, including the lateral recesses where the collaterals originate. Degenerative changes in the articular cartilage are treated by mechanical resection of cartilage fibrillation, loose or unstable fragment excision, and radiofrequency annealing of the lesion edges to limit further flaking. Full-thickness cartilage loss can be managed by drilling the subchondral bone and encouraging the formation of fibrocartilage.

After the pathology is identified and appropriately addressed, the arthroscope is removed, and portals are closed with a skin adhesive such as Benzoin and Steri-Strips only. Suturing of portals will lead to scars that will be apparent on the dorsum of the hand or thumb. The thumb MCP is protected with a short arm thumb spica splint in extension, and the other digits usually require a dorsal MCP block splint in flexion. This arrangement allows the collateral ligaments to heal in their most taut, elongated position so that there is no resultant extension contracture. The period of immobilization is determined by the type and extent of pathology found during the arthroscopic procedure. Postoperative therapy is usually minimal and focuses on regaining range of motion and muscle strength (Figs. 4 to 6).

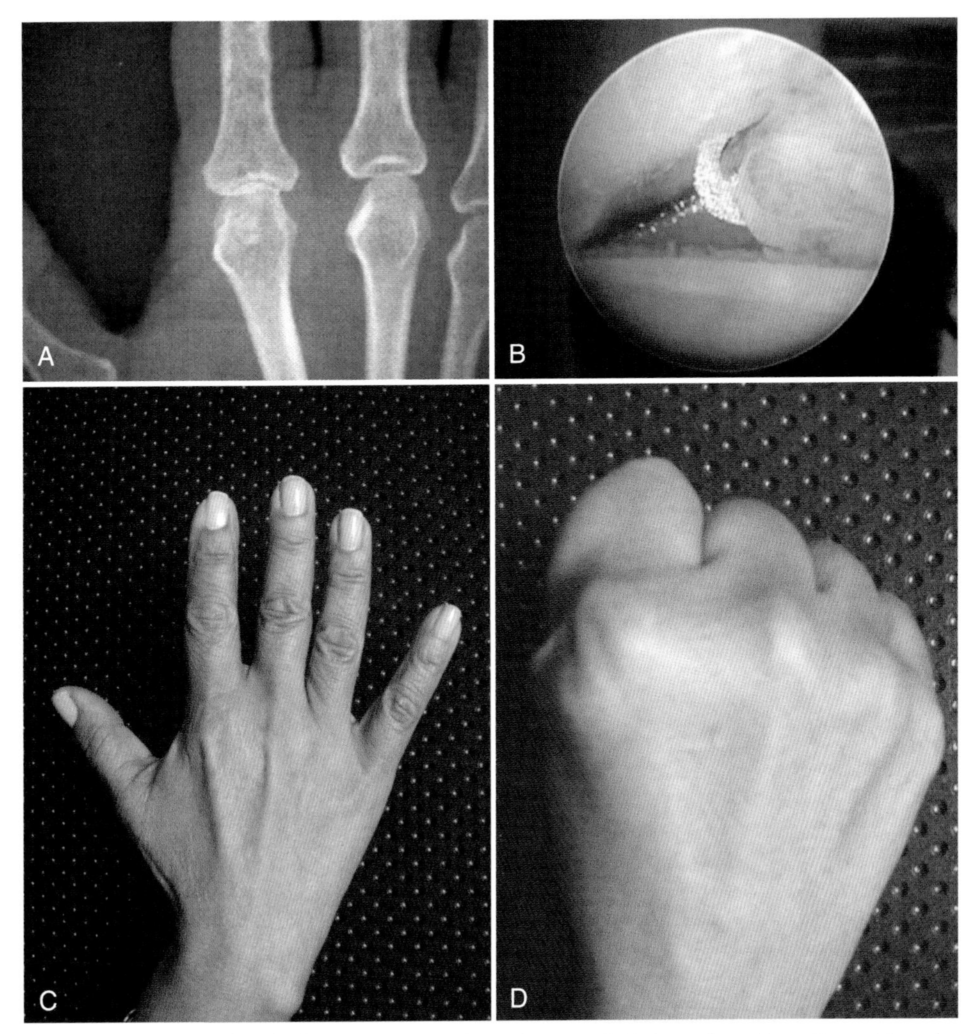

FIGURE 32-4 A–D, Isolated index metacarpophalangeal osteoarthritis is confirmed by radiographic and arthroscopic findings and by postoperative range-of-motion photographs. In many cases, portal scars are not visualized.

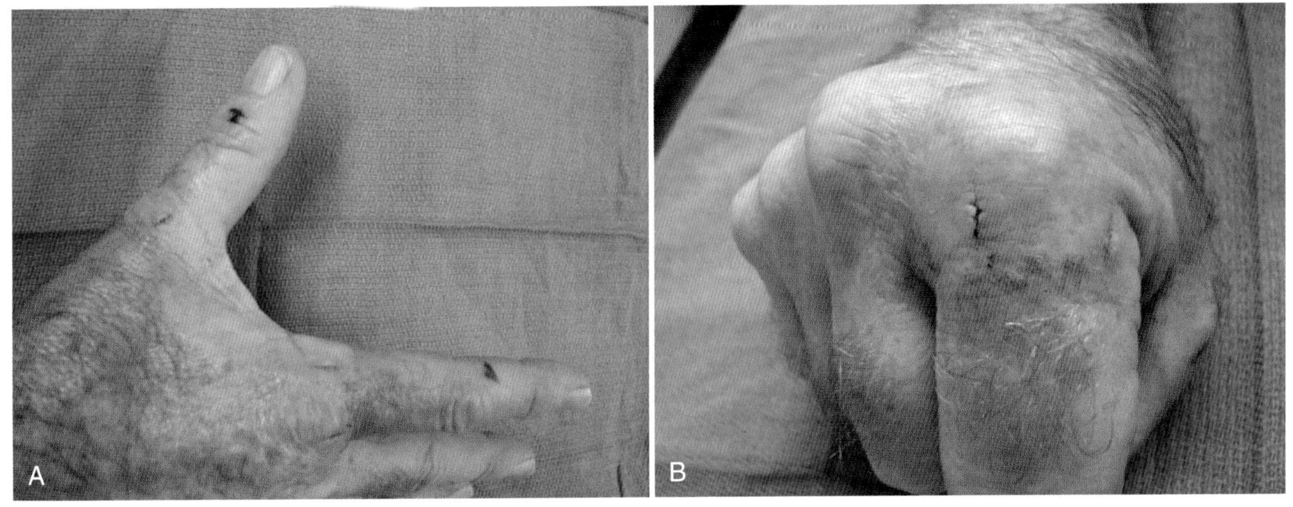

FIGURE 32-5 A and **B,** Postoperative photographs 2 days after thumb and index metacarpophalangeal débridements for osteoarthritis. Therapy began almost immediately, and the patient had excellent pain relief and range of motion at this early stage.

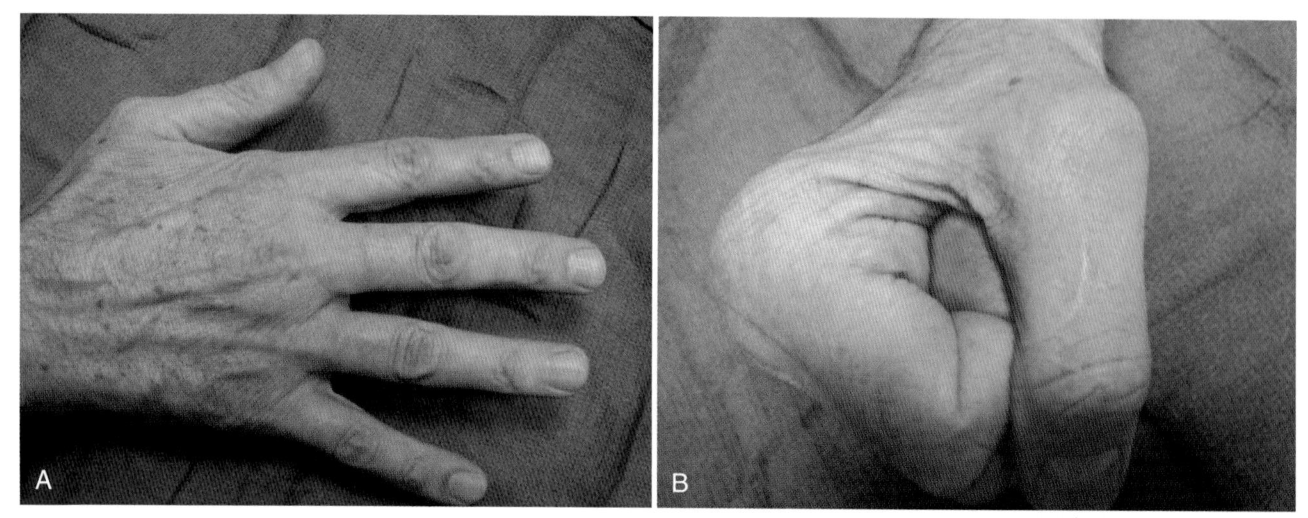

FIGURE 32-6 A and **B,** At the 7-year follow-up assessment after arthroscopic rheumatoid thumb and middle finger metacarpophalangeal synovectomy, there was no recurrence of synovitis, and the patient continues to have pain relief.

PROXIMAL INTERPHALANGEAL JOINT ARTHROSCOPY

Background

PIP joint arthroscopy is still considered an experimental procedure, and little has been written about it. However, Chen's landmark paper described one clinical case and eight cadaveric studies using small joint arthroscopy of the PIP joint.[1] The sole clinical case was use of the procedure in a patient with rheumatoid arthritis.

The only paper devoted solely to PIP joint arthroscopy was published by Thomsen and colleagues in a 2002 volume of the *Journal of Hand Surgery*.[3] They described their findings, including suggested portal placement, in eight cadaveric PIP joints and in two clinical cases. They concluded that the technique was possible, although technically demanding, and that indications for the procedure needed to be defined. They suggested that synovectomy, infection, and loose body removal would likely constitute the main indications. One of the case studies involved a patient with rheumatoid arthritis, and the other was a patient who required removal of a loose body with a synovectomy.

Sekiya and coworkers analyzed the use of MCP and PIP arthroscopy in 21 patients with rheumatoid arthritis.[4] Twenty-seven PIP joints and 16 MCP joints underwent rheumatoid synovectomy. The investigators concluded that it was a worthwhile procedure because biopsies could easily be performed and that synovectomies yielded clinical improvement. It was thought that small joint arthroscopy would become a standard procedure in the future, but the technique was limited by joint morphology and by the equipment available. The rigid nature and size of the arthroscope did not allow visualization of the palmar half of the middle phalanx base, and the condyles could be seen only by flexing the joint. Vertical traction was not used; instead, the finger was held horizontally while the arthroscope was introduced in the interval between central slip and lateral band. The study focused on rheumatoid disease, but the PIP joint is involved more often by osteoarthritis. A study assessing this more common pathology is needed.

Treatment

Indications and Contraindications

Indications are limited for PIP arthroscopy. The relatively large size and rigidity of the arthroscope is a limiting factor within this bicondylar joint.

The technique is limited to mostly dorsal synovectomy, predominantly in patients with rheumatoid arthritis or osteoarthritis. This procedure should be done with mechanical shaving, because the joint is directly subcutaneous, and radiofrequency could be risky at this level.

Joint lavage for infection can be considered, as can the rare loose or foreign body excision. Drilling of focal chondral lesions may warrant further exploration.

Arthroscopic Technique

The anatomic constrictions of the PIP joint require that arthroscopy be done horizontally and with free motion of the digit during the procedure to allow the surgeon to visualize different segments of the joint. Traction would not facilitate joint flexion.

Using a dorsal approach, the joint is insufflated with about 2 mL of lidocaine after adequate digital block anesthesia is achieved. The dorsal recesses are distended, allowing a 1.9- or 1.5-mm arthroscope to be inserted. The portals are on either side of the central slip, usually between that critical structure and the lateral bands. Sekiya and coworkers described a more lateral portal, passing through the transverse retinacular ligament and 1 to 2 mm dorsal to the midaxial line.[4] Regardless, the palmar aspect of the joint is not visualized adequately, and flexible micro-arthroscopes may allow passing over the condyles to gain better visualization. This challenging approach necessitates smaller shavers to enter the confined space. The current 2.0-mm shavers provide limited tissue resection because of the small level of suction that can be generated. PIP joint arthroscopy is technically in its infancy.

PEARLS & PITFALLS

- Arthroscopic procedures are indicated for joints with mild deformity that do not respond to conservative measures.
- A 1.9-mm arthroscope, small shavers, and a radiofrequency device are essential.
- Insufflation of the joint with fluid minimizes the possibility of iatrogenic injury during trocar or sheath insertion.
- Lateral recesses must be explored to detect additional synovitis and loose bodies.
- Longitudinal, small portal incisions are used to avoid dorsal sensory nerve injury.
- MCP joints are immobilized in flexion to minimize postoperative swelling and hemarthrosis and to maximize recovery of the range of motion.

Postoperative Rehabilitation

Rehabilitation usually begins in 2 to 7 days after small joint arthroscopy. The MCP joints are transiently protected by a block-type splint applied intraoperatively; it holds the MCP joints in flexion but allows the PIP joints to move freely. This hyperflexion position also limits postoperative joint swelling and hemarthrosis, because the dorsal recess of the joint is diminished. The collateral ligaments are under maximum tautness with the MCP flexion posture, and extension is easily recovered.

Inflammatory modalities are immediately initiated by the hand therapist, but portal care is minimal because stitches are not used. Portals are closed by a skin adhesive (e.g., Benzoin, Mastisol) and Steri-Strips. After the range of motion is recovered or maximized, strengthening is emphasized. Therapy is minimal compared with that for open arthroplasty, which is another advantage of this minimally invasive approach.

CONCLUSIONS

Arthroscopic synovectomy and débridement of degenerative joint disease constitute a useful technique for treating both the MCP and PIP joints. The small size of the joints encourages further exploration of this technique because open débridement is particularly difficult without destabilizing the joints. Arthroscopic synovectomy represents a more effective and long-lasting technique than a steroid injection, which has a limited half-life and does not prevent recurrence of the underlying problem.

Arthroscopy allows identification of the extent of degenerative disease and treatment with a combination of synovectomy, which removes the source of inflammatory cytokines, and débridement of unstable articular cartilage, which can minimize the underlying problem. Although osteoarthritis is most often seen in the PIP joint and rheumatoid arthritis is most commonly seen in MCP joints, post-traumatic arthritis is seen in both joints and may be the best indication for this technique, because the only other options are arthrodesis and joint replacement.

The efficacy of this technique should be established with prospective, randomized studies, perhaps comparing arthroscopic synovectomy and débridement with injection of corticosteroid. Long-term assessment also is needed to further refine the clinical indications and clarify the results.

REFERENCES

1. Chen YC. Arthroscopy of the wrist and finger joints. *Orthop Clin North Am*. 1979;10:723-733.
2. Vaupel GL, Andrews JR. Diagnostic and operative arthroscopy of the thumb metacarpophalangeal joint: a case report. *Am J Sports Med*. 1985;13:139-141.
3. Thomsen NO, Nielsen NS, Jørgensen U, Bojsen-Møller F. Arthroscopy of the proximal interphalangeal joints of the finger. *J Hand Surg Br*. 2002;27:253-255.
4. Sekiya I, Kobayashi M, Taneda Y, Matsui N. Arthroscopy of the proximal interphalangeal and metacarpophalangeal joints in rheumatoid hands. *Arthroscopy*. 2002;18:292-297.
5. Wilkes LL. Arthroscopic synovectomy in the rheumatoid metacarpophalangeal joint. *J Med Assoc Ga*. 1987;76:638-639.
6. Leclercq G, Schmitgen G, Verstreken J. Arthroscopic treatment of metacarpophalangeal arthropathy in haemochromatosis. *J Hand Surg Br*. 1994;19:212-214.
7. Ryu J, Fagan R. Arthroscopic treatment of acute complete thumb metacarpophalangeal ulnar collateral ligament tears. *J Hand Surg Am*. 1995;20:1037-1042.
8. Rozmaryn LM, Wei N. Metacarpophalangeal arthroscopy. *Arthroscopy*. 1999;15:333-337.
9. Slade JF 3rd, Gutow AP. Arthroscopy of the metacarpophalangeal joint. *Hand Clin*. 1999;15:501-527.
10. Ostendorf B, Dann P, Wedekind F, et al. Miniarthroscopy of metacarpophalangeal joints in rheumatoid arthritis. Rating of diagnostic value in synovitis staging and efficiency of synovial biopsy. *J Rheumatol*. 1999;26:1901-1908.
11. Wei N, Delauter SK, Erlichman MS, et al. Arthroscopic synovectomy of the metacarpophalangeal joint in refractory rheumatoid arthritis: a technique. *Arthroscopy*. 1999;15:265-268.
12. Badia A. Arthroscopy of the trapeziometacarpal and metacarpophalangeal joints. *Chir Main*. 2006;25(suppl 1):S259-S270.
13. Badia A. Arthroscopic reduction and internal fixation for bony gamekeeper's thumb. *Orthopedics*. 2006;29:675-678.

CHAPTER

33

Volar Carpal Ganglion Cysts

Jeffrey A. Greenberg

Use of the arthroscope for diagnosis and management of wrist disorders has evolved significantly since Roth first described the technique of wrist arthroscopy in 1988.[1] The development of sophisticated optical systems and instruments specific for small joint applications has enabled the experienced wrist arthroscopist to perform complex reconstructive procedures. Wrist arthroscopy facilitates visualization of intra-articular anatomy, whereas small, motorized shavers enable resection and elimination of intra-articular and capsular lesions.

In 1995, Osterman and Raphael presented a technique for the arthroscopic treatment of ganglion cysts arising from the dorsal portion of the scapholunate interosseous ligament and manifesting as dorsal space-occupying lesions.[2] The initial skepticism regarding treatment of this lesion has been quelled, and arthroscopic treatment of dorsal cysts has become routine for experienced arthroscopists. Although the anatomic origin of volar carpal ganglions has not been as well defined as for their dorsal counterparts and the location is not as consistent as for the dorsal ganglion, many of these cysts do have an intra-articular capsular origin.[3-5] Arthroscopic resection of volar ganglia is an effective technique with potential advantages when compared with traditional open techniques.

ANATOMY

Ganglion cysts are saclike structures that do not have a true cellular lining. They are benign soft tissue tumors that are most commonly found in the wrist but may occur adjacent to or originating from any joint. Approximately 10% of the time, they form from tendon sheaths. They are filled with a viscous fluid that contains glucosamine, albumin, globulin, and hyaluronic acid.[6] The origin of most ganglion cysts is idiopathic. Occasionally, a traumatic event precedes the development of a cyst, lending support to a possible traumatic origin of these lesions. Mathoulin's histologic analysis of ganglion cysts indicates that the base of the cyst arises in the histologic layer between the synovium and the joint capsule.[7] His group postulates that this area is exposed to stress that initiates histologic degenerative lesions, particularly mucoid degeneration. These masses are not inflammatory, and they do not arise as simple herniations from the joint capsule.[6,8] Other causative factors are capsular rents caused by preexisting joint pathology, synovial fluid leakage with secondary cyst formation, and mucoid degeneration or mucin secretion stimulated by joint stress or other degenerative processes. Occult volar ganglia may also contribute to volar wrist pain without a visible or palpable mass. Symptoms may be caused by capsular injury, inflammatory changes, or local pressure.

The anatomic origin of the volar ganglion cyst is not as well defined as that of its dorsal counterpart. The literature suggests a radioscaphoid, scaphotrapezial, or trapeziometacarpal (TM) joint origin.[9] Volar cysts may also arise from the flexor carpi radialis (FCR) tendon sheath or other aberrant locations. Aydin and colleagues studied open excision of volar ganglions and reported that 45% arose from the radiocarpal joint, 40% from the scaphotrapeziotrapezoid (STT) joint, and 5% from the FCR sheath.[10] Most arise from the radiocarpal joint, and when they do, they have a volar capsular origin from the relatively deficient area between the radioscaphocapitate (RSC) and long radiolunate (LRL) ligaments.[4,11] The ligaments represent the volar extrinsic components that work in conjunction with the intrinsic and extrinsic dorsal ligaments and with the interosseous ligaments to provide wrist stability. Starting radially and proceeding in an ulnar direction, they are the RSC, the LRL, and the short radiolunate (SRL) ligaments (Fig. 33-1). When they are visualized arthroscopically, distinct clefts can be seen between these ligaments. The volar ganglion cyst can be identified in the clefts between the extrinsic radiocarpal ligaments. Ho and associates, in their study on arthroscopic resection of volar carpal ganglia, observed that 75% of the cysts arose from the interval between the RSC and LRL, and 25% originated between the LRL and SRL.[3] The capsular origin can be visualized arthroscopically (Fig. 33-2).

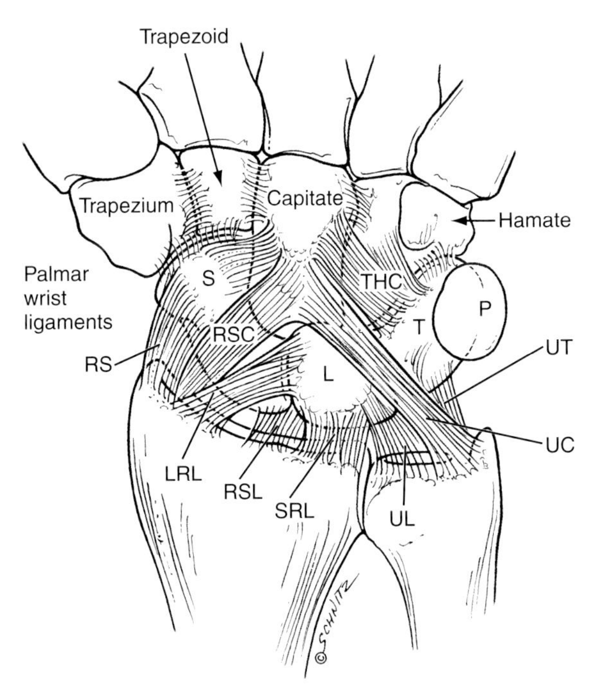

FIGURE 33-1 Artist's rendition of the volar extrinsic ligaments of the wrist. From radial to ulnar, the ligaments are the radioscaphocapitate (RSC), long radiolunate (LRL) and short radiolunate (SRL).

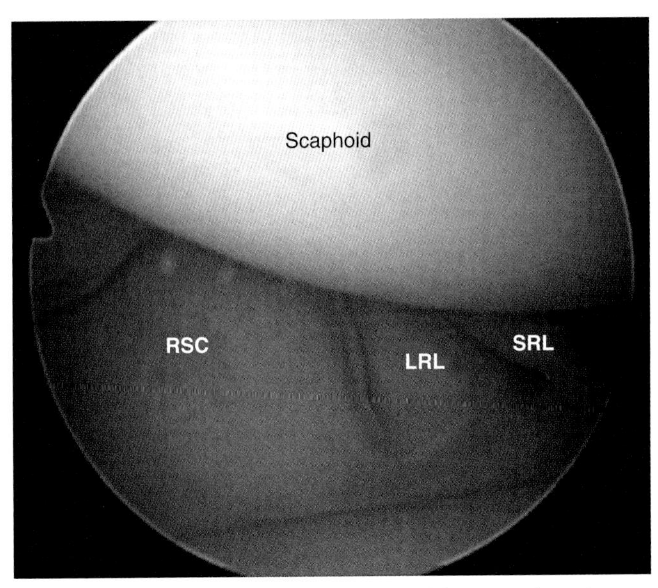

FIGURE 33-2 Arthroscopic view of the intervals between the volar extrinsic ligaments. Radiocarpal volar ganglions originate from capsular intervals between the radioscaphocapitate (RSC) and long radiolunate (LRL) ligaments or ulnar to the LRL, between the LRL and short radiolunate (SRL) ligament.

PATIENT EVALUATION

History and Physical Examination

Most ganglion cysts occur in women in their second, third, or fourth decade of life. The onset is usually insidious, with a progressive increase in size occurring over many years. The ganglion usually manifests as a visible and palpable mass. Patients may relate a traumatic event, such as a wrist hyperextension injury, that occurred before the cyst appeared; however, most cannot recall an event or activity related to the development or appearance of the mass. The masses may be painful, and the symptoms usually are described as an aching discomfort in the region of the mass. Cosmetic dissatisfaction and concern that the mass represents a malignancy are associated complaints. A painless mass is the most frequent presenting complaint.[12] Westbrook's study of 50 patients indicated that a minority of patients presented with pain, 38% presented because of the cosmetic appearance of the mass, and 28% were concerned that the ganglion was malignant.[13]

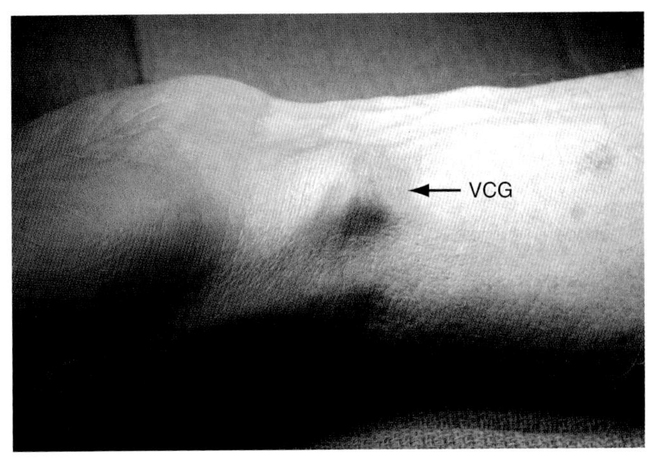

FIGURE 33-3 A volar carpal ganglion cyst (VCG) manifests as a mass on the volar wrist in the interval between the radial artery and the flexor carpi radialis tendon.

The diagnosis is easily made with visual inspection (Fig. 33-3). A 1- to 2-cm, round or ovoid mass usually manifests as a visible fullness in the interval between the FCR tendon and the radial artery. It may be unilobular or multilobular. Palpation reveals a mass that may be slightly tender. The consistency is usually soft and compressible, although chronic lesions may be quite firm. Transillumination with a penlight usually confirms the diagnosis. The differential diagnosis includes vascular lesions of the radial artery, and it is important to determine whether the mass is pulsatile or the pulsations of the radial artery can be distinguished from the mass itself. Despite the relatively easy diagnosis, it is important to exclude other causes of wrist discomfort, such as radiocarpal arthrosis, STT arthrosis, TM arthrosis, DeQuervain's tendonitis, and FCR tendonitis. Isolated loading and stress testing of the individual joints should not produce any pain if the joint is not arthritic. The result of a Finkelstein maneuver should be negative, and there should be no tenderness of the first dorsal compartment tendons. Resisted wrist flexion should produce no pain over the FCR tendon. In patients with an occult volar ganglion cyst, the only positive physical finding may be fullness in the FCR–radial artery interval and pain with pressure in the region. Exclusion of other potential causes of volar radial wrist pain is essential.

Diagnostic Imaging

If the diagnosis is certain and the physical examination presents no confounding findings, imaging is not necessary. Wong and colleagues showed that radiographic abnormalities were diagnosed in only 13% of patients with ganglion cysts, and treatment was affected in only 1% of the cases in their study. They concluded that routine radiographs are not cost-effective.[14] When desired, plain radiographs are usually sufficient as an imaging study to exclude arthrosis of the STT or TM joint. Arthroscopic management of volar ganglions is indicated only for capsular radiocarpal origins; preoperative radiographs that demonstrate arthrosis raise suspicion that the cyst may arise from a location other than the radiocarpal joint. If the nature of the mass is unclear, ultrasound or magnetic resonance imaging is useful. Ultrasound is a cost-effective study that demonstrates the mass as a hypoechoic lesion. Wang and associates were able to localize the stalk-like origin of the ganglion emanating from the volar radiocarpal joint in 7 of 15 cysts. They also found that small cysts can be hypoechoic or anechoic, and not all fulfill the ultrasound criteria for simple cysts.[5]

TREATMENT

Indications and Contraindications

Indications for arthroscopic ganglionectomy are relative. Patients desire excision of the ganglion cyst to improve cosmesis, to eliminate pain, and for absolute diagnosis and exclusion of potential malignancy. The procedure is recommended for the typical volar ganglion that manifests in the interval between the FCR and the radial artery and is not located distal to the distal wrist flexion crease. Distal lesions may be associated with the STT or TM joint and therefore not accessible to radiocarpal arthroscopic techniques. The procedure is technically much more challenging than open excision but cosmetically more appealing. Patients should be warned that even small arthroscopy portal incisions can form hypertrophic scar. Theoretically, there is less capsular damage, because the only capsule being excised is that associated with the stalk-like origin of the mass; however, some patients develop significant stiffness that requires extensive rehabilitation despite the arthroscopic approach. If conservative management has failed to bring about symptom resolution or elimination of the mass, surgical treatment is recommended.

Arthroscopic management of volar ganglions is contraindicated for masses that may be coming from locations other than the radiocarpal joint capsule, such as the STT joint or the FCR sheath. Wrists that have sustained prior trauma or are excessively stiff and may present difficulty in visualization of the volar extrinsic ligaments should have their ganglia excised in an open fashion. Unusual or atypical masses that are likely not ganglions should also be treated by open excision. Recurrent ganglion cysts should be treated in an open fashion, although some surgeons have reported success in treating recurrent lesions arthroscopically.[3]

Conservative Management

Conservative treatment of symptomatic volar ganglion cysts is somewhat limited. Historically, conservative treatment of ganglions has included external pressure with a variety of topical agents and mechanical devices, external rubbing or massage, and closed rupture with the use of digital pressure or more violent means, such as striking the mass with a heavy book, which accounts for the designation *Bible cyst*. These techniques are associated with recurrence rates as high as 64%.[6,15] Spontaneous resolution of ganglia occurs in approximately 50% of patients but can take many years.[16] Cysts that have developed acutely or after an identifiable traumatic event should be treated with a period of splint immobilization, because the initial symptoms and the mass may resolve. More frequently, patients present with a cyst of insidious origin with a duration of many months or even years, and splinting is not an effective treatment.

Aspiration of wrist ganglia has a success rate of only 30% to 50%. The poorest results for aspiration are associated with volar ganglion cysts, and most surgeons caution against aspiration because of the risk of injury to adjacent neurovascular structures such as the radial artery and the palmar cutaneous branch of the median nerve.[12,17,18] A 47% recurrence rate after aspiration was reported in Dias and Buchs' study, but recurrence did not correlate with patients' satisfaction with treatment.[16] Aspiration is offered to patients who desire cyst resolution but want to avoid a more involved surgical procedure. Physicians should be certain that adjacent neurovascular structures are separate from the mass and that there is no possibility that the volar mass represents a lesion of vascular origin. Patients should be warned that the failure rate with aspiration is high and that recurrence is likely.

Arthroscopic Technique

Arthroscopic excision of volar ganglion cysts starts with a standard arthroscopic setup. The arm is exsanguinated, and a proximal tourniquet is used. Traction is applied by means of sterile finger traps (Fig. 33-4). The method used to provide traction should not interfere with the ability to convert to an open procedure. A sterile traction tower offers full access to the dorsal and volar wrist, and if the need to convert to open ganglionectomy arises, the tower can be removed and an open procedure performed without compromising sterility.

After traction is applied, standard arthroscopic portals are marked (Fig. 33-5). The outer margins of the volar ganglion

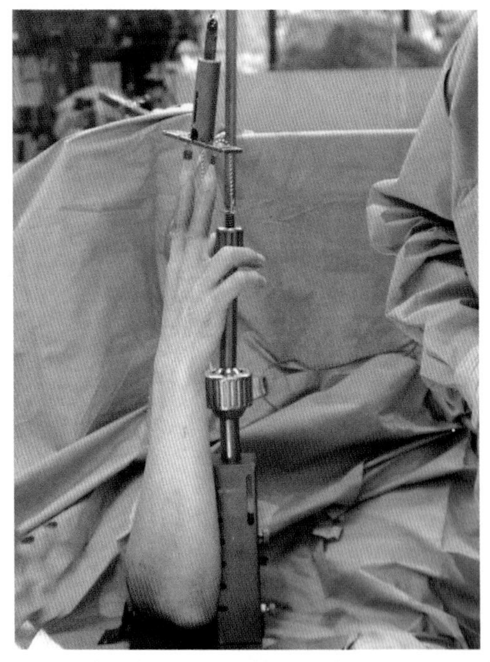

FIGURE 33-4 The hand is supported in an arthroscopy tower. The distraction facilitates instrument manipulation within the radiocarpal joint. Sterile access to the entire hand facilitates localization of the ganglion and conversion to an open procedure if necessary.

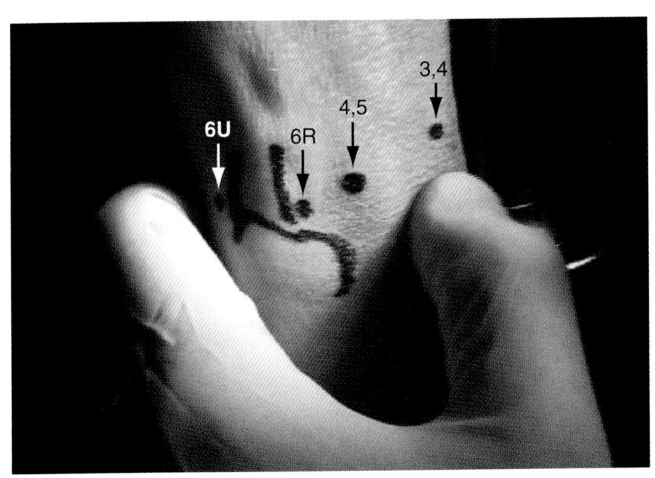

FIGURE 33-5 Standard arthroscopic portals are used for the procedure. Marking is done after traction is applied. The surgeon's thumb is on Lister's tubercle.

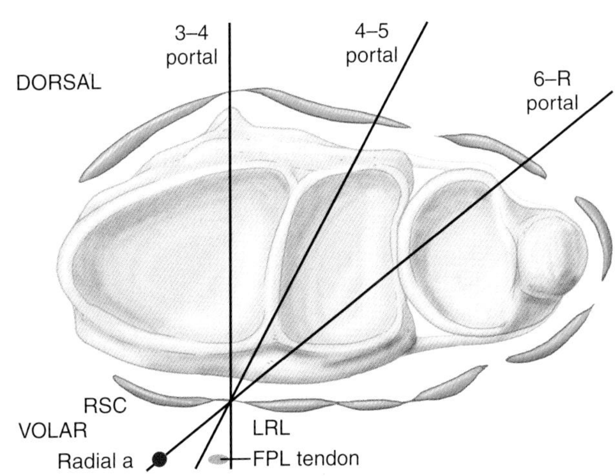

FIGURE 33-7 In cadaveric experiments, the combination of the 3-4 portal as a viewing portal and the 4-5 portal as a working portal was safest in terms of relative distance from neurovascular and tendon structures on the volar aspect of the wrist. The 4-5 portal provided good shaver access to the stalk of the mass for decompression and resection.

should be palpated and marked (Fig. 33-6). The skin landmarks are outlined to confirm that the mass has been eliminated and decompressed.

This procedure is commonly performed with the 3-4 portal as a viewing portal and a 4-5 portal as an operative portal. In cadaver experiments, this combination was identified as being most effective for access to the volar capsular origin of the cyst (Fig. 33-7), and it was safest in regard to injury to neurovascular and tendon elements volar to the wrist capsule (Vella and Greenberg, unpublished data).

The joint is insufflated with saline through the 3-4 portal. During insufflation of the joint, the needle used to inject the joint should mimic the path of the arthroscope. The angle should reflect the volar inclination of the distal radius. Portal incisions are made through the skin, and spreading of soft tissue with a hemostat exposes the joint capsule. The scope is placed gently into the wrist to avoid articular cartilage injury. A 4-5 portal is established by direct arthroscopic visualization. The angle of the portal is of paramount importance, because a portal that is placed too proximal or too distal will make access to the volar capsular origin of the cyst very difficult. Initially, diagnostic arthroscopy of the radiocarpal joint is performed to rule out or assess additional pathology. In most cases, diagnostic arthroscopy reveals no additional pathology. Occasionally, there is synovial proliferation, and a synovectomy is necessary to enable visualization.

After the diagnostic portion of the procedure is completed, a full-radius resector is introduced into the 4-5 portal. The shaver is used to remove any proliferative synovium that is present. Frequently, the ligamentous interval between the RSC and LRL ligaments is obscured by the vascular leash known as the radioscapholunate ligament or ligament of Testut. The shaver is used to resect this vascular leash so that the volar capsule can be easily seen (Fig. 33-8).

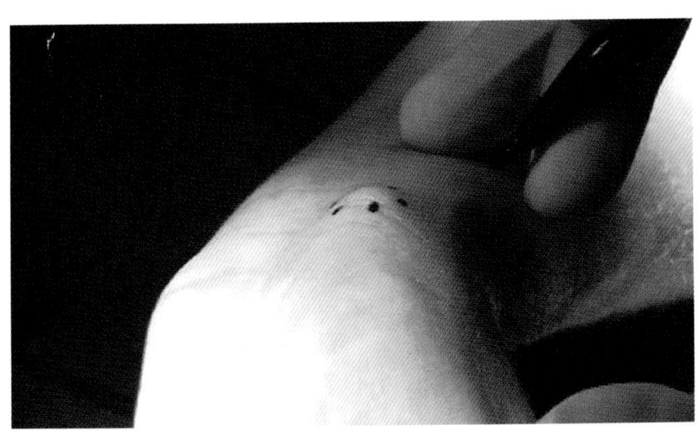

FIGURE 33-6 The outline of the ganglion is marked. This facilitates localization of the mass during the procedure and confirmation that the mass has been adequately decompressed.

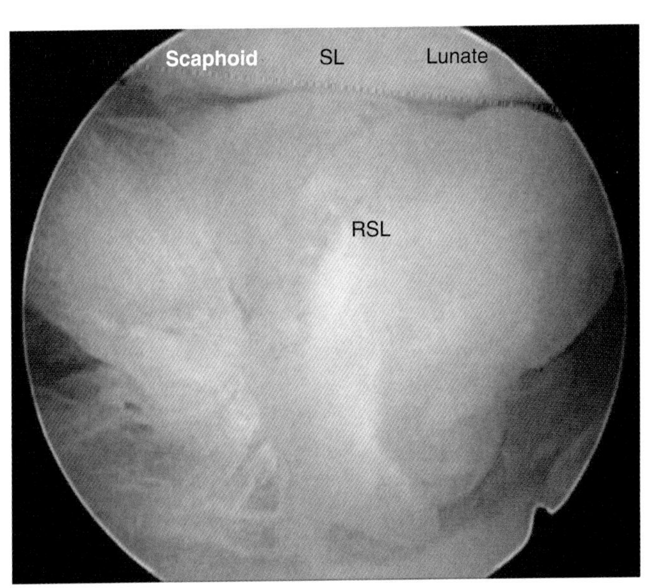

FIGURE 33-8 The ligament of Testut or radioscapholunate (RSL) ligament is a vascular leash that may obscure visualization of the capsular origin of the cyst. It should be resected so that the origin of the cyst can be seen.

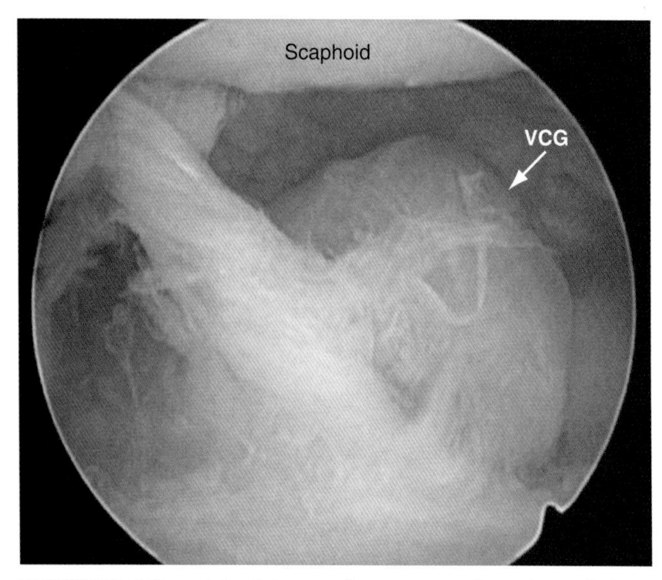

FIGURE 33-9 The origin of the ganglion emanates from the extrinsic ligament interval as a volar outpouching into the radiocarpal joint.

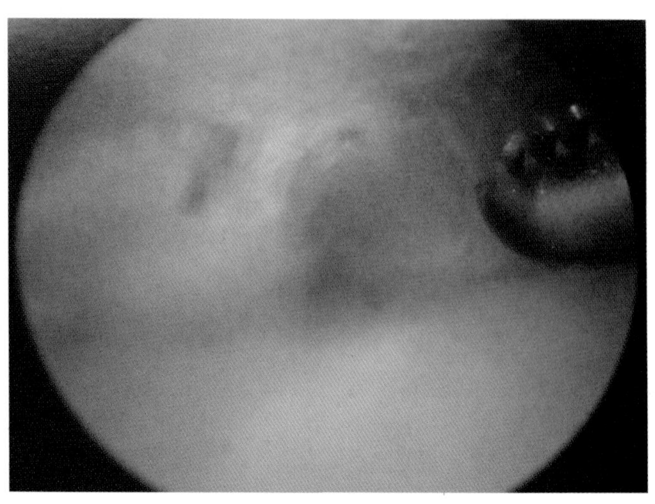

FIGURE 33-11 Frequently, a fluid blush of yellowish liquid can be seen entering the radiocarpal joint as the sac of the ganglion decompresses its contents into the joint.

At this point, a lobular structure representing the origin of the ganglion is visualized (Fig. 33-9). This is usually in the ligamentous interval on the volar capsule. Xanthomatous changes consistent with degeneration or mucinous changes may be present. If the cyst is not obvious, external pressure on the volar mass usually produces an outpouching that can be dynamically seen entering the joint in the RSC and LRL interval. This is especially true in cases of occult volar ganglion cysts.

After the origin is identified, the full-radius resector is used to carefully resect the capsular origin of the mass (Fig. 33-10). As the cyst base is removed, a distinct fluid blush is seen as the ganglion fluid decompresses into the radiocarpal joint (Fig. 33-11). This fluid movement can be enhanced by external pressure on the cyst. Resection continues until a window measuring approximately 1 × 1 cm is created (Fig. 33-12). The flexor pollicis longus tendon is visualized. A blunt probe can be passed through the created capsular defect into the cyst body and can be palpated. Passage of an instrument along this course safely avoids neurovascular structures.

After the cyst is decompressed, the procedure is complete. Arthroscopic equipment is removed. Portal incisions are closed with nonabsorbable suture. A dressing is applied to place compression on the volar radial wrist. The postoperative dressing and splint are removed at 2 weeks postoperatively. Range-of-motion exercises and modalities to control edema are initiated, with resumption of activities as tolerated. Most patients are back to full, unrestricted use at 6 weeks postoperatively.

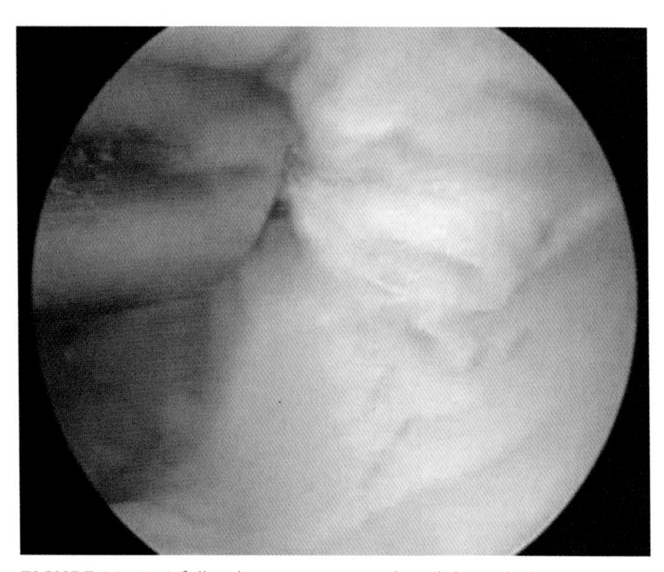

FIGURE 33-10 A full-radius resector introduced through the 4-5 portal has excellent access to the origin of the ganglion cyst.

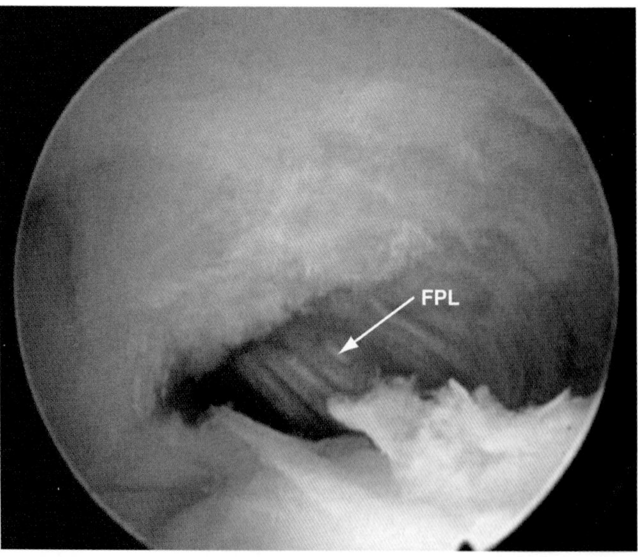

FIGURE 33-12 A capsular defect is created after resection of the origin of the volar ganglion. The flexor pollicis longus (FPL) tendon can be visualized through this defect.

PEARLS & PITFALLS

- Mark portals after traction is applied so that their relation to surface markings is not distorted. Outline the ganglion, so that its exact location can be identified after it is decompressed.
- Introduce instrumentation from the 4-5 portal to minimize injury to neurovascular elements and volar flexor tendons.
- Portal placement is paramount. Replicate the volar inclination of the radius with the working portal to facilitate access to the volar capsule. A synovectomy may be necessary to visualize the capsule and the stalk of the ganglion.
- If the ganglion cannot be readily seen, external pressure on the cyst usually brings the ganglion stalk into view.
- When performing the resection, keep the shaver blade in view at all times. Do not plunge the shaver deep to the capsule, because this puts the radial artery and volar flexor tendons at risk.

Postoperative Rehabilitation

Patients remove their postoperative dressing and start gentle range-of-motion exercises as tolerated. Suture removal is performed at 10 days postoperatively. Patients who demonstrate excessive stiffness or swelling during this time should start a supervised therapy program that emphasizes range-of-motion exercises and edema control. Most patients require minimal supervised therapy. The level of patient satisfaction with the outcome of the procedure is typically high.[3,7,20,21]

COMPLICATIONS

Recurrence of the ganglion cyst is the most common complication. In 2003, Ho's group published their initial results on arthroscopic resection of volar ganglia; there were no recurrences in the first five patients.[11] Their subsequent publication, which summarized the treatment of 21 patients, documented two recurrences.[3] This compares favorably with the reported recurrence rate for open excision, which ranges from 2% to 40% in the literature, and it is similar to recurrence rates reported for arthroscopic dorsal ganglia excisions. The 2003 study of open volar ganglionectomy by Aydin and colleagues identified a 22% recurrence rate,[10] whereas Jacobs and Govaers reported a recurrence rate of 28% after open excision.[19] Greenberg reported only one recurrence among his first 12 patients.[20]

Other potential complications related to arthroscopic volar ganglion excision are injury to neurovascular structures, notably the median nerve and the palmar cutaneous branch of the median nerve, and the radial artery. Tendon injuries may occur because of the proximity of the FPL during the procedure. Capsular injury may produce stiffness. Paying close attention to technique, especially keeping the shaver visualized at all times and not plunging deep to the capsule, should eliminate complications. Minor neurovascular injuries have been reported for volar ganglia excisions. In the series reported by Rocci and coworkers, arthroscopic resection of radiocarpal ganglia compared favorably with open excision, with significantly more rapid recovery times and earlier return to work.[21] There were no neurovascular or tendon complications in this series.

CONCLUSIONS

Arthroscopic management of intra-articular wrist pathology, including treatment of volar ganglion cysts, is an integral part of the practice of the wrist arthroscopist. Development of high-quality optical devices and joint-specific instrumentation has facilitated operative wrist arthroscopy, although the procedure is technically demanding.

Surgeons have a deep appreciation of the normal ligamentous anatomy and pathologic changes that occur and can lead to ganglion cysts. Arthroscopic ganglion cyst excision is recommended because of its advantages over open treatment, including less scar formation, less capsular injury, rapid rehabilitation and return to activities, and a lower recurrence rate.

REFERENCES

1. Roth, JH, Poehling GG, and Whipple TL. Arthroscopic surgery of the wrist. *Instr Course Lect*. 1988;37:183-194.
2. Osterman AL, Raphael J. Arthroscopic resection of dorsal ganglion of the wrist. *Hand Clin*. 1995;11:7-12.
3. Ho PC, Law BK, Hung LK. Arthroscopic volar wrist ganglionectomy. *Chir Main*. 2006;25(suppl 1):S221-S230.
4. Kuhlmann JN, Luboinski J, Baux S, Mimoun M. Ganglions of the wrist: proposals for topographical systematization and natural history. *Rev Chir Orthop Reparatrice Appar Mot*. 2003;89:310-319.
5. Wang G, Jacobson JA, Feng FY, et al. Sonography of wrist ganglion cysts: variable and noncystic appearances. *J Ultrasound Med*. 2007;26:1323-1328; quiz 1330-1331.
6. Gude W, Morelli V. Ganglion cysts of the wrist: pathophysiology, clinical picture, and management. *Curr Rev Musculoskelet Med*. 2008; 1:205-211.
7. Mathoulin C, Hoyos A, Pelaez J. Arthroscopic resection of wrist ganglia. *Hand Surg*. 2004;9:159-164.
8. Psaila JV, Mansel RE. The surface ultrastructure of ganglia. *J Bone Joint Surg Br*. 1978;60:228-233.
9. Greendyke SD, Wilson M, Shepler TR. Anterior wrist ganglia from the scaphotrapezial joint. *J Hand Surg Am*. 1992;17:487-490.
10. Aydin A, Kabakas F, Erer M, et al. Surgical treatment of volar wrist ganglia. *Acta Orthop Traumatol Turc*. 2003;37:309-312.
11. Ho PC, Lo WN, Hung LK. Arthroscopic resection of volar ganglion of the wrist: a new technique. *Arthroscopy*. 2003;19:218-221.
12. Thornburg LE. Ganglions of the hand and wrist. *J Am Acad Orthop Surg*. 1999;7:231-238.
13. Westbrook AP, Stephen AB, Oni J, Davis TR. Ganglia: the patient's perception. *J Hand Surg Br*. 2000;25:566-567.
14. Wong AS, Jebson PJ, Murray PM, Trigg SD. The use of routine wrist radiography is not useful in the evaluation of patients with a ganglion cyst of the wrist. *Hand (N Y)*. 2007;2:117-119.
15. Nelson CL, Sawmiller S, Phalen GS. Ganglions of the wrist and hand. *J Bone Joint Surg Am*. 1972;54:1459-1464.
16. Dias J, Buch K. Palmar wrist ganglion: does intervention improve outcome? A prospective study of the natural history and patient-reported treatment outcomes. *J Hand Surg Br*. 2003;28:172-176.
17. Nahra ME, Bucchieri JS. Ganglion cysts and other tumor related conditions of the hand and wrist. *Hand Clin*. 2004;20:249-260, v.
18. Wright TW, Cooney WP, Ilstrup DM. Anterior wrist ganglion. *J Hand Surg Am*. 1994;19:954-958.
19. Jacobs LG, Govaers KJ. The volar wrist ganglion: just a simple cyst? *J Hand Surg Br*. 1990;15:342-346.
20. Greenberg JA. Arthroscopic treatment of volar carpal ganglion cysts. In: Slutsky DJ, Nagle DJ, eds. *Techniques in Hand and Wrist Arthroscopy*. Philadelphia, PA: Churchill Livingstone/Elsevier; 2007:188-190.
21. Rocchi L, Canal A, Fanfani F, Cantalano F. Articular ganglia of the volar aspect of the wrist: arthroscopic resection compared with open excision. A prospective randomised study. *Scand J Plast Reconstr Surg Hand Surg*. 2008;42:253-259.

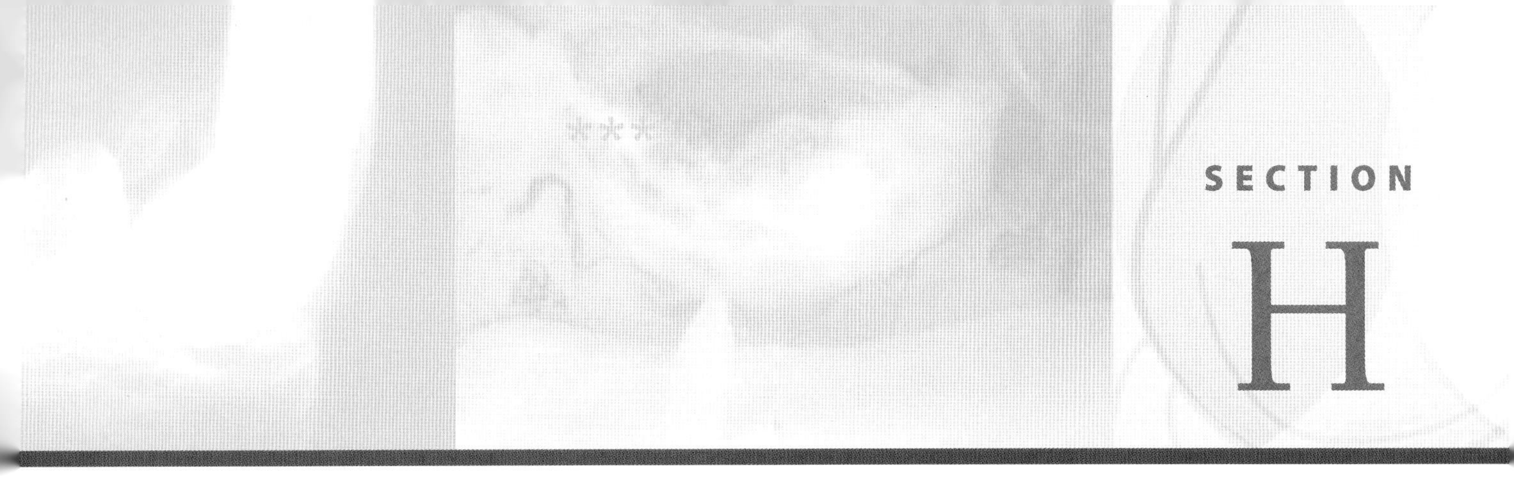

SECTION H

Carpal Tunnel Release

CHAPTER

34

Endoscopic Carpal Tunnel Release: Chow Technique

James C.Y. Chow • James Campbell Chow • Athanasios A. Papachristos

Sir James Paget first described median nerve compression after a distal radius fracture in 1854.[1,2] In 1880, James Putman, a neurologist from Boston, reported similar symptoms in a group of his patients.[3] The first formal description of surgical decompression for treatment of this condition was reported in 1933; this was followed by Phalen's classic article in 1950.[4] Since then, open carpal tunnel release has been established as the gold standard for surgical treatment of carpal tunnel syndrome.

James C.Y. Chow began working on an endoscopic release of the transverse carpal ligament in 1985, unaware that Ichiro Okutsu in Japan and John Agee in California were concurrently and separately working toward similar goals. The primary motivation of Chow's concept was to create a method for surgical treatment of carpal tunnel syndrome that could preserve the unaffected surrounding normal anatomic structures of the wrist and hand. Through these pursuits, Chow developed the slotted cannula late in 1986. After a thorough cadaveric trial period, the procedure was completed in May of 1987, and it was first performed in a patient in September of that year.

The first two reports in the literature on the topic of endoscopic carpal tunnel release (ECTR), written separately by Chow and by Okutsu and colleagues, were published in the March issue of *Arthroscopy* in 1989.[5,6] In the following year, Chow presented a paper describing his clinical results after ECTR in 149 cases at the 1990 Arthroscopy Association of North America (AANA) Annual Meeting in Orlando, Florida. In the fall of 1990, Agee and associates[7] reported to the American Society for Surgery of the Hand Annual Meeting in Toronto, Canada, the clinical results of a multicenter study of the use of Agee's technique for endoscopic release of the carpal ligament. Since the publication of these three endoscopic carpal ligament release techniques, there has been increasing interest and much debate among surgeons regarding the safety and efficacy of the endoscopic procedures compared with the open technique. Several modifications and variations of the three original ideas have been made since their initial demonstration.

ANATOMY

The carpal tunnel is bounded deeply by the volar surface of the distal radius, ulnarly by the hook of the hamate, radially by the scaphoid, and superficially by the confluence of the rather stout transverse carpal ligament, palmar aponeurosis, and antebrachial fascia. The carpal tunnel contains the median nerve and nine tendons (i.e., the flexor digitorum sublimus and profundus tendons to all four fingers and the flexor pollicis longus).

Superficial to the transverse carpal ligament lies a sling of vascular and nervous connective tissue, subcutaneous fat, and densely innervated palmar dermis and epidermis. This sling of soft tissue is an interthenar soft tissue band (ISTB) (Fig. 34-1A and B) that bridges the thenar and hypothenar musculature. It is a histologically distinct structure (see Fig. 34-1C) that lies volar to the transverse carpal ligament. The ISTB and the palmaris brevis muscle should be preserved. The ISTB prevents bowstringing of the flexor tendons after surgery, thereby maintaining their strength during contraction.[8-10] It is the goal of ECTR to preserve this natural anatomy while selectively releasing only the transverse carpal ligament.

Carpal tunnel syndrome is a compressive neuropathy of the median nerve at the wrist. It can result from any condition that increases intra–carpal tunnel pressure, such as irritation and swelling of any of the nine flexor tendons and their tenosynovium, edema of the median nerve, anatomic abnormality or scarring of any of the bordering structures of the carpal tunnel, anomalous lumbrical anatomy, an intra–carpal tunnel mass (e.g., a deep ganglion cyst), or stiffening and contracture of the transverse carpal ligament itself.

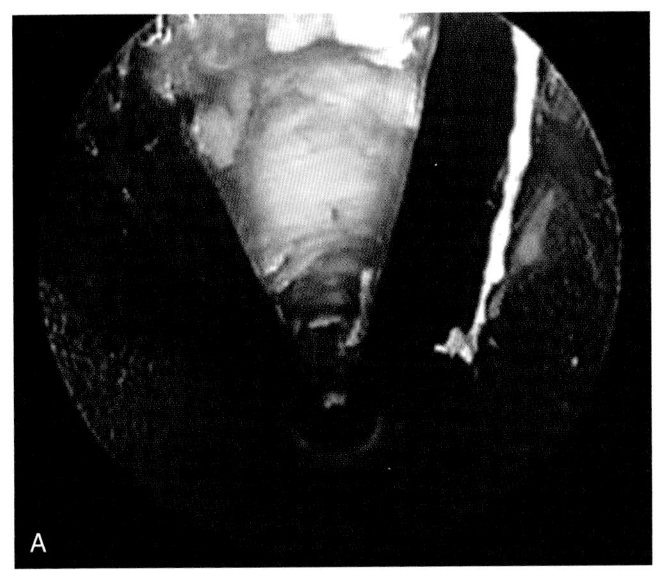

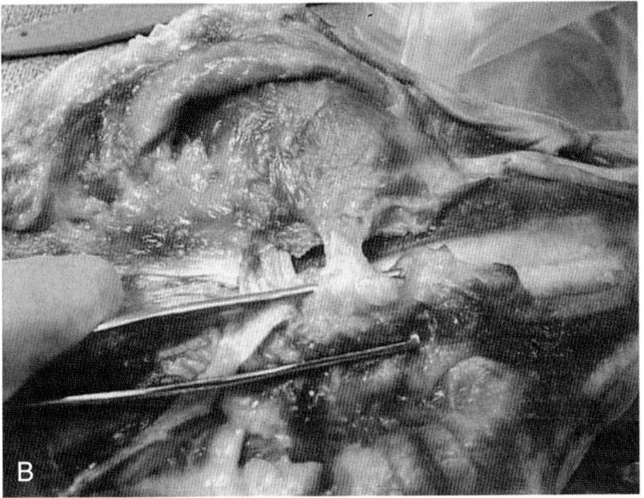

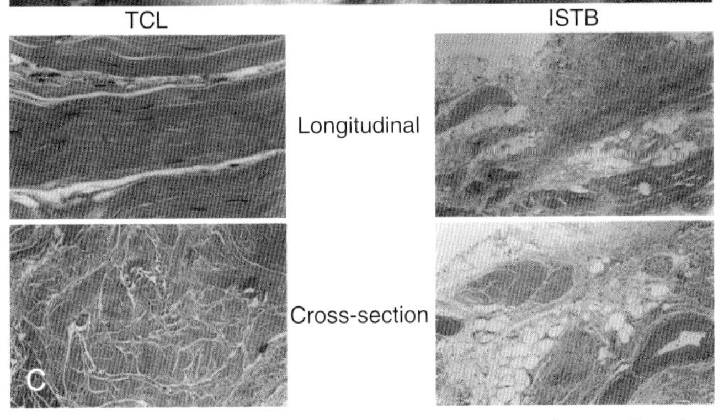

FIGURE 34-1 A, Endoscopic view of the interthenar soft tissue band (ISTB). **B,** Gross view of the ISTB. **C,** Histologic examination of the transverse carpal ligament (TCL) and the ISTB in longitudinal and cross-sectional views.

PATIENT EVALUATION

History and Physical Examination

Carpal tunnel syndrome accounts for approximately 463,673 carpal tunnel releases performed annually in the United States.[11] Patients who have developed this syndrome usually present with a history of characteristic symptoms, such as nocturnal pain, paresthesias, and numbness in the median nerve distribution distal to the wrist, and thenar muscular weakness. The physician should be aware of the patient's general health condition and family history. Congenital diseases or anomalies, connective tissue diseases, systemic and metabolic disorders, and previous injury to the distal forearm or wrist should be taken into consideration.

The physical examination is critical for accurate diagnosis. In an acute case, there is tenderness along the carpal canal area. Light percussion over the median nerve at the wrist produces a sensation of an electric current that radiates to the median nerve distribution; this is known as Tinel's sign. Phalen's sign is evoked by holding the wrists at maximum flexion with the dorsal aspects of the hands in full contact (i.e., reverse praying position). This position narrows the carpal canal; if it reproduces the paresthesias in the fingers within 60 seconds, the sign is considered positive. As the pathologic condition advances, less time is necessary to evoke a response. Other indicators include the monofilament test, two-point discrimination, the reverse Phalen's test, and the tourniquet test. In the late stages, with thenar muscle atrophy, the examiner can observe the muscle wasting in the thenar area.[12] Muscle weakness is tested subjectively by resisted palmar abduction of the thumb against the examiner's index finger and comparison of one hand with the other.

A carefully performed history and physical examination can help the physician distinguish between an isolated compression neuropathy at the wrist and a double crush syndrome. The double crush phenomenon clinically correlates with a high incidence of concurrent carpal syndrome in patients with cervical radiculopathy. An equally high incidence of associated carpal tunnel syndrome with more proximal entrapment of the median nerve has been reported. The physician must concomitantly exclude thoracic outlet syndrome, pronator compression syndrome in the forearm, and central nervous system disease.

Diagnostic Tests and Imaging

Electromyography and nerve conduction velocity tests aid in the detection of carpal tunnel syndrome. Indications for surgery should not be decided or altered according to the results of nerve conduction velocity tests, especially when the results are normal but the patient has the clinical signs and symptoms of the syndrome.[13-15] A delay in the distal latency of the median nerve of 7.0 msec or longer represents significant compression of the median nerve; if such a delay is present, surgery should be considered immediately. The most important aspects in diagnosing carpal tunnel syndrome are the history and the physical examination results. Electrodiagnostic studies of the median nerve are used adjunctively to confirm the diagnosis and perhaps to suggest how the patient will respond to surgery.

Wrist radiography can rule out the possibility of congenital or acquired bone or joint deformity, abnormality, or pathology. Previously sustained fractures of the distal forearm and wrist should be taken into account. A malunited fracture of the distal radius, previously performed surgery in the wrist area, or a hypoplastic or aplastic hook of the hamate[16] can produce difficulties for the surgeon during placement of and operation through the slotted cannula. Standard anteroposterior and lateral views of the distal forearm and wrist and a tunnel view of the wrist are required. If a more extensive study is indicated, magnetic resonance imaging (MRI), computed tomography (CT), ultrasound, bone scanning, or arthrography of the wrist may be necessary.[17,18]

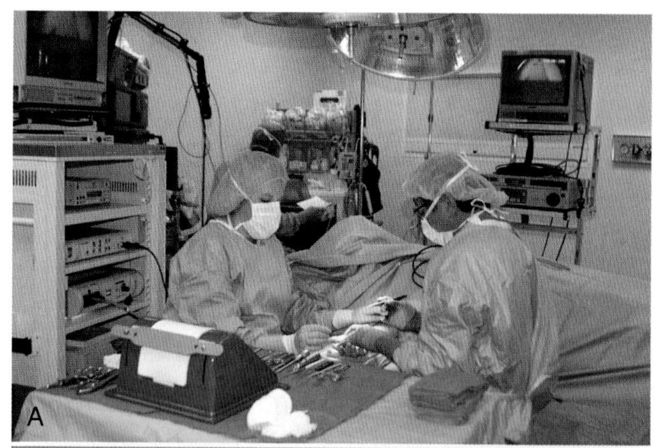

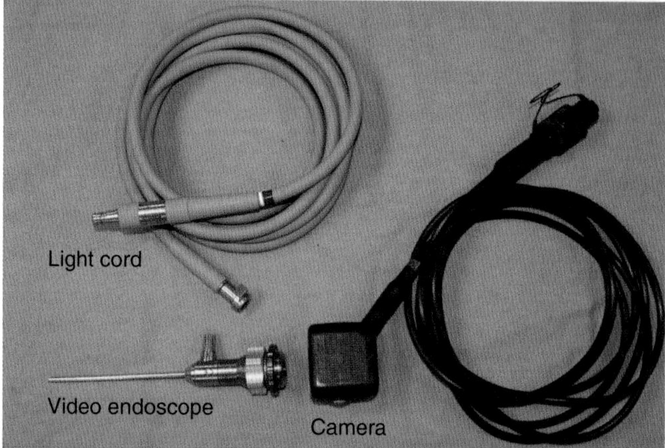

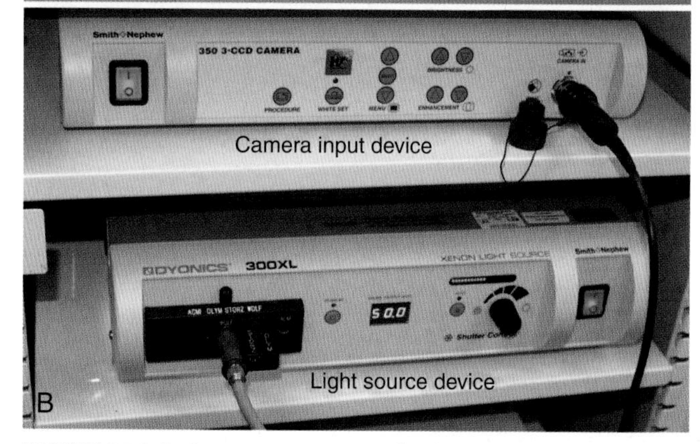

FIGURE 34-2 A, Operating room setup for the endoscopic carpal tunnel release using the Chow dual-portal technique. **B,** Arthroscopic equipment that is appropriate for the performance of this technique.

TREATMENT

Conservative Management

Conservative management includes daily or nightly wrist splinting, alteration of daily activities, physical therapy, and nonsteroidal anti-inflammatory oral medication. Intra–carpal tunnel steroid injections have been used with various degrees of success.

Open Versus Arthroscopic Management

The indications for the open surgical release of transverse carpal tunnel ligament have been well established, and in most cases they apply to ECTR. The advantages of endoscopic over open carpal tunnel release include no hypertrophic scar or scar tenderness, no pillar pain, less compromise of pinch or grip strength, and an earlier return to work and daily activities. However, ECTR can become a dangerous procedure if it is performed by an inexperienced surgeon.[19-21] Significant intraoperative complications have been reported throughout the United States,[22-24] raising questions about the value of ECTR. However, ECTR can be performed safely by experienced surgeons. Despite its steep learning curve, the results of ECTR can be satisfying for the patient and the surgeon.[25] As the knowledge, technique, and instrumentation have evolved, the safety of ECTR has improved.

Arthroscopic Technique

The original technique was described by Chow as a transbursal approach to the carpal tunnel requiring penetration of the ulnar bursa.[5,26] After a multicenter study,[27,28] the original technique was modified in an attempt to decrease the complications and improve the learning curve. Conversion to an extrabursal technique made the surgical procedure much easier and safer because it offered better visualization of the proximal transverse carpal ligament.[29-31] The following paragraphs describe the extrabursal, dual-portal technique.

Operating Room Setup

The patient is placed in a supine position, and a hand table is used. Two video monitors are preferred, although some surgeons can manage the procedure with only one. One of the two monitors should face the surgeon, and the other should face the assistant. The surgeon sits on the ulnar side of the patient, and the assistant faces the surgeon (Fig. 34-2A). The arthroscopic equipment consists of a short, 4.0-mm, 30-degree video endoscope. The light post is on the same side as the direction of view, the camera apparatus, the light cord, the camera input device, and the light source (see Fig. 34-2B). Optional equipment includes a digital video recorder and a video printer for the printing of any captured images. Water pump and shaver equipment are not used.

A standard handset should be available. Specific instrumentation for the procedure, designed by Chow, includes an ECTRA System Kit and an ECTRA Disposable Kit (Smith & Nephew Endoscopy, Andover, MA). The ECTRA System Kit includes a video endoscope, slotted cannula, dissecting obturator, curved blunt dissector, palmar arch suppressor, probe, retractors, and hand holder (Fig. 34-3). The dissecting obturator is attached with a detachable handle that can also take some other types of obturators included in the kit (e.g., conical, boat-nose obturator), but the latter are not used routinely. The ECTRA Disposable Kit includes a probe knife, triangle knife, retrograde knife, hand pad, and swabs (Fig. 34-4). These knives allow the surgeon to determine the direction and depth of the cut.

Standard preparations and draping are performed as usual, without the application of a tourniquet. Before local anesthesia is introduced, a skin marker is used to map landmarks for the entry and exit portals.

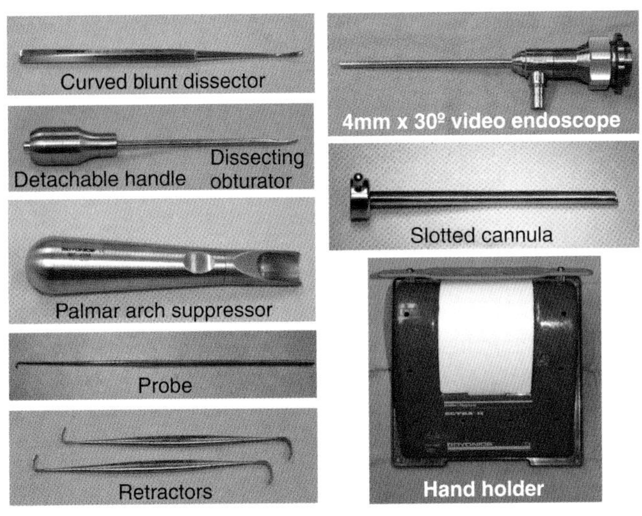

FIGURE 34-3 Instrumentation included in the ECTRA System Kit (Smith & Nephew Endoscopy, Andover, MA).

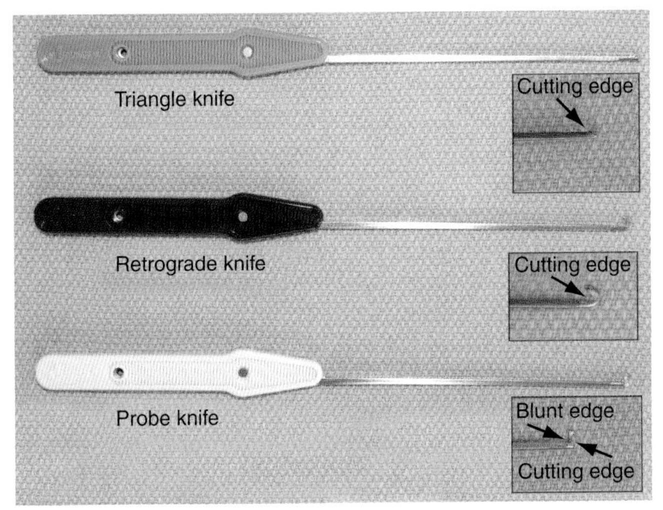

FIGURE 34-4 Specially designed knives for release of the transverse carpal ligament. The tip of each knife is shown in detail *(red square)* on the right side. This instrumentation is included in the ECTRA Disposable Kit (Smith & Nephew Endoscopy, Andover, MA).

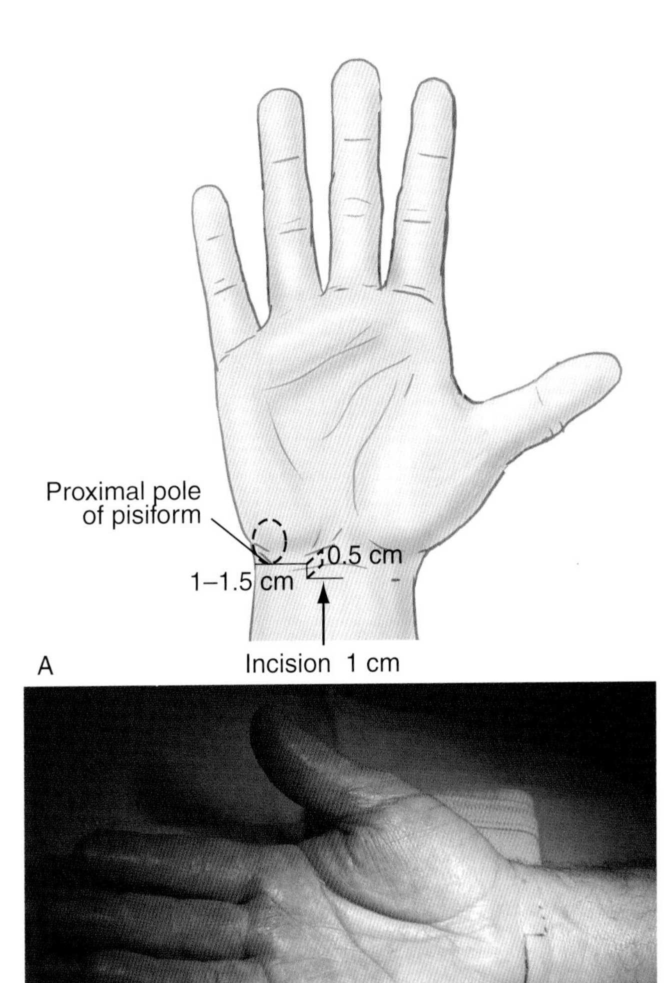

FIGURE 34-5 A and **B,** The entry portal is located by drawing a line 1 to 1.5 cm radially from the proximal pole of the pisiform bone and then drawing a second line of approximately 0.5 cm proximally from the end of the first one. A third line of approximately 1 cm is then drawn radially from the proximal end of the second line to create the entry portal.

Anesthesia

Local anesthesia combined with intravenous medication is recommended for the procedure, because it allows the patient and the surgeon to communicate. An alert patient can inform the surgeon during the procedure about any abnormal sensation in the hand, which can indicate a potential problem caused by a variance of nerve structure in the wrist and palm region.[32-38] Usually, when the patient first comes into the operating room, 100 μg of fentanyl citrate (Sublimaze, Baxter Healthcare Corporation, Westlake Village, CA) is given intravenously. This is a narcotic analgesic medication with an onset of 7 to 8 minutes and a peak action of approximately 30 minutes. Usually, the surgical time does not exceed 10 minutes. A 1% solution of Xylocaine (Astra, Westboro, MA) without epinephrine is injected, approximately 2 to 3 mL at the entry portal and 6 to 7 mL at the exit portal (because of the higher degree of sensitivity of the skin on the palmar region). Special care is taken to limit the injection to the skin and subcutaneous tissue and to avoid affecting the nerve by penetrating deeply.

Positioning the Entry Portal

The proximal end of the pisiform bone is palpated on the volar surface of the wrist within the flexor carpi ulnaris tendon at the distal wrist flexor crease and is marked with a small circle. A line from the proximal pole of the pisiform is drawn radially and is approximately 1.0 to 1.5 cm long. From that point, a second, 0.5-cm line is drawn proximally. A third dotted line, approximately 1.0 cm long, is drawn radially from the proximal end of the second line to create the entry portal (Fig. 34-5). If the palmaris longus muscle is present, the center of the entry portal should be located at the ulnar border of its tendon, almost at the level of the proximal wrist flexor crease. Average dimensions of these lines vary slightly, depending on the overall size of the hand.

Positioning the Exit Portal

The patient's thumb is placed in full abduction. A line is drawn across the palm from the distal border of the thumb to the approximate center of the palm, perpendicular to the long axis of the forearm. A second line is drawn from the third web space, parallel to the long axis of the forearm, to meet the first line. These two lines should form a right angle. A third line is drawn, bisecting this angle and extending approximately 1.0 cm proximally from its vertex, which establishes the site of incision for the exit portal (Fig. 34-6). The surgeon should be able to palpate the hook of the hamate. The exit portal should fall into the soft spot at the center of the palm and should line up with the ring finger, just slightly radial to the hook of the hamate.

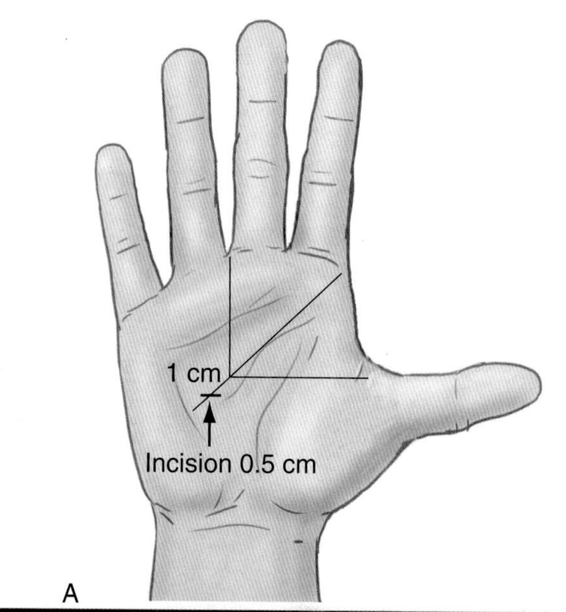

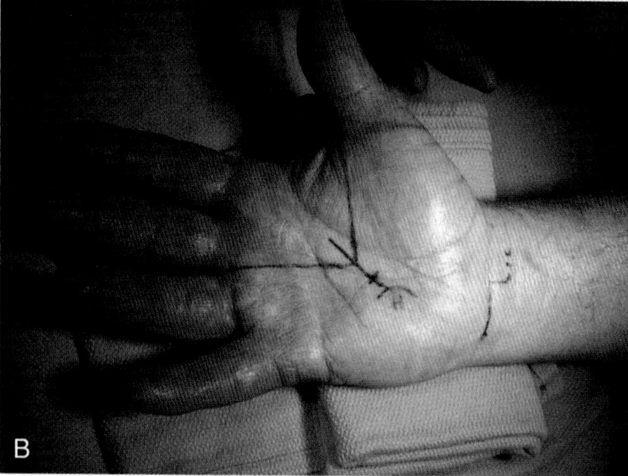

FIGURE 34-6 A and **B:** The exit portal is located by drawing a line from the distal border of the fully abducted thumb perpendicular to the long axis of the forearm. A second line is drawn from the third web space parallel to the long axis of the forearm. These two lines form a right angle. A third line is drawn, bisecting this angle and extending approximately 1.0 cm from its vertex to determine the exit portal.

Creation of Portals and Placement of the Cannula

The procedure begins with the creation of the entry portal. A transverse incision of approximately 1.0 cm (Fig. 34-7A) is made at the marked entry portal site, extending just through the skin. Subcutaneous tissue is bluntly dissected off the volar forearm fascia with the use of a hemostat and is retracted with the retractors. Care must be taken to avoid damage to the small subcutaneous blood vessels.

A knife is used to make a small, longitudinal opening of the antebrachial fascia that is extended distally with the use of a Stephen's tenotomy scissors (see Fig. 34-7B and C). If the palmaris longus muscle is present, the longitudinal cut should be along the ulnar border of palmaris longus tendon. Care should be taken, because sometimes there are two layers of fascia that must be cut. Retractors are passed just beneath the fascia, with one of them lifting the skin distally to create a vacuum that separates the transverse carpal ligament from the ulnar bursa. A blunt, curved dissector is gently slipped into the carpal tunnel, just under the transverse carpal ligament. A gentle "pop" of resistance should be felt as the blunt dissector punches through the bursal sheath at about midway past the transverse carpal ligament. Maneuvering the dissector back and forth should produce a type of washboard feeling because of the rough undersurface of the carpal ligament. The curved dissector is then removed.

A dissecting obturator and slotted cannula assembly unit can be guided into the space vacated by the curved dissector. The slotted cannula assembly is advanced into the carpal tunnel on the underside of the transverse carpal ligament to the level of the hook of the hamate, staying to the ulnar side of the carpal tunnel (see Fig. 34-7D). With the tip of this unit touching the hook of the hamate, the surgeon gently picks up and hyperextends the hand. The hand and cannula assembly are now moved as a unit (see Fig. 34-7E) and placed on the hand holder with the wrist and fingers in full hyperextension. The cannula assembly is advanced along the undersurface of the carpal ligament, while the assistant keeps the hand on the hand holder, until the tip of the cannula assembly can be easily palpated in the palm area where the mark for the exit portal was previously made.

A small, transverse or oblique incision is made just over the palpable cannula assembly tip, cutting only the skin (see Fig. 34-7F). The palmar skin and soft tissue are depressed with the palmar arch suppressor, and the cannula assembly is pushed into the receptacle of the palmar arch suppressor to exit through the distal portal (see Fig. 34-7G). The obturator is then removed from the cannula, which should lie just below the transverse carpal ligament, and the hyperextended hand is strapped onto the hand holder (see Fig. 34-7H and I). Hyperextension of the wrist brings the superficial palmar arch to a level lower than the exiting point of the slotted cannula assembly, thereby protecting it from injury. The creation of two portals is essential, because they stabilize the slotted cannula while it passes through the portals, ensuring the reproducibility of the technique. The slotted portion of the cannula allows a safe cutting zone, whereas delicate structures such as the

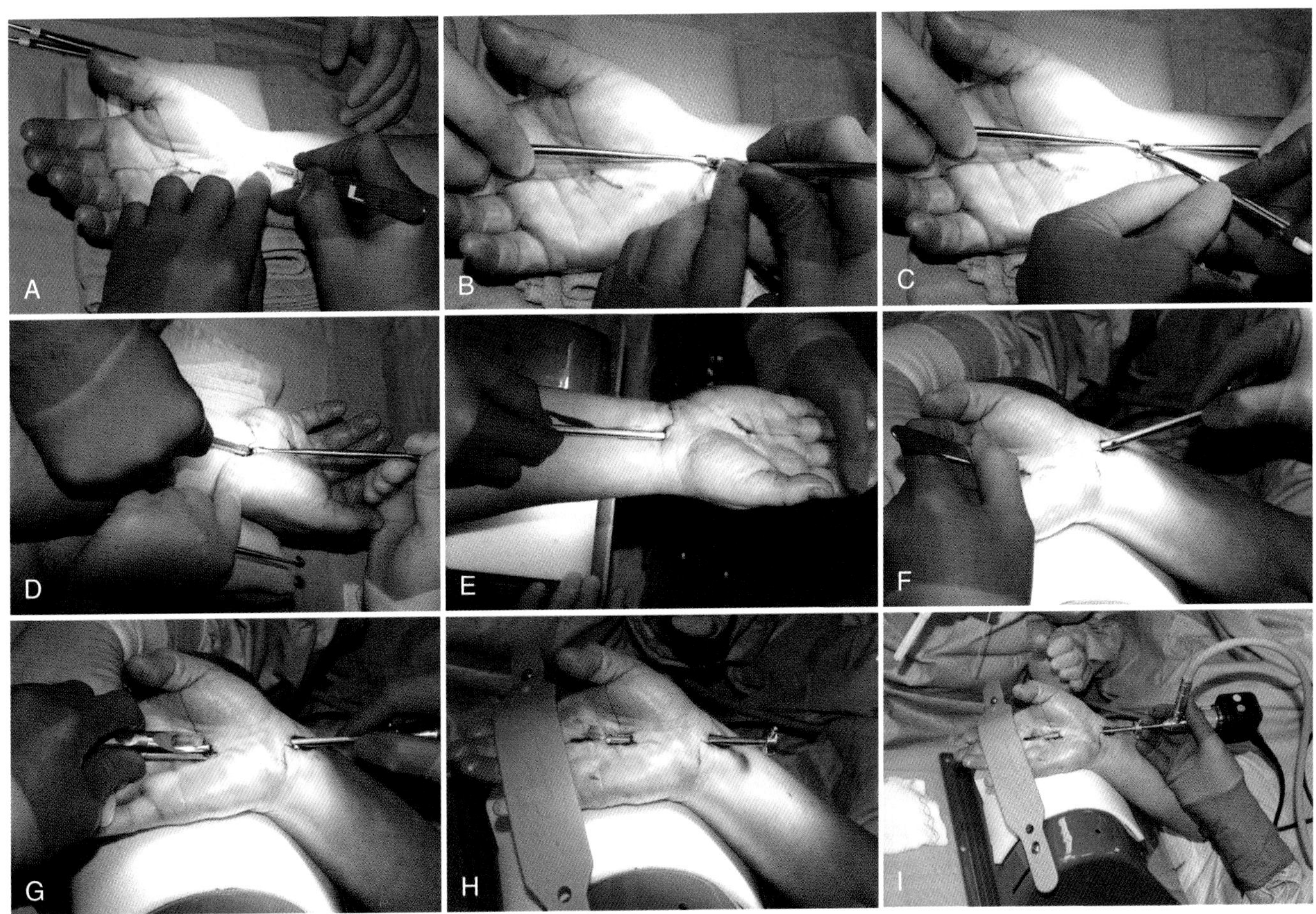

FIGURE 34-7 Step-by-step procedure for the creation of portals and placement of the slotted cannula. **A,** Skin incision. **B** and **C,** A small, longitudinal opening of the antebrachial fascia is created and is extended distally with the use of a tenotomy scissors. **D,** Insertion of the dissecting obturator and slotted cannula assembly into the carpal canal. **E,** Placement of the hand onto the hand holder. **F** and **G,** Skin incision and use of the arch suppressor to allow the cannula assembly to exit through the distal portal. **H,** The dissecting obturator has been removed, leaving the slotted cannula in the carpal canal. **I,** The scope is inserted into the carpal canal through the proximal portal.

median nerve and flexor tendons are protected by the walls of the cannula.

Endoscopic Examination

The video endoscope is inserted into the slotted cannula at the proximal portal. The camera and scope should rest comfortably in the first web space of the surgeon's hand. A cotton swab can be inserted into the tube from the distal portal to clean the lens while focus is adjusted to the best visualization. A blunt probe is inserted to palpate the undersurface of the transverse carpal ligament proximally to distally; if a thin bursal membrane is seen above the cannula's slotted opening, it is carefully dissected with the probe to gain access to the ligament, which has an ivory-white appearance and fibers that run transversely (Fig. 34-8A and B). If the median nerve is present in the field (see Fig. 34-8C), the patient will feel sharp pain radiating to the fingers when the nerve is probed; this response should alert the surgeon to the presence of the nerve. If abundant soft tissue is identified in the opening of the cannula, the procedure should not be performed. The slotted cannula may need to be reinserted to ensure better visualization; however, to avoid irreversible damage, surgery should not be carried out if tendons or other important structures are entrapped between the slotted cannula and the undersurface of the carpal ligament (see Fig. 34-8D).

If there is only a minimal amount of synovium obstructing the view, the obturator is replaced into the slotted cannula. The slotted cannula assembly unit can then be rotated radially about 355 to 360 degrees to provide the visualization and protection required. Surgeons should not hesitate to convert an endoscopic procedure to an open one if they are not able to obtain adequate visualization.

Technique for Release of the Transverse Carpal Ligament

With the scope in the proximal portal and the probe in the distal portal, the distal border of the transverse carpal ligament is identified. The probe knife, which permits forward cutting only, is inserted into the distal portal. The blunt edge of the knife can be used to probe proximally to distally along the ligament. The cut-

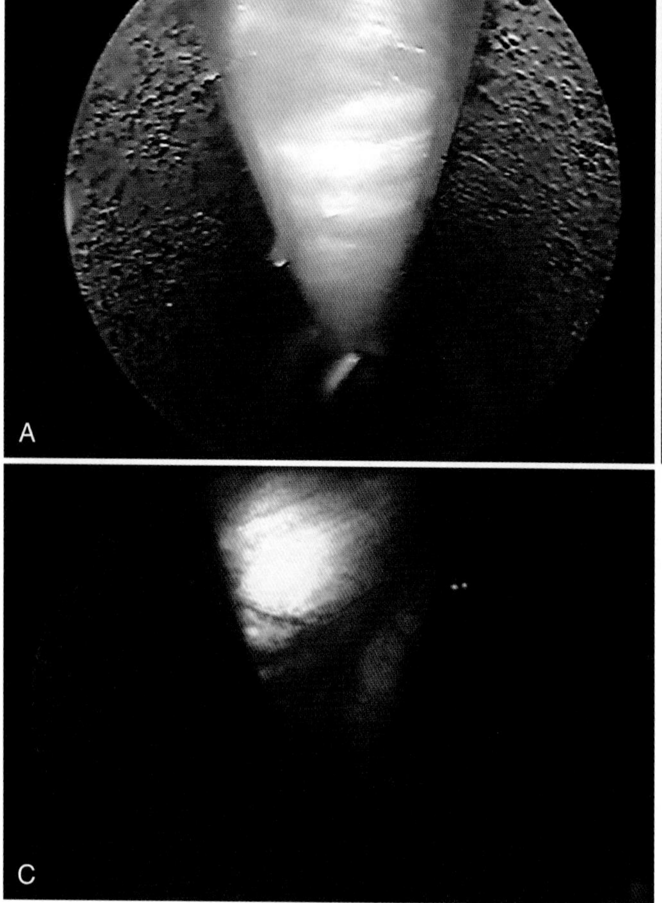

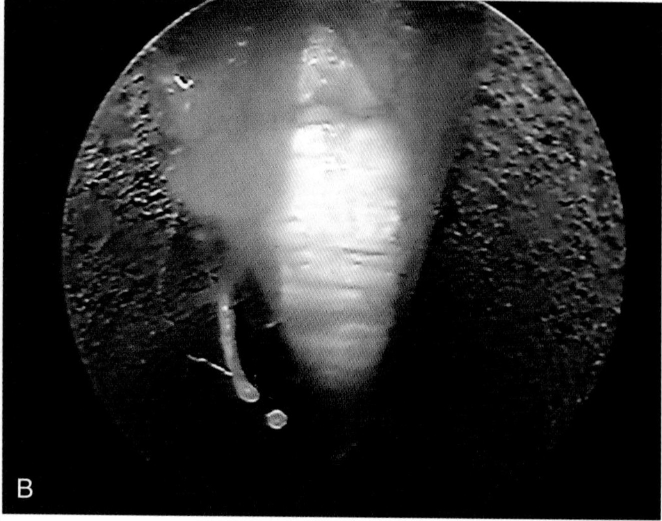

FIGURE 34-8 A, Endoscopic normal appearance of the transverse carpal ligament with its fibers running transversely. **B,** The thicker bursal membrane that sheaths the undersurface of the proximal portion of the carpal ligament has been probed proximally, depicting the fibers of the ligament. **C,** The median nerve is present in the field. **D,** Tendon is present in the field.

ting edge is then used to release the distal border of the ligament by drawing the knife distally to proximally (Fig. 34-9A). Anything beyond the distal border of the carpal ligament should not be excised. The scope is withdrawn proximally about 1 cm, and the triangle knife is used to make a small upward cut in the midsection of the ligament (see Fig. 34-9B). The retrograde knife is then inserted through the distal portal, and its blunt tip is gently positioned at the incision made by the triangle knife (Fig. 34-10). The proximal cutting edge of the retrograde knife is drawn distally, making an incision that joins the previous two cuts, thereby completing the release of the distal portion of transverse carpal ligament (see Fig. 34-10).

The scope is removed from the proximal opening and inserted into the distal opening of the slotted cannula. The camera view on the screen then forms a mirror effect, with the previous ulnar side now being the radial side. By moving the scope proximally and distally, the previous distal cut is identified. The probe knife is inserted into the proximal portal and is drawn toward the level of the previous distal cut with its blunt tip touching the underside of the transverse carpal ligament, just before the beginning of the distal cut (Fig. 34-11). From that point, the blunt edge of the knife is used to retract the thick bursal membrane, which sheaths the proximal portion of the carpal ligament, distally to proximally along the ligament's undersurface (see Fig. 34-11). After the cutting edge of the knife has engaged the proximal border of the ligament, the knife is advanced distally to make an incision that joins the previous cut, accomplishing the release of the transverse carpal ligament (see Fig. 34-11). This is a slight modification of the technique in which the retrograde knife is used to complete the release of the ligament.[31,39] The thick bursal membrane contains small vessels, and it should be preserved to avoid bleeding into the carpal canal. The slotted cannula is gently rotated about a few degrees, clockwise and counterclockwise sequentially, enabling the surgeon to view the edges of the transected carpal ligament. If additional fibers remain, the triangle knife, or any other knife that feels appropriate, can be used to release these fibers until the surgeon is satisfied.

Because of the position of the patient's hand, the cut edges of the transverse carpal ligament should spring apart and disappear from the slotted opening of the cannula. If the edges can still be seen through the opening, the release is incomplete. While the assistant fully abducts the patient's thumb, the uncut portion of the ligament can be identified, and the surgeon can complete the transection.

Only one suture is required for closure of each portal. Immediately after the procedure, the surgeon should clinically examine the patient while still in a sterilized environment. If there is any dysfunction indicating intraoperative damage to the median nerve or tendons, exposure and exploration of the carpal tunnel can be performed at that time.

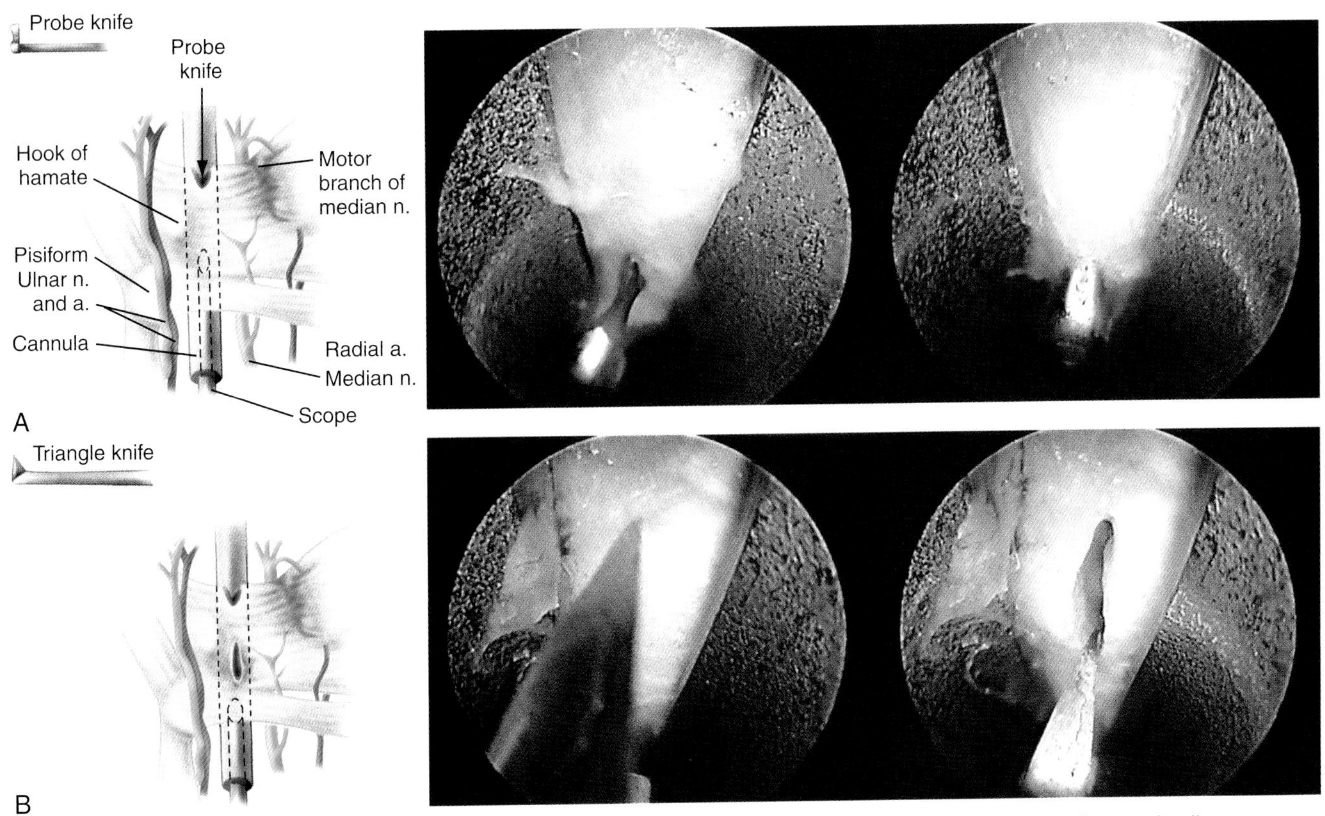

FIGURE 34-9 A, After the distal border of the transverse carpal ligament is identified, the probe knife is used to make the first cut distally to proximally. **B,** The scope is withdrawn proximally about 1 cm, and the triangle knife is used to make a small cut in the midsection of the transverse carpal ligament.

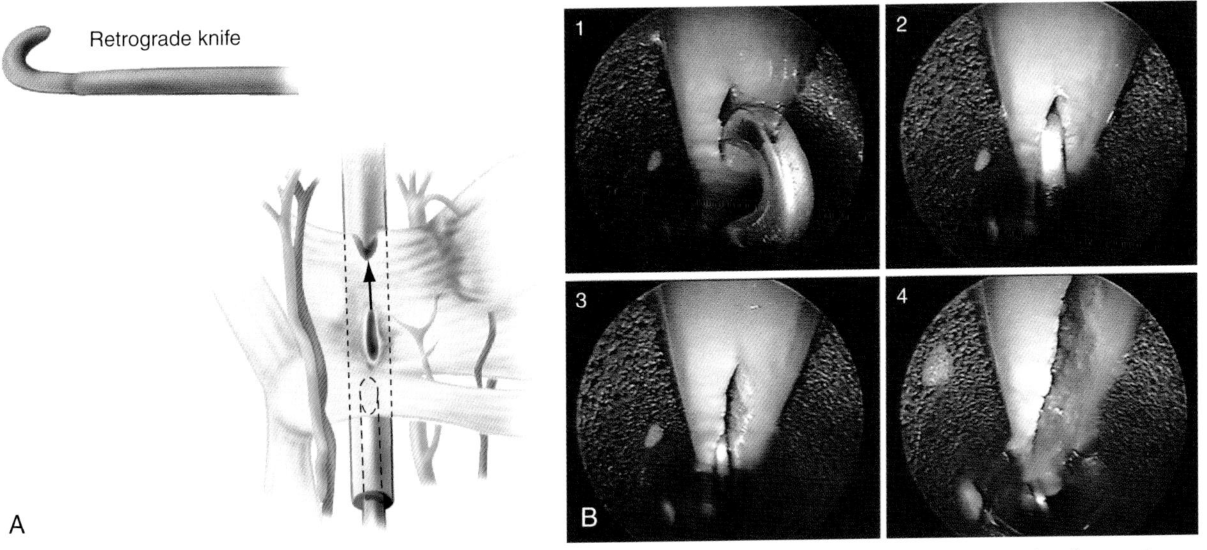

FIGURE 34-10 A and **B,** The retrograde knife is placed in the incision made by the triangle knife (B1, B2). It is drawn distally to make an incision that joins the previous two cuts (B3, B4).

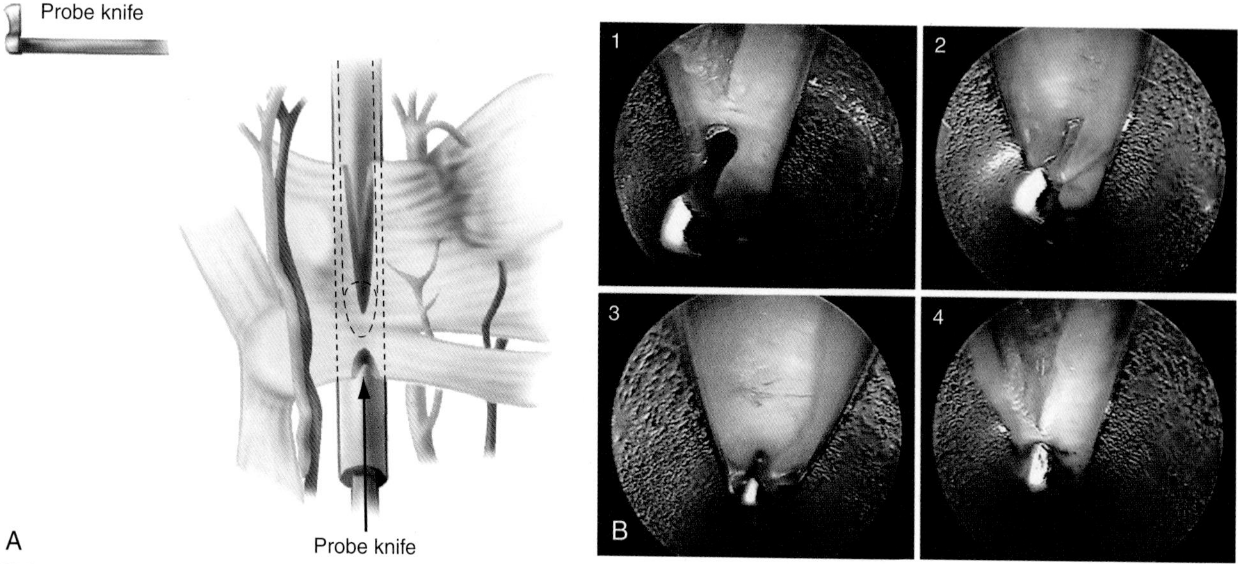

FIGURE 34-11 A and **B,** After the scope has been switched from the proximal to the distal opening of the slotted cannula, the tip of the probe knife is placed just before the beginning of the distal cut (B1). From that point, the knife's blunt edge is used to retract the thick bursal membrane distally to proximally (B2). After the knife has engaged to the proximal border of transverse carpal ligament, it is advanced distally to complete the release of the ligament (B3, B4).

PEARLS & PITFALLS

PEARLS

- When administering local anesthetic, preference is given to the subcutaneous regions proximally at the entry portal and distally at the exit portal. These are the areas of greatest pressure from the slotted cannula.
- To best visualize the fibers of the transverse carpal ligament, the light source often must be dimmed. Chow routinely turns off the "auto" function on his light source and dims it according to the available picture. This can markedly improve visualization and thereby increase the safety of the procedure.
- Because of the symmetric nature of the visual field, it is easy to lose orientation when operating through the slotted cannula. To avoid this, Chow always introduces instrumentation into the cannula with the blade facing ulnarly.
- It is safest to not use a tourniquet. This allows palpation of the ulnar artery before the skin incision for the entry portal is made, so that the ulnar neurovascular bundle can be protected.
- If necessary, the assistant can provide direct pressure to the palm between the two portals over the slotted cannula to control bleeding during the operation.

PITFALLS

- As with any endoscopic procedure, visualization is paramount. Regardless of the circumstance, if the surgeon is unable to obtain a clear view of the undersurface of the carpal ligament, the endoscopic procedure should be abandoned.
- A common pitfall is ulnar placement of the entry portal. To avoid this situation, the following steps should be taken:
  1. Watch the entire width of the wrist to ensure the central location of the entry portal.
  2. Make sure that the landmarks of the entry and exit portals are aligned along the long axis of forearm.
  3. Palpate and mark the hook of the hamate. Both portals should be located radially to the hook.
  4. During the entire procedure, surgical instruments that are introduced in the wrist and hand should follow the long axis of the forearm.

Postoperative Rehabilitation

Active range of motion is encouraged immediately after the effects of local anesthesia have subsided. The patient is advised to avoid heavy lifting or pressure on the palm region until the discomfort disappears, usually in 2 to 3 weeks. Active movement of the fingers decreases the formation of scar tissue in the wrist region, preventing adhesions on the tendons and nerves at the surgical site. Sutures are removed after 1 week. If the patient engages in hard occupational activities, such as heavy lifting, too soon after surgery, there may be swelling and prolonged pain in the palm region. If these occur, fluidized therapy (Fluidotherapy) for 20 minutes daily helps to decrease these symptoms within 1 week.

COMPLICATIONS

Several complications after ECTR by the Chow technique have been reported in the literature. Nagle and colleagues[28] performed a multicenter, prospective review study on a total of 640 cases. The initial transbursal technique was used in 110 cases, and the modified extrabursal technique was used in 530 cases. An overall (perioperative and late) complication rate of 11% was found with the transbursal technique, compared with 2.2% with the extrabursal technique. In 21 (3.3%) of the 640 cases, perioperative complications occurred. Fourteen of these 21 cases involved neurapraxia, all of which resolved without sequelae, and no nerves were lacerated or transected. One laceration of the superficial flexor tendon of the ring and small fingers, four incomplete releases, and one case with hematoma, and one laceration of the superior palmar arch were reported. Late complications included three cases of reflex sympathetic dystrophy (0.5%). This complication resolved in all cases without the use of sympathetic nerve blocks. The study authors concluded that ECTR performed by the extrabursal, dual-portal technique reliably decompresses the carpal tunnel and can be effectively performed with low perioperative and late complication rates.

Malek and Chow,[24] in a national study of the complications of 10,246 procedures in 9562 patients treated with the dual-portal Chow technique, found a complication rate of 2.3% (240 cases with complications were reported). Of these, there were 154 nerve-related complications (i.e., median or ulnar nerve neurapraxias, lacerations, or transections), 38 complications related to blood vessels, 15 tendon injuries, 18 incomplete releases of the transverse carpal ligament, and 6 cases of reflex sympathetic dystrophy. The remaining 9 cases were listed as miscellaneous complications, including hematoma and superficial wound infection. Most of the intraoperative nerve injuries occurred in cases in which general or regional anesthesia was used.

The reported complication rates of ECTR compare favorably with published series of open carpal tunnel release. Complications of the latter include incomplete ligament release, nerve injuries, palmar hematomas, bowstringing of the flexor tendons, adhesions between nerves and tendons, reflex sympathetic dystrophy, deep wound infections, scar tenderness, pillar pain, tendon lacerations, and vascular injuries.[40-48] The damage to the surrounding anatomic structures that occurs during open or endoscopic carpal tunnel surgery usually requires a second surgical procedure to be repaired.

OUTCOMES

Chow has successfully performed more than 4350 ECTR procedures since September 1987. During the past 21 years, his experience has included a failure rate of 0.83% (36 cases), a complication rate of 0.11% (5 cases), and a recurrence rate of 0.41% (18 cases). He converted two (0.045%) endoscopic procedures to open procedures. There were no instances of laceration or transection of any neural, vascular, or tendinous structure during treatment of 4353 hands. Superficial infection in the proximal surgical wound (entry portal) developed in three cases and was treated with oral antibiotics and local wound care.

Chow has encountered the anatomic variant of an extreme ulnar transligamental motor branch of the median nerve in 24 cases (0.55%), or approximately 1 of every 200 patients (Fig. 34-12). This variant is easily visualized and accommodated only by ECTR. This anatomic variant is thought to account for the higher rate of nerve injury and nerve-related complications reported for the open procedure.

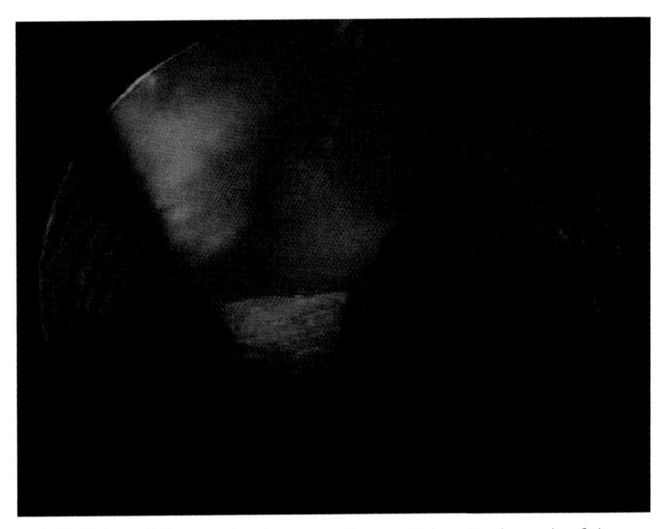

FIGURE 34-12 Extremely ulnar transligamental motor branch of the median nerve.

CONCLUSIONS

The advantages of endoscopic over open carpal tunnel release include no hypertrophic scar or scar tenderness, no pillar pain, less compromise to the pinch or grip strength, and an earlier return to work and daily activities. However, the surgeon may face unexpected difficulties (e.g., ganglion, neurofibroma, neurilemmoma) that limit visualization in the carpal canal. As with any surgical procedure, safety and success depend on a thorough knowledge of the anatomy of the area, adequate training, and familiarity with the instrumentation. Surgeons who are not familiar with endoscopes and arthroscopic techniques may experience major iatrogenic complications.

Data gathered from the experience of past 21 years strongly indicate that, because the normal anatomic structures of the hand (especially the ISTB) are preserved, clinical results of ECTR are better than those of the standard open procedure. ECTR with the Chow dual-portal technique is a reliable method of treating carpal tunnel syndrome and can be performed safely by a well-trained surgeon. Although debate among surgeons still exists, endoscopic release of the transverse carpal ligament has become established as an accepted minimally invasive surgical technique.

REFERENCES

1. Pfeffer GB, Gelberman RH, Boyes JH, Rydevik B. The history of carpal tunnel syndrome. *J Hand Surg Br*. 1988;13:28.
2. Paget J. *Lectures on Surgical Pathology delivered at the Royal College of Surgeons of England*. 2nd American ed. Philadelphia, PA: Lindsay & Blakiston; 1860.
3. Putman JJ. A series of paresthesia, mainly of the hand, of periodical recurrence, and possibly of vaso-motor origin. *Arch Med (New York)*. 1880;4:147-162.
4. Phalen GS, Gardner WJ, Lalonde AA. Neuropathy of the median nerve due to compression beneath the transverse carpal ligament. *J Bone Joint Surg Am*. 1950;32:109-112.
5. Chow JCY. Endoscopic release of the carpal ligament: a new technique for carpal tunnel syndrome. *Arthroscopy*. 1989;5:19-24.
6. Okutsu I, Nonomiya S, Takatori Y, Ugawa Y. Endoscopic management of carpal tunnel syndrome. *Arthroscopy*. 1989;5:11.
7. Agee JM, Tortsua RD, Palmer CA, Berry C. Endoscopic release of the carpal tunnel: a prospective randomized multicenter study. Paper presented at the 45th Annual Meeting of the American Society for Surgery of the Hand, September 24-27, 1990; Toronto, Canada.
8. Viegas S, Pollard A, Kaminski K. Carpal arch alteration and related clinical status after endoscopic carpal tunnel release. *J Hand Surg Am*. 1992;17:1012-1016.

9. Garcia-Elias M, Sanches-Freijo J, Salo J, et al. Dynamic changes of the transverse carpal arch during flexion-extension of the wrist: effects of sectioning the transverse carpal ligament. *J Hand Surg Am*. 1992;17: 1017-1019.
10. Richman JA, Gelberman RH, Rydevik BL, et al. Carpal tunnel syndrome: morphologic changes after release of transverse carpal ligament. *J Hand Surg Am*. 1989;14:852-857.
11. Duncan KH, Lewis RC, Foreman KA, Nordyke MD. Treatment of carpal tunnel syndrome by members of the American Society for Surgery of the Hand: results of a questionnaire. *J Hand Surg Am*. 1987;12:384-391.
12. Phalen GS. The carpal tunnel syndrome: clinical evaluation of 598 hands. *Clin Orthop*. 1972;(83):29-40.
13. Grundberg AB. Carpal tunnel decompression in spite of normal electromyography. *J Hand Surg Am*. 1983;8:348-349.
14. Jackson DA, Clifford JC. Electrodiagnosis of mild carpal tunnel syndrome. *Arch Phys Med Rehabil*. 1989;71:199-204.
15. Cioni R, Passero S, Paradiso C, et al. Diagnostic specificity of sensory and motor nerve conduction variables in early detection of carpal tunnel syndrome. *J Neurol*. 1989;236:208-213.
16. Chow JC, Weiss MA, Gu Y. Anatomic variations of the hook of hamate and the relationship to carpal tunnel syndrome. *J Hand Surg Am*. 2005; 30:1242-1247.
17. Murphy RX, Chernofsky MA, Osborne MA, Wolson AH. Magnetic resonance imaging in the evaluation of persistent carpal tunnel syndrome. *J Hand Surg Am*. 1993;18:113-120.
18. Richman JG, Gelberman RH, Rydevik B, Gylys-Morin V. Carpal tunnel volume determination by magnetic imaging 3-D reconstruction. *J Hand Surg Am*. 1987;12:712.
19. Rotman MB, Manske PR. Anatomical relationships of an endoscopic carpal tunnel device to surrounding structures. *J Hand Surg Am*. 1993; 18:442-450.
20. Seiler JG III, Barnes K, Gelberman RH, Chalidapong P. Endoscopic carpal tunnel release: an anatomic study of the two-incision method in human cadavers. *J Hand Surg Am*. 1992;17:996-1002.
21. Schwartz JT, Waters PM, Simmons BP. Endoscopic carpal tunnel release: a cadaveric study. *Arthroscopy*. 1993;9:209-213.
22. Chow JCY, Malek M, Nagle D. Complications of endoscopic release of the carpal ligament using the Chow technique. Paper presented at the 47th Annual Meeting of the American Society for Surgery of the Hand, November 11-24, 1992; Phoenix, AZ.
23. Chow JCY, Malek MM. Complications of endoscopic release of the carpal ligament using the Chow technique. Paper presented at the 60th Annual Meeting of the American Academy of Orthopaedic Surgeons, February 18-23, 1993; San Francisco, CA.
24. Malek MM, Chow JCY. National study of the complications of over 10,000 cases of endoscopic carpal tunnel release. Paper presented at the 61st Annual Meeting of the American Academy of Orthopaedic Surgeons, February 24–March 1, 1994; New Orleans, LA.
25. Chow JC, Hantes ME. Endoscopic carpal tunnel release: thirteen years' experience with the Chow technique. *J Hand Surg*. 2002;27:1011-1018.
26. Chow JCY. Endoscopic release of the carpal ligament for carpal tunnel syndrome: 22-month clinical results. *Arthroscopy*. 1990;6:288-296.
27. Nagle DJ, Fischer T, Hastings H, et al. A multicenter prospective study of 640 endoscopic carpal tunnel releases using the Chow extrabursal technique. Paper presented at the 47th Annual Meeting of the American Society for Surgery of the Hand, November 11-14, 1992; Phoenix, AZ.
28. Nagle D, Fischer T, Harris G, et al. A multi-center prospective review of 640 endoscopic carpal tunnel releases using the Chow technique. *Arthroscopy*. 1996;12:139-143.
29. Chow JCY. The Chow technique of endoscopic release of the carpal ligament for carpal tunnel syndrome: four years of clinical results. *Arthroscopy*. 1993;9:301-314.
30. Chow JCY. Endoscopic carpal tunnel release. *Clin Sports Med*. 1996;15: 769-784.
31. Chow JCY. Endoscopic carpal tunnel release. In: Chow JCY, ed. *Advanced Arthroscopy*. New York, NY: Springer-Verlag; 2001:271-286.
32. Mannerfelt L, Hybbinette CH. Important anomaly of the thenar motor branch of the median nerve. *Bull Hosp Joint Dis*. 1972;33:15.
33. Caffee HH. Anomalous thenar muscle and median nerve: a case report. *J Hand Surg*. 1979;4:446.
34. Ogden J. An unusual branch of the median nerve. *J Bone Joint Surg Am*. 1972;54:1779-1781.
35. Papathanassiou BT. A variant of the motor branch of the median nerve in the hand. *J Bone Joint Surg Br*. 1968;50:156.
36. Lanz U. Anatomical variations of the median nerve in the carpal tunnel. *J Hand Surg Am*. 1977;2:44.
37. Johnson RK, Shrewsbury MM. Anatomical course of the thenar branch of the median nerve, usually in a separate tunnel through the transverse carpal ligament. *J Bone Joint Surg Am*. 1970;52:269.
38. Seradge H, Seradge E. Median innervated hypothenar muscle: anomalous branch of median nerve in the carpal tunnel. *J Hand Surg Am*. 1990;15: 356-359.
39. Chow JCY. Carpal tunnel release. In: McGinty JB, ed. *Operative Arthroscopy*. 3rd ed. Philadelphia, PA: Lippincott Williams & Wilkins; 2003: 798-818.
40. Das SK, Brown HG. In search of complications in carpal tunnel decompression. *Hand*. 1976;8:243-249.
41. MacDonald RI, Lictman DM, Hanlon JJ, et al. Complications of surgical release for carpal tunnel syndrome. *J Hand Surg*. 1978;3:70-76.
42. Lilly CJ, Magnell TD. Severance of the thenar branch of the median nerve as a complication of carpal tunnel release. *J Hand Surg Am*. 1985; 10:399-402.
43. Louis DS, Green TL, Noellert RC. Complications of carpal tunnel surgery. *J Neurol*. 1985;62:352-355.
44. Kessler FB. Complications of the management of carpal tunnel syndrome. *Hand Clin*. 1986;2:401-406.
45. Gartsman GM, Kovach JC, Crouch CC, et al. Carpal arch alteration after carpal tunnel release. *J Hand Surg Am*. 1986;11:372-374.
46. Terrino AL, Belskey MR, Feldon PG, et al. Injury to the deep motor branch of the ulnar nerve during carpal tunnel release. *J Hand Surg Am*. 1993;18:1038-1040.
47. May JW, Rosen H. Division of the sensory ramus communicans between the ulnar median nerves: a complication following carpal tunnel release. *J Bone Surg Am*. 1981;63:836.
48. Brown RA, Gelberman RH, Seiler JG III, et al. Carpal tunnel release: a prospective randomized assessment of open and endoscopic methods. *J Bone Joint Surg Am*. 1993;75:1265-1275.

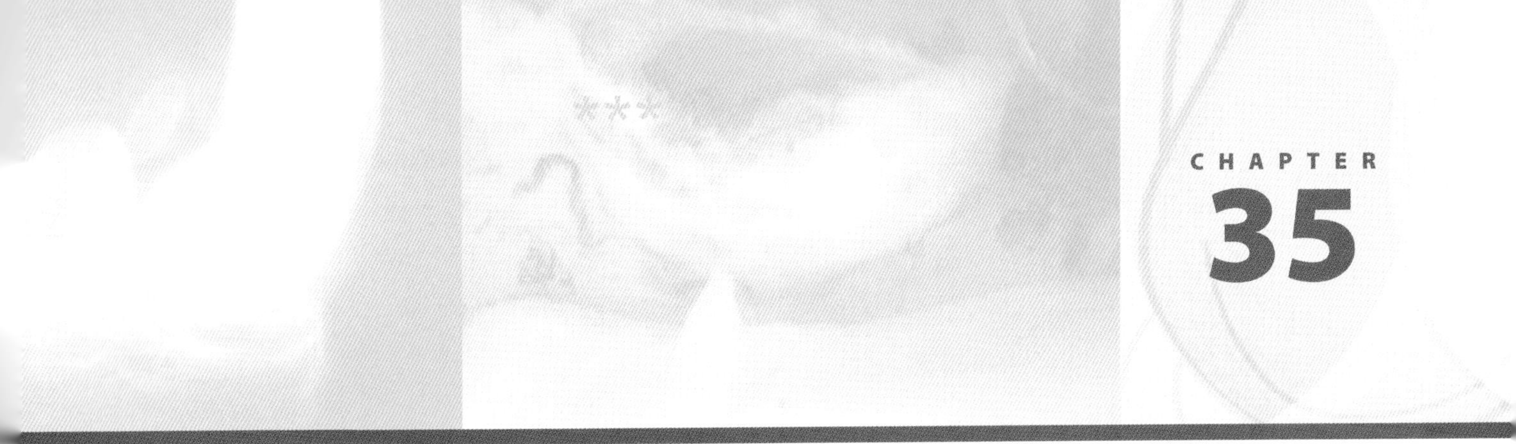

Wrist Arthroscopy: The Future

Adam C. Watts • Gregory I. Bain • Kush Shrestha • Justin Alexander

Wrist arthroscopy, first described by Chen in 1979,[1] was popularized by Roth and colleagues in an instructional course lecture of the American Academy of Orthopaedic Surgeons almost a decade later.[2] Since then, it has undergone substantial developments and has become an essential diagnostic and therapeutic tool for surgeons addressing a multitude of conditions affecting the wrist.

With improved techniques and equipment, procedures that were once performed as open surgery can be undertaken arthroscopically. Although initial therapeutic wrist arthroscopy focused on basic reparative procedures, some of the more complex reconstructive and salvage procedures are being performed with this procedure (Table 35-1), and the indications for wrist arthroscopy continue to expand. This chapter reviews some of the latest advances and discusses future directions for wrist arthroscopy.

ASSESSMENT

Arthroscopic examination of the wrist should include the radiocarpal and midcarpal joints and, if indicated, the distal radioulnar joint (DRUJ). Visualization of the pisotriquetral joint can be achieved through a fenestration communicating with the radiocarpal joint (which is present in approximately 50% of the population).[3] Traditionally, dorsal 3-4, 4-5, 6-R, and midcarpal portals have been used as diagnostic and working portals (Table 35-2). These portals limit access to the dorsal wrist capsule and impose restrictions on the surgeon's ability to treat dorsal pathology. The development of volar portals[4-6] has provided freedom to explore newer arthroscopic techniques to address certain pathologic conditions such as dorsal wrist ganglion[7] or capsular restriction.[8]

TABLE 35-1 Expanding Indications for Wrist Arthroscopy

Procedures	Soft Tissue	Bone
Diagnostic	Wrist pain of unknown origin Synovial biopsy	Assessment of instability Staging of Kienböck's disease Staging before limited wrist fusion
Removal ("ectomy")	Bacterial sampling, drainage and joint lavage Dorsal and volar ganglia Intraosseous ligaments Synovectomy TFCC tears Articular cartilage lesions Volar capsular release Dorsal capsular release	Distal pole of scaphoid Distal ulnar (wafer procedure) Hamate Lunate Os central carpi Pisiform Proximal pole of scaphoid Proximal row carpectomy STT débridement Ulnar styloid
Stabilization	Dorsal radiocarpal ligament Lunotriquetral instability Scapholunate instability TFCC suture Radiofrequency capsule or ligament shrinkage	Distal radius fractures Perilunate dislocation Scaphoid fractures Scapholunate instability
Reconstructive	Scapholunate ligament reconstruction DRUJ stabilization	Bone graft to scaphoid non-union Limited wrist fusion Full wrist fusion
Salvage		Proximal row carpectomy Limited wrist fusion Total wrist fusion

DRUJ, distal radioulnar joint; STT, scaphotrapeziotrapezoid; TFCC, triangular fibrocartilage complex.

TABLE 35-2 Arthroscopic Wrist Portals: Technique and Comment

Portals	Technique	Comment
Dorsal Portals		
1-2	Inserted in the extreme dorsum of the snuffbox just radial to the EPL tendon to avoid the radial artery[48,49]	Gives access to the radial styloid, scaphoid, lunate, and articular surface of the distal radius
3-4	Portal is 1 cm distal to Lister's tubercle between the tendons of the third and fourth compartment	Main working portal; gives a wide range of movement and view
4-5	Between the common extensor fourth compartment and the EI in the fifth compartment	Usually, the 6-R portal is preferred
6-R	Located distal to the ulnar head and radial to the ECU tendon; portal is established under direct vision through the arthroscope with a needle and avoids damage to the TFCC	Main working portal
6-U	Established under direct vision, similar to the 6-R portal; always use blunt dissection to avoid the dorsal branches of the ulnar nerve	6-U and 6-R portals allow visualization back toward the radial side and access to the ulna-sided structures
DRUJ	Forearm supinated to relax the dorsal capsule; arthroscope is introduced into the axilla between radius and ulna underneath the TFCC	Gives a view of the DRUJ articulation
Midcarpal Portals		
MCR	Soft depression palpated between proximal and distal carpal rows, 1 cm distal to the 3-4 portal along a line bordering the radial edge of the third metacarpal	Can be used to get across to the STT joint, scapholunate articulation, and distal pole of scaphoid
MCU	Soft depression palpated between proximal and distal carpal rows 1 cm distal to 4-5 portal and in line with the fourth metacarpal	Allows visualization of the distal lunate, lunotriquetral, and triquetral hamate articulation
STT	Between EPL and ECRB in the midcarpal row; on the ulnar margin of the EPL tendon; terminal branches of the radial sensory nerve are at risk	Used with the MCR portal for STT débridement
Volar Portals		
VR	A 2-cm longitudinal incision is made over the FCR on radial side of volar proximal wrist crease, and the FCR is retracted ulnarly. Radiocarpal joint is identified with a needle, and the port is expanded with artery forceps.[3] An inside-out technique also can be used. Work between the RSC and LR ligaments, staying to the radial side of the FCR tendon to avoid the median nerve.[2]	Safe zone of 3 mm in all directions with respect to the palmar cutaneous branch of the median nerve (ulnarly) and radial artery (radially)[2,3]
VU	A 2-cm longitudinal incision is made; the FCU is identified and retracted ulnarly with the ulnar nerve. Working in the interval between the FCU and common flexor tendons, inserting needle into the joint and then expanding the area with an artery forceps[4]	Both volar portals are used to assist in reduction of distal radius fracture and to view the dorsal articular surface and dorsal ligaments
DRUJ	Use the same mini-open approach as for a VU portal; take care to stay below the TFCC	Gives a view of the DRUJ and deep-sided TFCC tears

DRUJ, distal radioulnar joint; ECRB, extensor carpi radialis brevis; ECRL, extensor carpi radialis longus; ECU, extensor carpi ulnaris; EDC, extensor digitorum communis; EI, extensor indicis; EPB, extensor pollicis brevis; EPL, extensor pollicis longus; FCR, flexor carpi radialis; FCU, flexor carpi ulnaris; LR, long radiolunate; MCR, midcarpal radial; MCU, midcarpal ulnar; RSC, radioscaphocapitate ligament; STT, scaphotrapeziotrapezoid; TFCC, triangular fibrocartilage complex; VR, volar radial; VU, volar ulnar.
From Bain GI, Munt J, Turner PC. New advances in wrist arthroscopy. Arthroscopy. *2008;24:355-367.*

The wrist can be visualized as a box with access through four sides (Fig. 35-1). The arthroscope can be introduced to provide the optimal view of pathology, and any number of portals can be used for instrumentation. The use of multiple portals does not increase the surgical insult significantly as long as standard precautions are taken to protect soft tissue structures, but it can ensure that the surgeon has optimal placement of instruments and the arthroscope.

Most investigators describe arthroscopy of the wrist in a manner similar to large joint arthroscopy, with infiltration of the joint with fluid (i.e., lactated Ringer's solution). Dry arthroscopy of the wrist has not been associated with undue procedural difficulty.[9] It provides a different perspective of tissue and chondral surfaces. Other benefits of the dry technique include a decreased risk of compartment syndrome and the availability of dry tissue planes in the event of conversion to open surgery. The main role of dry wrist arthroscopy is in the management of intra-articular distal radial fractures,[10] but indications may broaden to include carpal fracture management and other reconstructive procedures.

The value of arthroscopy can be augmented by the use of fluoroscopy, which enables accurate intraosseous placement of drills and implants. It also can be used to confirm reduction of fractures or joint diastasis.[11]

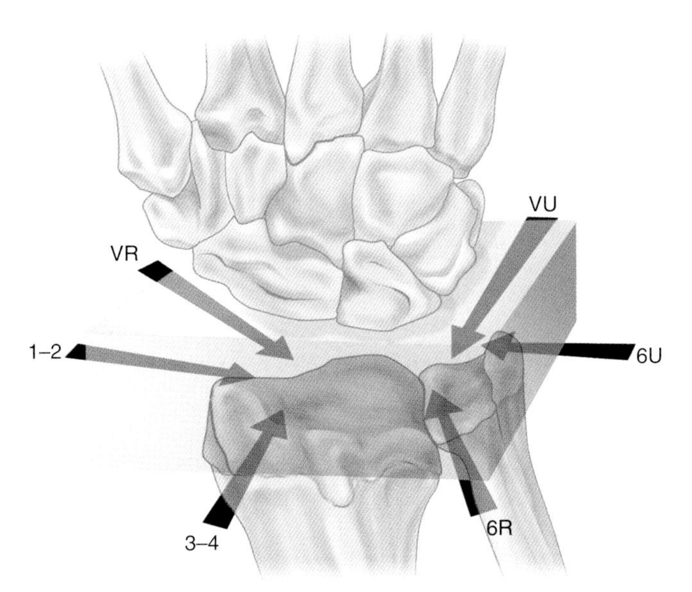

FIGURE 35-1 The box concept of wrist arthroscopy. *(Modified from Bain GI, Munt J, Turner PC. New advances in wrist arthroscopy.* Arthroscopy. *2008; 24:355-367.)*

> **PEARLS & PITFALLS**
>
> **PEARLS**
> - The use of multiple portals can facilitate technically demanding procedures.
> - Dry arthroscopy can be performed if there is concern about fluid extravasation.
> - Fluoroscopy can assist in the assessment of joint stability, reduction, and positioning of implants.
>
> **PITFALLS**
> - Some portals, such as the 1-2 portal, should be established with a mini-open approach to protect branches of the superficial radial nerve and the dorsal branch of the radial artery.

SPECIFIC AREAS OF ADVANCEMENT

Carpal Instability

Assessment of Instability

Numerous radiologic investigations are used to assess carpal instability, including plain radiographs, fluoroscopy, arthrography, computed tomography (CT), and magnetic resonance imaging (MRI). Although three-compartment arthrography can identify intercarpal ligament perforations, it is inadequate for localizing these lesions.[12] CT is less sensitive than MRI for detecting intercarpal ligament tears and triangular fibrocartilage complex (TFCC) injuries.[13]

Arthroscopy is the gold standard for the diagnosis of carpal instability. It has the benefit of giving surgeons direct visualization of the scapholunate and lunotriquetral ligaments and allows them to assess the state of the ligament, the extent of the ligament injury, and whether it is reparable. Associated problems such as hemorrhage, synovitis, chondral damage, and degenerative changes can be assessed at the time of arthroscopy.

Repair Procedures

Arthroscopic débridement alone has been used in the management of scapholunate interosseous ligament (SLIL) and lunotriquetral interosseous ligament (LTIL) injuries. Good results have been achieved from arthroscopic débridement of partial tears of the SLIL and LTIL.[14,15] Weiss and colleagues described arthroscopic débridement as sole treatment for complete tears of the SLIL and LTIL.[15]

There has been interest in the use of ligament and capsular thermal shrinkage in the treatment of interosseous ligament injuries, and early results are promising. Good results have been achieved with arthroscopic débridement and thermal shrinkage of Geissler grade I or II injuries (Table 35-3).[16-18] Battistella and coworkers compared outcomes of débridement alone and thermal shrinkage as a sole treatment of Geissler I SLIL injuries.[19] They also compared the results of débridement and pinning with those of thermal shrinkage and pinning for Geissler II and III injuries. In both comparisons, superior outcomes were achieved with thermal shrinkage.[19] However, the use of thermal shrinkage techniques remains controversial, and no long-term studies have been published to confirm its safety and efficacy.

In patients with significant instability (Geissler grades II through IV), arthroscopic débridement and percutaneous pinning have produced mixed results.[20-22] Whipple's series supported the concept that the chronicity of the lesion and the degree of instability affect the eventual outcomes.[20] In that study, SLIL tears were treated with arthroscopically assisted reduction and percutaneous pinning, and outcomes were compared for patients with less than 3 months' history and less than 3 mm of scapholunate displacement and for those with symptoms of more than 3 months' duration and more than 3 mm of displacement. Eighty-five percent of patients in the first group maintained comfort and stability at 2 to 7 years, and 53% of patients in the second group remained symptom free at 1 to 3 years.

The reduction-association scapholunate (RASL) procedure is often performed as an open procedure for chronic scapholunate

TABLE 35-3 Geissler Arthroscopic Classification of Carpal Instability

Grade	Description
I	Attenuation or hemorrhage of interosseous ligament as seen from the radiocarpal joint. No incongruence of carpal alignment in the midcarpal space.
II	Attenuation or hemorrhage of interosseous ligament as seen from the radiocarpal joint. Incongruence or step-off as seen from midcarpal space. A slight gap (less than width of a probe) between the carpal bones may be present.
III	Incongruence or step-off of carpal alignment is seen in the radiocarpal and midcarpal space. The probe may be passed through the gap between the carpal bones.
IV	Incongruence or step-off of carpal alignment is seen in the radiocarpal and midcarpal space. There is gross instability with manipulation. A 2.7-mm arthroscope may be passed through the gap between the carpal bones.

From Geissler WB. Intra-articular distal radius fractures: The role of arthroscopy. Hand Clin. *2005;21:407-416.*

instability. An arthroscopically assisted method of RASL has been described, with arthroscopy facilitating anatomic reduction and precise placement of the cannulated screw, with the advantage of a three-portal rather than a two-incision approach.[23]

The future role of arthroscopy in treating carpal instability is likely to include arthroscopically assisted tendon graft reconstruction procedures, such as the modified Brunelli procedure.[24]

Preferred Technique

Alexander has performed an arthroscopically assisted scapholunate ligament reconstruction; however, research continues in this area. The procedure is performed in four stages. The flexor carpi radialis (FCR) tendon is split, and one half of the tendon is harvested through three small transverse incisions at the wrist and forearm. The distal attachment is maintained.

The second step is to pass the ligament through the scaphoid. This can be performed by passing a guidewire percutaneously from the palpable scaphoid tubercle through to the dorsum of the scaphoid with fluoroscopic guidance. Alternatively, the guidewire can be introduced into the radiocarpal joint through a volar radial portal created with the use of an inside-out technique, after which the wire is walked distally onto the distal pole of the scaphoid with arthroscopic guidance and then advanced through to the dorsum of the scaphoid with fluoroscopic control. The guidewire is overdrilled with a 3.5-mm cannulated drill. A Beath pin, which is passed through this bone tunnel to the 3-4 portal, is used to pass the FCR graft through the scaphoid.

In the third step, the graft must be positioned across the dorsum of the scapholunate and lunotriquetral joints. To do this, the FCR graft is passed between the capsule and the fourth and fifth extensor compartments, using the blunt end of a Mayo needle or a fine artery clip, to the 6-R portal. The graft is passed to the midcarpal ulnar portal under a slip of dorsal wrist capsule with the reversed Mayo needle or clip and then to the midcarpal radial portal in the extracapsular layer. The Mayo needle is passed out of the skin on the radial side of the wrist. The graft can then be tensioned.

The fourth step is to stabilize the scapholunate interval and secure the graft. Alexander has used two 1.6-mm Kirschner wires passed under fluoroscopic control from the scaphoid to the lunate. Other options include an arthroscopically assisted RASL procedure and the use of Opus suture anchors (ArthroCare Corporation, Austin, TX). The graft can also be secured with the Opus anchors. If there is a marked dorsal intercalated segment instability (DISI) deformity, 1.6-mm Kirschner wires can be introduced under fluoroscopic guidance and used as joysticks for reduction of the osseous elements. Eight weeks of cast immobilization is recommended.

For advanced carpal collapse with degenerative changes, salvage procedures, including proximal row carpectomy, limited wrist fusion, or total wrist fusion, may be indicated. These procedures have been performed arthroscopically, although not routinely. Arthroscopic proximal row carpectomy was first described in 1997.[25] Ho described techniques for arthroscopic limited wrist fusion and applied these techniques to scaphotrapeziotrapezoid (STT) fusion, scaphoidectomy and four-corner fusion, radioscapholunate fusion, radiolunate fusion, and lunotriquetral fusion.[26] The common steps include assessment of radiocarpal and midcarpal articular surfaces to ensure that the joints to be preserved have articular cartilage that can maintain normal wrist movement and loading; cartilage denudation with an arthroscopic burr; correction of carpal deformity with joysticks; provisional fixation with Kirschner wires under fluoroscopic control; arthroscopic bone grafting using autogenous graft or bone graft substitutes introduced through the arthroscope cannula; and definitive fixation with cannulated compression screws. Ho described the use of Foley catheters at the time of grafting to contain graft in the joints where it is wanted. In the future, this may become mainstream practice.

PEARLS & PITFALLS

PEARLS

- Thermal shrinkage may help in the treatment of Geissler grade I, II, and III lesions.
- Good fluid inflow and outflow is required to dissipate excess thermal energy.

PITFALLS

- Lesions present for longer than 3 months are associated with poorer outcomes, compared with those treated within 3 months, rega rdless of treatment method.
- After thermal shrinkage, the biomechanical strength of collagen is reduced for 6 to 12 weeks, and restretching of the collagen fibers can occur if the joint is not immobilized after the procedure.
- Reported complications of thermal shrinkage include tendon rupture, damage to hyaline cartilage, and skin burns.

Midcarpal Instability

Midcarpal instability (MCI) is a poorly understood entity, and there is no consensus on underlying pathomechanics, nomenclature, or optimal treatment.[27] It is characterized by pain and clicking in the wrist, especially during ulnar deviation (i.e., dart thrower's motion). This can be reproduced clinically under video fluoroscopy; abnormal movement at the midcarpal joint is observed and results in dynamic displacement of the distal carpal row (volarly or dorsally), as described by Lichtman and colleagues.[28] The importance of the dorsal radiocarpal ligament and the ulnar arm of the volar arcuate ligament has been demonstrated in anatomic and biomechanical studies.

Management of MCI has been based largely on nonoperative measures, including analgesia, activity modification, and splinting. Operative management techniques have included various soft tissue reconstruction procedures, which have enjoyed limited success, and limited carpal fusion as a salvage procedure.

Arthroscopic thermal shrinkage "capsulorrhaphy" has been described.[29] In Mason and Hargreave's study, 13 patients (15 wrists) were treated for palmar midcarpal instability with arthroscopic thermal shrinkage of the ulnar and radial arms of the arcuate ligament and the accessible parts of the dorsal capsule at the radiocarpal and midcarpal levels.[29] Clinical instability improved in all patients postoperatively, as did functional scores. These were early reports, and larger trials with consistent surgical techniques are needed before this technique can be adopted more widely.

PEARLS & PITFALLS

PEARLS

- A volar radial portal may be useful for access to the dorsal radiocarpal ligament.

PITFALLS

- A static VISI deformity and combined palmar and dorsal MCI are not amenable to arthroscopic treatment.

Triangular Fibrocartilage Complex Lesions

One of the major areas of interest in wrist arthroscopy is the diagnosis and treatment of TFCC tears. Arthroscopy is the gold standard for investigation of a suspected TFCC tear; with this technique, the size of the TFCC lesion, its effect on DRUJ stability, and associated synovitis and chondral or ligament lesions can be assessed.

The role of arthroscopy goes well beyond diagnosis of TFCC tears, and several techniques have been described for the treatment of injuries in this region. When assessing the technical options, Palmer's classification, which separates tears into degenerative and traumatic lesions, should be considered. Most interest is focused on the management of traumatic injury to the TFCC, and as our understanding of the anatomy of the TFCC improves, the role of the TFCC in DRUJ stability will be more clearly defined.

Type 1b TFCC lesions are described as tears from the distal ulna attachment with or without ulnar styloid fracture. The dorsal and volar radioulnar ligaments have two elements, superficial (distal) and deep (proximal). Various arthroscopic techniques have been described for repair of a superficial tear by suture ligation to the extensor carpi ulnaris (ECU) subsheath and joint capsule. One study looked at the use of holmium:yttrium-aluminium-garnet (Ho:YAG) laser to treat traumatic TFCC lesions, primarily Palmer type 1a central disk rupture and meniscal homologue tears. The advantage of using the Ho:YAG laser for débridement in the wrist joint is that surrounding tissue does not become too hot. Heat is transmitted less than 3 mm in water, and flexible probes are available. The reported results for a cohort of 79 patients were promising, but the report provided no comparative sample and no preoperative functional or symptom data to validate the results.[30] Further work is required in this interesting area, including comparison with conventional techniques of arthroscopic débridement.

Injury to the deep elements of the radioulnar ligaments most commonly occurs at the foveal insertion, although radial avulsion has been described. These elements form important primary ligamentous stabilizers of the DRUJ.[31] Volar or dorsal dislocation of the ulnar head may be seen, depending on the additional stabilizers that are injured, and is likely to be related to the position of the wrist at the time of injury.

The patient typically complains of ulnar-sided wrist pain after a fall onto an outstretched hand or a violent twisting injury. Clicking may be experienced on forearm rotation. Tenderness may be elicited by palpation over the fovea with the arm in full supination. The deep TFCC lesion may be diagnosed on MRI with gadolinium contrast. In our practice, if clinical examination indicates instability of the DRUJ, a CT scan is performed with the wrist in full supination and in full pronation to assess the osseous architecture of the sigmoid notch and the instability of the ulnar head.[32] Further assessment can be performed at the time of arthroscopy. With the arthroscope in the 3-4 portal, the trampoline test can be performed to assess the taughtness of the TFCC. Another useful test is to pass a hook probe through the 6-R portal and under the TFCC through the ulnar-sided tear; if the deep elements are disrupted, the TFCC can be pulled upward and radially.[33] DRUJ arthroscopy can be used to directly assess the deep elements of the TFCC and to examine the chondral surface of the distal ulna. A classification specific to traumatic peripheral tears has been described that may guide treatment (Table 35-4).

The important elements that guide treatment decisions are the anatomic structures injured (i.e., distal or proximal elements, or both), the chronicity or retraction of the tear (i.e., how reparable it is), and the presence of arthrosis. For class 1 reparable distal element tears, arthroscopic suture ligation is acceptable. Atzei and colleagues described a technique for treatment of class 2 and 3 reparable complete and deep tears.[33] It employed a suture anchor placed in the fovea through a small arthrotomy located 1 cm proximal to the 6-U portal. Positioning of the forearm in full supination moves the styloid dorsally and facilitates access. Curettage and drilling is performed as a mini-open procedure. With arthroscopic assistance, the sutures from the anchor are passed through the TFCC dorsally and palmarly with the aid of a Touhy needle and secured with the use of knot pushers. This technique has produced 95% good or excellent results, as measured with the Mayo wrist score, in 18 patients treated by the originator.[33]

An alternative technique for treatment of reparable Palmer 1b peripheral lesions is the suture welding technique described by Badia and coworkers,[34] who have achieved excellent results in 23 patients. This knotless technique employs an ultrasonic device (Axya Suture Welding System, Axya Inc., Houston, TX) to weld prepositioned 2-0 nylon sutures through the periphery of the TFCC.

Preferred Technique

Our preferred technique for type 2 and 3 lesions, which is also suitable for treatment of type 4 nonreparable deep or combined tears, is a palmaris longus tendon autograft with an arthroscopically assisted mini-open technique that is an extension of the foveal repair concept. The indication for this procedure is DRUJ instability due to a foveal tear. If there is a radial-sided tear, this reconstruction is contraindicated, and an Adams procedure[35] is the preferred reconstructive option.

With the patient under general anesthesia, standard wrist arthroscopy is performed. After the pathology is confirmed by the techniques described earlier, a 3-cm longitudinal incision is made on the subcutaneous border of the distal ulna. The dorsal branch of the ulnar nerve is identified and protected. Dissection is continued to the ulna. A 3.5-mm tunnel is made in the ulna, exiting at the fovea, with the use of a guidewire and a cannulated drill. A Touhy needle is passed through the tunnel from proximal to distal with arthroscopic guidance and pierces the TFCC at the volar margin. Through this, a Prolene loop suture can be introduced and the needle withdrawn, leaving the loop in situ. The

TABLE 35-4 Classification of Peripheral Triangular Fibrocartilage Complex Tears

	Clinical DRUJ Instability	Involved TFCC Component		TFCC Healing Potential	Stratus of DRUJ Cartilage	Treatment
		Distal	Proximal			
Class 1 Repairable *distal tear*	None or slight	Torn	Intact	Good	Good	**Repair** *Suture (Lig-to-capsule)*
Class 2 Repairable complete tear	Mild or severe	Torn	Torn	Good	Good	**Repair** *Foveal refixation*
Class 3 Repairable proximal tear	Mild or Severe	Intact	Torn	Good	Good	
Class 4 Non-repairable	Severe	Torn	Torn	Poor	Good	**Reconstruction** *Tendon graft*
Class 5 Arthritic DRUJ	Mild or severe	§	§	§	Poor	**Salvage** *Arthroplasty or joint replacement*

From Atzei A, Rizzo A, Luchetti R, Fairplay T. Arthroscopic foveal repair of triangular fibrocartilage complex peripheral lesion with distal radioulnar joint instability. Tech Hand Up Extrem Surg. *2008;12:226-235.*

loop can then be delivered through the 6-R portal with sugar tong forceps. The procedure is repeated to place a loop through the dorsal part of the TFCC. If it is available, a palmaris longus graft is then harvested from the ipsilateral forearm.

A plantaris graft is an alternative. Sutures are placed in either end of the graft with a Bunnell technique for grasping the tendon. These sutures are then brought back through the 6-R portal, TFCC, and bone tunnel with the Prolene loop shuttles. Care must be taken to ensure that no soft tissue is interposed between the two at the 6-R portal. A bridge of TFCC must remain between the two limbs as the graft is pulled through the bone tunnel. With an adequate grasp of the TFCC, the two ends of the graft can be tensioned in the bone tunnel and an interference screw inserted to maintain the tension. If there is dorsal instability, the graft is secured and subsequently immobilized in supination. For volar instability, the graft is secured, and the wrist is immobilized in pronation. After wound closure, the patient is placed in a forearm cast for 8 weeks. Results have been promising in the small number of patients treated with this technique, but further investigation is needed, and this remains a technically demanding procedure.

The advantage of this technique over the Adams procedure is that it can be combined with a sigmoid notch osteoplasty when there is an osseous contribution to DRUJ instability.

PEARLS & PITFALLS

PEARLS

- When deciding on the treatment for peripheral TFCC injury, the surgeon must consider the anatomy of the tear, the possibility of repair, and degenerative wear.

PITFALLS

- Failure to address tears of the deep elements of the TFCC will result in persistent DRUJ instability.

Joint-Based Approach to Kienböck's Disease

Lichtman's radiologic classification system provides an assessment of the osseous structure of the lunate. It has been used historically to classify Kienböck's disease, but it proved to have poor reliability.[36] Arthroscopy has the benefit of direct visualization of the pathologic changes through the radiocarpal and midcarpal joints. It enables a joint-based approach to the assessment and management of Kienböck's disease. As reported by Bain and coworkers, plain radiographs often underscore the severity of the articular surface involvement that can be seen arthroscopically.[37]

We developed an arthroscopic classification system for the assessment of Kienböck's disease (Fig. 35-2). It is based on the number of nonfunctional articular surfaces that display extensive

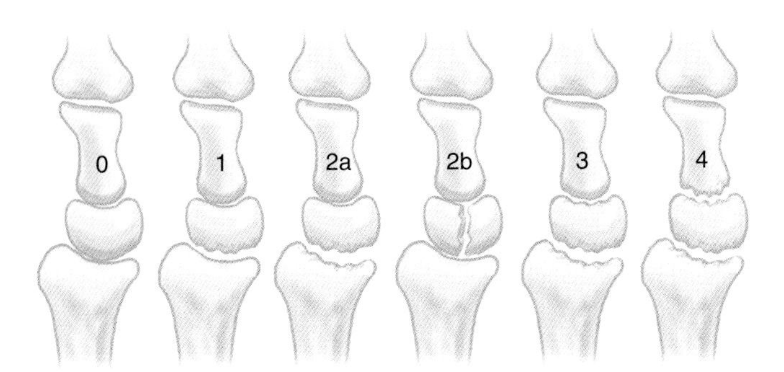

FIGURE 35-2 Arthroscopic classification of Kienböck's disease. The grade for each wrist depends on the number of articular surfaces that are defined as nonfunctional. Grade 0 indicates Kienböck's disease identified on imaging (e.g., a magnetic resonance imaging scan); it may be associated with synovitis identified on wrist arthroscopy, but the articular surfaces are intact. The usual progression of articular damage is from the proximal aspect of the lunate (grade 1) to the lunate facet of the radius (grade 2a). If there is a coronal fracture in the lunate, the proximal and distal aspects of the lunate (grade 2b) will be involved. In grade 3 disease, further progression involves the proximal and distal aspects of the lunate and the lunate facet of the radius. Grade 4 disease involves all four articular surfaces, including the proximal capitate. *(Modified from Bain GI, Begg M. Arthroscopic assessment and classification of Kienböck's disease.* Tech Hand Up Extreme Surg. *2006;10:8-13.)*

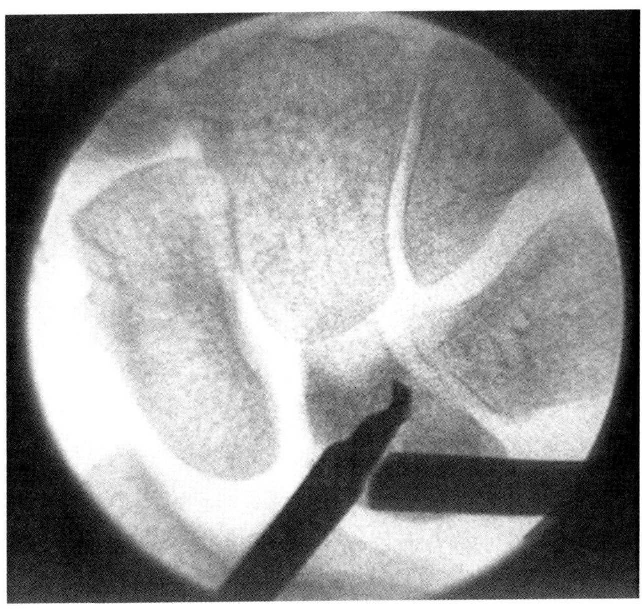

FIGURE 35-3 Core decompression of the lunate for precollapse Kienböck's disease. *(From Bain GI, Smith ML, Watts AC. Arthroscopic assisted forage for Kienböck's disease of the lunate.* J Hand Surg Am. *In press.)*

fibrillation, fissuring, articular cartilage loss, loose articular cartilage fragments, or osteochondral fractures. Although other changes such as synovitis are not included in the classification system, their presence can help indicate the severity of the chondral damage. This joint-based approach provides an algorithm for assessment of the nonfunctioning joints in a wrist with Kienböck's disease, and it guides the reconstructive approach to removal of nonfunctioning articulations and restoration of function through mobilization of the unaffected carpal joints.

Preferred Technique

Our grading system for Kienböck's disease can help guide the management of these cases. Grade 0 disease can be managed with extra-articular procedures such as joint leveling or a revascularization procedure of the lunate. Intraosseous hypertension is a putative cause of Kienböck's disease. Alexander performed a technique of lunate forage (i.e., core biopsy) for the precollapse lunate, and early results were promising. Using a standard wrist arthroscopy setup and fluoroscopic control, the surgeon passes a 2-mm drill into the lunate through the 6-R portal to perform core decompression (Fig. 35-3). Further investigation of this technique is required to assess its efficacy in preventing progression to collapse and arthrosis.

Radioscapholunate fusion can be appropriate treatment for grade 1 or 2a changes, whereas grade 1 or 2b disease can be managed with a proximal row carpectomy. The higher grades of Kienböck's disease (i.e., grades 3 and 4) require salvage procedures, such as wrist arthrodesis or arthroplasty. The use of arthroscopic débridement in the management of this condition was reported in one series to give excellent pain relief and improve the range of motion after 2 years of follow-up.[38]

The future role of arthroscopy in the management of Kienböck's disease is encouraging. Leblebicioglu and colleagues[39] reported in a small, prospective, randomized study that arthroscopic scaphocapitate fusion and capitate pole excision in stage IIIA and IIIB Kienböck's disease resulted in shorter operating time, shorter hospital stay, earlier return to unrestricted daily activities, and equal range of motion and grip strength compared with open scaphocapitate fusion and lunate revascularization.

Ulnar Styloid Carpal Impaction

Ulnar styloid carpal impaction is an uncommon condition that is typically managed with open excision of the ulna styloid.[40] Arthroscopic excision of the ulnar styloid can be successfully performed for stylocarpal impaction.[41] Fluoroscopy can be used to confirm the correct positioning of the burr, which is then used to débride the ulnar styloid under arthroscopic vision. The TFCC is not violated, and recovery is rapid.

Wrist Ganglia

Ganglia can be excised arthroscopically to reduce scarring and to avoid the capsular wrist stiffness associated with an open resection.[42] We have found that rehabilitation is more rapid after arthroscopic excision. Arthroscopy also provides the opportunity to assess any underlying instability of the intrinsic scapholunate ligament, which is implicated as a causative factor for dorsal and volar ganglia.

Initial cohort studies of ganglion excision have been encouraging. Osterman and Raphael reported one recurrence in their series of 150 patients. Rizzo and associates,[43] in their series of 41 patients undergoing arthroscopic resection of a dorsal wrist ganglion, reported increased postoperative range of motion and grip strength with no intraoperative and postoperative complications. They had two recurrences requiring two attempts at open excision. They concluded that this was a safe and reliable procedure. Ho and associates[44] reported successful evacuation of volar ganglion contents by means of wrist arthroscopy in five cases, with no complications or recurrences reported after 1.6 months of follow-up. A prospective, randomized study of arthroscopic versus open dorsal ganglion excision for 72 patients (41 arthroscopic, 31 open procedures) found no significant difference in rate of recurrence.[45] The study suggests that additional long-term comparative studies are needed.

Painful intraosseous carpal ganglia can be treated arthroscopically. Ashwood and Bain reported results of arthroscopic débridement of intraosseous ganglia of the lunate using fluoroscopic guidance through a volar or dorsal portal, depending on the position identified by CT. This technique was found to be safe, with minimal morbidity and recurrence of symptoms during a follow-up period of 1 year.[46]

Preferred Technique

Our preferred method is that described by Osterman and Raphael.[42] The ganglion and the portals are marked preoperatively. The arthroscope is placed in the 6-R portal, and the 1-2 portal is used for instrumentation. In approximately two thirds of patients, a pearl-like stalk can be visualized[42]; if this stalk is not seen, it is assumed that the origin is from the dorsal capsule, and these cases usually have associated synovitis. A needle is passed into the ganglion externally and advanced to the stalk.

A ganglion portal, which usually corresponds approximately to the 3-4 portal, is established. The ganglion, along with a 1-cm diameter of dorsal capsule at the ganglion origin, is resected with a full-radius resector or basket punch. Resection is continued to the dorsum of the scapholunate ligament with care taken to avoid damaging this structure and the extensor tendons that are visible in about one third of cases. Associated dorsal synovitis can also be débrided arthroscopically. It is important to ensure that the extra-articular portion of the ganglion has been fully ruptured, and the wrist should be re-examined after removal from the traction tower. In one approach, a nylon tape was railroaded from the 3-4 portal to the 6-R portal. An artery clip was used to perform the blunt dissection between the extensor tendons and joint capsule; this clip can be used as a retractor to protect the extensor tendons.

A volar wrist ganglion is excised through the 1-2 and 3-4 portals. The instruments and arthroscope can be switched between the two portals, but we find it easier to use the chondrotome shaver through the 3-4 portal. The volar ganglion usually arises from the cleft between the radioscaphocapitate and long radiolunate ligaments. At the time of arthroscopy, gentle pressure over the volar ganglion my reveal its location, sometimes with ganglion contents seen emptying into the radiocarpal joint. Field resection of the capsule between the two ligaments is performed. Pressure is placed on the volar ganglion to expel fluid into the joint, confirming the location of the stalk, and to aid débridement.

Post-traumatic Contractures and Wrist Arthrofibrosis

Lee and Hausmann proposed a classification for wrist arthrofibrosis based on pathologic anatomic location, in which type I represents intrinsic adhesions and type II represents extrinsic contracture.[29] The types are subdivided according to the location of the pathology (Box 35-1). The causes also can be considered as intra-articular, capsular, and extracapsular, and these designations can determine the appropriate method of surgical treatment. Intra-articular and capsular pathology may be best addressed with arthroscopic techniques, whereas extracapsular pathology mandates open surgical approaches.[47]

Box 35-1 Classification of Wrist Arthrofibrosis

Type I: Intrinsic (adhesions)
- A. Radiocarpal joint
- B. Midcarpal joint
- C. Distal radioulnar joint (DRUJ)
- D. Combination of previous subtypes

Type II: Extrinsic (capsular fibrosis)
- A. Dorsal
- B. Palmar
- C. Distal radioulnar joint (DRUJ)
- D. Combination of above

From Geissler WB. Wrist arthrofibrosis. *Hand Clin*. 2006;22:529-538.

Arthroscopic arthrolysis of adhesions in the radiocarpal and midcarpal joints (type IA and IB) is well described, and satisfactory results have been achieved with this procedure. In Luchetti's series, arthroscopic débridement was performed for patients with pain and restricted range of motion after distal radius fractures. Débridement included arthrolysis, excision of scar tissue on the volar aspect of the radiocarpal joint, leveling of intra-articular steps, and débridement of TFCC and interosseous ligament tears.

Arthroscopic release of dorsal[8] and volar capsular[47] contractures has been associated with good patient outcomes. However, the indications must be clear. The ideal patient has a post-traumatic contracture with intact joint surfaces and no carpal instability. Significant preexisting post-traumatic osteoarthritis limits any gains from this procedure and is considered a relative contraindication. Frank carpal instability pattern is considered an absolute contraindication to volar or dorsal release, because the procedure is likely to exacerbate the instability. Likewise, in patients who have conditions that predispose to ulnar translocation (e.g., rheumatoid arthritis, previous radial styloid resection), release of the radioscaphocapitate and the long and short radiolunate ligaments should be performed with caution.

Preferred Technique

When performing arthroscopic volar capsular release, the proximity of the major neurovascular structures must be considered because they are at risk for injury. The procedure is performed through the 3-4 and 6-R portals. At least part of the radioscaphocapitate ligament should be left intact to reduce the risk of ulnar translocation, and instruments should not be used through the volar periarticular fat to avoid neurovascular injury.[47]

Dorsal capsular release is also performed through the 3-4 and 6-R portals. A nylon tape passed though the 3-4 portal can be railroaded between the extensor tendons, and the dorsal capsule can be used to retract the tendons dorsally (Fig. 35-4).[8] This maneuver lessens the risk of injury to the extensor tendons as

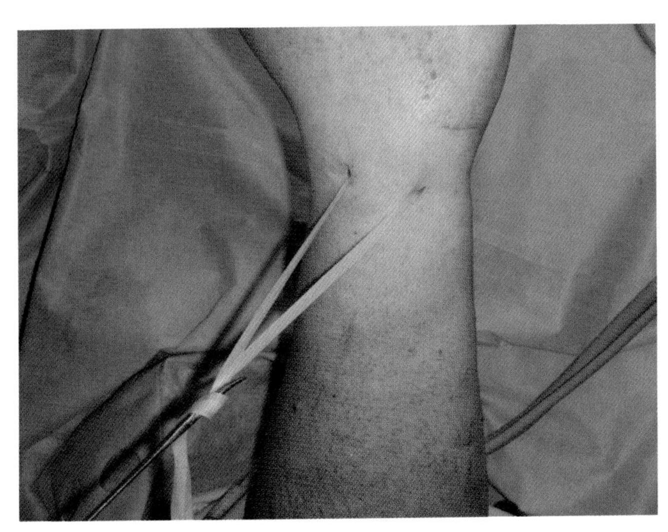

FIGURE 35-4 Dorsal capsulectomy may be assisted with tape to retract the tendons. *(From Bain GI, Munt J, Turner PC. New advances in wrist arthroscopy.* Arthroscopy. *2008;24:355-367.)*

capsular excision is performed. Resection is carried out with basket forceps introduced through the 3-4 portal.

PEARLS & PITFALLS

PEARLS

- The use of a nylon tape between the extensor tendons and the dorsal capsule can protect the tendons during excision of the dorsal capsule.
- Volar portals can be useful for visualization and for resection of adhesions in the dorsal aspects of the joint.

PITFALLS

- Complete release of the radioscaphocapitate ligament can result in ulnar translocation of the carpus, especially in predisposed patients, such as those with rheumatoid arthritis or previous radial styloidectomy.
- Frank carpal instability is a contraindication to release of extrinsic ligaments.
- Significant coexisting post-traumatic osteoarthritis limits any gains from the procedure.

CONCLUSIONS

Wrist arthroscopic techniques are being expanded and refined. Many of the procedures discussed in this chapter require advanced techniques, which have evolved from those used in established open techniques. However, as enthusiasts, we must be prepared to examine the benefits of these new techniques with rigorous scientific study.

REFERENCES

1. Chen YC. Arthroscopy of the wrist and finger joints. *Orthop Clin North Am*. 1979;10:723-733.
2. Roth JH, Poehling GG, Whipple TL. Arthroscopic surgery of the wrist. *Instr Course Lect*. 1988;37:183-194.
3. Arya AP, Kulshreshtha R, Kakarala GK, et al. Visualisation of the pisotriquetral joint through standard portals for arthroscopy of the wrist: a clinical and anatomical study. *J Bone Joint Surg Br*. 2007;89:202-205.
4. Abe Y, Doi K, Hattori Y, et al. A benefit of the volar approach for wrist arthroscopy. *Arthroscopy*. 2003;19:440-445.
5. Slutsky DJ. Wrist arthroscopy through a volar radial portal. *Arthroscopy*. 2002;18:624-630.
6. Tham S, Coleman S, Gilpin D. An anterior portal for wrist arthroscopy: anatomical study and case reports. *J Hand Surg Br*. 1999;24:445-447.
7. Edwards SG, Johansen JA. Prospective outcomes and associations of wrist ganglion cysts resected arthroscopically. *J Hand Surg Am*. 2009;34:395-400.
8. Bain GI, Munt J, Turner PC, Bergman J. Arthroscopic dorsal capsular release in the wrist: a new technique. *Tech Hand Up Extrem Surg*. 2008;12:191-194.
9. del Pinal F, Garcia-Bernal FJ, Pisani D, et al. Dry arthroscopy of the wrist: surgical technique. *J Hand Surg Am*. 2007;32:119-123.
10. del Pinal F. Dry arthroscopy of the wrist: its role in the management of articular distal radius fractures. *Scand J Surg*. 2008;97:298-304.
11. Bain GI, Hunt J, Mehta JA. Operative fluoroscopy in hand and upper limb surgery: one hundred cases. *J Hand Surg Br*. 1997;22:656-658.
12. Chung KC, Zimmerman NB, Travis MT. Wrist arthrography versus arthroscopy: a comparative study of 150 cases. *J Hand Surg Am*. 1996;21:591-594.
13. Morley J, Bidwell J, Bransby-Zachary M. A comparison of the findings of wrist arthroscopy and magnetic resonance imaging in the investigation of wrist pain. *J Hand Surg Br*. 2001;26:544-546.
14. Ruch DS, Poehling GG. Arthroscopic management of partial scapholunate and lunotriquetral injuries of the wrist. *J Hand Surg Am*. 1996;21:412-417.
15. Weiss AP, Sachar K, Glowacki KA. Arthroscopic débridement alone for intercarpal ligament tears. *J Hand Surg Am*. 1997;22:344-349.
16. Darlis NA, Weiser RW, Sotereanos DG. Partial scapholunate ligament injuries treated with arthroscopic débridement and thermal shrinkage. *J Hand Surg Am*. 2005;30:908-914.
17. Hirsh L, Sodha S, Bozentka D, et al. Arthroscopic electrothermal collagen shrinkage for symptomatic laxity of the scapholunate interosseous ligament. *J Hand Surg Br*. 2005;30:643-647.
18. Shih JT, Lee HM. Monopolar radiofrequency electrothermal shrinkage of the scapholunate ligament. *Arthroscopy*. 2006;22:553-557.
19. Battistella F, Golano P, Taverna E. Arthroscopic thermal shrinkage for scapholunate injuries. In: Slutsky DJ, Nagle D, eds. *Techniques in Wrist and Hand Arthroscopy*. Philadelphia, PA: Elsevier; 2007:86-92.
20. Whipple TL. The role of arthroscopy in the treatment of scapholunate instability. *Hand Clin*. 1995;11:37-40.
21. Osterman AL, Seidman GD. The role of arthroscopy in the treatment of lunatotriquetral ligament injuries. *Hand Clin*. 1995;11:41-50.
22. Darlis NA, Kaufmann RA, Giannoulis F, Sotereanos DG. Arthroscopic débridement and closed pinning for chronic dynamic scapholunate instability. *J Hand Surg Am*. 2006;31:418-424.
23. Aviles AJ, Lee SK, Hausman MR. Arthroscopic reduction-association of the scapholunate. *Arthroscopy*. 2007;23:105 e101-e105.
24. Van Den Abbeele KL, Loh YC, Stanley JK, Trail IA. Early results of a modified Brunelli procedure for scapholunate instability. *J Hand Surg Br*. 1998;23:258-261.
25. Culp RW, Lee Osterman A, Talsania JS. Arthroscopic proximal row carpectomy. *Tech Hand Up Extrem Surg*. 1997;1:116-119.
26. Ho PC. Arthroscopic partial wrist fusion. *Tech Hand Up Extrem Surg*. 2008;12:242-265.
27. Lichtman DM, Wroten ES. Understanding midcarpal instability. *J Hand Surg Am*. 2006;31:491-498.
28. Lichtman DM, Bruckner JD, Culp RW, Alexander CE. Palmar midcarpal instability: results of surgical reconstruction. *J Hand Surg Am*. 1993;18:307-315.
29. Mason WT, Hargreaves DG. Arthroscopic thermal capsulorrhaphy for palmar midcarpal instability. *J Hand Surg Eur* 2007;32:411-416.
30. Infanger M, Grimm D. Meniscus and discus lesions of triangular fibrocartilage complex (TFCC): treatment by laser-assisted wrist arthroscopy. *J Plast Reconstr Aesthet Surg*. 2009;62:466-471.
31. Nakamura T, Makita A. The proximal ligamentous component of the triangular fibrocartilage complex. *J Hand Surg Br*. 2000;25:479-486.
32. Lo IK, MacDermid JC, Bennett JD, et al. The radioulnar ratio: a new method of quantifying distal radioulnar joint subluxation. *J Hand Surg Am*. 2001;26:236-243.
33. Atzei A, Rizzo A, Luchetti R, Fairplay T. Arthroscopic foveal repair of triangular fibrocartilage complex peripheral lesion with distal radioulnar joint instability. *Tech Hand Up Extrem Surg*. 2008;12:226-235.
34. Badia A, Khanchandani P. Suture welding for arthroscopic repair of peripheral triangular fibrocartilage complex tears. *Tech Hand Up Extrem Surg*. 2007;11:45-50.

35. Adams BD, Berger RA. An anatomic reconstruction of the distal radioulnar ligaments for posttraumatic distal radioulnar joint instability. *J Hand Surg Am*. 2002;27:243-251.
36. Goldfarb CA, Hsu J, Gelberman RH, Boyer MI. The Lichtman classification for Kienböck's disease: an assessment of reliability. *J Hand Surg Am*. 2003;28:74-80.
37. Bain GI, Begg M. Arthroscopic assessment and classification of Kienböck's disease. *Tech Hand Up Extrem Surg*. 2006;10:8-13.
38. Menth-Chiari WA, Poehling GG, Wiesler ER, Ruch DS. Arthroscopic débridement for the treatment of Kienböck's disease. *Arthroscopy*. 1999; 15:12-19.
39. Leblebicioglu G, Doral MN, Atay AA, et al. Open treatment of stage III Kienböck's disease with lunate revascularization compared with arthroscopic treatment without revascularization. *Arthroscopy*. 2003;19: 117-130.
40. Topper SM, Wood MB, Ruby LK. Ulnar styloid impaction syndrome. *J Hand Surg Am*. 1997;22:699-704.
41. Bain GI, Bidwell TA. Arthroscopic excision of ulnar styloid in stylocarpal impaction. *Arthroscopy*. 2006;22:677e1-677e3.
42. Osterman AL, Raphael J. Arthroscopic resection of dorsal ganglion of the wrist. *Hand Clin*. 1995;11:7-12.
43. Rizzo M, Berger RA, Steinmann SP, Bishop AT. Arthroscopic resection in the management of dorsal wrist ganglions: results with a minimum 2-year follow-up period. *J Hand Surg Am*. 2004;29:59-62.
44. Ho PC, Lo WN, Hung LK. Arthroscopic resection of volar ganglion of the wrist: a new technique. *Arthroscopy*. 2003;19:218-221.
45. Kang L, Akelman E, Weiss AP. Arthroscopic versus open dorsal ganglion excision: a prospective, randomized comparison of rates of recurrence and of residual pain. *J Hand Surg Am*. 2008;33:471-475.
46. Ashwood N, Bain GI. Arthroscopically assisted treatment of intraosseous ganglions of the lunate: a new technique. *J Hand Surg Am*. 2003; 28:62-68.
47. Verhellen R, Bain GI. Arthroscopic capsular release for contracture of the wrist: a new technique. *Arthroscopy*. 2000;16:106-110.
48. Bain GI, Richards R, Roth J. Wrist arthroscopy: indications and technique. In: Peimer CA, ed. *Surgery of the Hand and the Upper Extremity*. New York, NY. McGraw-Hill; 1996:867-882.
49. Abrams RA, Petersen M, Botte MJ. Arthroscopic portals of the wrist: an anatomic study. *J Hand Surg Am*. 1994;19:940-944.

SECTION

I

Complications

CHAPTER

36

Complications of Wrist Arthroscopy

D. Nicole Deal • Gary G. Poehling

The use of arthroscopy has enabled direct visualization and diagnosis of intra-articular wrist pathology.[1-3] It is widely used in the treatment of wrist injuries, such as triangular fibrocartilage complex tears, scapholunate and lunatotriquetral tears, and synovitis, and the excision of dorsal ganglia and débridement of arthritic lesions.[4-10] Wrist arthroscopy has proved to be an excellent way to examine intra-articular pathology[11-14] and to treat these pathologic conditions.[15-27]

PREVENTING COMPLICATIONS

Arthroscopy has justifiably been touted as a safe and effective method for examining the intra-articular components of the radiocarpal and midcarpal joints,[28] and it is considered a relatively low-risk procedure.[29-33] As with any surgical procedure, complications may be encountered, including tendon injury from inappropriately placed portals, skin slough from traction devices, nerve injury, complex regional pain syndrome,[34-36] and rare conditions such as one case involving fistula formation after wrist arthroscopy.[37] Associated with each portal are certain anatomic structures with which the surgeon must be familiar to prevent portal-specific complications from occurring.[38] This chapter seeks to familiarize the wrist surgeon with these structures and techniques for preventing injury to them. Portal anatomy and the risks associated with each portal based on surrounding anatomic structures are addressed, along with the general risks associated with wrist arthroscopy. The Pearls and Pitfalls section describes common errors made when learning wrist arthroscopy and the techniques employed to avoid those errors.

One commonly employed technique to facilitate wrist arthroscopy is to place the wrist into traction with slight flexion that distracts the joints, making the portal intervals more easily palpable and allowing easier and less traumatic trocar and cannula entry into the joint. One portal is established to allow visualization during placement of the other portals. Most commonly, it is the 3-4 portal. Insufflation of the joint using lactated Ringer's solution through an 18-gauge needle placed in the 3-4 portal allows distention of wrist joint capsule. This portal is located just distal to Lister's tubercle and radial to the extensor digitorum communis at the radiocarpal joint line.

For making portal skin incisions, we recommend using a no. 11 scalpel blade in the longitudinal orientation just into the skin with traction on the skin itself, thereby making a skin incision without the trauma of an in-and-out sawing motion, which places deeper structures at risk.

RISKS AND COMPLICATIONS BY PORTAL SITE

Wrist arthroscopy portals are based on the extensor compartments of the wrist. Figure 36-1 provides an overview of the dorsal arthroscopy portals with associated structures.

1-2 Portal

The structures most at risk by placement and use of the 1-2 portal (i.e., extensor pollicis brevis–extensor carpi radialis longus [EPB-ECRL] portal) are the radial artery and superficial radial nerve. The radial artery lies deep to the first dorsal compartment and therefore should be out of harm's way if the portal is placed correctly. However, if the portal is placed too radially or too distally, this structure is at risk for injury. The easiest way to avoid damage to the radial artery as it passes deep to the tendons is to make a small portal incision, bluntly dissect down to capsule, and insert the trocar through the capsule after ensuring that the artery is not directly under the trocar.

The superficial radial nerve is also at risk because its dorsal branch lies over the 1-2 portal. The most effective way to avoid laceration or traction of this nerve as the medial branch of the superficial radial nerve arborizes ulnarly is to make the portal skin incision with a no. 11 blade knife inserted only through the skin layer and then by traction on the skin itself, rather than us-

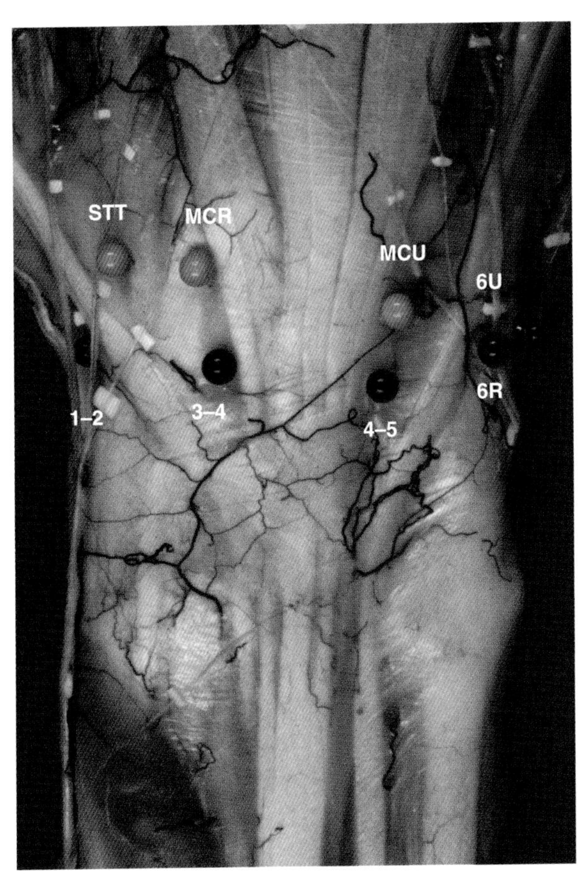

FIGURE 36-1 Dorsal arthroscopy portals 3-4, 4-5, and 6-R are safe to use because they are clear of the dorsal sensory nerves. *(Photograph courtesy of Pau Galano, MD, Barcelona, Spain.)*

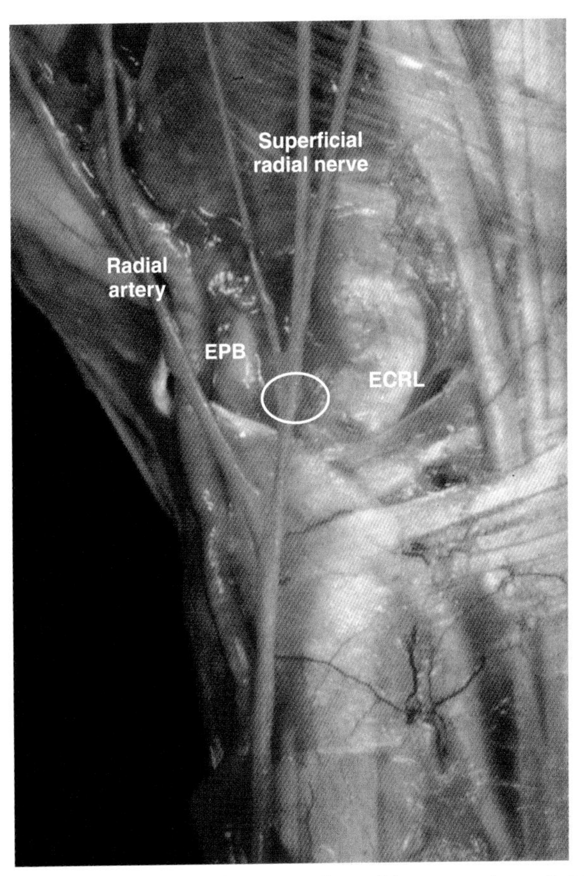

FIGURE 36-2 The 1-2 portal is near to the radial artery and superficial radial nerve. *(Photograph courtesy of Pau Galano, MD, Barcelona, Spain.)*

ing the blade, to enlarge the portal. Blunt dissection down to the capsule is recommended to ensure preservation of this dorsal branch as it crosses the portal site (Fig. 36-2).

3-4 Portal

The structures most at risk during placement of the 3-4 portal (i.e., extensor pollicis longus/extensor carpi radialis brevis–index extensor digitorum communis [EPL/ECRB-index EDC] portal) are the tendons of the EPL, ECRB, and EDC. This portal should be placed just distal to Lister's tubercle, around which the EPL tendon passes.

The 3-4 portal is most commonly the first portal established and is most easily established by inserting an 18-gauge needle into the wrist joint just distal to Lister's tubercle and insufflating the joint with as much solution as the joint can hold comfortably. At that point, the needle and syringe may be removed from the joint while maintaining the capsular distention. The information from needle insertion and palpation of the capsular distention guides placement of the 3-4 portal directly over the radiocarpal joint between the ECRB/EPL and the EDC. The skin is pulled over the tip of the blade to establish the portal, lessening the risk of inadvertently lacerating one of the tendons. After the skin incision is made, the blunt trocar and cannula are inserted, moving the tip in a medial and lateral direction to have tactile feedback and ensuring guidance into the joint without injury to the articular cartilage (Fig. 36-3).

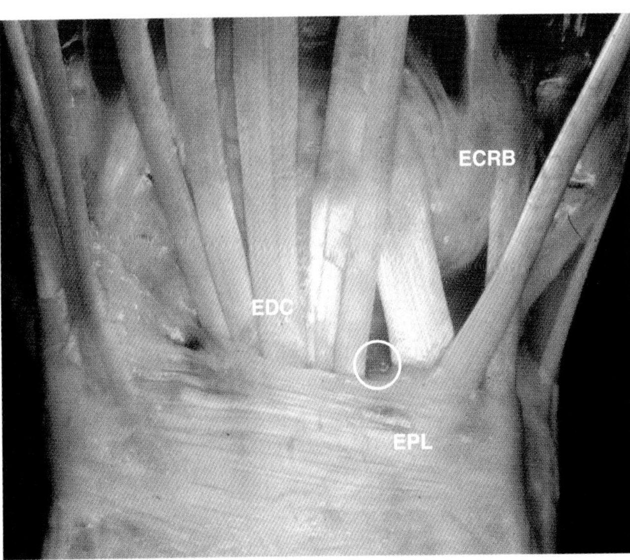

FIGURE 36-3 The 3-4 portal provides excellent, safe access to the extensor pollicis longus, extensor carpi radialis brevis, and extensor digitorum communis tendons in the wrist. *(Photograph courtesy of Pau Galano, MD, Barcelona, Spain.)*

4-5 Portal

The structures most at risk during placement of the 4-5 portal (i.e., extensor digitorum communis–extensor digiti quinti [EDC-EDQ] portal) are the terminal branch of the posterior interosseous nerve

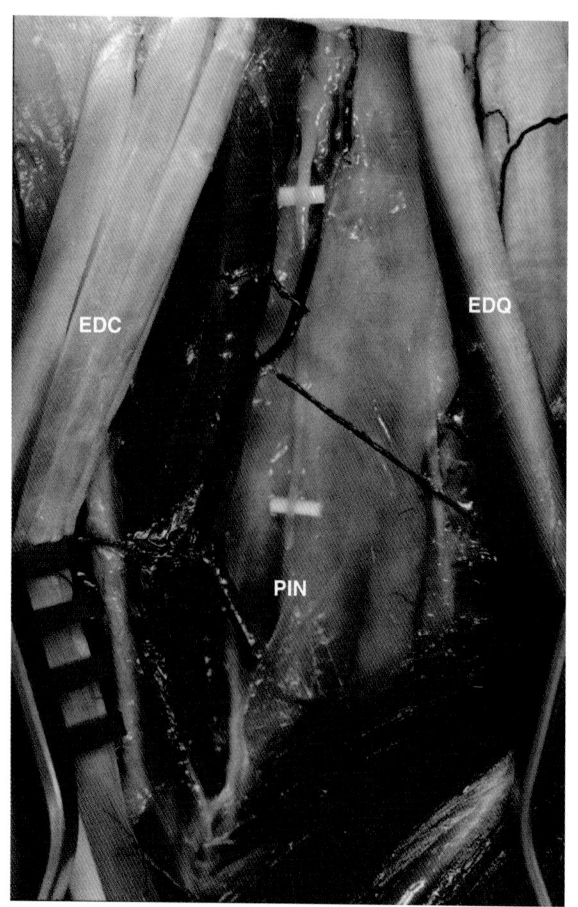

FIGURE 36-4 The 4-5 interval is close to the terminal branch of the posterior interosseous nerve. Most think this nerve supplies only sensation to the wrist joint itself and is of little consequence if sacrificed. *(Photograph courtesy of Pau Galano, MD, Barcelona, Spain.)*

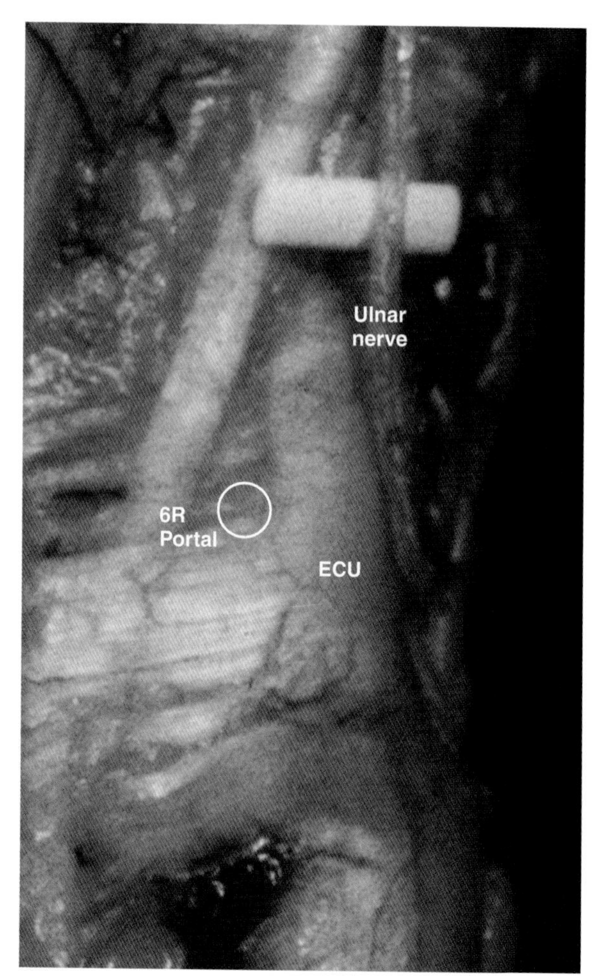

FIGURE 36-5 The 6-R portal can be used safely as long as it is on the radial side of the extensor carpi ulnaris. *(Photograph courtesy of Pau Galano, MD, Barcelona, Spain.)*

and the dorsal sensory branch of the ulnar nerve. The posterior interosseous nerve passes deep to the fourth dorsal compartment on the ulnar side dorsal to the wrist to provide sensation to the wrist joint. The risk of damage to this nerve during placement of the 4-5 portal is lessened by placement of the portal in a slightly ulnar position with relation to the EDC tendon. The portal should be placed just radial to the EDQ tendon. From a practical point of view, the loss of the function of this nerve causes no functional deficit, and some think that it diminishes pain in the wrist joint.

The transverse branch of the ulnar dorsal sensory nerve is also at risk during placement of this portal. The transverse branch of this nerve passes distal to the portal, and risk of injury may be lessened by placing the portal as proximal as possible in the wrist joint. We recommend longitudinal portal placement followed by blunt insertion into the joint to ensure preservation of the nerve (Fig. 36-4).

6-R Portal

The structures at most risk during placement of the 6-R portal (i.e., radial to the extensor carpi ulnaris [ECU] tendon) are the extensor tendons and branches of the dorsal sensory branch of the ulnar nerve. This nerve passes ulnar to the portal, and we stress portal placement on the radial side of the ECU tendon with blunt dissection to the joint, thereby preventing damage to this superficial nerve. We recommend making the skin incision in a longitudinal fashion with careful dissection down to capsule, at which point the trocar may be safely placed bluntly on the radial side of the ECU tendon (Fig. 36-5).

6-U Portal

The structure at most risk during placement of the 6-U portal (i.e., ulnar to the ECU tendon) is the main dorsal sensory branch of the ulnar nerve. We do not recommend the use of this portal unless there is no other alternative. This nerve passes over the portal, and we stress portal placement with blunt dissection to the joint, thereby preventing damage to this superficial nerve. We recommend making the skin incision and then carefully dissecting down to capsule to ensure that the nerve is not lacerated or entrapped during portal placement. After the nerve has been protected, the trocar may be placed bluntly on the ulnar side of the ECU tendon (Fig. 36-6).

Midcarpal Radial Portal

The structures most at risk in the midcarpal radial (MCR) portal (i.e., 1 cm distal to the 3-4 portal and in line with the radial border

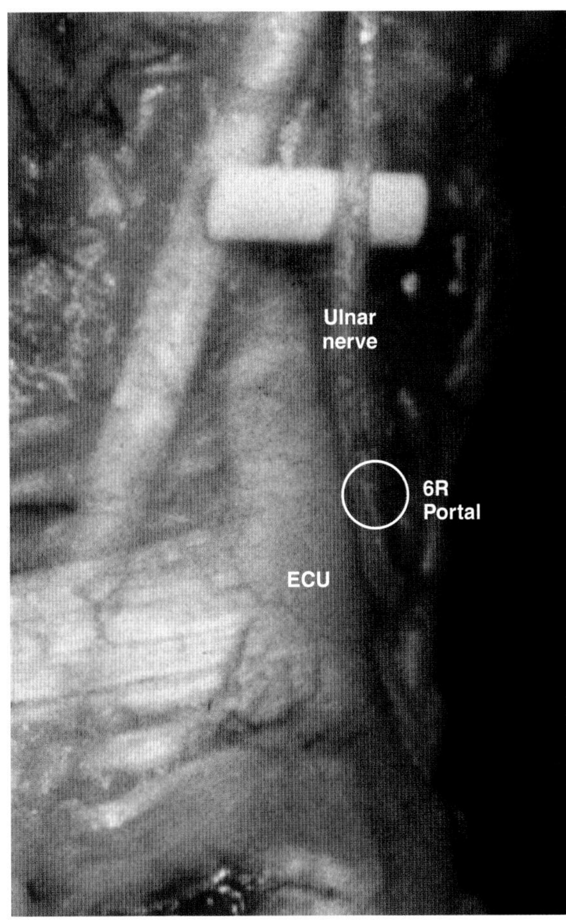

FIGURE 36-6 The 6-U portal is close to the main dorsal sensory branch of the ulnar nerve. If this portal must be used, dissection and retraction of the nerve must be performed before portal placement. *(Photograph courtesy of Pau Galano, MD, Barcelona, Spain.)*

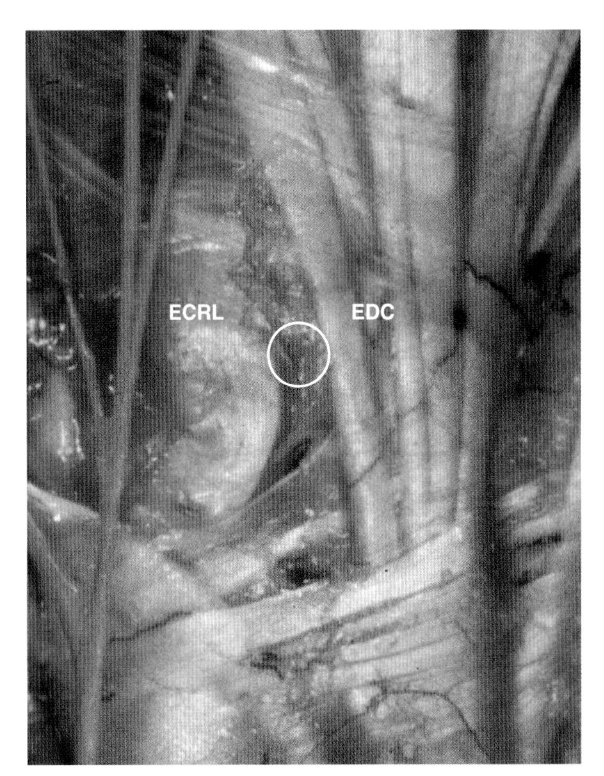

FIGURE 36-7 The midcarpal radial portal is 1 cm distal to the 3-4 portal and is bordered by the extensor carpi radialis longus and extensor digitorum communis tendons. There are no adjacent nervous or vascular structures. *(Photograph courtesy of Pau Galano, MD, Barcelona, Spain.)*

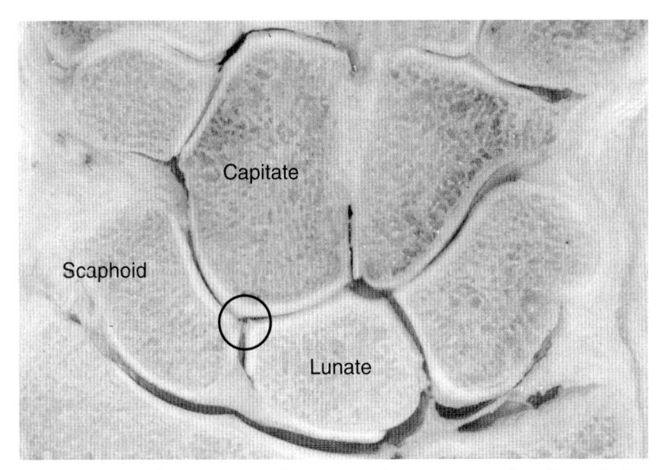

FIGURE 36-8 This intra-articular section demonstrates that the articular cartilage is at risk with placement of the midcarpal radial portal because of the small space available for instrumentation. *(Photograph courtesy of Pau Galano, MD, Barcelona, Spain.)*

of the long metacarpal) are the extensor tendons (Fig. 36-7) and the articular cartilage. The space available for portal placement is smaller in the MCR portal compared with the midcarpal ulnar (MCU) portal (Fig. 36-8). For smaller patients, we recommend the use of a 1.8-mm arthroscope in all of the portals of the midcarpal joint because of the small potential space.

Midcarpal Ulnar Portal

The structures most at risk in the MCU portal (i.e., 1 cm distal to the 4-5 radiocarpal portal and in line with the axis of the ring metacarpal) are the extensor tendons (Fig. 36-9) and the articular cartilage. This portal has more room than the MCR portal, especially in patients who have a significant hamate facet of the lunate (Fig. 36-10).

Scaphotrapeziotrapezoid Portal

The structures most at risk with placement and use of the scaphotrapeziotrapezoid (STT) portal (i.e., EDC-EPL distal portal) are the radial artery and superficial radial nerve. The radial artery passes deep to the extensors through the anatomic snuffbox to lie between the two heads of the first dorsal interosseous muscle, and it is therefore directly at risk during placement of this portal (Fig. 36-11). The easiest way to avoid damage to the radial artery is to approach the space between the ECRL and the ECRB and ulnar to the EPL. This approach ensures that the artery and the radial nerve are palmar and radial to the portal.

Palmar Portal

The palmar portal is the most precarious of all the portals discussed, because it lies between the radial artery, the median nerve, and the palmar cutaneous nerve (Fig. 36-12). Whether

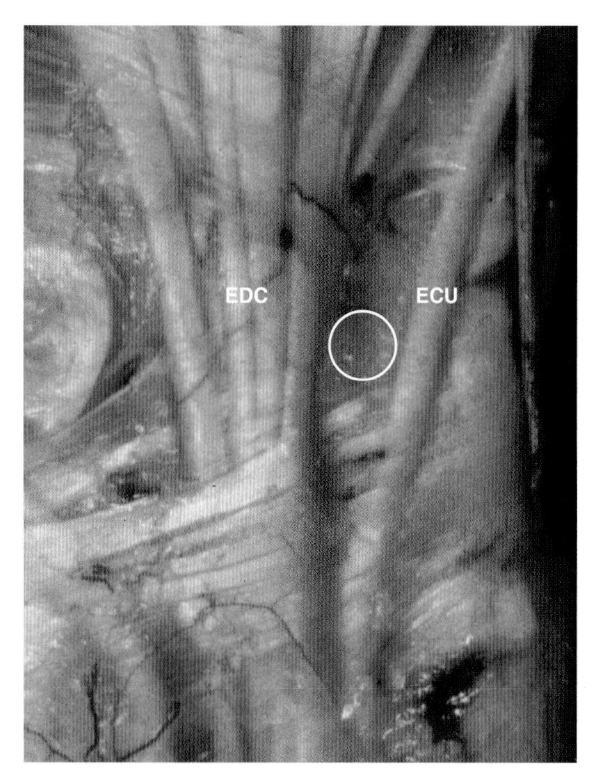

FIGURE 36-9 The midcarpal ulnar portal is 1 cm distal to the 4-5 radiocarpal portal and is bordered by the extensor digitorum communis and extensor carpi ulnaris tendons. There are no adjacent nervous or vascular structures. *(Photograph courtesy of Pau Galano, MD, Barcelona, Spain.)*

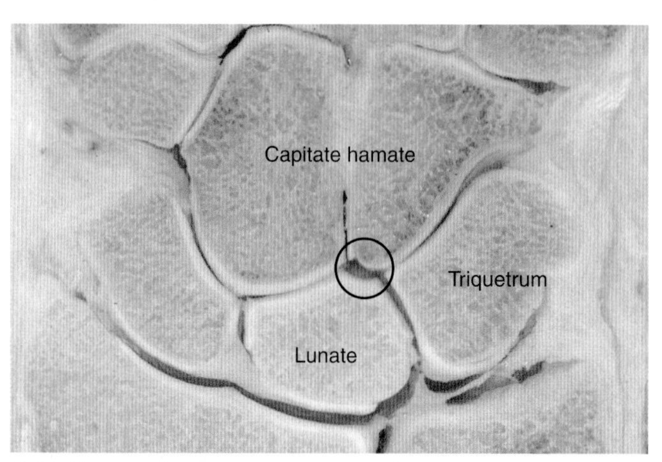

FIGURE 36-10 This intra-articular section demonstrates the relatively larger space in the midcarpal ulnar portal compared with the midcarpal radial portal. *(Photograph courtesy of Pau Galano, MD, Barcelona, Spain.)*

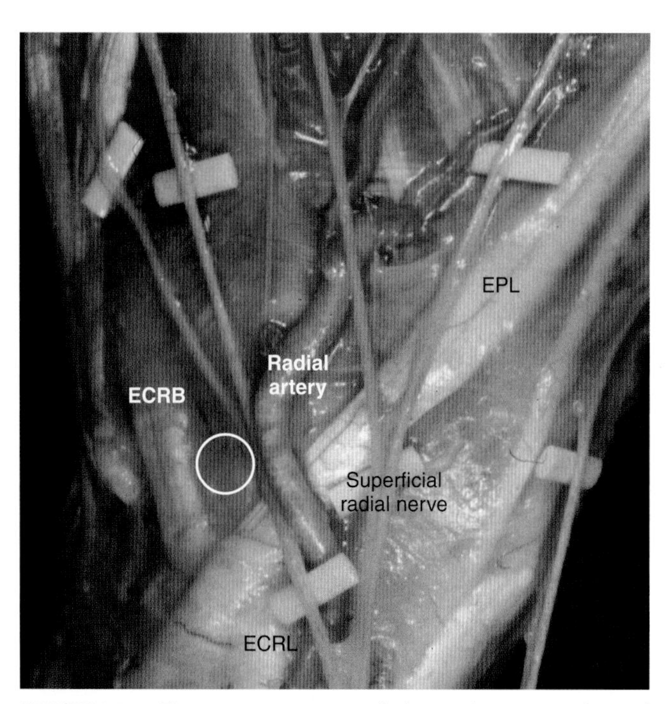

FIGURE 36-11 The structures most at risk during placement and use of the scaphotrapeziotrapezoid (STT) portal are the radial artery and superficial radial nerve. It is safest if the STT portal is made on the radial border of the extensor carpi radialis brevis tendon. *(Photograph courtesy of Pau Galano, MD, Barcelona, Spain.)*

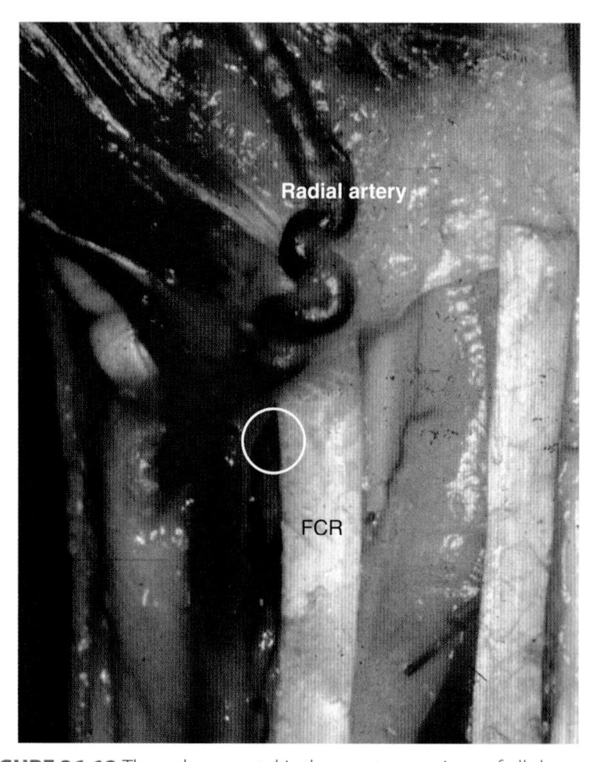

FIGURE 36-12 The palmar portal is the most precarious of all the portals discussed because it lies just adjacent to the radial artery. Open dissection is recommended if this portal is used. *(Photograph courtesy of Pau Galano, MD, Barcelona, Spain.)*

placed inside-out or outside-in, care must be taken to preserve the radial artery, which lies radial to the flexor carpi radialis (FCR) tendon; the palmar cutaneous nerve, which lies superficially between the FCR and palmaris longus tendons; and the median nerve, which lies deep to the palmaris longus and ulnar to the FCR. If placing the portal with an inside-out technique, the switching stick should be placed through the 3-4 portal between the radioscaphocapitate ligament and the long radiolunate ligaments with an incision radial to the FCR tendon on the volar aspect of the wrist. It is crucial to identify the radial artery and protect it during insertion of the cannula. If the outside-in technique is used with an incision made on the ulnar aspect of the FCR tendon, as described by Slutsky, care must be taken to protect the palmar cutaneous and median nerve proper.[39]

CONCLUSIONS

Wrist arthroscopy is a safe and effective technique for treating intra-articular wrist pathology. Complications are rare, and most can be prevented by using proper technique as described in this chapter.

PEARLS & PITFALLS

PEARLS

- Know the anatomic landmarks around potential portals, and remember that small variations in portal placement may injury adjacent structures.
- Distend the joint before portal placement.
- Place a needle in the proposed portal sites before establishing the portal.
- Make skin incisions longitudinally using a no. 11 blade scalpel, and apply traction on the skin rather than using a sawing motion with the blade to enlarge the portal.

PITFALLS

- For thin or frail skin, use caution when applying finger traps, and watch carefully for skin tearing.
- Use caution when placing portals to avoid articular cartilage damage, particularly in the midcarpal joints.
- When evaluating wrist pain, be aware of patients with constant pain, especially if they experience a burning sensation and have difficulty sleeping. They should be treated for complex regional pain syndrome (formerly called reflex sympathetic dystrophy) before any operative procedure to correct mechanical problems.
- The risk of infection is low with the use of proper sterile technique.
- Use described techniques to avoid injury to the many superficial nervous structures around the wrist and prevent neuroma formation.
- Use described techniques to avoid injury to tendons.
- Bluntly dissect down to the capsule, and identify at-risk structures before portal placement.

REFERENCES

1. Geissler W, Walsh JJ. Wrist arthroscopy. Available at http://emedicine.medscape.com/article/1241370-overview (accessed August 2007).
2. North ER, Thomas S. An anatomic guide for arthroscopic visualization of the wrist capsular ligaments. *J Hand Surg Am*. 1988;13:815-822.
3. Whipple TL, Marotta JJ, Powell JH. Techniques of wrist arthroscopy. *Arthroscopy*. 1986;2:244-252.
4. Bain GI, Munt J, Turner PC. New advances in wrist arthroscopy. *Arthroscopy*. 2008;24:355-367.
5. Beredjiklian PK, Bozentka DJ, Leung YL, Monaghan BA. Complications of wrist arthroscopy. *J Hand Surg Am*. 2004;29:406-411.
6. Bernstein MA, Nagle DJ, Martinez A, et al. A comparison of combined arthroscopic triangular fibrocartilage complex débridement and arthroscopic wafer distal ulna resection versus arthroscopic triangular fibrocartilage complex débridement and ulnar shortening osteotomy for ulnocarpal abutment syndrome. *Arthroscopy*. 2004;20:392-401.
7. Chloros GD, Wiesler ER, Poehling GG. Current concepts in wrist arthroscopy. *Arthroscopy*. 2008;24:343-354.
8. Chloros GD, Shen J, Mahirogullari M, Wiesler ER. Wrist arthroscopy. *J Surg Orthop Adv*. 2007;16:49-61.
9. McAdams TR, Hentz VR. Injury to the dorsal sensory branch of the ulnar nerve in the arthroscopic repair of ulnar-sided triangular fibrocartilage tears using an inside-out technique: a cadaver study. *J Hand Surg Am*. 2002;27:840-844.
10. Tsu-Hsin CE, Wei JD, Huang VW. Injury of the dorsal sensory branch of the ulnar nerve as a complication of arthroscopic repair of the triangular fibrocartilage. *J Hand Surg Br*. 2006;31:530-532.
11. Chung KC, Zimmerman NB, Travis MT. Wrist arthrography versus arthroscopy: a comparative study of 150 cases. *J Hand Surg*. 1996;21:591-594.
12. Cooney WP. Evaluation of chronic wrist pain by arthrography, arthroscopy, and arthrotomy. *J Hand Surg Am*. 1993;18:815-822.
13. Johnstone DJ, Thorogood S, Smith WH, Scott TD. A comparison of magnetic resonance imaging and arthroscopy in the investigation of chronic wrist pain. *J Hand Surg Br*. 1997;22:714-718.
14. Pederzini L, Luchetti R, Soragni O, et al. Evaluation of the triangular fibrocartilage complex tears by arthroscopy, arthrography, and magnetic resonance imaging. *Arthroscopy*. 1992;8:191-197.
15. Adolfsson L. Arthroscopic diagnosis of ligament lesions of the wrist. *J Hand Surg Br*. 1994;19:505-512.
16. Aviles AJ, Lee SK, Hausman MR. Arthroscopic reduction-association of the scapholunate. *Arthroscopy*. 2007;23:105.
17. Geissler WB. Arthroscopically assisted reduction of intra-articular fractures of the distal radius. *Hand Clin*. 1995;11:19-29.
18. Geissler WB, Freeland AE. Arthroscopically assisted reduction of intraarticular distal radial fractures. *Clin Orthop Relat Res*. 1996;(327):125-134.
19. Geissler WB. Arthroscopic excision of dorsal wrist ganglia. *Tech Upper Extrem Surg*. 1998;2:196-201.
20. Levy HJ, Glickel SZ. Arthroscopic assisted internal fixation of volar intraarticular wrist fractures. *Arthroscopy*. 1993;9:122-124.
21. Osterman AL. Arthroscopic débridement of triangular fibrocartilage complex tears. *Arthroscopy*. 1990;6:120-124.
22. Osterman AL, Raphael J. Arthroscopic resection of dorsal ganglion of the wrist. *Hand Clin*. 1995;11:7-12.
23. Osterman AL, Seidman GD. The role of arthroscopy in the treatment of lunatotriquetral ligament injuries. *Hand Clin*. 1995;11:41-50.
24. Slade JF 3rd, Gutow AP, Geissler WB. Percutaneous internal fixation of scaphoid fractures via an arthroscopically assisted dorsal approach. *J Bone Joint Surg Am*. 2002;84(suppl 2):21-36.
25. Whipple TL. The role of arthroscopy in the treatment of intra-articular wrist fractures. *Hand Clin*. 1995;11:13-18.
26. Whipple TL. The role of arthroscopy in the treatment of scapholunate instability. *Hand Clin*. 1995;11:37-40.
27. Wolfe SW, Easterling KJ, Yoo HH. Arthroscopic-assisted reduction of distal radius fractures. *Arthroscopy*. 1995;11:706-714.
28. Viegas SF. Midcarpal arthroscopy: anatomy and portals. *Hand Clin*. 1994;10:577-587.
29. Bettinger PC, Cooney WP, Berger RA. Arthroscopic anatomy of the wrist. *Orthop Clin North Am*. 1995;26:707-719.
30. Botte MJ, Cooney WP, Linscheid RL. Arthroscopy of the wrist: anatomy and technique. *J Hand Surg Am*. 1989;14(2 pt. 1):313-316.
31. Buterbaugh GA. Radiocarpal arthroscopy portals and normal anatomy. *Hand Clin*. 1994;10:567-576.
32. Ekman EF, Poehling GG. Principles of arthroscopy and wrist arthroscopy equipment. *Hand Clin*. 1994;10:557-566.
33. Roth JH, Poehling GG, Whipple TL. Hand instrumentation for small joint arthroscopy. *Arthroscopy*. 1988;4:126-128.

34. Culp RW. Complications of wrist arthroscopy. *Hand Clin*. 1999;15:529-535.
35. DelPinal F, Herrero F, Cruz-Camara A, San Jose J. Complete avulsion of the distal posterior interosseous nerve during wrist arthroscopy: a possible cause of persistent pain after arthroscopy. *J Hand Surg Am*. 1999;24:240-242.
36. DeSmet L. Pitfalls in wrist arthroscopy. *Acta Orthop Belg*. 2002;68:325-329.
37. Shirley DSL, Mullet H, Stanley JK. Extensor tendon sheath fistula formation as a complication of wrist arthroscopy. *Arthroscopy*. 2008;24:1311-1312.
38. Yu HL, Chase RA, Strauch B. *Atlas of Hand Anatomy and Clinical Implications*. St. Louis, MO: Mosby; 2004.
39. Slutsky DJ. Wrist arthroscopy through a volar radial portal. *Arthroscopy*. 2002;18:624-630.

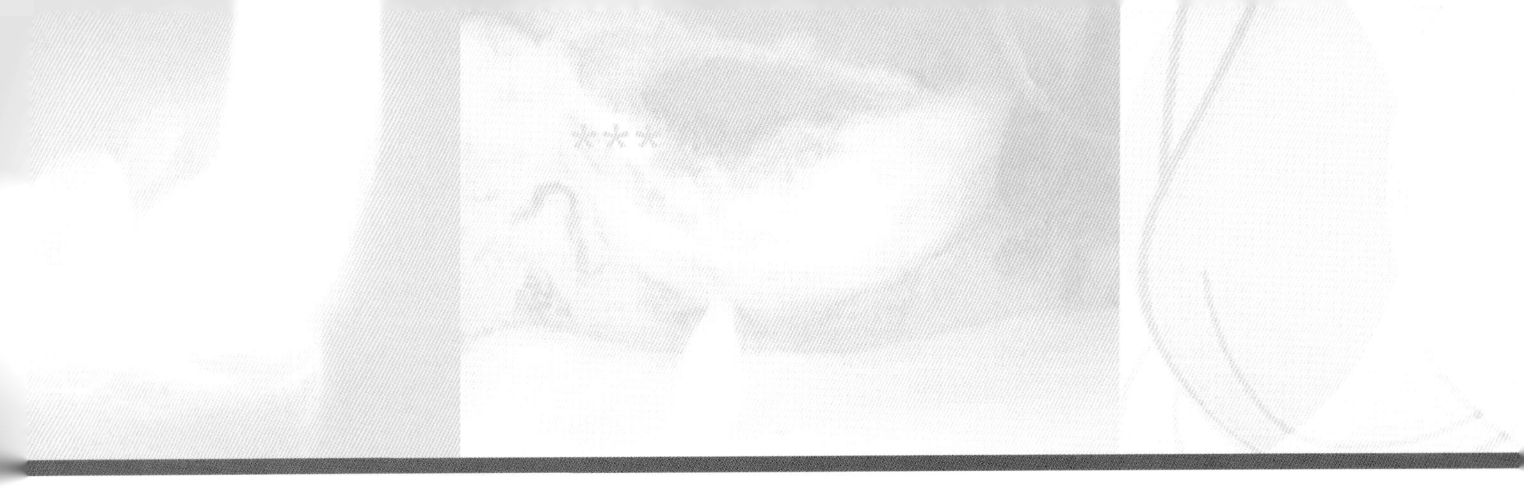

Index

Note: Page numbers followed by f refer to figures; page numbers followed by t refer to tables; page numbers followed by b refer to boxes.

M

N

O

P

W